Informatik aktuell

T0207493

Herausgegeben
im Auftrag der Gesellschaft für Informatik (GI)

Weitere Bände in dieser Reihe:
http://www.springer.com/series/2872

Heinz Handels · Thomas M. Deserno
Hans-Peter Meinzer · Thomas Tolxdorff
Herausgeber

Bildverarbeitung
für die Medizin 2015

Algorithmen – Systeme – Anwendungen

Proceedings des Workshops
vom 15. bis 17. März 2015 in Lübeck

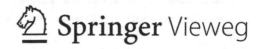

Herausgeber

Heinz Handels
Universität zu Lübeck
Institut für Medizinische Informatik
Ratzeburger Allee 160, 23562 Lübeck

Hans-Peter Meinzer
Deutsches Krebsforschungszentrum
Abteilung für Medizinische
und Biologische Informatik
Im Neuenheimer Feld 280, 69120 Heidelberg

Thomas Martin Deserno, geb. Lehmann
Uniklinik RWTH Aachen
Institut für Medizinische Informatik
Pauwelsstr. 30, 52074 Aachen

Thomas Tolxdorff
Charité – Universitätsmedizin Berlin
Institut für Medizinische Informatik
Hindenburgdamm 30, 12200 Berlin

ISSN 1431-472X
Informatik aktuell
ISBN 978-3-662-46223-2   ISBN 978-3-662-46224-9   (eBook)
DOI 10.1007/978-3-662-46224-9

CR Subject Classification (1998): A.0, H.3, I.4, I.5, J.3, H.3.1, I.2.10, I.3.3, I.3.5, I.3.7, I.3.8, I.6.3

Die Deutsche Nationalbibliothek verzeichnet diese Publikation in der Deutschen Nationalbibliografie; detaillierte bibliografische Daten sind im Internet über http://dnb.d-nb.de abrufbar.

Springer Vieweg

Springer-Verlag GmbH Berlin Heidelberg ist Teil der Fachverlagsgruppe Springer Science+Business Media (www.springer.com)

Bildverarbeitung für die Medizin 2015

Veranstalter

IMI   Institut für Medizinische Informatik, Universität zu Lübeck

Unterstützende Fachgesellschaften

BVMI	Berufsverband Medizinischer Informatiker
CURAC	Deutsche Gesellschaft für Computer- und Roboterassistierte Chirurgie
	Fachgruppe Medizinische Informatik der
DGBMT	Deutschen Gesellschaft für Biomedizinische Technik im
VDE	Verband Deutscher Elektrotechniker
DAGM	Deutsche Arbeitsgemeinschaft für Mustererkennung
GMDS	Gesellschaft für Medizinische Informatik, Biometrie und Epidemiologie
IEEE	Joint Chapter Engineering in Medicine and Biology, German Section und der
GI	Gesellschaft für Informatik

Tagungsvorsitz

Prof. Dr. rer. nat. habil. Heinz Handels
Institut für Medizinische Informatik, Universität zu Lübeck

Tagungssekretariat

Susanne Petersen
Institut für Medizinische Informatik, Universität zu Lübeck
Postanschrift: 23562 Lübeck
Lieferanschrift: Ratzeburger Allee 160, Gebäude 64
Telefon: +49 451 500 5601
Telefax: +49 451 500 5610
Email: bvm2015@imi.uni-luebeck.de
Web: http://bvm-workshop.org

Lokales BVM-Komitee

Prof. Dr. H. Handels (Leitung)
Prof. Dr. J. Barkhausen, Klinik für Radiologie und Nuklearmedizin
Prof. Dr. T. Buzug, Institut für Medizintechnik
Prof. Dr. J. Modersitzki, Fraunhofer MEVIS Lübeck

Verteilte BVM-Organisation

Prof. Dr. Thomas M. Deserno, Jan Dovermann
Rheinisch-Westfälische Technische Hochschule Aachen (Tagungsband)

Prof. Dr. Heinz Handels, Dr. Jan-Hinrich Wrage
Universität zu Lübeck (Beitragsbegutachtung)

Prof. Dr. Hans-Peter Meinzer, Michael Brehler
Deutsches Krebsforschungszentrum Heidelberg (Anmeldung)

Prof. Dr. Thomas Tolxdorff, Dr. Thorsten Schaaf
Charité – Universitätsmedizin Berlin (Internetpräsenz)

Programmkomitee

Prof. Dr. Dr. Johannes Bernarding, Universität Magdeburg
Prof. Dr. Oliver Burgert, Universität Leipzig
Prof. Dr. Thorsten Buzug, Universität zu Lübeck
Prof. Dr. Thomas Deserno, RWTH Aachen
Prof. Dr. Hartmut Dickhaus, Universität Heidelberg
Dr. Jan Ehrhardt, Universität zu Lübeck
Prof. Dr. Nils Forkert, University of Calgary, Kanada
Prof. Dr. Rolf-Rainer Grigat, TU Hamburg-Harburg
Prof. Dr. Heinz Handels, Universität zu Lübeck
Priv.-Doz. Dr. Peter Hastreiter, Universität Erlangen
Jun.-Prof. Dr. Mattias Heinrich, Universität zu Lübeck
Dr. Tobias Heimann, Siemens Corporate Technology Erlangen
Prof. Dr. Joachim Hornegger, Universität Erlangen
Prof. Ron Kikinis, MD, Fraunhofer MEVIS Bremen
Dr. Cristian Lorenz, PHILIPS Hamburg
Dr. Klaus Maier-Hein, DKFZ Heidelberg
Priv.-Doz. Dr. Lena Maier-Hein, DKFZ Heidelberg
Prof. Dr. Hans-Peter Meinzer, DKFZ Heidelberg
Prof. Dr. Dorit Merhof, RWTH Aachen
Prof. Dr. Alfred Mertins, Universität zu Lübeck
Prof. Dr. Jan Modersitzki, Fraunhofer MEVIS Lübeck
Prof. Dr. Heinrich Müller, Technische Unversität Dortmund
Prof. Dr. Henning Müller, Université Sierre Schweiz
Prof. Dr. Nassir Navab, Technische Universität München
Prof. Dr. Arya Nabavi, International Neuroscience Institute, Hannover
Prof. Dr. Heinrich Niemann, Universität Erlangen
Prof. Dr. Christoph Palm, OTH Regensburg
Prof. Dr. Bernhard Preim, Universität Magdeburg
Priv.-Doz. Dr. Karl Rohr, Universität Heidelberg
Priv.-Doz. Dr. Dennis Säring, Universitätsklinikum Hamburg
Prof. Ingrid Scholl, Fachhochschule Aachen
Dr. Stefanie Speidel, KIT Karlsruhe

Prof. Dr. Thomas Tolxdorff, Charité-Universitätsmedizin Berlin
Dr. Gudrun Wagenknecht, Forschungszentrum Jülich
Dr. Stefan Wesarg, Fraunhofer IGD Darmstadt
Prof. Dr. Herbert Witte, Universität Jena
Priv.-Doz. Dr. Thomas Wittenberg, Fraunhofer IIS Erlangen
Dr. Stefan Wörz, Universität Heidelberg
Prof. Dr. Ivo Wolf, Hochschule Mannheim

Sponsoren des Workshops BVM 2015

Die BVM wäre ohne die finanzielle Unterstützung der Industrie in ihrer so erfolgreichen Konzeption nicht durchführbar. Deshalb freuen wir uns sehr über langjährige kontinuierliche Unterstützung mancher Firmen sowie auch über das neue Engagement anderer. Dies gilt insbesondere für unsere Platinsponsoren.

Platin-Sponsor

Agfa HealthCare
Konrad-Zuse-Platz 1-3, D-53227 Bonn
http://www.agfa.com/healthcare

OLYMPUS SURGICAL TECHNOLOGIES EUROPE
Olympus Winter und Ibe GmbH
Kuehnstrasse 61, D-22045 Hamburg
http://www.olympus-oste.eu

Sponsoren

CHILI GmbH
Burgstr. 61, D-69121 Heidelberg
http://www.chili-radiology.com

Haption GmbH
Technologiezentrum am Europaplatz Dennewartstr. 25, D-52068 Aachen
http://www.haption.de

MiE GmbH
Hauptstrasse 112, D-23845 Seth
http://www.miegermany.de

Springer Verlag GmbH
Tiergartenstr. 17, D-69121 Heidelberg
http://www.springer.com

VISUS Technology Transfer GmbH
Universitätsstr. 136, D-44799 Bochum
http://www.visus.com

Preisträger des BVM-Workshops 2014 in Aachen

Auf der BVM 2014 wurde der mit 1.000 € dotierte BVM-Award an eine herausragende Diplom-, Bachelor-, Master- oder Doktorarbeit aus dem Bereich der Medizinischen Bildverarbeitung gesplittet. Die mit einem Preisgeld von je 333,33 € dotierten BVM-Preise zeichnen besonders hervorragende Arbeiten aus, die auf dem Workshop präsentiert wurden.

BVM-Award 2014 für eine herausragende Dissertation

Dagmar Kainmüller (Universität zu Lübeck)
Deformable Meshes for Accurate Automatic Segmentation of Medical Image Data
Nils D. Forkert (Universität Hamburg)
Model-Based Analysis of Cerebrovascular Diseases Combining 3D and 4D MRA Datasets

BVM-Preis 2014 für die beste wissenschaftliche Arbeit

Thomas Köhler (Friedrich-Alexander University Erlangen-Nürnberg)
Outlier Detection for Multi-Sensor Super-Resolution in Hybrid 3D Endoscopy

BVM-Preis 2014 für den besten Vortrag

Sandy Engelhardt mit *Bastian Graser, Raffaele De Simone, Norbert Zimmermann, Matthias Krack, Hans-Peter Meinzer, Diana Nabers, Ivo Wolf* (DKFZ Heidelberg)
Vermessung des Mitralapparats mit einem optisch getrackten Zeigeinstrument für die virtuelle Annuloplastie

BVM-Preis 2014 für die beste Posterpräsentation

Julian Schröder mit *Andre Mastmeyer, Dirk Fortmeier, Heinz Handels* (Universität zu Lübeck)
Ultraschallsimulation für das Training von Gallengangspunktionen

Vorwort

In diesem Jahr wird die Tagung Bildverarbeitung für die Medizin (BVM 2015) vom Institut für Medizinische Informatik an der Universität zu Lübeck ausgerichtet. Nach der erfolgreichen Durchführung der BVM 2001 und 2011 findet diese zentrale Tagung zu neuen Entwicklungen in der Medizinischen Bildverarbeitung in Deutschland nun zum dritten Mal in der traditionsreichen Hansestadt Lübeck statt.

Die Bedeutung des Themas Bildverarbeitung für die Medizin hat über die Jahre deutlich zugenommen. Die Bildverarbeitung ist eine Schlüsseltechnologie in verschiedenen medizinischen Bereichen wie der Diagnoseunterstützung, der OP-Planung und der bildgeführten Chirurgie. An der Universität zu Lübeck bilden die Medizinische Bildgebung und Bildverarbeitung einen zentralen Forschungsschwerpunkt, der in den letzten Jahren systematisch ausgebaut wurde. Vor diesem Hintergrund ist es eine besondere Freude, die BVM 2015 in Lübeck ausrichten zu dürfen.

Die BVM konnte sich in den letzten Jahren als ein zentrales interdisziplinäres Forum für die Präsentation und Diskussion von Methoden, Systemen und Anwendungen im Bereich der Medizinischen Bildverarbeitung etablieren. Ziel der Tagung ist die Darstellung aktueller Forschungsergebnisse und die Vertiefung der Gespräche zwischen Wissenschaftlern, Industrie und Anwendern. Die BVM richtet sich ausdrücklich auch an Nachwuchswissenschaftler, die über ihre Bachelor-, Master-, Promotions- und Habilitationsprojekte berichten wollen.

Die BVM 2015 wird unter der Federführung von Prof. Dr. rer. nat. habil. Heinz Handels, Direktor des Instituts für Medizinische Informatik der Universität zu Lübeck, ausgerichtet. Die Organisation ist wie in den letzten Jahren auf Fachkollegen aus Aachen, Berlin, Heidelberg und Lübeck verteilt, so dass die Organisatoren der vergangenen Jahre ihre Erfahrungen mit einfließen lassen können.

Anhand anonymisierter Bewertungen durch jeweils drei Fachgutachter wurden 86 Beiträge zur Präsentation ausgewählt: 48 Vorträge, 34 Poster und 4 Softwaredemonstrationen. Die Qualität der eingereichten Arbeiten war insgesamt sehr hoch. Die besten Arbeiten werden auch im Jahr 2015 mit BVM-Preisen ausgezeichnet. Die schriftlichen Langfassungen der Beiträge werden im Tagungsband abgedruckt, der auch dieses Jahr wieder im Springer Verlag in der Reihe Informatik aktuell zur BVM erscheint.

Höhepunkte der BVM 2015 bilden die Gastvorträge von *Prof. Dr. Julia Schnabel*, Institute of Biomedical Engineering der University of Oxford (UK) und von *Prof. Dr. Thorsten Buzug*, Institut für Medizintechnik der Universität zu Lübeck, die neueste Methoden und Trends in der medizinischen Bildregistrierung und Modellierung sowie aktuelle und zukünftige Entwicklungen der neuen Bildgebungstechnik Magnetic Particle Imaging vorstellen.

Die Internetseiten des Workshops bieten ausführliche Informationen über das Programm und organisatorische Details rund um die BVM 2015. Sie sind abrufbar unter der Adresse:

XII

http://www.bvm-workshop.org

Am Tag vor dem wissenschaftlichen Programm werden zwei Tutorials angeboten:

Prof. Dr. Bernhard Preim, Institut für Simulation und Graphik der Otto-von-Guericke-Universität Magdeburg, hält unterstützt von seinen Mitarbeiterinnen und Mitarbeitern ein Tutorial zum Thema „Visualisierung und Virtual-Reality-Techniken in der Medizin". Neben grundlegenden Methoden der medizinischen Visualisierung wie dem Volume Rendering und der Oberflächenvisualisierung werden ihre Anwendungsmöglichkeiten in verschiedenen medizinischen Bereichen vorgestellt. Weiterhin werden ausgewählte Anwendungsbeispiele aus der Operations- und Interventionsplanung sowie Methoden zur intraoperativen Visualisierung mit Virtual-Reality-Techniken präsentiert.

Das zweite Tutorial trägt den Titel „Medizinische Bildregistrierung". *Prof. Dr. Jan Modersitzki*, Fraunhofer MEVIS Lübeck, erläutert hier unterstützt von seinen Mitarbeiterinnen und Mitarbeitern wichtige medizinische Bildregistrierungsmethoden, beleuchtet ihren mathematischen Hintergrund und zeigt anhand von Beispielen ihre vielfältigen medizinischen Anwendungsmöglichkeiten auf.

Die Herausgeber dieser Proceedings möchten allen herzlich danken, die zum Gelingen der BVM 2015 beigetragen haben. Den Autoren für die rechtzeitige und formgerechte Einreichung ihrer qualitativ hochwertigen Arbeiten, dem Programmkomitee für die gründliche Begutachtung, den Gastrednern und den Referenten der Tutorials für Ihre aktive Mitgestaltung und inhaltliche Bereicherung der BVM 2015. *Herrn Dr. Thorsten Schaaf* vom Institut für Medizinische Informatik der Charité Universitätsmedizin Berlin danken wir für die engagierte Mithilfe bei der Erstellung und Pflege der Internetpräsentation. Herrn *Michael Brehler* von der Abteilung Medizinische und Biologische Informatik am Deutschen Krebsforschungszentrum in Heidelberg möchten wir herzlich für seine engagierte Tätigkeit bei der Umsetzung der WWW-basierten Tagungsanmeldung und der Pflege des BVM-Email-Verteilers danken. Herrn *Jan Dovermann* vom Institut für Medizinische Informatik der RWTH Aachen danken wir für die tatkräftige Mitarbeit bei der Erstellung des Proceedingsbandes. Für die webbasierte Durchführung des Reviewingprozesses gebührt Herrn *Dr. Jan-Hinrich Wrage*, für die Programmerstellung Herrn *Dr. Jan Ehrhardt* und *Jun.-Prof. Dr. Mattias Heinrich* vom Institut für Medizinische Informatik der Universität zu Lübeck unser Dank. Weiterhin danken wir der Tagungssekretärin Frau *Susanne Petersen* und allen übrigen Mitarbeiterinnen und Mitarbeitern des Instituts für Medizinische Informatik der Universität zu Lübeck für ihre tatkräftige Unterstützung bei der Organisation und Durchführung der BVM 2015. Unser Dank gilt auch den Mitgliedern des lokalen Lübecker BVM-Komitees für die Unterstützung bei Werbemaßnahmen und der Gewinn von Industriesponsoren für die BVM 2015. Für die finanzielle Unterstützung bedanken wir uns bei den Fachgesellschaften und der Industrie.

Wir wünschen allen Teilnehmerinnen und Teilnehmern der BVM 2015 lehrreiche Tutorials, viele anregende Vorträge, Gespräche an den Postern und in der Industrieausstellung sowie interessante neue Kontakte zu Kolleginnen und Kollegen aus dem Bereich der Medizinischen Bildverarbeitung.

Januar 2015

Heinz Handels (Lübeck)
Thomas Deserno (Aachen)
Hans-Peter Meinzer (Heidelberg)
Thomas Tolxdorff (Berlin)

Inhaltsverzeichnis

Die fortlaufende Nummer am linken Seitenrand entspricht den Beitragsnummern, wie sie im endgültigen Programm des Workshops zu finden sind. Dabei steht V für Vortrag, P für Poster und S für Softwaredemonstration.

Eingeladene Vorträge

Segmentierung I

Bildgebung I

Navigation & Visualisierung

Registrierung I

Bildgebung (Poster)

Bildrekonstruktion (Poster)

Navigation & Tracking (Poster)

Registrierung (Poster)

Physiologische Modellierung (Poster)

Mikroskopie & Optische Verfahren

Bildvorverarbeitung & Bildgestützte Dokumentation

Segmentierung II

Physiologische Modellierung

Segmentierung (Poster)

Klassifikation (Poster)

Parallelverarbeitung & Lehre (Poster)

Mikroskopie (Poster)

Visualisierung (Poster)

Klassifikation & Lernbasierte Verfahren

Bildgebung II

Complex Motion Modelling in Cancer Imaging

Julia Schnabel

Department of Engineering Science, University of Oxford
julia.schnabel@eng.ox.ac.uk

Abstract of Invited Talk

In this talk I will present our recent research efforts and advances in the field of motion modelling of complex organs in oncological applications, as part of the Cancer Research UK / EPSRC Cancer Imaging Centre at Oxford. I will focus on a number of novel non-linear image registration methodologies developed for motion compensation in single- and multi-modality lung imaging, which is a particularly challenging application due to the physiological complexity of the respiration process, such as the interaction between rigid structures, interfacing organs, and large deformations involved. We are currently working on two major challenges in this field: 1. Correcting for the sliding motion of the lungs, by modelling locally discontinuous deformations, and 2. Formulating computational tractable solutions for image alignment between different types of imaging modalities.

About the Presenter

Julia Schnabel is Professor in Engineering Science (Medical Imaging) at the Institute of Biomedical Engineering, University of Oxford, and a Fellow of St. Hilda's College, Oxford. She received her MSc in Computer Science in 1993 from the Technical University of Berlin, and her PhD in Computer Science in 1998 from University College London (UCL). Before taking up her academic post at Oxford in 2007, Julia was Research Associate at the Image Sciences Institute at the University Medical Centre Utrecht, Research Fellow at the Imaging Science Division at King's College London and at the Centre for Medical Image Computing at UCL. Julia's research in her 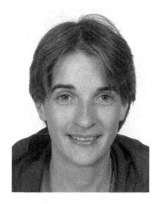 Biomedical Image Analysis (BioMedIA) laboratory focuses on developing innovative and translational imaging solutions for applications in oncology and

neurosciences. Julia has published over 130 peer-reviewed journal and confer-
ence articles, is Associate Editor for IEEE Transactions on Medical Imaging,
IEEE Transactions on Biomedical Engineering, and Editorial Board member for
Medical Image Analysis.

Magnetic Particle Imaging
Chancen und Herausforderungen einer neuen Modalität

Thorsten M. Buzug

Institut für Medizintechnik, Universität zu Lübeck
buzug@imt.uni-luebeck.de

Kurzfassung

Magnetic Particle Imaging (MPI) ist ein neues Bildgebungsverfahren, mit dem sich die lokale Konzentration von magnetischen Nanopartikeln quantitativ sowohl mit hoher Empfindlichkeit, als auch mit hervorragender räumlicher Auflösung in Echtzeit darstellen lässt [1]. Diese Vorteile gegenüber etablierten Verfahren, die oft nur einen der Bereiche abdecken können oder nicht quantitativ sind, lassen ein hohes klinisches Potenzial in vielen Anwendungen erwarten. Die Grundidee besteht in der Nutzung der nichtlinearen Magnetisierungskurve der Partikel [2]. Das Verfahren nutzt dazu zwei überlagernde Magnetfelder, zum einen ein statisches Selektionsfeld, zum anderen ein dynamisches Wechselfeld. Werden die Nanopartikel in das Wechselfeld gebracht, erzeugen sie eine nichtlineare Magnetisierung, die mit einer Empfangsspule gemessen werden kann. Aufgrund der Nichtlinearität enthält das gemessene Signal neben der Grundfrequenz des Wechselfelds auch Harmonische, also Schwingungen mit einem Vielfachen der Grundfrequenz. Nach Separation der Harmonischen von dem eingespeisten

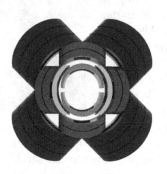
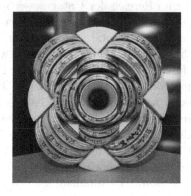

Abb. 1. Simulation (links) und Spulenrealisierung (rechts) eines 2D MPI-Scanners mit dynamisch rotier- und verschiebbarer feldfreier Linie [3].

Grundsignal, kann die Konzentration der Nanopartikel ermittelt werden. Eine örtliche Kodierung wird durch das statische Selektionsfeld erreicht. Als Tracer kommen nanopartikuläre Systeme aus Eisenoxid zum Einsatz. Die Rekonstruktion besteht beim Magnetic Particle Imaging in der Lösung des inversen Problems, bei dem zu den gemessenen induzierten Spannungen, die Konzentrationsverteilung der Nanopartikel bestimmt werden muss. Die Beziehung zwischen beiden Größen wird durch eine entsprechende Systemfunktion beschrieben. Aktuelle Entwicklungen in der Instrumentierung fokussieren insbesondere auf Spulenoptimierungen [4] (Abb. 1) sowie Konzepte für die Ganzkörpertomographie [5].

1. Buzug TM, Bringout G, Erbe M et al. Magnetic particle imaging: introduction to imaging and hardware realization. Z Med Phys. 2012;22(4):323-34
2. Lüdtke-Buzug K, Haegele J, Biederer S et al. Comparison of commercial iron oxide-based MRI contrast agents with synthesized high-performance MPI tracers. Biomed Eng. 2013;58(6): 527-33
3. Bente K, Weber M, Gräser M et al. Electronic field free line rotation and relaxation deconvolution in magnetic particle imaging. IEEE Trans Med Imaging. 2014, [Epub ahead of print], DOI: 10.1109/TMI.2014.2364891
4. Wojtczyk H, Bringout G, Tenner W et al. Toward the optimization of D-shaped coils for the use in an open magnetic particle imaging scanner. IEEE Trans Magn 2014;50(7):
5. Kaethner C, Ahlborg M, Bringout G et al. Axially elongated field-free point data acquisition in magnetic particle imaging. IEEE Trans Med Imaging. 2015;34(2):1-7

Über den Vortragenden

Prof. Buzug promovierte 1993 im Fach Angewandte Physik an der Universität zu Kiel. Nach einer postdoktoralen Position an der Forschungsanstalt der Bundeswehr für Wasserschall- und Geophysik (FWG) in Kiel, wo er im Bereich der Unterwasserbildgebung an SONAR-Systemen arbeitete, wechselte er 1994 zu den Philips Forschungslaboratorien Hamburg. Als Leiter des Forschungsclusters Bildverarbeitung war Prof. Buzug dort für Projekte der medizinischen Bildverarbeitung verantwortlich. Prof. Buzug wurde 1998 auf eine C3-Professur für Physik und Medizintechnik an den RheinAhrCampus Remagen berufen. 2006 wurde er 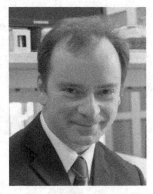 in seine derzeitige Position als Direktor des Instituts für Medizintechnik an der Universität zu Lübeck berufen. Prof. Buzug ist unter anderem Vizepräsident der Universität zu Lübeck, Sprecher des Kompetenzzentrums für Medizintechnik TANDEM und Vorstandsmitglied des Life-Science Nord e.V. (LSN).

Data-Driven Spine Detection for Multi-Sequence MRI

Daniel Kottke[1], Gino Gulamhussene[1], Klaus Tönnies[2]

[1]Otto-von-Guericke-University Magdeburg (equal contributors)
[2]Computer Vision Group, Otto-von-Guericke-University Magdeburg
parsos@gmx.de

Abstract. Epidemiology studies on vertebra's shape and appearance require big databases of medical images and image processing methods, that are robust against deformation and noise. This work presents a solution of the first step: the vertebrae detection. We propose a method that automatically detects the central spinal curve with 3D data-driven methods in multi-sequence magnetic resonance images (MRI). Additionally, we use simple edge operations for vertebra border detection that can be used for a statistical evaluation with help of some fast user interaction. Our automatic vertebrae detection algorithm fits a polynomial curve through the spinal canal, that afterwards is shifted towards the vertebra centers. An edge operator gives a first approximation of the vertebra borders, that can be evaluated and corrected by some user interaction within 12 seconds. We show, that our algorithm automatically detects more than 90% of all spines correctly, and present a preliminary analysis of vertebrae sizes.

1 Introduction

Huge field studies using medical images are a trade-off between the number of participants and the cost of each. Normally, computer science studies on magnetic resonance imaging (MRI) consist of a small number of subjects, and high quality images. The "Study of Health in Pomerania" (SHIP) [1] produced approximately 3300 datasets of human spine images. In contrast to many other studies, the number of available data is huge and enables statistical analysis of human anatomy in the normal population. However, the image sampling rate was reduced which complicates the image processing task.

Studying the anatomy of spine and vertebrae and thus generating anatomical norms for the normal population is one of the goals of SHIP. This work proposes a spine detection algorithm and gives an outlook on vertebra identification. The merit of our method lies in its data-driven nature, which ensures robustness towards vertebrae deformation and prevents model induced biases. The automatic process is divided into three phases: spinal canal extraction, spine curve calculation and vertebra border detection. Furthermore, we provide a graphical user interface, that allows validation and correction with fast user interaction.

Source code is available at: https://bitbucket.org/dkottke/parsos

The most challenging problem on medical images is the image quality. Hence, research on spinal detection and segmentation relies on top-down (model-based) methods. To cope with vertebrae deformation, one can use model descriptions (e.g. vertebra size ratios) or capture representative variations in a complex model. We observed that researchers preferred using more complex models in recent years. Specialized models only detect parts of the spine [2, 3, 4, 5, 6] whereas others use the full spine [7, 8]. 3D methods (e.g. [2, 4, 5]) allow more complex models.

One recent paper on segmentation of vertebrae in CT images was proposed by Kadoury et al. [3]. They segmented 12 thoracic and 5 lumbar vertebral bodies (VB) with help of a previously learned articulated deformable model and higher order markov random fields. MRI based algorithms rely on model-based segmentation and detection i.e. statistical shape models [4, 8], or graphical models [5]. Other methods build complex learning algorithms, e.g., Huang et al. [7] used an AdaBoost algorithm on wavelet transformed vertebrae, followed by a normalized cut segmentation. Some algorithms require initial user input, as they need key markers for an approximate detection [3, 5]. Others replaced this step by locating a central line through the spine or the spinal canal [4, 9, 7]. Neubert et al. [4] and Stern et al. [9] use a method based on the work by Vrtovec [10]. Here, a curve through the vertebra centers defines a local coordinate system of the spine, that facilitate to transform the whole spine into a straight one with more simple properties. Pohle-Frölich et al. [6] uses symmetry transformation to detect the spine position.

The next section provides a detailed description of our method in Sec. 2. In Sec. 3, we discuss our results and finally conclude our work in Sec. 4.

2 Materials and methods

Our data comprises 3D registered T1 and T2 weighted MR images of 3300 subjects that took part in the "Study of Health in Pomerania" (SHIP) [1]. The images cover the whole spine in 15 sagittal slices (1.11 mm x 1.11 mm x 4.4 mm) and contain a marker line in the center that locates the slice where the upper spine image was connected to the corresponding lower part. This is recognized and removed because we process the complete spine.

Our method does not use a spine model and consists of five phases (Fig. 2). First, we generate a mask for the spinal canal region that is used as a global region of interest (ROI) for all subjects. The main part contains three automatic phases: the extraction of the spinal canal using the pre-calculated ROI, the calculation of the polynomial through the vertebra centers (spine curve), and the detection of the vertebra borders. The fifth phase is interactive and ensures correct results with help of a graphical user interface.

2.1 Mask generation

To create a global mask, we manually segmented the cerebrospinal fluid from 10 randomly selected subjects. Due to varying body positions and shapes among the subjects, we did not use the absolute coordinates of the segmentation. Each transverse image plane was shifted such that the back was moved to the image border. We used the logical OR operator to combine the different transformed masks, that finally are dilated separately for every spine part. The dilation degree depends on the variance between the different segmentations. Thus, we have a mask that defines the region of interest relative to the subject's back position.

2.2 Spinal canal extraction

To find the spinal canal, we used the mask from the previous step. It is placed relatively to the subject's back, which is localized by an intensity comparison, as the rightmost visible structure in our MR images (Fig. 2 (a)). This region of interest (ROI) ensures that structures i.e. fluids, that are far from the spine, will not be considered. To create an estimate of the bias field, we used a maximum filter with infinite kernel depth and width and a height of 16mm. Each sequence (T1 and T2-weighted MRI) is multiplied with the inverse of the bias field estimate to remove this artifact. Since cerebrospinal fluid appears dark in T1 and bright in T2 weighted MR images, subtracting the T1 weighted from the T2 weighted image, generates an image where only fluids are bright. To find tubelike structures these images are convolved with kernels filled with ones of 20x2x2mm size and $\pm15°$ and $\pm30°$ orientation. To detect outliers, we use information of volume and variance of each connected segment in the binary image after thresholding. Fitting a polynomial curve on the means of the axial slice, we produce a non-linear transformation such as in Vrtovec [10] (Fig. 2 (b)). This simplifies the future operations: the detection of the central spinal curve and vertebrae borders.

2.3 Spine curve calculation

The polynomial curve from the previous step can be used to create a curved planar reconstruction (CPR) [10]. This provides a straight spinal canal and a approximate straight spine (Fig. 2 (c)), which simplifies subsequent steps.

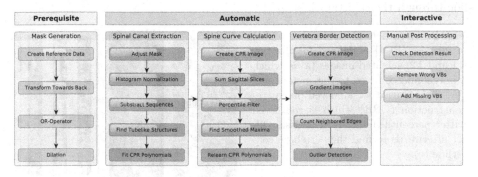

Fig. 1. Graphical summary of the complete algorithm.

Since vertebral bodies, intervertebral discs and other neighboring structures cannot be distinguished only by intensity, the most valuable information are the edges between vertebral bodies and intervertebral discs. Near the spine centers ($[-8mm, 8mm]$) these edges do not vary in the sagittal plane because of the CPR. Summing the derivatives of the image slices sagittally produces a noise reduced edge image (Fig. 2 (c) left). Using a percentile filter with a kernel that overlaps at least one vertebra edge and smoothing the result with a Gaussian filter, we get an image with the highest values along the centerline of the spine (Fig. 2 (c) center and right). Tracking the local maximums produces the shifted polynomial.

2.4   Vertebrae border detection

To detect the borders between vertebral bodies and intervertebral discs, we search for significant edges. In order to minimize the noise we add the first derivative of both T1 and T2 weighted MR images pixel-wise. This is equivalent to the mean derivative of both images. Then, we distinguish between strong rising (start of a vertebral body (VB)) and falling edges (end of VB) with a zero crossing at the second derivative of the mean image. Hence, we can generate a first estimation of vertebral body borders by assigning starting and ending edges according to their order. In an iterative process we eliminate inconsistencies by assuming that the vertebral body length and the intervertebral disc thickness change linearly with its position on the spine. We estimate this model iteratively by linear regression and distinguish outlying data points. When segments are abnormally large, additional edges are searched, and edges are deleted if segments are abnormally small. The process ends when no more outliers are detected.

2.5   Manual post processing

In order to assess the results, we implemented a graphical user interface, providing a 2D sagittal view of the spine with its polynomial curve and the detected vertebrae with their borders. Furthermore, this tool allows the user to remove wrongly detected vertebrae and add missing ones, while being able to zoom and slide through the sagittal slices.

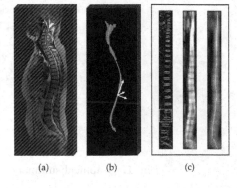

Fig. 2. With help of the mask a region of interest (ROI) is defined for the raw T1 and T2 weighted images (a) in which a polynomial is fitted to the spinal canal (b). This is used for a curved planar reconstruction (CPR) which is convolved with a percentile filter and a Gaussian filter afterwards to find the vertebrae centerline (c).

(a)   (b)   (c)

Table 1. Relative frequency of manual removing/adding of vertebral bodies.

Number of VBs deleted	0	1	2	3	4	5	6	7+
Relative frequency	0.18	0.13	0.24	0.18	0.15	0.05	0.03	0.03
Number of VBs added	0	1	2	3	4	5	6	7
Relative frequency	0.60	0.13	0.12	0.08	0.00	0.01	0.02	0.02

3   Results

To evaluate our algorithm we randomly selected 100 data sets, which have never been seen during development to minimize the probability of overfitting. The automatic detection takes approximately 30 seconds per data on a normal customer PC. Determined by human inspection, the algorithm's success rate for correctly detecting the spine centerline was 92%. A trial was marked as correct, if the polynomial line crossed all vertebral bodies. In 5 out of the 8 erroneous results the detected spine centerline was to short, in 2 cases the mask did not match the subject's exceptionally body width and in 1 case the T1 and T2 weighted MR images have been wrongly registered. As the algorithm is based on basic data-driven operations, the performance was not sensitive to small parameter changes. The mean execution time for the interactive step and hence the correction was 11.4s. In 73% of the cases not more then 3 vertebral bodies had to be removed, and in 93% no more than 3 vertebral bodies had to be added (Tab. 1).

We used the corrected results for a preliminary epidemiological analysis of vertebra heights. So, we created a boxplot for each vertebra (Fig. 3). Notice, that C1 and C2 are plotted together as it was not possible to distinguish them. Using our method with all 3300 data sets of the SHIP study, it can be possible to derive epidemiological models for the healthy Pomeranian population. A preliminary analysis of the 100 randomly selected subjects shows the distribution of relative vertebra heights. 3 shows that the thickness does not increase linearly (as assumed for border detection, see section 2.4). Hence, inclusion of a better vertebra thickness model may improve detection of vertebrae borders.

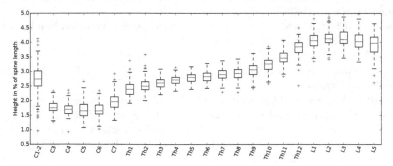

Fig. 3. Boxplots of relative vertebra sizes.

4 Discussion

This paper proposes a new data-driven method for robust spine detection using three automatic phases, namely spinal canal extraction, spine curve calculation and vertebra border detection, a initial mask generation step and a final post-processing phase. We are able to get a success rate higher than 90% for the spine centerline detection with solely bottom-up methods. Furthermore, the vertebrae border detection approach with a consecutive fast ($\approx 12\,$s) user interaction enables statistical vertebrae lengths analysis. Using only a few and not sensitive parameters (like tube kernels or other filters), the method is very robust.

Applying a robust segmentation algorithm will create a huge database of vertebral bodies and intervertebral discs that can be used to reliably classify spine pathologies. Our algorithm already allows robust analysis on spine shapes and can be used in medical applications.

Acknowledgement. The work presented in this paper has been funded by DFG, grant TO 166/13-2.

References

1. Völzke H, Alte D, Schmidt CO, et al. Cohort profile: the study of health in Pomerania. Int J Epidemiol. 2011;40(2):294–307.
2. Tönnies KD, Rak M, Engel K. Deformable part models for object detection in medical images. Biomed Eng Online. 2014;13:S1.
3. Kadoury S, Labelle H, Paragios N. Spine segmentation in medical images using manifold embeddings and higher-order MRFs. IEEE Trans Med Imaging. 2013;32(7):1227–38.
4. Neubert A, Fripp J, Engstrom C, et al. Automated detection, 3D segmentation and analysis of high resolution spine MR images using statistical shape models. Phys Med Biol. 2012;57(24):8357–76.
5. Dong X, Lu H, Sakurai Y, et al. Automated intervertebral disc detection from low resolution, sparse MRI images for the planning of scan geometries. Lect Notes Computer Sci. 2010;6357:10–7.
6. Pohle-Fröhlich R, Brandt C, Koy T. Segmentierung der lumbalen bandscheiben in MRT-bilddaten. Proc BVM. 2013; p. 63–8.
7. Huang SH, Chu YH, Lai SH, et al. Learning-based vertebra detection and iterative normalized-cut segmentation for spinal MRI. IEEE Trans Med Imaging. 2009;28(10):1595–605.
8. Schmidt S, Kappes J, Bergtholdt M, et al. Spine detection and labeling using a parts-based graphical model. Inf Process Med Imaging. 2007;20:122–33.
9. Stern D, Likar B, Pernus F, et al. Automated detection of spinal centrelines, vertebral bodies and intervertebral discs in CT and MR images of lumbar spine. Phys Med Biol. 2010;55(1):247–64.
10. Vrtovec T, Ourselin S, Gomes L, et al. Automated generation of curved planar reformations from MR images of the spine. Phys Med Biol. 2007;52(10):2865–78.

Automated Breast Volume of Interest Selection by Analysing Breast-Air Boundaries in MRI

Tatyana Ivanovska[1], Lei Wang[2], Henry Völzke[1], Katrin Hegenscheid[1]

[1]University Medicine, Ernst-Moritz-Arndt University Greifswald
[2]Fraunhofer MeVis, Bremen
tiva@uni-greifswald.de

Abstract. The first step in automated breast density estimation is to extract breast volume of interest, namely, the start and end slice numbers from the whole sequence. We evaluated results produced by two radiologists and developed an automatic strategy for the start and end slice detection. The result comparison showed that it is usually more straightforward to find the breast start than the breast end, where the tissue gradually disappears. In general, the results produced by the algorithm are sufficiently accurate, and our solution will be integrated into a fully automatic breast segmentation pipeline.

1 Introduction

Breast density is one of the important risk factors for breast cancer development [1]. Manual delineation of breast and parenchymal tissues is an observer dependent and extremely time-consuming procedure, which makes processing of numerous datasets acquired, for example, within epidemiological research studies, practically infeasible. Therefore, automated segmentation algorithms are required.

The first subtask in automated breast density estimation is detecting a breast volume of interest (VOI): one needs to find a region, where the breast actually presents, and exclude unnecessary slices from further processing. Whereas there are several methods for automatic breast segmentation or breast density estimation presented in the literature [2, 3, 4, 5], this subtask has been usually solved either manually, when for each dataset the user selects the start and end slices, or semi-automatically, for instance, by setting a threshold on the distance between the top breast-air boundary and breast cavity in each slice. Such approaches require user interaction (such as selecting different parameter settings for dense and fatty breasts), which is not optimal for processing of numerous data. In this paper, we evaluate breast VOI selection results from two independent observers and propose a fully automated strategy for such detection.

2   Materials and methods

2.1   Materials

Breast MR data were acquired at 1.5 Tesla on a whole-body MR imager (Magnetom Avanto; Siemens Medical Solutions, Erlangen, Germany). In our tests an unenhanced non-fat-suppressed T1-weighted time-resolved sequence with stochastic trajectories (TWIST) with $0.9 \times 0.7 \times 1.5$ mm voxels in the axial plane was used. Forty cases of healthy subjects were selected randomly from four breast density groups (10 datasets from each group). The volume resolution is $512 \times 512 \times 128$. "Breast start" and "breast end" anatomically represent the lower breast boundary, which is located close to liver, and the upper breast boundary, which is located close to lung, respectively.

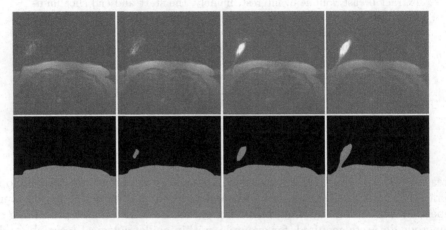

Fig. 1. Several consecutive slices taken in the breast start region from original data (dataset 10) and the correspondent breast-air masks. Slice numbers are marked red.

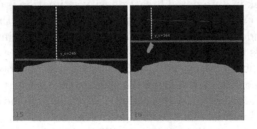

Fig. 2. A difference between minimum bounding box's upper boundaries of the mask is computed for each pair of consecutive slices. In slice 15, $y_{s_{15}} = 245$ and in slice 16, $y_{s_{16}} = 164$. The difference is $diff_{16} = |245 - 164|$.

2.2 Methods

Manual detection Two experienced radiologists (R_1 and R_2) evaluated the images independently. They scrolled through each dataset and named two slice numbers indicating the breast start and end positions.

Automated detection For the automated detection we utilized positions of breast-air boundaries in each slice. It is a rather straightforward task to detect these boundaries, since the air produces a signal close to 0, and the breast-air boundary is the first boundary with a significant gradient in the image. Here, multiple approaches can be applied. For example, Wu et al. [3] applied thresholding, image morphological opening [6], and contour extraction; Wang et al. [2] used a Hessian-based filter; Nie et al. [5] utilized the Fuzzy C-Means [6]. We apply Expectation Maximization for Gaussian mixture model [6], extract the class with the lowest intensity level, and smooth contours with the fast implicit active contours [7]. As a result, the breast-air boundary mask is obtained. Such a mask can be further utilized for multiple purposes, e. g., for simultaneous bias field correction and segmentation [8] on a selected VOI.

We use the breast-air mask to identify the breast start and end slices:

- *Breast start detection:* The breast start usually appears in the slice, where one or both breast regions overhang significantly from the body part (Fig. 1). The radiologists marked the start slice as „the first slice, where the breast is significantly visible ". We formalize this statement as follows. For each slice $z_i \in [Z_1, \ldots, Z_m]$, where $[Z_1, Z_m]$ is a slice interval in the beginning of the sequence, we compute the minimum bounding rectangle of the breast mask defined by the upper left and lower right points $(x_s, y_s, z_s)_{z_i}$ and $(x_e, y_e, z_e)_{z_i}$. Thereafter, we compute the difference between y_s-values for each pair of slices $\text{diff}_{z_{i+1}} = |y_{s_{z_i}} - y_{s_{z_{i+1}}}|$. In Fig. 2, an example for a pair of slices is shown. Finally, we select the slice z_{start} with the maximal difference $\{\forall z_i \in [Z_1, \ldots, Z_m]\ \text{diff}_{z_{\text{start}}} = \max(\text{diff})\}$ as the breast start slice.
- *Breast end detection:* The breast end is usually more complicated to detect, since the tissue decreases gradually. The radiologists define the breast end

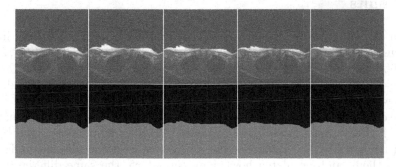

Fig. 3. Several consecutive slices taken in the breast end region from original data (dataset 33) and the correspondent breast-air masks. Slice numbers are marked red.

Fig. 4. Processing steps for breast end slice detection. Left: the central breast VOI is marked red, and the lowest breast cavity point is marked green. Right: in each slice the distance between y_s and Y_{bcp} is computed.

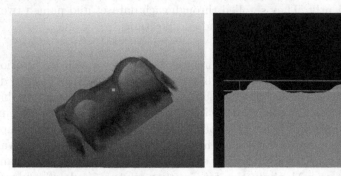

as "the last slice, where the breast is still visible". In Fig. 3, several slices from another test dataset are shown.

We observe that a measure, similar to the one used for the breast start detection, is not reliable enough for the cases where breast tissue decreases gradually, so we extend it as follows. First, we compute the central breast VOI, so that it covers the top points, located close to nipples, and detect y coordinate of the lowest breast cavity point (denoted as Y_{bcp}) within this VOI (Fig. 4).

Second, for slices $z_i \in [Z_1, \dots, Z_k]$, where $[Z_1, Z_k]$ is a slice interval in the end of the sequence, we compute the axis-aligned bounding box of the breast mask in the same manner as for the breast start. Thereafter, we compute two difference values and associate them with each z_i value:

1. between the upper points for each pair of slices $\text{diff}_{z_i} = |y_{s_{z_i}} - y_{s_{z_{i+1}}}|$,
2. between the upper point and the cavity point $\text{cDiff}_i = |Y_{bcp} - y_{s_{z_i}}|$.

Finally, the breast end slice is detected as $z_{\text{end}} = \min(z_{\text{end}_1}, z_{\text{end}_2})$, where z_{end_1} is the slice with $\{\forall z_i \in [Z_l, \dots, Z_k]\ \text{diff}_{z_{\text{end}_1}} = \max(\text{diff})\}$, and z_{end_2} is the slice, where the values cDiff reach the first local minimum.

3   Results

For our target sequence, we empirically selected $60\,mm$ slice intervals in the beginning and the end of the sequence and set $[Z_1, Z_m] = [10, 50]$ and $[Z_l, Z_k] = [80, 120]$.

The detection is computationally inexpensive and takes about a second. The scripts were implemented in Python and run in MeVisLab (mevislab.de).

The comparison results are presented as histograms (Fig. 5) and summarized in Tab. 1. For 40 test datasets, we compared the slice numbers selected by the human readers and the automatic detector, computed the absolute difference between them, and calculated how many cases have the same difference. For example, in breast start detection two radiologists fully agreed only in 5 cases (the difference equals 0).

Table 1. Summary of start and end slice selections by two human observers (R_1 and R_2) and the automatic detector (*Auto*).

Methods	Breast start			Breast end		
	Min	Max	$\mu \pm \sigma$	Min	Max	$\mu \pm \sigma$
R_1 vs R_2	0	10	1.825 ± 1.66	0	18	2.85 ± 4.15
Auto vs R_1	0	5	1.95 ± 0.98	0	21	4.9 ± 3.6
Auto vs R_2	0	14	1.2 ± 2.3	0	17	3.68 ± 2.52

4 Discussion

Our goal is to replace manual or semi-automatic breast VOI selection with an automated procedure, which would produce results similar to the human experts' ones. We observed, for instance, that the approach utilized by Wang et al. [2], which accepted a slice for processing, if the distance between the central breast cavity point and the breast-air boundary was less than a user-defined threshold, required careful selection of the threshold value. Otherwise, even in the cases where the experts had a difference interval of $[0, 2]$ slices, the method produced up to $[6, 10]$ slice difference in comparison to the observers' results. On the other hand, the presented method produces the results that are similar to the observers' ones.

In general, the detection of breast start appeared more straightforward than the breast end detection. The experienced radiologists produce, on average, a difference of 2 ± 1.66 and 3 ± 4 slices for the breast start and end, respectively. For the automatic detector's results, the average difference lies in the interval of $[1, 2]$ with the standard deviation in $[1, 2.3]$ for the breast start and for the breast end the difference is $[3, 4]$ slices with the standard deviation in $[3.6, 4.9]$. Taking the example in Fig. 1, the radiologists selected slices 18 and 15, respectively,

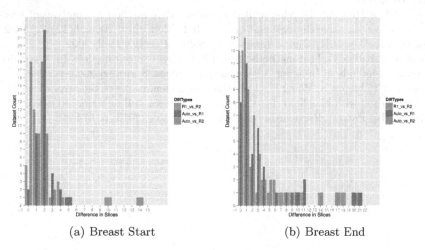

(a) Breast Start   (b) Breast End

Fig. 5. Histograms of the slice differences produced by two human observers and the algorithm.

whereas the automatic detector took slice 16. In Fig. 3, the experts selected slices 102 and 109, and the algorithm chose slice 104. There are also outliers both in start and end detection (Fig. 5), which are the cases, where the tissue increases or decreases gradually. Here, no good agreement between the experts is noticeable. For example, in dataset 39 the differences in breast start and end values between the human observers are 10 and 18, correspondingly. Hence, the same dataset becomes an outlier for the automatic detector.

The presented approach is rather general and relies on the extracted breast-air boundaries. It can be applied to any data, where the boundaries are clearly visible and not affected by such artefacts as complicated tumors or mastectomy. However, the slice intervals $[Z_1, Z_m]$ and $[Z_l, Z_k]$ need to be adapted dependent on the volumetric resolution of a specific sequence.

Our automatic procedure produces sufficiently accurate results. When compared to the values produced by the radiologists, the differences lie close to the inter-reader variability. The proposed method will be used as the first step in automated breast density evaluation pipeline.

References

1. Boyd N, Guo H, et al. Mammographic density and the risk and detection of breast cancer. N Engl J Med. 2007;356(3):227–36.
2. Wang L, Platel B, Ivanovska T, et al. Fully automatic breast segmentation in 3D breast MRI. Proc ISBI. 2012; p. 1024–7.
3. Wu S, Weinstein S, Conant E, et al. Automated fibroglandular tissue segmentation and volumetric density estimation in breast MRI using an atlas-aided fuzzy C-means method. Med Phys. 2013;40(12):122302.
4. Gubern-Mérida A, Kallenberg M, Mann R, et al. Breast segmentation and density estimation in breast MRI: A fully automatic framework. J Biomed Health Inform. 2014;To appear.
5. Nie K, Chen JH, et al. Development of a quantitative method for analysis of breast density based on three-dimensional breast MRI. Med Phys. 2008;35(12):5253–62.
6. Gonzales R, Woods R. Digital Image Processing. Prentice Hall; 2002.
7. Weickert J, Kühne G. Fast methods for implict active contour models. In: Geometric Level Set Methods in Imaging, Vision, and Graphics. Springer; 2003. p. 43–57.
8. Ivanovska T, Laqua R, Wang L, et al. Fast implementations of the levelset segmentation method with bias field correction in MR images: full domain and mask-based versions. In: Pattern Recognition and Image Analysis; 2013. p. 674–81.

Automatische Detektion von Okklusionen zerebraler Arterien in 3D-Magnetresonanzangiographiedaten

Albrecht Kleinfeld[1], Oskar Maier[1], Nils Forkert[2], Heinz Handels[1]

[1]Institut für Medizinische Informatik, Universität zu Lübeck
[2]Department of Radiology, University of Calgary, Canada
kleinfea@miw.uni-luebeck.de

Kurzfassung. Eine schnelle und präzise Detektion verschlossener Hirn-arterien ist für die Therapie des ischämischen Schlaganfalls ausschlag-gebend. In diesem Beitrag wird eine automatische Methode vorgestellt, um okkludierte Blutgefäße in 3D-TOF-MRA-Bildsequenzen aufzufinden. Hierbei werden unter Verwendung verschiedener Schwellwertparameter, auf Grundlage von Vesselnesswerten, alle Endarme des Gefäßskeletts hin-sichtlich einer möglichen Okklusion untersucht. Erste Ergebnisse zeigen, dass der vorgestellte Ansatz mit einer Sensitivität von über 85% eine Auf-findung verschlossener Arterien ermöglicht und somit eine gute Grund-lage für weiterführende Algorithmen darstellt.

1 Einleitung

Der Schlaganfall gilt als die dritthäufigste Todesursache in den Industrielän-dern [1]. Jährlich erleiden etwa 150.000 bis 200.000 Einwohner Deutschlands einen Gehirnschlag, deren Zahl mit steigendem Durchschnittsalter weiter zuneh-men wird. In 80% − −85% dieser Fälle sind ischämische Hirninfarkte, die durch einen Verschluss oder eine starke Verengung zerebraler Arterien hervorgerufen werden, deren schnelle Auffindung für den Erfolg einer Therapie entscheidend ist. Ein bei der Detektion unterstützendes, automatisches Verfahren kann daher ein wichtiges Hilfsmittel in der Früherkennung ischämischer Schlaganfälle sein.

Bildgebende Verfahren, wie die Computer- (CT) oder Magnetresonanzto-mographie (MRT), sind wichtige diagnostische Mittel bei der Erkennung zere-braler Infarkte. Die mit diesen Verfahren generierten 3D-Übersichtsaufnahmen ermöglichen eine Einstufung und Lagebestimmung ischämischer Läsionen. Wei-terhin erlaubt die CT- oder MRT-Angiographie eine Lokalisation verschlossener Blutgefäße, wobei die gewonnenen Bilddaten weitestgehend manuell ausgewertet werden müssen. Automatisierte Segmentierungen und Klassifizierungen betrof-fener Hirnareale wurden bereits vorgestellt und von Rekik et al. [2] kürzlich zusammengefasst. Ein automatisches Verfahren hinsichtlich der Stenosefindung in Herzgefäßen wurde von Teßmann et al. [3] entwickelt und wäre für die Detek-tion verengter, kranialer Arterien denkbar. Computergestützte Bestimmungen zerebraler Okklusionen sind nach bestem Wissen des Autors nicht bekannt. Der hier vorgestellte, regelbasierte Algorithmus, auf Grundlage von Time-of-Flight-Magnetresonanzangiographie und Vesselnessdaten, ist ein neues, automatisches Verfahren zur Erkennung komplett verschlossener Gefäße.

2 Material und Methoden

2.1 Bilddaten

Die bei der Okklusionsbestimmung verwendeten 3D-Bilddaten beruhen auf der Time-of-Flight (TOF)-Magnetresonanzangiographie (MRA), die Abbildungen zerebraler Arterien erzeugen kann. Eine klare Differenzierung zwischen Hirngewebe und Blutbahnen ist dabei ohne Einsatz von Kontrastmitteln möglich. Für die Evaluation des hier vorgestellten Detektionsalgorithmus standen fünf TOF-MRA-Bildsequenzen mit eindeutigen Okklusionen verschiedener Arterien zur Verfügung. Als Grundlage für die Phantomerstellung dienten drei weitere Datensätze ohne vorhandene Verschlüsse.

2.2 Phantomgenerierung

Ein zur Erstellung künstlicher Okklusionen entwickelter Algorithmus ermöglicht eine variationsreiche Generierung von Test- und Validierungsdaten. Hierbei wird unter Verwendung des segmentierten Arterienbaumes einer TOF-Aufnahme die Mittelachslinie des zu verschließenden Gefäßes berechnet und unter Angabe von Durchmesser, Füllstartpunkt und Richtung ein künstlicher Verschluss durch Dilatation der Centerline erzeugt. Der entstehende Bereich wird mit Grauwerten gefüllt, die auf einer Gaußschen Normalverteilung der originalen Hirnwerte basieren, welche durch Maskierung der TOF-Bilder ermittelt werden. Wie in Abb. 1(a) und (b) zu sehen, ist nach Überlagerung des berechneten Areals auf die 3D-Bildsequenz ein Verschluss simulierbar.

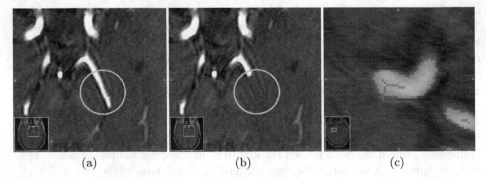

(a)   (b)   (c)

Abb. 1. Hirngefäß vor (a) und nach (b) der Phantomerstellung. (c) Abzweigung der Centerline (rot), die nicht auf einer echten Bifurkation der Arterie beruht und durch einen vermeintlichen Ausläufer der Segmentierung (orange) entsteht.

2.3   Segmentierung und Skelettierung des Gefäßbaumes

Grundlage für die Segmentierung des Arterienbaumes bildet der von Sato et al. [4] vorgestellte Vesselness-Filter. Der auf den Eigenwerten einer Hessematrix basierende Algorithmus ermöglicht eine Bestimmung tubulärer Strukturen und ist in der Lage auch kleinere, oft weniger kontrastreiche Arterien zu detektieren. Unter Verwendung der erhaltenen Vesselnessdaten und der originalen TOF-Bildsequenz wird mit dem von Forkert et al. [5] entwickelten Fuzzy-Schwellwertverfahren ein dreidimensionaler Arterienbaum segmentiert. Entstehende Hohlräume werden automatisch gefüllt und detektiertes Knochen- und Augengewebe durch eine Hirnmaskierung eliminiert. Das von Homan [6] entwickelte Skelettierungsverfahren, basierend auf einer Methode von Lee et al. [7], ermöglicht die Berechnung der Centerline der segmentierten Gefäße. Unter Berücksichtigung der topologischen Euler-Charakteristik werden durch diese Methode dreidimensionale Strukturen iterativ ausgedünnt. Die Anzahl der im Bild enthaltenen Komponenten bleibt hierbei unverändert und eine symmetrische Lage der Centerline in Bezug auf den Arterienverlauf wird erzeugt.

2.4   Nachbearbeitung der Centerline

Vor Beginn der Okklusionsmarkierung werden einzelne Komponenten und Lücken des Skelettbaumes verbunden bzw. geschlossen. Hierfür werden Skelettenden durch eine Nachbarschaftsanalyse bestimmt, wobei ein bestehendes Endvoxel genau ein benachbartes Centerlinevoxel besitzt. Innerhalb eines Kugelsektors mit einem Öffnungswinkel von 120° und einer Höhe von 5 mm wird nach potentiellen Fortsetzungspunkten gesucht und beginnend mit dem dichtesten Voxel eine mögliche Verbindung entlang der höchsten Vesselness erstellt. Hierbei darf der Winkel zwischen dem Vektor der jeweiligen letzten beiden Astpunkte und dem Vektor vom temporären Endpunkt zum Fortsetzungspunkt maximal 60° groß sein. Dies verhindert ein Zurücklaufen der Centerline in die Arterie. Um weitere fehlerhafte Lückenfüllungen zu vermeiden, müssen die Vesselnesswerte entlang der entstehenden Verbindung mindestens 30% des Mittelwertes der ursprünglichen Astvoxel betragen.

Sehr kurze Seitenarme mit einer Länge von unter 1 mm werden gelöscht, da diese häufig durch den Skelettierungsalgorithmus entstehen und nicht auf reellen Gefäßabzweigungen basieren. Des Weiteren müssen Skelettarme mit einer Maximallänge von 10 mm entlang ihrer letzten 3 mm eine verbleibende Vesselness von mindestens 30% des durchschnittlichen Hauptastwertes aufweisen, da diese durch kleine Ausläufer der Segmentierung entstehen und fehlerhaft als Okklusion erkannt werden. Ein Beispiel hierfür ist in Abb. 1(c) dargestellt.

2.5   Okklusionsdetektion

Alle nach der Bearbeitung des Skelettbaumes bestehenden Endäste werden als potentielle Okklusionskandidaten betrachtet und in weiteren Schritten untersucht. Abrupt endende Arterien weisen hohe Vesselnesswerte auf, die im Verschlussbereich stark abfallen. Um diesen Gradienten zu ermitteln, wird die Centerline jeder endenden Hirnarterie entlang der höchsten Vesselness um durchschnittlich 10 mm verlängert. Dadurch entstehen zwei Abschnitte, die der inneren und äußeren Centerline. Eine schematische Darstellung dieser Bereiche ist in Abb. 2 zu finden. Die Richtung der hinzugefügten Voxel wird dabei durch die jeweiligen letzten beiden Punkte des Skelettastes bestimmt. Der Vektor dieser zwei und der Vektor zwischen neuem und letztem Voxel dürfen einen maximalen Winkel von 60° aufspannen. Auf diese Weise wird ein Zurücklaufen der verlängerten Centerline in das Gefäß verhindert. Unter Verwendung der ursprünglichen und der hinzugefügten Astpunkte werden auf Basis gaussgefilterter Vesselnesswerten alle Skelettarme analysiert. Eine als verschlossen eingestufte Arterie muss hierbei vier wesentlich Schwellwertparameter erfüllen.

- *Vesselnessgradient:* Für jeden Endarm wird entlang der verlängerten Centerline der maximale Vesselnessabfall zwischen seinen benachbarten Voxeln bestimmt und über alle erhaltenen Maximumgradienten des Skelettbaumes der Durchschnittswert ermittelt. Diesen Schwellwert muss ein als verschlossen eingeordnetes Gefäß mit seinem maximalen Vesselnessabfall überschreiten.
- *Vesselnessdurchschnitt:* Des Weiteren wird über alle endenden Skelettarme, ohne Berücksichtigung der Verlängerungsvoxel, der mittlere Vesselnesswert berechnet. Auch diesen muss eine als okkludiert eingestufte Arterie entlang ihrer initialen Astpunkte im Durchschnitt übersteigen.
- *Vesselnessmedian:* Weiterhin werden für jedes Gefäß die Vesselnessmediane der inneren und der äußeren Centerline bestimmt. Weisen diese Werte einen Unterschied von mindestens 70% auf, so wird die zugehörige Arterie als nicht durchblutet erkannt.
- Durchmesserschätzung: Um fehlerhaft segmentiertes Gewebe und sehr kleine auslaufende Arterien ausschließen zu können, wird unter Verwendung der Segmentierung eine Durchmesserschätzung der Gefäße durchgeführt. Entlang der originalen Centerline muss hierbei eine durchschnittliche Segmentdicke von mindestens 1 mm bestehen.

Diese Parameter ermöglichen eine Unterscheidung von kontinuierlich und abrupt endenden Arterien. Gefäße, die über den Bildrand hinaus verlaufen und bei Ver-

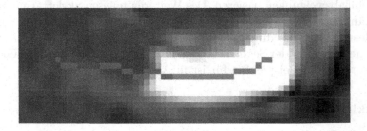

Abb. 2. Schematische Darstellung einer verlängerten Centerline. Abgebildet sind innere, originale Skelettvoxel (grün) und äußere, hinzugefügte Astpunkte (rot).

Tabelle 1. Quantitative Ergebnisse der Evaluation auf Grundlage von fünf Datensätzen mit realen Okklusionen und 9 Phantomen, erstellt auf Grundlage dreier TOF-Bildsequenzen. Aufgelistet ist die Anzahl aller untersuchten Endpunkte des Skelettbaumes und die Zahl der als verschlossen eingestuften Arterien sowie richtig-positiv (RP) detektierte Okklusionen. Weiterhin ist die Art der verschlossenen Arterie angegeben.

Datensatz	Endpunkte	Okklusionen	RP	Arterienart
Original 1	120	3	1	A. cerebri media
Original 2	99	3	1	A. cerebri media
Original 3	117	1	0	A. cerebri media
Original 4	232	3	1	A. cerebri media
Original 5	271	8	1	A. cerebri posterior
Phantom 1.01	111	3	1	A. cerebri media
Phantom 1.02	126	4	1	A. carotis interna
Phantom 1.03	123	4	1	A. vertebralis
Phantom 2.01	143	4	1	A. cerebri posterior
Phantom 2.02	148	4	1	A. cerebri posterior
Phantom 2.03	147	3	0	Abzweigung der A. basilaris
Phantom 3.01	86	2	1	A. cerebri media
Phantom 3.02	87	2	1	A. cerebri posterior
Phantom 3.03	89	2	1	A. vertebralis

längerung der Centerline einen hohen Vesselnessgradienten aufweisen, werden nicht bei der Verschlussdetektion berücksichtigt.

3 Ergebnisse

Für die Validierung des Detektionsalgorithmus wurden 9 Phantome mit verschiedenen Arterienverschlüssen erstellt. Zusätzlich standen fünf Aufnahmen mit originalen Okklusionen zur Verfügung. Nach Berechnung und Bearbeitung des Gefäßbaumes wurde die Anzahl der zu untersuchenden Astenden ermittelt und

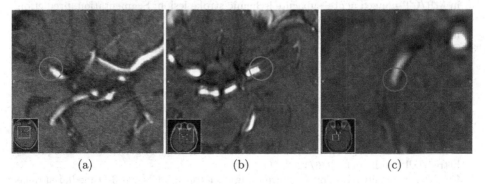

(a)	(b)	(c)

Abb. 3. Dargestellt sind richtig detektierte Arterien mit (a) originaler und (b) simulierter Okklusion. Unter (c) ist ein nicht erkannter, künstlicher Verschluss abgebildet.

jede hinsichtlich einer potentiellen Verstopfung untersucht. Die Zahlen der als verschlossen eingestuften Arterien mit Angabe der richtig ermittelten Okklusionen ist in Tab. 1 aufgelistet. Beispiele verschiedener Bilddaten mit richtig und falsch ermittelten Okklusionen sind in Abb. 3 dargestellt.

4 Diskussion

In der vorliegenden Arbeit wurde eine Methode zur Auffindung okkludierter, zerebraler Gefäße vorgestellt und unter Verwendung verschiedener TOF-MRA-Datensätze getestet. Eine erste Validierung ergab, dass 4 von 5 echt verschlossene Arterien und 8 von 9 simulierte Verstopfungen richtig erkannt wurden. Hierbei konnte eine Spezifität von über 98% erreicht werden. Die Arterienverschlüsse wurden durch den Median-, Gradienten- und Vesselnessdurchschnittsfilter stets ermittelt, wohingegen in zwei Fällen aufgrund einer nur schmalen Segmentierung die Okklusion durch die Durchmesserschätzung aus der Ergebnismenge gelöscht wurde. Eine verbesserte Durchmesserüberprüfung könnte auch hier ein Auffinden der Verschlüsse ermöglichen. Okklusionen die direkt an einer arteriellen Bifurkation liegen, können aufgrund einer nicht vorhandenen oder nur sehr kurzen Centerline nicht detektiert werden. Ebenso können die Verlängerungsvoxel eines Endarmes in benachbarte Arterien führen und so die Auffindung eines Verschlusses verhindern.

Der vorgestellte Algorithmus ist mit einer Detektionswahrscheinlichkeit von über 85% ein erster guter Ansatz zur Auffindung verschlossener Hirnarterien. Für die Weiterentwicklung dieses Verfahrens ist eine Evaluation basierend auf verschiedenen Originaldaten echt okkludierter Gefäße wünschenswert. Durch erweiterte Schwellwertparameter und unter Verwendung hochauflösender TOF-Bildsequenzen ist eine Verbesserung von Spezifität und Sensitivität denkbar.

Literaturverzeichnis

1. Poeck K, Hacke W. Neurologie. Berlin: Springer; 2006.
2. Rekik I, Allassonnière S, Carpenter TK, et al. Medical image analysis methods in MR/CT-imaged acute–subacute ischemic stroke lesion: Segmentation, prediction and insights into dynamic evolution simulation models. a critical appraisal. NeuroImage Clin. 2012;1(1):164–78.
3. Teßmann M, Vega-Higuera F, Fritz D, et al. Learning-based detection of stenotic lesions in coronary CT data. Vision Mod Vis. 2008; p. 189–98.
4. Sato Y, Nakajima S, Atsumi H, et al. 3D multi-scale line filter for segmentation and visualization of curvilinear structures in medical images. Lect Notes Computer Sci. 1997;1205:213–22.
5. Forkert N, Säring D, Wenzel K, et al. Fuzzy-based extraction of vascular structures from time-of-flight MR images. Proc MIE. 2009; p. 816–20.
6. Homann H. Implementation of a 3D Thinning Algorithm. Insight J, http://hdl.handle.net/1926/1292; 2007.
7. Lee TC, Kashyap RL, Chu CN. Building skeleton models via 3-D medial surface axis thinning algorithms. Graph Models Image Process. 1994;56(6):462–78.

Robust Identification of Contrasted Frames in Fluoroscopic Images

Matthias Hoffmann[1], Simone Müller[1], Klaus Kurzidim[2], Norbert Strobel[3], Joachim Hornegger[1,4]

[1]Pattern Recognition Lab, Friedrich-Alexander-Universität Erlangen-Nürnberg, Erlangen, Germany
[2]Klinik für Herzrhythmusstörungen, Krankenhaus Barmherzige Brüder, Regensburg, Germany
[3]Siemens AG, Healthcare, Forchheim, Germany
[4]Erlangen Graduate School in Advanced Optical Technologies (SAOT), Erlangen, Germany
matthias.hoffmann@cs.fau.de

Abstract. For automatic registration of 3-D models of the left atrium to fluoroscopic images, a reliable classification of images containing contrast agent is necessary. Inspired by previous approaches on contrast agent detection, we propose a learning-based framework which is able to classify contrasted frames more robustly than previous methods. Furthermore, we performed a quantitative evaluation on a clinical data set consisting of 34 angiographies. Our learning-based approach reached a classification rate of 79.5%. The beginning of a contrast injection was detected correctly in 79.4%.

1 Introduction

Atrial fibrillation (AF) is a heart rhythm disorder characterized by fast and chaotic electrical excitation of the atria [1]. It is the most common heart disease with about two million of the US population affected. A common catheter based therapy of AF is the electrical isolation of the pulmonary veins performed in electro-physiology (EP) labs [2]. EP-labs are typically equipped with a C-arm X-ray system that is used to acquire fluoroscopic images of the left atrium (LA). To get a better 3-D impression in the projective X-ray images, biplane C-arm systems can be used, to acquire images from two different directions at the same time. Contrary to catheters, the LA is only visible in fluoroscopic images, if a contrast agent is injected. In order to provide the surgeon with a permanent overview of the heart's shape, a 3D-model may be superimposed on the fluoroscopy [3]. If such 3-D models are gained pre-operatively by CT or MRI, a registration to the C-arm coordinate system has to be performed.

Nowadays the registration is mostly performed manually [4], but recently, also automatic approaches based on contrast agent were proposed [5, 6]. Both require an uncontrasted and a contrasted frame to obtain the contrast agent by means of a Digital Subtraction Angiography (DSA), see Fig. 1 for an example.

So far, only Zhao et al. [6] published an approach for automatic detection of contrasted frames for LA angiographies.

Approaches to contrast agent detection for different anatomical structures were proposed by Condurache et al. [7], Chen et al. [8] and Liao et al. [9]. Condurache et al. [7] used the 98-percentile of image intensities to classify contrasted images of coronary arteries, Chen et al. [8] applied for this task a learning-based framework. Liao et al. [9] published an approach for detecting contrast agent in images of the aortic root by calculating the similarity of histograms. However, this method was designed to decide if a sequence contains contrast agent at all and not to detect the first contrasted frame.

The detection of contrasted frames in LA angiographies is more complicated: As the LA is a large object, the density of contrast agent is lower. Additionally, the large movement of catheters in the LA may introduce artifacts in subtraction images and their histograms. We present a robust identification of contrasted frames in fluoroscopic images which extends the methods of Zhao et al. and Condurache et al. and combines them into a learning based framework using a support vector machine (SVM). As there exists no quantitative evaluation of the method by Zhao et al., we evaluate our novel approach as well as the approach by Zhao et al. and an adaption of the method by Condurache et al. using a set of 34 clinical fluoroscopic sequences.

2   Materials and methods

All methods described here require a sequence of fluoroscopic images I_k, $k = 1, \ldots, n$ of n containing contrasted and uncontrasted frames. They make all use of DSA: To obtain the injected contrast agent, an uncontrasted reference frame I_r is subtracted from a contrasted frame k, $I_{\mathrm{DSA},k} = I_k - I_r$.

As our method takes up some ideas of the methods by Zhao et al. and Condurache et al., we first describe them briefly in Sec. 2.1. Then, we present in Sec 2.2 how we integrate and extend them into a learning-based framework. Finally, in Sec. 2.3 we present our evaluation material and error measures.

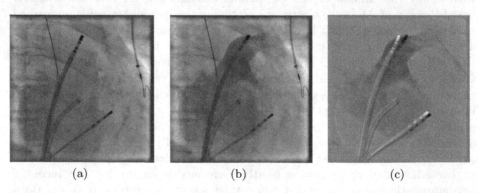

(a)   (b)   (c)

Fig. 1. Example of a reference frame (a), a contrasted frame (b) and a computed DSA-image of one acquisition (c).

2.1 State of the art

Approach according to Zhao et al. [6] First, a Difference Digital Subtraction Angiography (DDSA) $I_{\mathrm{DDSA},k}$ is calculated by subtracting two neighboring fluoroscopic frames to estimate how the amount of contrast agent changes

$$I_{\mathrm{DDSA},k} = I_{\mathrm{DSA},k} - I_{\mathrm{DSA},k-1} = I_k - I_{k-1} \qquad (1)$$

A threshold T_{Z}, determined by e.g. a training step, is applied to $I_{\mathrm{DDSA},k}$ to detect the region with newly contrasted pixels. The number of pixels p, with $I_{\mathrm{DDSA},k}(p) < T_{\mathrm{Z}}$ is denoted by n_k. Given a second threshold value N_{pixel}, the first frame with $n_k > N_{\mathrm{pixel}}$ is taken as first contrasted frame. The value of N_{pixel} was empirically set as 1000 in a 256×256 image, i.e. 1.53% of the image size.

Approach according to Condurache et al. [7] First, a tophat-filter is applied to the images to highlight vessel-like structures. Then, the 98-percentile value $x(k)$ of the pixel intensities is computed over all frames k. To denoise the curve $x(k)$ it is low-pass filtered resulting in $y(k)$. The distribution of $y(k)$ in uncontrasted images in this sequence is modeled as a Gaussian $\mathcal{N}_0(\mu_0, \sigma_0^2)$. μ_0 and σ_0 are estimated using frames which are known to be uncontrasted. Based on the concept of a significance test, they compute a threshold $T_{\mathrm{C}} = \mu_0 + l \cdot \sigma_0$. A frame k is considered to be contrasted if $y(k) > T_{\mathrm{C}}$.

To adapt this method to angiographies of the LA, we replace the tophat-filter by a DSA as a tophat filter is not suitable to enhance large contrasted areas which appear in LA angiographies. We estimate μ_0 and σ_0 using the first three frames which are always uncontrasted. l is estimated in a training step.

2.2 Learning-based framework

We use a linear SVM [10] to combine several features which are partially inspired by the methods described in Sec. 2.1. Before computing the features, the image borders which are covered by shutters are removed. The first part of the features is based on pixel intensity percentiles as proposed by Condurache et al. To enhance the contrasted area we used subtraction images $I_{\mathrm{DSA},k}$ with I_0 as reference frame instead of a tophat-filter. Furthermore, we used not only the 98-percentile but chose 15 percentiles, namely the 0-, 2-, 5-, 10-, 20-, 30-, 40-, 50-, 60-, 70-, 80-, 90-, 95-, 98-, 100-percentiles of DSA images. These features for frame k are denoted by f_1^k to f_{15}^k. Like Zhao et al. [6], we used features based on the computation of DDSA-images, see Eq. 1. They are referred to as f_{16}^k to f_{20}^k. These features are the sums of pixels below a certain threshold. We use the values 0, -50, -100, -150, -200 as thresholds.

In most cases, the contrast state of a frame is the same as for its neighboring frames. So, the features f_1^{k-1} to f_{20}^{k-1} of the previous frame and the features f_1^{k+1} to f_{20}^{k+1} of the following frame are included. To set the feature values in relationship to the overall brightness which varies from patient to patient, the mean value of the 98-percentile of I_2 and I_3 is added as feature f_{21} which is constant for all frames of a sequence. The feature vector for frame k includes 64 features: $\boldsymbol{f}^k = (f_1^{k-1}, \ldots f_{21}^{k-1}, f_1^k, \ldots f_{21}^k, f_1^{k+1}, \ldots f_{21}^{k+1}, f_{21})^T$. If a biplane system is used as in our case, the information of both views can be combined ending up in 128 features per frame. A feature selection is done by a three-fold crossvalidation on training data in order to get an insight into the importance of the different features.

2.3   Evaluation

We evaluated our SVM-based approach on 34 biplane angiographic sequences from 15 patients. The image series had a resolution of 1024×1024 pixels, 7 fps and different maximal frame numbers from 8 up to 57. Furthermore, an evaluation of the approach by Zhao et al. and Condurache et al. was performed. To allow a fair comparison, the parameters T_Z and l were trained in a leave-one-out manner as well as the SVM. So, the feature selection was performed as three-fold crossvalidation nested into the leave-one-out crossvalidation. The parameter C of the SVM was set to $\frac{n_c+n_u}{2n_c}$ and $\frac{n_c+n_u}{2n_u}$ for the training samples of n_c constrasted and n_u uncontrasted frames, respectively. The first frame was used as uncontrasted reference frame and was excluded from training and evaluation as well as the second frame which uses features from the first frame, too. Also frames where contrast agent flows out from the LA are not used for training as it is often difficult to decide whether they should be labeled contrasted or not. However, these ambiguous frames were used for evaluation but marked separately.

We performed two types of evaluation: For automatic contrast based registration [5, 6] it is important to identify the first contrasted frame. Therefore we calculated the difference between the position of the first contrasted frame and the position of the first frame which was classified as contrasted. Sequences with a difference of -1, 0 or 1 were considered as detected correctly. Second,

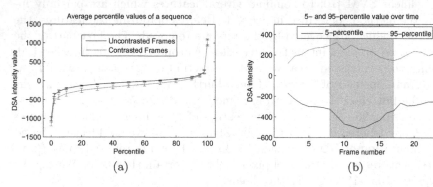

(a)   (b)

Fig. 2. (a) Mean value and standard deviation of the percentiles for contrasted and uncontrasted frames. (b) Value of the 5- and 95-percentile. It becomes clear that the 5-percentile is better suited to distinguish contrasted frames (gray area) from uncontrasted frames.

Table 1. Confusion matrices for the results of our evaluation.

Frames		All				Unambigous			
Approach		Condurache		SVM-based		Condurache		SVM-based	
Class		contr.	uncontr.	contr.	uncontr.	contr.	uncontr.	contr.	uncontr.
Class	contr.	240	90	295	35	142	25	145	22
	uncontr.	110	131	82	159	36	80	9	107

we measured the classification rate. This evaluation was not performed for the method by Zhao et al. [6] as it can only find the first contrasted frame.

3   Results

Results for the first frame detection are provided in Fig. 3. The confusion matrix is given in Tab. 1 for the approach based on Condurache et al. and the SVM based algorithm. In 79.4% of all sequences, the SVM-based approach was able to find the first contrasted frame, the approach by Zhao et al. found in 58.8% the first frame and the adaption of Condurache's approach found in 41.2% the first frame correctly. The classification rate was 79.5% for the SVM-based approach and 65.0% for the adaption of Condurache's method. If only clearly contrasted and clearly uncontrasted frames were evaluated, the classification rate was 89.0% for the SVM-based approach and 78.4% for the approach according to Condurache et al.

4   Discussion

It turns out that the approach by Condurache et al. does not perform well, probably as the first three frames are not sufficient to estimate μ_0 and σ_0 reliably.

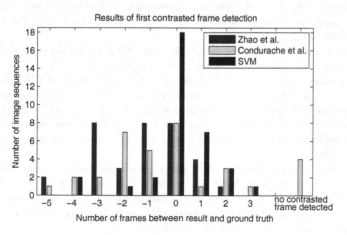

Fig. 3. Difference between the first contrasted frame and first frame classified as contrasted. A negative difference indicates a too early detected contrast injection.

Also the approach by Zhao et al. yields unsatisfying results as it compares each frame only to its previous frame and relies on a strong diffusion of contrast agent from one to the next frame. This is, however, not always given, especially for higher frame rates. The SVM-based approach can take much more information into account to distinguish contrasted from uncontrasted frames. Also additional information, e.g. from previous frames or from a second image plane, could easily be integrated to achieve more reliable results. This results in a high classification rate and a more reliable detection of the first contrasted frame. The features selected most often in the feature selection were the 2-, 50- and 90-percentile values, the number of pixels in the DSA image below an intensity of -150 and the mean of the 98-percentile of the first two frames.

Acknowledgement. This work was supported by the German Federal Ministry of Education and Research (BMBF) in the context of the initiative Spitzencluster Medical Valley – Europäische Metropolregion Nürnberg, project grant No. 12EX1012A. Additional funding was provided by Siemens AG, Healthcare. The concepts and information presented in this paper are based on research and are not commercially available.

References

1. Calkins H, Brugada J, Packer D, et al. HRS/EHRA/ECAS expert consensus statement on catheter and surgical ablation of atrial fibrillation: recommendations for Personnel, Policy, Procedures and Follow-Up. Europace. 2007;9(6):335 – 79.
2. Dilling-Boer D, van der Merwe N, Adams J, et al. Ablation of focally induced atrial fibrillation. J Cardiovasc Electrophysiol. 2004;15(2):200–5.
3. Brost A, Raab J, Kleinoeder A, et al. Medizinische Bildverarbeitung für die minimalinvasive Behandlung von Vorhofflimmern. DZKF. 2013;17(6):36 – 41.
4. Bourier F, Vukajlovic D, Brost A, et al. Pulmonary vein isolation supported by MRI-derived 3D-augmented biplane fluoroscopy: a feasibility study and a quantitative analysis of the accuracy of the technique. J Cardiovasc Electrophysiol. 2007;115:3057–63.
5. Thivierge-Gaulin D, Chou CR, Kiraly A, et al. 3D-2D registration based on mesh-derived image bisection. Lect Notes Computer Sci. 2012; p. 70–78.
6. Zhao X, Miao S, Du L, et al. Robust 2-D/3-D registration of CT volumes with contrast-enhanced x-ray sequences in electro-physiology based on a weighted similarity measure and sequential subspace optimization. Proc ICASSP. 2013; p. 934–8.
7. Condurache A, Aach T, Eck K, et al. Fast detection and processing of arbitrary contrast agent injections in coronary angiopgraphy and fluoroscopy. Procs BVM. 2004; p. 5–9.
8. Chen T, Funka-Lea G, Comaniciu D. Robust and fast contrast inflow detection for 2D x-ray fluoroscopy. Lect Notes Computer Sci. 2011; p. 243–50.
9. Liao R, You W, Liu Y, et al. Integrated spatiotemporal analysis for automatic contrast agent inflow detection on angiography and fluoroscopy during transcatheter aortic valve implantation. Med Phys. 2013;40(4).
10. Cortes C, Vapnik V. Support-vector networks. Mach Learn. 1995;20(3):273–97.

Interaktive und skalierungsinvariante Segmentierung des Rektums/Sigmoid in intraoperativen MRT-Aufnahmen für die gynäkologische Brachytherapie

Tobias Lüddemann[1], Jan Egger[2]

[1]Institut für Mechatronik, TU München
[2]Institut für Maschinelles Sehen und Darstellen, TU Graz
egger@tugraz.at

Kurzfassung. Gynäkologische Tumore sind die vierthäufigste Art karzinogener Krankheiten. Eine Behandlung besteht i.A. aus Chemotherapie, externer Bestrahlung und interner Strahlentherapie (Brachytherapie). Im Gegensatz zur externen Bestrahlung wird bei der Brachytherapie radioaktives Material direkt in den Tumor oder in seiner unmittelbaren Nähe platziert. Vorher müssen allerdings Tumor und umliegende Organe für eine optimale Strahlendosis segmentiert werden, was – manuell durchgeführt – sehr zeitintensiv ist. In diesem Beitrag stellen wir einen interaktiven, graphbasierten Ansatz zur Segmentierung des Rektums/Sigmoid als ein Risikoorgan (also als Gewebe, das möglichst nicht/wenig bestrahlt werden sollte) der gynäkologischen Brachytherapie vor. Der Ansatz verwendet zur Graphkonstruktion eine benutzerdefinierte Vorlage zur anschließenden interaktiven und skalierungsinvarianten Segmentierung; er wurde anhand von manuellen Segmentierungen von 7 Datensätzen evaluiert, wobei er einen mittleren DSC von 83.85±4.08% und eine mittlere Hausdorff-Distanz von ca. 11 Voxeln erreichte. Im Gegensatz zu einer manuellen Segmentierung, die im Schnitt 5 Minuten dauerte, konnte ein Datensatz mit unserem Ansatz in 2 Minuten segmentiert werden.

1 Einleitung

Unter allen Krebsarten sind gynäkologische Tumore die vierthäufigste Art karzinogener Krankheiten [1]. Neben Chemotherapie und externer Bestrahlung gilt die Brachytherapie als Standardbehandlung für Krankheiten dieser Art. Im Verlauf der Therapieplanung ist es nötig, die relative Lage des Tumors und benachbarter Organe durch Segmentierung zu erfassen, um die verabreichte Strahlung möglichst genau platzieren zu können, wobei der Tumor zerstört, aber umliegende Organe geschont werden sollen. Die Segmentierung wird manuell durchgeführt und stellt einen höchst zeitaufwendigen Schritt im Verlauf der Therapieplanung dar. Dieser Beitrag konzentriert sich auf die Segmentierung des Rektums/Sigmoid (Colon sigmoideum) als ein Risikoorgan in der gynäkologischen Brachytherapie (Abb. 1). Aufgrund der patientenindividuellen Variabilität des

Rektums (was vor allem die Größe, die Form und auch die schlechte Abgrenzung zum umliegenden Gewebe angeht) ist eine automatische Segmentierung äußerst schwierig. Den Autoren ist kein vollautomatischer Ansatz bekannt, der zuverlässige und robuste Ergebnisse für einen klinischen Einsatz liefert. Besonders dies ist die Motivation, in diesem Beitrag einen interaktiven Ansatz zur Konturierung des Rektums vorzustellen, bei dem ein Benutzer unterstützend in den semi-automatischen Segmentierungsprozess eingreift. Zwei neuere Arbeiten, die sich mit der Segmentierung des Rektums in Magnetresonanztomographie (MRT)-Daten befassen, sind von Namías et al. [2] und Ma et al. [3]. Bei [2] liegt der Schwerpunkt allerdings auf einer automatischen Detektion des Rektums/Sigmoid in den Aufnahmen mit anschließender (automatischer) Bestimmung der Rektum-Obergrenze. Ma et al. [3] dagegen segmentieren in ihrer Arbeit neben dem Rektum noch weitere Strukturen, z.B. die Blase. Allerdings wurde der Ansatz nur anhand zweier Aufnahmen evaluiert und erforderte eine präzise Parameterdefinition durch den Benutzer. In diesem Beitrag dagegen wird ein interaktiver graphbasierter Algorithmus zur Segmentierung des Rektums in intraoperativen MRT-Aufnahmen vorgestellt. Der Algorithmus stützt sich dabei auf eine benutzerdefinierte Vorlage, um den Graphen aufzubauen. Die Vorlage wird durch die manuelle Segmentierung des Rektums in einer ersten Schicht erzeugt und danach zur Segmentierung des Rektums in den folgenden Schichten verwendet.

2   Material und Methoden

Zum Ausarbeiten und Evaluieren der Methoden aus diesem Beitrag standen gynäkologische MRT-Daten aus der interstitiellen Brachytherapie zur Verfügung, die mit einem 3-Tesla-Scanner von Siemens erzeugt wurden. Alle Datensätze stehen der Community für eigene Forschungszwecke frei zur Verfügung [4].

Die Segmentierung basiert auf der Konstruktion eines Graphen $G(K, W)$ in der Patientenaufnahme mit anschließendem minimalen s-t-Schnitt [5], um das Rektum/Sigmoid von den umliegenden Strukturen zu trennen. Dabei orientiert sich der prinzipielle Aufbau des Graphen (bestehend aus Kanten mit dazugehörigen Kantengewichten W) an Li et al. [6], wobei unser Ansatz zwei elementare Erweiterungen aufweist: (1.) kann ein Benutzer die Form des Graphen vorgeben und (2.) ist es möglich, die Segmentierung interaktiv zu steuern. Dadurch können auch anspruchsvolle Strukturen wie das Rektum zumindest semi-automatisch segmentiert werden. Abb. 2 zeigt, wie ein patientenindividueller Segmentierungsgraph $G(K, W)$ erstellt wird. Dazu konturiert der Benutzer zuerst das Rektum in

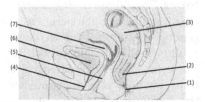

Abb. 1. Darstellung des weiblichen Beckens: Analkanal (1), Rektum (2), Sigmoid (3), Harnröhre (4), Vagina (5), Blase (6) und Uterus (7). Illustration basiert auf *Drake et al. Gray's anatomy for students, Elsevier, 2005.*

einer 2D-Schicht (gelb, obere Reihe). Diese Kontur definiert die Vorlage $V \in R^3$ und besteht aus einer diskreten Anzahl von Markern $M_t = (m_x, m_y, m_z)$

$$V = \{M_0, ..., M_n\} : 0 \leq n \leq \infty \tag{1}$$

Aus dieser Kontur wird der Mittelpunkt $MP = (\sum_{t=0}^{n} M_t)/n$ (blau, linkes Bild unten) aus Abb. 2 automatisch bestimmt. Als nächstes werden die Knoten K des Graphen (rote Punkte, mittleres Bild unten) anhand von Strahlen $s_i = 1 \leq i \leq k$, die von $MP = (mp_x, mp_y, mp_z)$ ausgesandt werden, abgetastet [7] und für alle s_i wird der Schnittpunkt SP_i mit der Vorlage V berechnet. Die Längen der einzelnen Strahlen ergeben sich aus der Distanz zwischen MP und $SP_i(|s_i| = |SP_i - MP|)$. Für einen vollständigen Graphen werden dann die Kanten mit ihren ∞-Kantengewichten zwischen den Knoten (rot, rechtes Bild unten in Abb. 2) und Kanten von den Knoten zu einer Quelle s und einer Senke t (im Bild nicht dargestellt) erzeugt. Die Kantengewichte zur Quelle bzw. Senke berechnen sich hierbei aus einem mittleren Grauwert MG im Bereich des Mittelpunktes MP aus dem Datensatz. Solch ein vollständiger Graph kann anschließend zur interaktiven Segmentierung des kompletten Rektums eingesetzt werden, wie es in Abb. 3 beispielhaft für mehrere 2D-Schichten veranschaulicht wird. Der Ansatz wurde innerhalb von MeVisLab realisiert, und der C++ Quellcode für die eigenen Module wurde mit Microsoft Visual Studio 2008 (Version 9) kompiliert.

3   Ergebnisse

Die Berechnungen der Segmentierungen wurden auf einem Windows 7 PC mit Intel Prozessor (Intel® Core™ i3 CPU M330 mit 2.13 GHz Dual Core) und 4 GB Arbeitsspeicher durchgeführt. Die automatische Trennung von Rektum/Sigmoid und Hintergrund erfolgt in jeder Schicht durch einen minimalen s-t-Schnitt. Ein

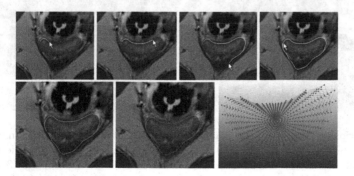

Abb. 2. Erstellung eines patientenindividuellen Segmentierungsgraphen; der Benutzer konturiert das Rektum in einer 2D-Schicht (gelb, obere Reihe). Aus der Kontur werden anschließend automatisch der Mittelpunkt (blau, linkes Bild unten), die Knoten des Graphen (rote Punkte, mittleres Bild unten) und der Segmentierungsgraph (rot, rechtes Bild unten) generiert.

Vergleich mit rein manuellen Schicht-für-Schicht-Segmentierungen ergab einen mittleren DSC [8] von ca. 84% und eine mittlere Hausdorff-Distanz von ca. 11 Voxeln, bei einer Zeitersparnis von etwa drei Minuten für jeden Datensatz. Dadurch liegt die ermittelte Segmentierungszeit für ein komplettes Rektum im Bereich der von Haas et al. [9] anvisierten zwei Minuten für eine automatische Segmentierung ohne Korrekturen [10]. Tab. 1 listet detailliert die Evaluationsergebnisse (Min., Max., Mittelwert μ und Standardabweichung σ) für sieben Datensätze auf. IS steht dabei für die interaktive Segmentierung, und M1 und M2 sind zwei manuelle Expertensegmentierungen. Für einen direkten visuellen Vergleich zwischen manueller und semi-automatischer Segmentierung dient Abb. 4.

4 Diskussion

Der vorgestellte Ansatz zur Segmentierung des Rektums/Sigmoid basiert auf einer benutzerdefinierten Vorlage, um einen Graphen aufzubauen. Bei dieser Vorgehensweise bevorzugt ein s-t-Schnitt eine patientenindividuelle Anatomie. Unseres Wissens ist dies das erste Mal, dass bei einem graphbasierten Verfahren die Knoten des Graphen nicht gleichmäßig und äquidistant auf einem Bild verteilt wurden, sondern anhand einer individuellen benutzerdefinierten Vorlage. Zusätzlich ist der vorgestellte Ansatz durch den speziellen Graphaufbau skalierungsinvariant und kann dadurch Größenänderungen des Rektums/Sigmoid zwischen zwei Schichten handhaben. Durch die Interaktivität können Parameter wie der mittlere Grauwert in den Ansatz integriert werden. In einem nächsten Schritt soll das vorgestellte Verfahren zu einem 3D-Ansatz erweitert werden. Denkbar ist, dass der Benutzer drei initiale Konturen in einer axialen-, einer

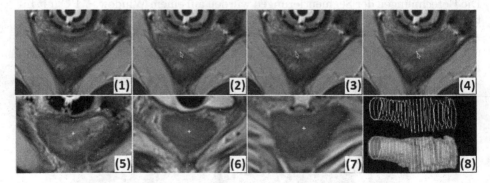

Abb. 3. Prinzipieller Ablauf der Segmentierung eines kompletten Rektums/Sigmoid: erste Originalschicht in 2D (1), Platzieren des Mauscursors (2), Segmentierung (rot) des Rektums durch die linke Maustaste an der Stelle des Mauscursors (3), interaktive Verfeinerung der Segmentierung durch Verschieben des Graphmittelpunkts (4), interaktive Segmentierung – äquivalent zu den Schritten (1) bis (4) – in angrenzenden Schichten in z-Richtung (5, 6 und 7), Segmentierungsergebnis des kompletten Rektums (8, oben) und anschließende Triangulierung (8, unten). Anmerkung: Die blauen Punkte beschreiben die benutzerdefinierte Vorlage, anhand derer der patientenindividuelle Segmentierungsgraph aufgebaut wird.

Tabelle 1. Evaluationsergebnisse: Minimum (Min.), Maximum (Max.), Mittelwert μ und Standardabweichung σ für sieben Datensätze (IS steht für interaktive Segmentierung und M1 und M2 sind zwei manuelle Segmentierungen).

Datensatz	DSC (%)		Hausdorff-Distanz (Voxel)	
	IS-M2	M1-M2	IS-M2	M1-M2
1	88,43	86,93	11,04	4,03
2	80,88	85,16	6,48	11,45
3	79,04	78,19	25,47	18,92
4	80,17	70,37	11,05	22,29
5	84,78	n.v.	9,34	n.v.
6	89,54	91,05	4,36	9,78
7	84,14	91,40	9,64	4,12
$\mu\pm\sigma$	83,85±4,08	83,97±8,08	11,05±6,81	11,76±7,54
Min.	79,04	70,37	4,36	4,03
Max.	89,54	91,40	25,47	22,29

sagittalen- und einer koronaren Schicht vorgibt, äquivalent zur Initialisierung

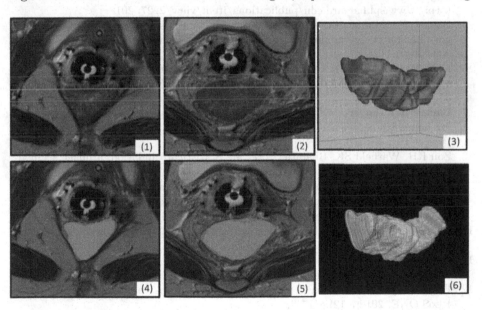

Abb. 4. Segmentierungsergebnisse des Rektums/Sigmoid in 2D und 3D: (1) und (2) sind zwei Originalschichten aus einem Magnetresonanztomographie (MRT)-Datensatz, (3) ist eine rein manuelle Segmentierung aller 2D-Schichten des Rektums/Sigmoid (grau), (4) und (5) sind die Ergebnisse der vorgestellten interaktiven Segmentierung (rot), einer rein manuellen Expertensegmentierung (grün) und der Übereinstimmung beider Segmentierungen (braun); (6) stellt das interaktive Segmentierungsergebnis aller 2D-Schichten in einer dreidimensionalen Visualisierung dar (gelb).

in [11, 12]. Anschließend soll ein 3D-Graph anhand dieser Vorgaben aufgebaut und zur interaktiven Segmentierung des kompletten Rektums genutzt werden, was die Praktikabilität des Ansatzes deutlich erhöhen würde.

Danksagung. Die Autoren danken Frau Edith Egger-Mertin für das Korrekturlesen des Beitrags. Videos der interaktiven Segmentierung finden sich unter dem YouTube-Kanal: http://www.youtube.com/c/JanEgger/videos

Literaturverzeichnis

1. Siegel R, Naishadham D, Jemal A. Cancer statistics 2012. CA Cancer J Clin. 2012;62(1):10–29.
2. NamÃas R, D'Amato JP, del Fresno M, et al. Three-dimensional imaging in gynecologic brachytherapy: a survey of the american brachytherapy society. Comput Med Imaging Graph. 2014;38(4):245–50.
3. Ma Z, Jorge RM, Mascarenhas T, et al. Segmentation of female pelvic organs in axial magnetic resonance images using coupled geometric deformable models. Comput Biol Med. 2013;43(4):248–58.
4. Egger J, Kapur T, Viswanathan A. GYN Data Collection. NCITG. http://www.spl.harvard.edu/publications/item/view/2227; 2012.
5. Boykov Y, Kolmogorov V. An experimental comparison of min-cut/max-flow algorithms for energy minimization in vision. IEEE Trans Pattern Anal Mach Intell. 2004;26(9):1124–37.
6. Li K, Wu X, Chen DZ, et al. Optimal surface segmentation in volumetric images: a graphtheoretic approach. IEEE Trans Pattern Anal Mach Intell. 2006;28(1):119–34.
7. Bauer MHA, Egger J, O'Donnell T, et al. A fast and robust graph-based approach for boundary estimation of fiber bundles relying on fractional anisotropy maps. Proc ICPR. 2010; p. 4016–9.
8. Zou KH, Warfield SK, Bharatha A, et al. Statistical validation of image segmentation quality based on a spatial overlap index. Acad Radiol. 2004;2:178–89.
9. Haas B, Coradi T, Scholz M, et al. Automatic segmentation of thoracic and pelvic CT images for radio-therapy planning using implicit anatomic knowledge and organ-specific segmentation strategies. Phys Med Biol. 2008;53(6):1751–71.
10. Lüddemann T, Egger J. Rectum segmentation in MR-guided gynecologic brachytherapy data. Proc Bri Gynaecologic Cancer Soc Ann Sci Meet. 2013; p. 162–3.
11. Egger J, Kapur T, Fedorov A, et al. GBM volumetry using the 3D slicer medical image computing platform. Sci Rep. 2013;3(1364):1–7.
12. Egger J, Kapur T, Nimsky C, et al. Pituitary adenoma volumetry with 3D slicer. PLoS ONE. 2012;7(12):e51788.

Over-Exposure Correction in CT Using Optimization-Based Multiple Cylinder Fitting

Alexander Preuhs[1], Martin Berger[1,2], Yan Xia[1,3], Andreas Maier[1],
Joachim Hornegger[1], Rebecca Fahrig[4]

[1]Pattern Recognition Lab, FAU Erlangen-Nürnberg
[2]Research Training Group 1773 "Heterogeneous Image Systems"
[3]Erlangen Graduate School in Advanced Optical Technologies (SAOT)
[4]Department of Radiology, Stanford University, Stanford, CA, USA
alexander.preuhs@fau.de

Abstract. Flat-Panel Computed Tomography (CT) has found its commonly used applications in the healthcare field by providing an approach of examining 3D structural information of a human's body. The popular CT reconstruction algorithms are based on a filtered backprojection (FBP) scheme, which would face challenges when imaging the knee. This is because in some views, the X-rays are highly attenuated when traveling through both thigh bones. In the same view, X-rays also travel through soft tissue that absorbs much less energy with respect to bone. When these high intensity X-rays arrive at the detector they cause detector saturation and the generated sinogram suffers from overexposure. Reconstructing an overexposed sinogram results in images with streaking and cupping artifacts, which are unusable for diagnostics. In this paper, we propose a method to correct overexposure artifacts using an optimization approach. Parameters describing a specific geometry are determined by the optimization and then used to extrapolate the overexposed acquisition data.

1 Introduction

In X-ray imaging, overexposure typically refers to a situation where the intensity range of the traveled X-rays in projections are greater than the detector's inherent detectable range – that is a dynamic range of 14 Bit. In Flat-Panel CT these circumstances can arise when examining the knee and are amplified by an automatic tube current and voltage modulation.

The overexposure occurs in views where the X-rays travel through both femurs (thigh bones). Then certain X-rays are attenuated strongly by two thigh bones, while other X-rays are attenuated less by soft tissue. The resulting amplitude range of the incoming X-rays is greater then the detectable range of the detector. The pixels that measure the less attenuating soft tissue receive numerous X-ray photons which causes saturation. In these locations not all the data can be collected and the sinogram suffers from discontinuity between measured and unmeasured data.

In the sense of the resulting discontinuity, the overexposure problem is similar to a truncation occurring from an object extending the field of view. The high-pass-filtering during the FBP algorithms intensifies discontinuities and leads to cupping artifacts in the reconstructed image. In this manner, approaches concerning truncation correction can thus be used to correct overexposure artifacts.

That is often done by extrapolating the missing data, using an estimation model. Hsieh et al. [1] fit a water cylinder at the transitions between the measured- and unavailable data and use a mass constraint to post-fit them. Instead of water cylinders Ohnesorge et al. [2] use the mirrored values of the available data to extrapolate the missing areas. Ritschl et al. [3] use an additional low intensity scan for extrapolation. Gompel et al. [4] correct the discontinuity by fitting a single ellipse in the projections using consistency conditions as constraints. An implicit extrapolation scheme in the derivative domain was also investigated recently [5, 6].

In the proposed method, the missing data is extrapolated using multiple cylinder shapes that are fitted in the sinogram domain. The parameters describing these objects are estimated from the overexposed data using an optimization-based approach, by minimizing the least square error. This differs from the optimization approach proposed by Maier et al. [7], in which a water-cylinder was used to initialize the optimization but the objective function concentrates on high frequency artifacts and constant extrapolation in the reconstruction domain.

2   Materials and methods

2.1   Two-dimensional imaging geometry

The Radon transform of a 2D object function $f(x, y)$ in parallel-beam geometry is defined as

$$p(s, \theta) = \int_{-\infty}^{\infty} \int_{-\infty}^{\infty} f(x, y)\delta(x \cos \theta + y \sin \theta - s)\mathrm{d}x\mathrm{d}y \qquad (1)$$

where s is the distance from the central ray and θ defines the view angle of the system. By introducing a fan-angle γ and the view angle of a fan-beam system β, the equation can be expressed in fan-beam geometry by

$$p(s, \theta) = p(\gamma, \beta) \qquad \forall \theta \in \Theta \wedge \forall s \in S \qquad (2)$$

with $\Theta = \{\theta \mid \theta = \beta + \gamma\}$ and $S = \{s \mid s = D \sin \gamma\}$, where D defines the focal length.

2.2   Optimization-based multiple shape fitting

By its simple and smooth geometric properties, cylinder shapes are fitted in the sinogram domain. The forward transformation to the sinogram domain is given by equation (1). We use that equation and insert for $f(x, y)$ the formulation of a cylinder with radius r that has the density ρ inside the region $x^2 + y^2 \le r^2$. The resulting integration along a ray leads to a multiplication of the intersection length with the density of the cylinder positioned at the intersection. With the distance s between any ray and the central ray together with the radius of the cylinder r, the projection can be gained using simple trigonometry

$$p(s, \theta) = 2\rho\sqrt{r^2 - s^2} \tag{3}$$

Equation (3) is defined in parallel-beam geometry. To convert the equation to the fan-beam geometry and a general off centered case, with the new center coordinates (c_x, c_y), we substitute the distance parameter s with $(D \sin\gamma - c_x \sin\theta - c_y \cos\theta)$ constrained by $(\theta = \beta + \gamma)$, thus

$$p_{\text{cyl}}(c_x, c_y, r, \rho, \gamma, \beta) = 2\rho\sqrt{r^2 - (D \sin\gamma - c_x \sin\theta - c_y \cos\theta)^2} \tag{4}$$

Equation (4) provides the projection value of a cylinder along any ray defined by γ and β in fan-beam geometry. Defining a single cylinder with respect to its parameters and with the Radon transform providing the property of linearity, the projection resulting from a composition of cylinders is a summation. It can be calculated by

$$p(\gamma, \beta) = \sum_i p_{\text{cyl}}(c_{x_i}, c_{y_i}, r_i, \rho_i, \gamma, \beta) \tag{5}$$

In the proposed method, the knee should be approximated as a composition of cylinders. The goal is to extrapolate the overexposed areas with forward projections of fitted cylinders. Therefore, we minimize the difference between the projections of a set of fitted cylinders $\sum_i p_{\text{cyl}}(c_{x_i}, c_{y_i}, r_i, \rho_i, \gamma, \beta)$ and the measured data $p_{\text{meas}}(\gamma, \beta)$. The parameters describing cylinders are optimized, so that the least-squares are as small as possible over the available data. That gives the objective function

$$\underset{\sum_{i=1}^{N} c_{x_i}, c_{y_i}, r_i, \rho_i}{\text{argmin}} \sum_{\gamma \in \Omega} \sum_{\beta \in \Omega} \left| p_{\text{meas}}(\gamma, \beta) - \sum_{i=1}^{N} p_{\text{cyl}}(c_{x_i}, c_{y_i}, r_i, \rho_i, \gamma, \beta) \right|_2^2 \tag{6}$$

The set Ω includes all the parameter pairs (γ, β) that correspond to data that does not suffer from overexposure. It can be determined prior to the reconstruction by simple thresholding of the raw detector values.

Also note that any other geometric object desired can be plugged into the objective function, if an analytic formulation of its Radon transform is available.

2.3   Experimental setup

The used synthetic knee phantoms are a composition of cylindrical and elliptical shapes which are shown in Fig. 1(a) and 1(e), respectively. The two thigh bones are represented by two cylinders having the density of bones. The two knee caps (patellas) are simulated using two ellipses with the same density. The phantoms differ in the representation of the soft tissue. For the cylinder phantom, as shown in Fig. 1(a), two cylinders are used to simulate the soft tissue. The phantom shown in Fig. 1(e) uses two ellipses to simulate the soft tissue and is referred to as ellipse phantom. The density of soft tissue is approximated with the density of water. The shapes are placed such that they appear as close as possible to real knees.

In a next step, the phantoms are forward projected to the sinogram domain. During that step, a synthetic overexposure simulation is performed as follows: From each view the histogram is computed and all values that are beyond a pre-defined range are set to zero in the sinogram.

Using these overexposed sinograms, a state of the art and the proposed algorithms are applied. The ground truth is obtained using the filtered backprojection of the non-overexposed knee phantom. A quantitative comparison is performed using the root mean square error (RMSE) and relative root mean square error (rRMSE) with respect to the ground truth. We also investigated the performance of the standard water cylinder extrapolation [1] and compare it with our proposed method. At the position of discontinuity, i.e. the truncation edge, the projection of a water cylinder is fitted. The position and size of the fitted cylinder can be computed by fulfilling the continuity assumption of the truncation edge. In a second step, with the mass consistency the cylinders are adjusted so that the resulting extrapolated mass per view, is equal to the real/reference mass. In our algorithm, this is done by adjusting the slope, followed by a cosine-smoothing.

For the optimization approach, the first step is to initialize the cylinder parameters. By heuristics, we use two cylinders to estimate the thigh bones, two cylinders for the soft tissues and six cylinders for the patellas. That results in a total of ten cylinders and 40 parameters. The initial parameters are approximated empirically as follows: The greatest value of the whole sinogram is expected to be the ray, where both knee bones overlap most. In an orthogonal view, the two highest values are expected to mark the position of the two thigh bones. By finding the intersection of these rays, the centers of the two knees are approximated. Then the radius of the soft tissue is approximated with the slope and intensity value at the edges in the orthogonal view. In practice, the initial parameters can be computed by using an initial reconstruction and extracting the parameters from the overexposed image. After optimization, the areas where real data is missing due to overexposure are completed by the values that are extrapolated using the fitted shapes.

3   Results

The reconstruction results of the proposed method, compared with the reference, method without correction and the water cylinder extrapolation, are presented in Fig. 1. Both correction algorithms increase the image quality with respect to no correction, cf. Fig. 1(b) and 1(f). The water cylinder approach shown in Fig. 1(c) and 1(g) removes artifacts in the center-lateral direction but the upper

Table 1. Table of the RMSE, rRMSE and Improvement for the optimization approach, the water cylinder extrapolation and no correction applied on the cylinder- and ellipse phantom.

Correction Model	Phantom	RMSE	rRMSE	Improvement
Water Cylinder Extrapolation	Cylinder	0.1342	0.1119	66 %
Optimization with Cylinders	Cylinder	0.0300	0.0250	92 %
No Correction	Cylinder	0.3899	0.3249	0 %
Water Cylinder Extrapolation	Ellipse	0.1581	0.1318	66 %
Optimization with Cylinders	Ellipse	0.1643	0.1388	64 %
No Correction	Ellipse	0.4680	0.3900	0 %

and lower boarders of the knee still suffer from artifacts. With the optimization approach, the cylinder phantom can be reconstructed close to the ground truth, as shown in Fig. 1(d). Applied to the ellipse phantom, the streaking artifacts are removed but the original contour is not recovered. However within 1(d) and 1(h) the shape of the patella is reconstructed close to the ground truth.

The quantitative results are presented in Tab. 1. With both methods the RMSE and rRMSE are substantially lower compared to no correction. The cylinder optimization reduces the error by 92% within the cylinder phantom, whereas the water cylinder extrapolation reduces the error by 66%. The ability of the optimization to improve the image lowers when applied to the ellipse phan-

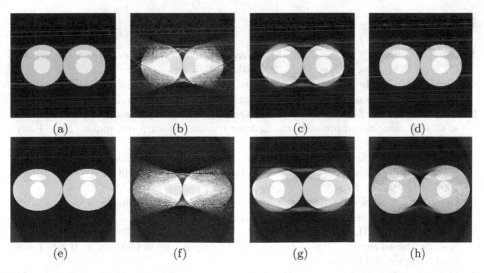

Fig. 1. Reconstructions for the cylinder and the ellipse phantom in the top and bottom row, respectively. From left to right: Ground truth, overexposed reconstructions without correction, the corrected reconstruction using mass constrained water cylinder extrapolation and the reconstructions of the proposed optimization-based approach. The visualization window was set to $[0, 1.2]$.

tom. The improvement of the water cylinder extrapolation remains unchanged at 66% when applied on the ellipse phantom.

4   Discussion

Both extrapolation approaches recover the central-lateral regions close to the ground truth. In these directions, the knees do not overlap in the projections and the extrapolation performed by the water cylinder correction is very precise. In the areas where the knees overlap, this algorithm cannot provide exact reconstructions. The extrapolation scheme consists of local continuity condition at the truncation edges and has not enough information to extrapolate more then one cylinder close to the ground truth. That information is provided by the optimization approach, which is thus capable to extrapolate a composite of cylinders. The only areas that differ from the ground truth, are the patella regions, where the transitions are blurred. The optimization approach faces challenges, when it comes to shapes that can not be modeled with cylinders. The fitted shape is either to small or to great to simulate the real object.

This may be handled when introducing more complex geometric shapes like ellipses, splines or level-sets. A further improvement to the proposed algorithm is increasing the number of fitted independent shapes. The future work involves the validation of the proposed method using real knee data.

References

1. Hsieh J, Chao E, Thibault J, et al. A novel reconstruction algorithm to extend the CT scan field-of-view. Med Phys. 2004;31(9):2385–91.
2. Ohnesorge B, Flohr T, Schwarz K. Efficient correction for CT image artifacts caused by objects extending outside the scan field of view. Med Phys. 2000;27(1):39–46.
3. Ritschl L, Knaup M, Kachelrieß M. Extending the dynamic range of flat detectors in CBCT using a compressed-sensing-based mulit-exposure technique. Proc Fully 3D. 2013; p. 26–9.
4. Van Gompel G, Defrise M, Van Dyck D. Elliptical extrapolation of truncated 2D CT projections using Helgason-Ludwig consistency conditions. Proc SPIE. 2006;6142:61424B–10.
5. Dennerlein F, Maier A. Region-of-interest reconstruction on medical C-arms with the ATRACT algorithm. Proc SPIE. 2012; p. 83131B–9.
6. Xia Y, Hofmann H, Dennerlein F, et al. Towards clinical application of a Laplace operator-based region of interest reconstruction algorithm in C-arm CT. IEEE Trans Med Imaging. 2014;33(3):593–606.
7. Maier A, Scholz B, Dennerlein F. Optimization-based extrapolation for truncation correction. Salt Lake City, Utah, USA; 2012.

B-Mode-gestützte zeitharmonische Leber-Elastographie zur Diagnose hepatischer Fibrose bei adipösen Patienten

Selcan Ipek-Ugay[1], Heiko Tzschätzsch[2], Manh Nguyen Trong[3],
Thomas Tolxdorff[1], Ingolf Sack[2], Jürgen Braun[1]

[1]Institut für Medizinische Informatik, Charité – Universitätsmedizin Berlin
[2]Institut für Radiologie, Charité – Universitätsmedizin Berlin
[3]Gampt mbH, Merseburg, Germany
selcan.ipek-ugay@charite.de

Kurzfassung. Die Leber-Elastographie ist ein etabliertes bildgebendes
Verfahren zur Diagnose hepatischer Fibrose. Limitationen bestehen bei
der Untersuchung adipöser Patienten oder Patienten mit Aszites. Daher wurde im Rahmen dieser Arbeit eine neue Methode entwickelt, um
anhand zeitharmonischer Ultraschallelastographie (USE) die viskoelastischen Gewebeparameter der Leber in großen und tiefen Messfenstern
durchzuführen und eine automatisierte Auswertung zu ermöglichen. Zur
Erzeugung von Scherwellen wurde eine Vibrationseinheit in die Patientenliege integriert. Zur Detektion der in die Leber eingekoppelter Scherwellen wurde ein modifizierter klinischer B-Mode-Scanner eingesetzt. Es
wurden mehrere Einzelmessungen mit einer Messtiefe von bis zu 14 cm
durchgeführt, um die effektive Scherwellengeschwindigkeit sowie den Di-
spersionsanstieg der Scherwellengeschwindigkeiten zu berechnen. Beide
Kenngrößen korrelieren mit der Viskoelastizität des untersuchten Gewebes. Zur Evaluation wurde die USE mit der Magnetresonanzelastographie
(MRE) verglichen. Dazu wurden 10 gesunde Freiwilligen mit beiden Verfahren untersucht. Die Resultate zeigen eine sehr gute Übereinstimmung.
Die USE wurde nachfolgend in einer klinischen Studie mit 10 weiteren
gesunden Freiwilligen und 22 Patienten mit klinisch bewiesener Zirrhose
durchgeführt. In Patientenlebern konnte eine signifikante Erhöhung der
Scherwellengeschwindigkeiten gegenüber der Kontrollgruppe festgestellt
werden. Hiermit wird Medizinern erstmals die nichtinvasive Diagnose der
hepatischen Fibrose auf der Grundlage der viskoelastischen Leberverän-
derungen in adipösen Patienten und bei Vorliegen von Aszites ermöglicht.

1 Einleitung

Ein neues, nichtinvasives Verfahren zur Diagnose der Leberzirrhose ist die Elastographie [1], welche im Prinzip auf die Palpation zurückgeht. Die leichte, qua-
sistatische Druckausübung der Hand des Arztes wird dabei durch eine extern
angeregte Vibration des Gewebes zur kontrollierten Scherdeformation ersetzt,
während die Detektion resultierender Gewebeverschiebungen mittels Ultraschall

oder Magnetresonanztomographie erfolgt. Daraus können Parameter wie z.B. Schermodul, Scherwellengeschwindigkeit und Dispersionsverhalten der Scherwellen rekonstruiert werden, um hepatische Fibrose sowie Leberzirrhose zu diagnostizieren. In den vergangenen Jahren wurden vielfältige Methoden der Elastographie erforscht, um den therapeutisch relevanten Grad der Leber-Fibrose zu bestimmen [2]. Bei den dynamischen Methoden der Ultraschallelastographie (USE) werden die Scherwellen entweder mittels transienter mechanischer Anregung erzeugt (Fibroscan) oder es werden Ultraschallsignale als Puls auf einen Punkt fokussiert (ARFI), um Scherwellen zu stimulieren [3]. Eine weitere Vorgehensweise ist die externe Erzeugung von zeitharmonischen Scherwellen mittels eines Lautsprechers [4]. Dieses Prinzip wurde für die Magnetresonanzelastographie (MRE) erfolgreich eingesetzt [5]. Die MRE gilt bislang als Standardmethode zur nichtinvasiven Graduierung der Leberfibrose [6]. Für die USE wurde das Prinzip von extern erzeugten Scherwellen mit niedrigen Frequenzen ($\leq$ 60 Hz) bereits am menschlichen Herz sowie an der menschlichen Leber angewendet [7]. Im Rahmen dieser Arbeit wurde die diagnostische Tauglichkeit einer neuen, B-Mode gestützten zeitharmonischen USE-Methode an Gesunden und übergewichtigen Patienten mit Leberzirrhose überprüft, welche zudem teilweise unter Aszites litten und für die klinische Diagnostik eine große Herausforderung darstellen. Bei diesen Patienten stießen bisherige USE-Techniken aufgrund limitierter Schallfenstern mit nur geringer Tiefenausleuchtung und Ausdehnung an ihre Grenzen. Zur Validierung der neuen, auf niederfrequenter, zeitharmonischer Vibrationsanregung basierenden Methode, wurden gesunde Freiwillige neben der USE auch mit der multifrequenten MRE als Referenzmethode untersucht.

2 Material und Methoden

Zur Validierung dieser Technik wurden im Rahmen einer klinischen Leber-Studie 10 gesunde Freiwillige (9 Männer und 1 Frau zwischen 18 und 52 Jahren, Durchschnittsalter 32) und 22 Patienten (15 Männer und 7 Frauen zwischen 36 und 80 Jahren, Durchschnittsalter 58) mit klinisch bestätigter Zirrhose und einem durchschnittlichen body-mass index (BMI) von 26.4 ± 5.3 untersucht. Bei 10 der Patienten lag Aszites vor. Als Kontrolle wurde eine Gruppe von 10 gesunden Freiwilligen mittels zeitharmonischer USE und multifrequenter MRE untersucht.

2.1 Erzeugung von Scherwellen

Es wurde eine Patientenliege mit integriertem Aktor entwickelt (Abb. 1a). Im Gegensatz zu unserem früheren Aktor ist der, als Vibrationsquelle agierende Lautsprecher direkt in das Bett montiert. Die mittels eines Wellengenerators erzeugten Sinussignale (f = 30, 35, 40, 45, 50, 55 und 60 Hz) (Abb. 1b) werden durch einen Audioverstärker verstärkt (Abb. 1a) und an den Lautsprecher weitergeleitet, der diese Signale in mechanische Anregungen transformiert, welche im Oberkörper der, auf dem Bett liegenden Patienten in Form von Vibrationen spürbar werden. Die vom Lautsprecher erzeugten Kompressionswellen werden über Moden-Konversion an den Gewebegrenzen zu Scherwellen umgewandelt.

2.2   Signalakquisition mit B-Mode gestützter zeitharmonischer USE

Um die gesuchten Scherwellen zu akquirieren wurde ein Standard B-Mode Ultraschall Scanner (Ultrasonix Touch, Vancouver, Canada) mit einer Phased-Array-
Sonde eingesetzt. Für eine gute Messposition im M-Mode wurde in der B-Mode
Darstellung ein möglichst homogener Bereich im rechten Leberlappen gesucht
(Abb. 1c). Die M-Mode Daten (40 MHz Abtastrate, 1kHz Wiederholrate, 7 bis
14 cm Messfenstergröße, 1 Sek. Aufnahmezeit) wurden bei angehaltenem Atem
aufgenommen. Diese Messung wurde an 40 unterschiedlichen Positionen wiederholt, um das Scherwellenfeld innerhalb der Leber in unterschiedlichen Projektio-
nen zu erfassen. Nach dieser Gesamtmessung (ca. 10 Minuten) wurden die Daten
an einem separaten Rechner in nahezu Echtzeit ausgewertet.

2.3   Datenauswertung und Visualisierung

Die einzelnen Signalverarbeitungsschritte der vollautomatischen Auswertung ist
in Abb. 2 dargestellt. Hierbei wurde für jede Einzelmessung zuerst die Ge-
webeverschiebung und darüber die Auslenkungsgeschwindigkeit ermittelt. Dazu wurde der Phase-root-seeking (PRS) Algorithmus [8] angewendet. Die zeitliche Fourier-Transformation der Gewebeauslenkungsgeschwindigkeit und ihre

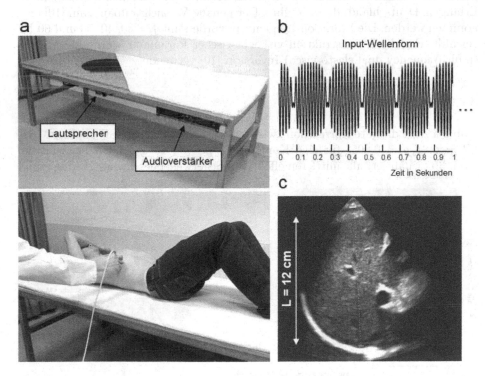

Abb. 1. Technisches Setup der USE: a) Patientenliege, b) zeitharmonische multifrequente Vibrationssignale, c) B-Mode Darstellung des rechten Leberlappens.

Betrachtung bei einer bestimmten Vibrationsfrequenz lieferte die komplexe Welle, bestehend aus einem Kompressions- und einem Scheranteil. Der Kompressionsanteil sowie die Rauschanteile dieses Signals wurden mit einem Bandpassfilter unterdrückt. Die resultierende zeitharmonische Scherwelle wurde mit dem Downhill-Simplex-Verfahren [9] gefittet. Damit wurde eine, dem gemessenen Schersignal bestmöglich angepasste Modellwelle kreiert und ihre Ausbreitungsgeschwindigkeit festgestellt. Um die Qualität dieses Modells zu bestimmen, wurde jeweils das Verhältnis zwischen gefitteter Scherwellenamplitude und Restsignal ermittelt. Messungen mit einem Qualitätsmaß kleiner als 0.65 wurden vom Algorithmus als stark verrauschte Daten erkannt und automatisch aussortiert. Als weiteres Ausschlusskriterium wurden die Scherwellenlängen im gemessenen Tiefenfenster der Länge L betrachtet. Messungen, bei denen die Wellenlängen den empirisch ermittelten Grenzwert von

2.4   Multifrequente MRE

Die multifrequente MRE wurde als Standard-Methode ausgewählt, um die Qualität der neuen zeitharmonischen USE-Methode zu validieren. Hierzu wurden 10 gesunde Freiwillige unmittelbar nach der USE mittels MRE untersucht. Die Experimente wurden an einem 1.5 Tesla MRT Scanner (Magnetom Sonata; Siemens Erlangen, Deutschland) durchgeführt. Der genaue Versuchsaufbau kann [10] entnommen werden. Die Vibrationsfrequenzen wurden mit $f = 30, 40, 50$ und 60 Hz gewählt. Für die Rekonstruktion viskoelastischer Paramater wurde die MDEV (multifrequency dual elasto-visco)-Inversion [10] verwendet.

3   Ergebnisse

Abb. 3a zeigt die gute Korrelation zwischen zeitharmonischer USE und der MRE ($R = 0.81, p = 0.005$) für eine Kontrollgruppe von 10 gesunden Freiwilligen. Abb. 3b visualisiert alle mittleren effektiven Scherwellengeschwindigkeiten $\bar{c}$ und

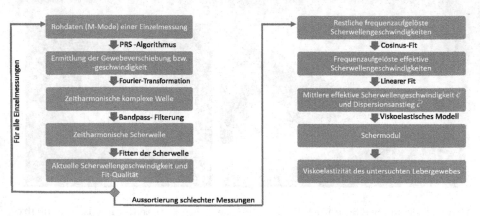

Abb. 2. Leber-USE: Gesamtauswertungsprozess.

das gemittelte Dispersionsverhalten $\bar{c}'$ für alle gesunden Freiwilligen und Patienten. Die gemittelten Werte für die Patienten sind $\bar{c} = 3.11 \pm 0.64$ m/s (im Bereich 2.14 bis 4.81 m/s) und $\bar{c}' = 39.1 \pm 32.2$ m/s/kHz. Die Kontrollgruppe hat deutlich geringere Werte von $\bar{c} = 1.74 \pm 0.10$ m/s (im Bereich 1.60 bis 1.91 m/s) und $\bar{c}' = 5.2 \pm 1.8$ m/s/kHz.

4 Diskussion

Im Rahmen dieser Arbeit wurde demonstriert, dass ein kombinierter B- und M-Mode US-Scanner eingesetzt werden kann, um die gesamte Leber durchdringende zeitharmonische Wellen zu detektieren und darauf basierend die Lebersteifigkeit auch bei adipösen Patienten mit Leberzirrhose nichtinvasiv zu diagnostizieren. Zudem wurden die Resultate dieser Technik mit dem elastographischen Goldstandard MRE validiert, indem eine Gruppe von weiteren Freiwilligen mittels beider Techniken untersucht wurde. Die gute Korrelation ($R = 0.81, p = 0.005$) beider Methoden bestätigt die Anwendbarkeit der kostengünstigeren und schnelleren Ultraschall-basierten Methode. Die Wellengeschwindigkeiten der mittels zeitharmonischer USE untersuchten Zirrhose-Patienten unterschieden sich signifikant ($p = 0.0025$) von der gesunden Kontrollgruppe. Im Gegensatz zu unseren bisherigen Arbeiten [7] konnte die Datenakquisitionen durch die B-Mode Darstellung besser positioniert durchgeführt werden, was die Signal-Qualität enorm gesteigert hat. Zudem konnte vor allem während der Untersuchung adipöser Patienten erstmals ein größeres Tiefenfenster gewählt werden. Des Weiteren wurde bei dieser Arbeit im letzten Auswertungsschritt die Aussortierung von Fehlruns vollautomatisch und benutzerunabhängig durchgeführt.

Zusammengefasst wurde eine klinisch einsetzbare nichtinvasive zeitharmonische USE-Technik entwickelt, welche es ermöglicht, auch bei adipösen Patienten

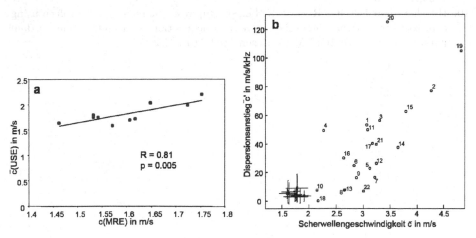

Abb. 3. Resultate: (a) Mittels USE und MRE ermittelte Scherwellengeschwindigkeit bei 10 Freiwilligen, (b) mittlere effektive Scherwellengeschwindigkeit und Dispersionsverhalten von 10 Gesunden (Kreuze) und alle 22 Patienten (Kreise).

zuverlässig Leberzirrhose zu diagnostizieren. Im nächsten Schritt muss die derzeit retrospektiv durchgeführte Datenauswertung in Echtzeit umgesetzt und die Funktionalität dieser Technik bei Patienten mit niedrigeren Fibrosegraden überprüft werden.

Literaturverzeichnis

1. Cui XW, Friedrich-Rust M, Molo CD, et al. Liver elastography, comments on EFSUMB elastography guidelines. World J Gastroenterol. 2013;19:6329–47.
2. Sarvazyan AP, Urban MW, Greenleaf JF. Acoustic waves in medical imaging and diagnostics. Ultrasound Med Biol. 2013;39:1133–46.
3. Chen S, Sanchez W, Callstrom MR, et al. Assessment of liver viscoelasticity by using shear waves induced by ultrasound radiation force. Radiology. 2013;266:964–70.
4. Krouskop TA, Dougherty DR, Vinson FS. A pulsed Doppler ultrasonic system for making noninvasive measurements of the mechanical properties of soft tissue. J Rehabil Res Dev. 1987;24:1–8.
5. Muthupillai R, Lomas D, Rossman P, et al. Magnetic resonance elastography by direct visualization of propagating acoustic strain waves. Science. 1995;269(5232):1854–7.
6. Bonekamp S, Kamel I, Solga S, et al. Can imaging modalities diagnose and stage hepatic fibrosis and cirrhosis accurately? J Hepatol. 2009;50:17–35.
7. Tzschatzsch H, Ipek-Ugay S, Guo J, et al. In vivo time-harmonic multifrequency elastography of the human liver. Phys Med Biol. 2014;59:1641–54.
8. Pesavento A, Perrey C, Krueger M, et al. A Time-efficient and accurate strain estimation concept for ultrasonic elastography using iterative phase zero estimation. IEEE Trans Ultrason Ferroelectr Freq Control. 1999;46:1057–67.
9. Nelder JA, Mead R. A simplex-method for function minimization. Comput J. 1965;7:308–13.
10. Hirsch S, Guo J, Reiter R, et al. MR elastography of the liver and the spleen using a piezoelectric driver, single-shot wave-field acquisition, and multifrequency dual parameter reconstruction. Magn Reson Med. 2013;71:267–77.

Discrete Estimation of Data Completeness for 3D Scan Trajectories with Detector Offset

Andreas Maier[1], Patrick Kugler[2], Günter Lauritsch[2], Joachim Hornegger[1]

[1]Pattern Recognition Lab and SAOT Erlangen, FAU Erlangen
[2]Siemens AG, Healthcare, Forchheim
andreas.maier@fau.de

Abstract. The sequence of source and detector positions in a CT scan determines reconstructable volume and data completeness. Commonly this is regarded already in the design phase of a scanner. Modern flat-panel scanners, however, allow to acquire a broad range of positions. This enables many possibilities for different scan paths. However, every new path or trajectory implies different data completeness. Analytic solutions are either designed for special trajectories like the Tam-window for helical CT scans or do not incorporate the actual detector size such as Tuy's condition. In this paper, we describe a method to determine the voxel-wise data completeness in percent for discretely sampled trajectories. Doing so, we are able to model any sequence of source and detector positions. Using this method, we are able to confirm known theory such as Tuy's condition and data completeness of trajectories using detector offset to increase the field-of-view. As we do not require an analytic formulation of the trajectory, the algorithm will also be applicable to any other source-detector-path or set of source-detector-path segments.

1 Introduction

Modern flat-panel CT scanners allow many scan configurations. In particular, multi-axis C-arm systems allow a broad range of application scenarios. For example, Herbst et al. identified novel opportunities to reduce the scan range for eliptical fields-of-view [1] and Xia et al. found that reduction of scan range and dose is possible for volume-of-interest scans [2]. Both studies, however, demonstrate these effects only in 2D imaging geometries and lack the analysis in 3D.

While the adjustment of the scan configuration for a specific task allows many different benefits ranging from image quality improvement [3] to novel applications such as long-volume imaging [4], data completeness is typically determined for each scan configuration analytically. This results in new analytic formulations for each new path. Important examples are Tuy's condition [5] and the Tam-window for helical scans [6]. While Tuy's condition holds for any cone-beam scan, it does not incorporate detector size and delivers thus a necessary but not sufficient condition. Tam's window applies only for helical scans.

Thus, there is a need for a method to compute data completeness for arbitrary trajectories. In the following, we describe such a method for discrete source and detector positions. Note that the method is conceptually very close previously published methods [7, 8] which have not been applied to off-center detector trajectories to the knowledge of the authors.

2   3D Radon space

While 2D Radon transform and 2D X-ray transform are identical, the 3D Radon transform differs from the 3D X-ray transform [5]. Fig. 1 shows this difference in a parallel geometry: The line integrals obtained by X-rays are indicated as arrows. The respective plane integral in 3D Radon space is obtained as line integral on the 2D X-ray detector at the intersection of the plane and the detector. Note that we assume that the object fits completely onto the X-ray detector.

For cone-beam geometries, the above relation is not entirely correct. The line integral on the 2D projector is not identical to a plane integral in object space as the rays generally form fans through the object. The fan integral is weighted with increasing magnification though the object [5]. While this is important for the reconstruction algorithm, it does not affect data completeness in general.

3   Point-wise data completeness in cone-beam geometry

We know that we are able to reconstruct the object of interest, if the 3D Radon data is completely acquired. In order to compute a local approximation of the amount of acquired Radon data, we investigate the coverage of Radon planes for every voxel. In order to do so, we investigate 3D coverage of Radon plane normals on a unit sphere, called Radon sphere in the following. In this context, we ignore object-dependent information such as truncation on the detector. Note that this formalism still allows to include the detector size into the data completeness estimation. Fig. 2 shows this process for a circular trajectory. In fact,

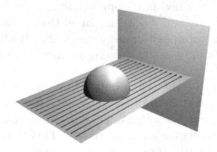

Fig. 1. While X-rays form integrals along individual rays (denoted as arrows), the 3D Radon transform evaluates plane integrals. Note that an integral along a line on the 2D X-ray detector evaluates exactly a plane integral in parallel geometry.

the requirement of complete sampling of the radon sphere is identical to Tuy's condition as Tuy postulates that every plane that intersects the object needs to intersect the source path. Given a detector that fits the entire object, this allows to compute the respective plane integral, because we are able to compute the respective line integral on the 2D detector. Thus if all planes that intersect the object also intersect the source trajectory, all plane integrals are measured and the Radon sphere is sampled completely at every point of the object.

4   Numerical data completeness estimation

So far we have only summarized known theory for data completeness and showed the relation between Tuy's condition and the Radon sphere sampling. As mentioned above, Tuy's condition does not incorporate the actual detector size. In

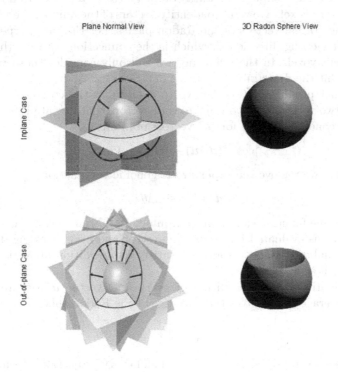

Fig. 2. Example for 3D Radon space sampling for a point of interest for a circular scan trajectory: The upper row shows the sampling for a point inside the acquisition plane. The normals of the Radon planes (denoted as arrows) that are measured lie on a plane that is aligned with the rotation axis for each projection image. By rotation, the entire Radon sphere is sampled. In the bottom row, a case is shown where the point of interest is below the reconstruction plane. In this case, the plane normals lie in a plane that is slant with respect to the rotation axis. Thus rotation misses planes aligned with the rotation axis. This leads to an incomplete sampling of the Radon sphere.

order to include this in our algorithm, we now determine the Radon sphere sampling at every voxel position in the volume under consideration.

First, we require a discrete sampling of the unit sphere in vectors $\boldsymbol{u}$. Here, we follow ideas of Saff et al. [9]. We approximate the unit sphere in intervals of the same angular step size $\Delta\theta$. For the elevation angle α, we sample the range $[-\pi/2, \pi/2]$ in steps of $\Delta\theta$ size. For the azimuth angle β, we determine a step size $\Delta\beta$ that is dependent on the elevation angle α

$$\Delta\beta = \sin^{-1}\left(\frac{\sin(\Delta\theta/2)}{\cos\alpha}\right) * 2 \tag{1}$$

Note that it is sufficient to sample only half of the unit sphere, as the plane integrals are symmetric for top and bottom (Fig. 2). In the following, we denote the total number of points sampled on the sphere as N_u.

Next, we need to compute the data completeness in terms of Radon sphere coverage for every voxel. We want to identify vectors of the unit sphere $\boldsymbol{u}$ that are covered by the normal vectors of the Radon planes, i.e. that are perpendicular to the current viewing direction $\boldsymbol{d}$, which is the connection between the source and the current voxel. In the following, we will only consider those vectors $\boldsymbol{d}$ that actually hit the detector.

As the inner product of two unit vectors describes the cosine of the angle between the two vectors and we want to find vectors that deviate less than $\Delta\theta$, the following condition is true for the vectors of interest

$$|\cos^{-1}(\boldsymbol{d}^\top\boldsymbol{u}) - 90°| < \Delta\theta \tag{2}$$

By rearranging, we remove the expensive trigonometric function

$$|\boldsymbol{d}^\top\boldsymbol{u}| < \sin\Delta\theta \tag{3}$$

Note that the sine function can be precomputed, as $\Delta\theta$ is a constant in our case. Above equation is evaluated for every unit vector and every viewing direction. The unique number of unit vectors that satisfy the condition above is denoted as N_c in the following.

After evaluation of this condition of every unit vector $\boldsymbol{u}$, we are able to compute a coverage c that gives the coverage of the Radon sphere

$$c = \frac{N_c}{N_u} \cdot 100\,\% \tag{4}$$

As above process is repeated for every voxel and every projection, the algorithm has a complexity of $\mathcal{O}(N^3 \cdot P \cdot N_u)$, if N^3 is the number of voxels and P the number of projections. Note that P should be sampled at least in angular intervals of $\Delta\theta$ and thus both P and N_u are dependent on this angular sampling, i.e. the smaller $\Delta\theta$ the higher the complexity.

5   Results

We investigated two types of trajectories: Helix scans with the detector centered, i.e. the principal ray passes the rotation axis and hits the detector in the center.

Furthermore, we investigated a configuration with an off-center detector. Here the configuration was that the principal ray passes the rotation axis and hits the detector at the most left pixel row. We simulated three rotations of the helix at different forward feed along the rotation axis. The detector was in landscape orientation and had a ratio of 4:3. Volumetric sampling was performed on a $64 \times 64 \times 128$ grid. $\Delta\theta$ was set to $1.5°$. We denote the forward motion per helical turn as h_{helix}. In order to normalize this independent of the detector size, we define a p value that is motivated by pitch in CT. However, we have to take into account, that perspective projection may magnify the current view in an arbitrary flat-panel system. Therefore, the detector height projected into the iso-center h_{iso} is taken into account. p is then found as $p = \frac{h_{\text{helix}}}{h_{\text{iso}}}$.

For visualization, we set a cut-off value of $c = 90\%$ and projected the reconstructable areas of the volume as line integrals to a virtual large detector to display all configurations. The visualizations were created using the CONRAD software framework [10]. Fig. 3 shows the results. The center configuration with $p = 1.0$ shows the longest coverage in rotation axis direction, however, there are areas that are not completely covered within the volume. The configuration with $p = 0.75$ delivers a complete coverage of the volume, i.e. there are no gaps in between. This result matches known theory for helical scans [6]. For the off-center cases, the coverage in rotation axis direction is shorter and their pitch values are respectively shorter. However, the field-of-view is almost doubled in inplane orientation. With $p = 0.5$ the off-center configuration is not able to cover a continuous volume. The configuration with $p = 0.33$ is able to cover the entire field-of-view with at least 99% completeness. However, this comes at a reduction of coverage in axial direction.

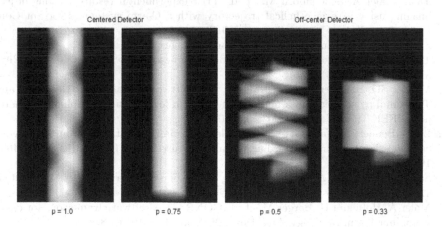

Centered Detector   Off-center Detector

p = 1.0   p = 0.75   p = 0.5   p = 0.33

Fig. 3. Integral projections the reconstructable volume for three turns of the helix. With off-center detector, the $p = 0.33$ configuration still lacks a very small amount of data that is moving along the helix.

6   Discussion and outlook

We presented an algorithm for the computation of data completeness at every voxel. Conceptually, the algorithm is very close to [7, 8]. We show that the algorithm is suited to analyze scan configurations with different detector offset. The results on the helical configuration match the theory known from literature. Furthermore, it is interesting to note, that the off-center configuration is close to complete, but still lacks small amounts of data ($< 1\,\%$). Limitations of the presented method are that it does not handle object truncation and it does not allow to recommend a specific reconstruction algorithm. However, source position and detector size are handled correctly.

Acknowledgement. The concepts and information presented in this paper are based on research and are not commercially available.

References

1. Herbst M, Schebesch F, Berger M, et al. Improved trajectories in C-arm computed tomography for non-circular fields of view. Proc Int Conf Image Form X-ray Comput Tomogr. 2014; p. 274–8.
2. Xia Y, Maier A, Berger M, et al. Region of interest reconstruction from dose-minimized super short scan data. Proc BVM. 2014; p. 48–53.
3. Stayman JW, Siewerdsen JH. Task-based trajectories in iteratively reconstructed interventional cone-beam CT. Proc Int Meet Fully Three-Dimens Image Reconstr Radiol Nucl Med. 2013; p. 257–60.
4. Yu Z, Maier A, Schoenborn M, et al. Frist experimental results on long-object imaging using a reverse helical trajectory with a C-arm system. Proc Int Conf Image Form X-ray Comput Tomogr. 2012; p. 364–8.
5. Zeng GL. Medical Image Reconstruction. Springer; 2010.
6. Tam KC, Samarasekera S, Sauer F. Exact cone beam CT with a spiral scan. Phys Med Biol. 1998;43(4):1015.
7. Metzler SD, Bowsher JE, Jaszczak RJ. Geometrical similarities of the Orlov and Tuy sampling criteria and a numerical algorithm for assessing sampling completeness. IEEE Trans Nuc Sci. 2003;50:1550–5.
8. Liu B, Bennett J, Wang G, et al. Completeness map evaluation demonstrated with candidate next-generation cardiac CT architectures. Med Phys. 2012;39(5):2405–16.
9. Saff EB, Kuijlaars ABJ. Distributing many points on a sphere. Math Intell. 1997;19(1):5–11.
10. Maier A, Hofmann H, Berger M, et al. CONRAD: a software framework for cone-beam imaging in radiology. Med Phys. 2013;40(11):111914–18.

Optimal C-arm Positioning for Aortic Interventions

Salvatore Virga[1], Verena Dogeanu[1],Pascal Fallavollita[1], Reza Ghotbi[2],
Nassir Navab[1], Stefanie Demirci[1]

[1]Computer Aided Medical Procedures, Technische Universität München
[2]Vascular Surgery Department, Klinikum München-West
salvo.virga@tum.de

Abstract. Due to the continuous integration of innovative interventional imaging modalities into vascular surgery rooms, there is an urgent
need for computer assisted interaction and visualization solutions that
support the smooth integration of technological solutions within the surgical workflow. In this paper, we introduce a new paradigm for optimal-
view controlled maneuvering of Angiographic C-arms during thoracic
endovascular aortic repair (TEVAR). This allows the semi-automatic
pre-computation of well-defined anatomy-related optimal views based on
pre-operative 3D image data and automatic interventional positioning of
the imaging device relative to the patient's anatomy through inverse
kinematics and CT to patient registration. Together with our clinical
partners, we have evaluated the new technique using 5 patient datasets
and are able to show promising results.

1 Introduction

Minimally-invasive interventions have replaced many conventional surgical procedures and, thereby, increased patient survival rate for various diseases. Endovascular procedures have become state-of-the-art interventions, and are among
routine skills of vascular surgeons and interventional radiologists. The continuous transformation of conventional surgery rooms into *hybrid ORs* have had
tremendous impact on the medical workflow. There is an urgent need for computer assisted interaction and visualization solutions that support the smooth
integration of technological solutions within the surgical workflow.

Thoracic endovascular aortic repair (TEVAR) describes the implantation of
stent grafts into the ascending or descending aorta. Due to the arch's anatomy,
the placement of a stent graft in the proximity of the left subclavian artery (LSA)
may lead to its partial or total occlusion. Here, it is crucial for surgeons and
interventionalists to acquire an optimal X-ray view that let them easily detect
the exact point where the LSA divides from the aortic arch. The efficient maneuvering of an integrated (robotic) C-arm into the surgeon's desired position is
a crucial phase that require an optimal interaction within the surgery team. The
current decision process of the surgeon or interventionalist is based on a mental

mapping between the 3D patient anatomy and intra-operative image data in order to gather information on how to reposition the C-arm gantry to their desired view. However, moving the C-arm into the best viewing projection in regard to the anatomy is time-consuming and requires a lot of skill. This is mainly due to the complex kinematic chain defining C-arms, the miscommunication among surgical staff members, and the lack of intelligent user interfaces facilitating C-arm positioning. Consequently, this leads to the acquisition of non-optimal X-ray images from additional gantry positions and thereby an increase in radiation and use of contrast agent.

Approaches towards providing computer-assistance for endovascular aortic repair procedures have been in the focus of research activities for quite some time. Until now, respective publications have mainly been concerned with the integration of pre-operative 3D image data into the interventional setup [1, 2, 3] in order to allow for 3D navigation of endovascular devices [4, 5]. The first efforts towards an integrated solution for Fluoroscopy guided procedures have recently been made by Brehler et al. [6] and Fallavollita et al. [7]. Inspired by these recent efforts, we introduce a new paradigm for optimal-view controlled maneuvering of angiographic C-arms during thoracic endovascular aortic repair (TEVAR).

2   Materials and methods

We have developed a framework to pre-compute the interventionalist's *desired views* to avoid the occlusion of the LSA – or other branches of the aortic arch – during TEVAR procedures. As specified in Fig 2, this is done by the extraction of geometrical features from pre-operative Computed Tomography Angiography (CTA) data routinely acquired for every patient for diagnosis and procedural

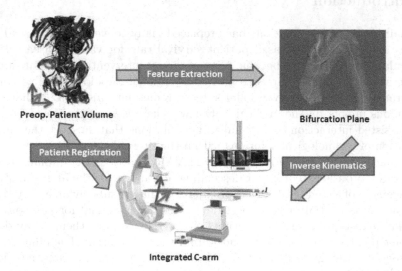

Fig. 1. Optimal-view controlled maneuvering of angiographic C-arms during TEVAR.

Fig. 2. Computation of optimal viewing plane: (a) segmentation of thoracic aorta and all branching vessels, (b) centerline and bifurcation points extraction, (c) optimal branching planes computation.

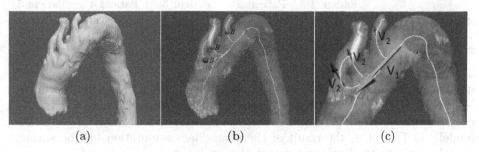

(a)   (b)   (c)

planning, and the automatic interventional positioning of the imaging device relative to the patient's anatomy through inverse kinematics. The accuracy of this process heavily relies on a correct patient registration to CTA. For this paper, we have considered a procedure-specific 2D/3D algorithm [3] that solves the challenging matching of pre-operative to intra-operative data via disocclusion and an intensity-based robust similarity measure.

2.1   Feature extraction

As the final goal of the proposed framework is to obtain clear views of the bifurcation points between the aortic arch and the LSA, the feature extraction consists in the computation of those 3D points from pre-operative CTA data. We first segment the main vessels – the aorta and its branches on the aortic arch – then we compute the centerlines and analyze related geometrical features to obtain the bifurcation points.

For the actual implementation of the framework, we have taken advantage of the VMTK[1] library, which is based on the well know ITK[2] and VTK[3] frameworks and extends some of their methods to achieve vessel segmentation, centerlines extraction and geometric analysis of the vessels. Its use allows easy implementation of other methods and features directly from ITK and VTK, such as the visualization of intermediate and final results within a graphical UI and the interaction of the end users – the clinical staff – with it.

3D vessel segmentation There is extensive literature on vessel segmentation [8] covering different approaches and mathematical frameworks. Our approach employs the ITK geodesic active contour level set segmentation method. Fig. 3(a) shows the result of the segmentation of the aortic arch and its branches from pre-operative CTA data as a surface model. Our own implementation requires the user to select random pixels (seed points) for every branch to be segmented.

---

[1] The Vascular Modeling Toolkit – http://www.vmtk.org
[2] The Insight Toolkit – http://www.itk.org
[3] The Visualization Toolkit – http://www.vtk.org

Table 1. Accuracy study results: RMSE in translation and rotation parameters respectively.

	Patient 1	Patient 2	Patient 3	Patient 4	Patient 5
Translation (mm)	0.0	0.0	0.0	0.0	0.0
Rotation (deg)	0.7	0.0	0.3	0.3	0.0

3D centerlines extraction Given the surface model of the aortic arch and its branches, centerlines are computed using the algorithm implemented in the VMTK library. Here, centerlines are computed as weighted shortest path between two seed points bounded to run on the Voronoi diagram of the vessel model. In Fig. 3(b), the result of the centerline computation for the surface model obtain by the level set segmentation is depicted.

3D bifurcation points Finally, the bifurcation points are extracted in two steps. First, the vessel model is decomposed in its constituent branches using the *slitting* algorithm [9] dividing the entire vasculature into segments. The 3D geometry of each vascular segment is then analyzed for the existence of bifurcation and its position in 3D [10] (Fig. 3(b)).

2.2   Optimal view

For every branch from the aortic arch, we obtain a description of its geometry in the form of a 3D point B that describes the position of the underlying bifurcation point, and two vectors V_1, V_2 directed along the centerlines of the aortic arch and its branches respectively (Fig. 3(c)). Having this information, the bifurcation plane $\Pi_{bifurcation}$ can easily be computed as the plane that is formed by vectors V_1 and V_2.

Having a correct patient registration to CT in place and $\Pi_{current}$ being the current plane of view of the imaging device, the matrix T describing the transformation to the desired plane $\Pi_{bifurcation}$ is computed using the normal vectors $u_{bifurcation}, u_{current}$ of the two planes. The transformation matrix T is computed so that

$$u_{bifurcation} = Tu_{current} \tag{1}$$

and serves as input for the inverse kinematics framework [7].

3   Results

We have validated our method on datasets of five patients undergoing thoracic aneurysm stenting procedure. Patient-specific CTA and intra-operative C-arm images were acquired for each one of them. Two dedicated experimental setups were created in order to focus on two different evaluation aspects.

Table 2. Questionnaire for clinical feasibility study. The Lickert Score is given in (min-median-max).

Question	Likert Score
1 Precomputation of optimal C-arm positions for aortic branches has an important clinical impact	(4-5-5)
2 Every surgeon should consider planning optimal viewpoints	(3-4-5)
3 I would use the precomputation of optimal views immediately during clinical practice	(4-5-5)
4 The current C-arm interaction workflow does not fit smoothly within the surgical workflow of aortic interventions.	(4-5-5)
5 Slight deviation from the optimal view is unacceptable	(1-1-2)

3.1 Accuracy study

For the first setup, we provided our clinical partner (chief vascular surgeon) with a tool that produces digitally reconstructed radiographs (DRR) from patient-specific CTA volumes and allows rotation and translation interaction. For each patient dataset, the optimal view computed by our proposed method was displayed. The task was to evaluate whether it actually represented the desired interventional view and, if not, to use the available interaction modes to yield such an optimal view. We then computed the deviation of the resulting view from the optimal view computed by our presented approach.

Tab. 1 shows the results of this study in terms of the root mean square error in translation and rotation parameters respectively.

3.2 Clinical feasibility study

In our second experimental setup, we aimed at evaluating the clinical feasibility of our proposed approach by a Likert scale-based questionnaire, which was filled out by our clinical partners (chief vascular surgeon and three resident surgeons with more than 4 yrs. experience). The 5-pt Likert scale was defined as follows: (1-strongly disagree; 2-disagree; 3-neutral; 4-agree; 5-strongly agree).

The average results depicted in Tab. 2 are very positive. All participants strongly agreed that our idea of precomputing the optimal C-arm positions for aortic branches had great potential to be translated in current clinical practice.

4 Discussion

Results of our evaluation studies are very promising and our partner clinicians approved the clinical feasibility of our proposed approach. Despite this very positive feedback, we will focus our future efforts on evaluating the clinical application in more detail. We are aware of the fact that the accuracy of maneuvering the C-arm to the precomputed optimal view highly depends on the accuracy and robustness of underlying patient-to-CTA registration. As already indicated by our questionnaire, clinicians would accept slight deviations from the optimal view (Question 5 in Tab. 2). It will be one of our main focuses to analyze this aspect in more detail.

In this paper, we have presented, for the first time, a new paradigm for optimal-view controlled maneuvering of angiographic C-arms during TEVAR. The optimal views are precomputed based on pre-operative patient-specific 3D image data and show clear views of the bifurcation points between the aortic arch and the LSA. Beside their overall very positive feedback to the proposed approach, our clinical partners confirmed the urgent need for innovative inter-action solutions that support the smooth integration of technological solutions within the surgical workflow of TEVAR.

References

1. Bauer S, Wasza J, Haase S, et al. Multi-modal surface registration for markerless initial patient setup in radiation therapy using microsoft's Kinect sensor. Proc ICCV. 2011; p. 1175–81.
2. Miao S, Liao R, Pfister M. Toward smart utilization of two X-ray images for 2-D/3-D registration applied to abdominal aortic aneurysm interventions. Comput Electr Eng. 2013;39(5):1485–98.
3. Demirci S, Baust M, Kutter O, et al. Disocclusion-based 2D-3D registration for angiographic interventions. Comput Biol Med. 2013;43(4):312–22.
4. Rietdorf U, Riesenkampff E, Schwarz T, et al. Planning of vessel grafts for recon-structive surgery in congenital heart diseases. Proc SPIE. 2010; p. 76252W–8.
5. Demirci S, Bigdelou A, Wang L, et al. 3D stent recovery from one x-ray projection. Proc MICCAI. 2011; p. 178–85.
6. Brehler M, Görres J, Wolf I, et al. Automatic standard plane adjustment on mobile c-arm CT images of the calcaneus using atlas-based feature registration. Proc SPIE. 2014; p. 90360E–6.
7. Fallavollita P, Winkler A, Habert S, et al. Desired-view controlled positioning of angiographic C-arms. Proc MICCAI. 2014; p. 659–66.
8. Lesage D, Angelini ED, Bloch I, et al. A review of 3D vessel lumen segmen-tation techniques: models, features and extraction schemes. Med Image Anal. 2009;13(6):819–45.
9. Antiga L, Steinman D. Robust and objective decomposition and mapping of bi-furcating vessels. IEEE Trans Med Imag. 2004;23(6):704–13.
10. Piccinelli M, Veneziani A, Steinman D, et al. A framework for geometric analysis of vascular structures: application to cerebral aneurysms. IEEE Trans Med Imag. 2009;28(8):1141–55.

Projection and Reconstruction-Based Noise Filtering Methods in Cone Beam CT

Benedikt Lorch[1], Martin Berger[1,2], Joachim Hornegger[1,2], Andreas Maier[1,2]

[1]Pattern Recognition Lab, FAU Erlangen-Nürnberg
[2]Research Training Group 1773 "Heterogeneous Image Systems"
benedikt.lorch@fau.de

Abstract. A reduction of the radiation dose in computed tomography typically leads to more noise in the acquired projections. Here filtering methods can help to reduce the noise level and preserve the diagnostic value of the low-dose images. In this work, six variants of Gaussian and bilateral filters are applied in both projection and reconstruction domain. Our comparison of noise reduction and image resolution shows that 2D and 3D bilateral filtering in the projection domain can reduce the noise level, but must be applied carefully to avoid streaking artifacts. By smoothing homogeneous regions while preserving sharp edges, the 3D bilateral filter applied in the reconstruction domain yielded the best results in terms of noise reduction and image sharpness.

1 Introduction

In cone beam computed tomography (CBCT), X-rays are used to acquire projection images of patient anatomies. A general goal in CBCT is to reduce the radiation dose while preserving the diagnostic value of the images. However, a low radiation dose typically leads to higher noise level in the reconstructions. In clinical practice reconstruction filter kernels are used that incorporate low-pass filters into the ramp filtering step during image reconstruction. This process is similar to Gaussian filtering, as the filtering operations are by definition linear and are therefore not able to preserve image resolution properly.

Non-linear filtering methods have been proposed that aim to keep sharpness and resolution as constant as possible while decreasing noise in homogeneous areas. In analytic reconstruction, adaptive weighting of the projection data can be used prior to reconstruction to reduce noise [1, 2]. A different approach is to apply noise filtering after reconstructing the 3D object, e.g. by bilateral or wavelet-based filtering [3, 4]. Less work has been done on non-linear filtering in the projection domain. Manduca et al. proposed to use an adaptive 2D bilateral filter on the projection images [5]. Further, 2D [6] as well as 3D [7] anisotropic filtering was applied in the projection domain, where the latter uses the view angles of a circular CBCT trajectory as a third dimension.

In this work, we also investigate a 3D bilateral filter in the projection domain along with convolution-based and non-linear, edge-preserving noise filtering methods on projections and reconstructions. Through comparison of all methods we identify which domain is best suited for the individual filtering approach.

2   Materials and methods

2.1   Filtering methods

In total, we evaluated six variants of 2D and 3D Gaussian and bilateral filtering. The Gaussian filter is a simple convolution of the input image with a Gaussian function used to reduce image noise and smooth edges. The filtered image function $\hat{f}$ is given by the convolution function

$$\hat{f}(\boldsymbol{x}, \sigma_g) = \sum_{\boldsymbol{\mu} \in \Omega} f(\boldsymbol{\mu}) \cdot c(\boldsymbol{x}, \boldsymbol{\mu})$$

$$c(\boldsymbol{x}, \boldsymbol{\mu}, \sigma_g) = \frac{1}{\sqrt{(2\pi\sigma_g)^d}} \exp\left(-\frac{1}{2\sigma_g^2}(\boldsymbol{x} - \boldsymbol{\mu})^{\mathrm{T}}(\boldsymbol{x} - \boldsymbol{\mu})\right) \qquad (1)$$

where $\boldsymbol{x}$ is the geometric position in the image, Ω is the set that defines the neighborhood of $\boldsymbol{x}$ and σ_g is the spherical standard deviation of the d-dimensional Gaussian filter kernel. An advantage of Gaussian filters is that they can be applied by a fast convolution, however they are also known to blur edge information.

We also used the non-linear bilateral filter [3], which combines the smoothing of a Gaussian with an edge-preserving component by adjusting the filter kernel based on the local intensities of the image. The filtered image $\widetilde{f}$ is computed by

$$\widetilde{f}(\boldsymbol{x}, \sigma_g, \sigma_p) = \frac{1}{k(\boldsymbol{x}, \sigma_p)} \sum_{\boldsymbol{\mu} \in \Omega} f(\boldsymbol{x}) \cdot c(\boldsymbol{x}, \boldsymbol{\mu}, \sigma_g) \cdot s(f(\boldsymbol{x}), f(\boldsymbol{\mu}), \sigma_p)$$

$$s(f(\boldsymbol{x}), f(\boldsymbol{\mu}), \sigma_p) = \exp\left(-\frac{1}{2\sigma_p^2}(f(\boldsymbol{x}) - f(\boldsymbol{\mu}))^2\right) \qquad (2)$$

where σ_p is the standard deviation used for the photometric distance. The kernel function is now given by $c(\boldsymbol{x}, \boldsymbol{\mu}, \sigma_g) \cdot s(f(\boldsymbol{x}), f(\boldsymbol{\mu}), \sigma_p)$, hence the normalization factor $k(\boldsymbol{x}, \sigma_p)$ is formed by the sum of all kernel values. If the intensity difference between $f(\boldsymbol{x})$ and $f(\boldsymbol{\mu})$ becomes high, e.g. due to an edge, the weight for $f(\boldsymbol{\mu})$ becomes low which prevents edges from being smoothed out.

In the projection domain, Gaussian (GP-2D) and bilateral filtering (BP-2D) were applied to all 2D projection images. To further reduce noise we also applied 3D Gaussian (GP-3D) and bilateral filtering (BP-3D) on the complete stack of projections. Note that in this case the third dimension refers to the view angle, as we aim to incorporate information from neighboring projections. Finally, these measurements were compared to 3D Gaussian (GV-3D) and 3D bilateral filtering (BV-3D) applied as pure post-processing on the volume which was reconstructed from the noisy projections.

2.2   Data and setup

To obtain the same projection data with different noise levels, we simulated an CBCT scan using the Forbild head phantom[1]. The focal length was set to

---

[1] http://www.imp.uni-erlangen.de/forbild

1200 mm and the phantom was centered at the rotation center at a distance of 600 mm to the X-ray source. The detector size was set to 640 × 480 pixels with an isotropic pixel size of 1.2 mm. We simulated a circular trajectory around the z-axis, acquiring a short-scan with 248 projections and an angular increment of 0.869°. For noise simulation a monochromatic absorption model was used, releasing 50 000 photons with an energy of 80keV for simulating a moderate noise level and 30 000 photons with an energy of 50 keV for an increased noise level. As ground truth we also generated a 3D volume of the Forbild phantom with a resolution of 1024 × 1024 × 1024 voxels and an isotropic voxel size of 0.25 mm.

The FDK method was used for reconstruction [8]. We applied a Ram-Lak filter without window function to ensure that the resolution is not influenced by the ramp-filtering step. Noise filtering on the projections was conducted at the beginning, filtering on the reconstruction was done at the end of the pipeline.

To quantify the noise level, we calculated the standard deviation σ_{sd} inside a box shaped homogeneous region with a side length of 16 mm. The central section of the box is depicted in Fig. 1. For measuring the residual resolution of the filtered images, we computed the modulation transfer function (MTF). Therefore, the mean of 150 line profiles was taken along the inner edge of the scull bone as shown in Fig. 1 to minimize the influence of streak and noise artifacts. Then the MTF is calculated by the Fourier transform of the derivative of the mean line profile. The achieved resolution was determined by the frequency that corresponds to a ten percent residual of the magnitude spectrum's maximum. In order to evaluate the filtering methods' performance w.r.t. their parameters, we

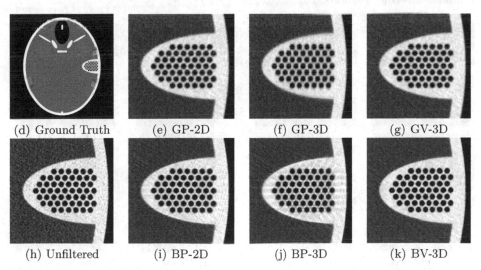

(d) Ground Truth   (e) GP-2D   (f) GP-3D   (g) GV-3D

(h) Unfiltered   (i) BP-2D   (j) BP-3D   (k) BV-3D

Fig. 1. Filtering methods with $\sigma_{sd} = 0.01$ on the 80keV dataset. The box in (a) depicts a section of the homogeneous region where σ_{sd} was calculated. The colored lines indicate the line profiles used for the MTF. Visualization window set to $[0.10, 0.52]$ cm^2/g.

Table 1. Resolution measured at 10% MTF for a fixed noise level σ_{sd}. Given an isotropic voxel size of 0.25mm, the theoretical maximum is given by 10 lp/cm.

10% MTF in lp/cm	GP-2D	GP-3D	BP-2D	BP-3D	GV-3D	BV-3D
80keV dataset ($\sigma_{sd} = 0.01$)	4.81	4.96	5.88	5.60	4.46	6.79
50keV dataset ($\sigma_{sd} = 0.07$)	5.01	5.08	6.11	5.95	4.81	7.34

used a grid search approach where the upper and lower bounds of the parameter range have been adjusted heuristically.

3   Results

In Fig. 1 and Fig. 2, the reconstructions are shown for the 80keV and the 50keV datasets, respectively. The residual noise σ_{sd} was fixed as denoted in Tab. 1. In both datasets, the BV-3D produces the best results with the highest resolution. The BP-2D gives the sharpest results of the projection domain approaches, closely followed by BP-3D. All Gaussian methods show a reduced sharpness compared to bilateral filtering. However, the BP-3D and the BP-2D reveal increased streaking artifacts especially in the 50keV dataset. Fig. 3 and Fig. 4 compare the achieved MTF values w.r.t. the measured noise level σ_{sd}. A high σ_p degenerates the bilateral filter to a Gaussian filter as depicted in Fig. 3a. In Fig. 3b, we can see that the Gaussian methods perform similarly well, yet, the projection based methods show a slightly higher MTF value. Fig. 4 displays the MTF results for bilateral filtering methods.

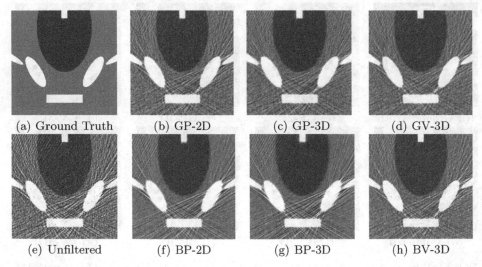

(a) Ground Truth   (b) GP-2D   (c) GP-3D   (d) GV-3D

(e) Unfiltered   (f) BP-2D   (g) BP-3D   (h) BV-3D

Fig. 2. Filtering methods with $\sigma_{sd} = 0.07$ on the 50keV dataset. Visualization window set to $[0.20, 0.80]$ cm^2/g.

Fig. 3. Comparison of resolution and noise level of Gaussian and bilateral filtering on the 80keV dataset.

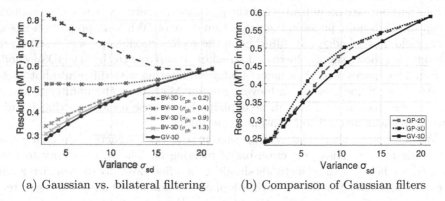

(a) Gaussian vs. bilateral filtering   (b) Comparison of Gaussian filters

By decreasing σ_p, results yield a higher resolution until a turning point, at which resolution as well as noise reduction do not vary anymore. Quantitative MTF measurements support the visual impressions and are given in Tab. 1.

4 Discussion

In this work, we compared Gaussian and bilateral filtering methods in projection and reconstruction domain. From Fig. 3b we can see that the projection-based Gaussian methods slightly exceed the GV 3D methods in terms of resolution, which can be due to the high-pass effect of the subsequent ramp filtering step. Nevertheless, BP-2D and BP-3D appear sharper than GP-2D and GP-3D. However, BP-3D reveals streak artifacts especially at sharp structures (Fig. 1 and Fig. 2), which might be caused by incorporating non-correct information of the neighboring projections. BP-2D is also affected by less dominant streak artifacts, whereas BV-3D showed good noise suppression while preserving sharp edges.

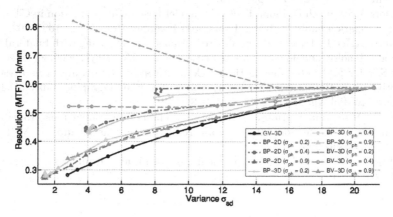

Fig. 4. Bilateral filtering with different σ_p on projections and reconstructions.

In the 50keV dataset all images reveal streaking artifacts caused by the high amount of noise. In case of BP-2D and BP-3D the smooth areas in homogeneous regions without streaks indicate that the photometric kernel was not wide enough to capture high-noise peaks in the projection domain. While all projection-based filters yield blurred edges, 3D filtering on the reconstructions preserves structure well but also shows slightly increased streaking compared to the GV-3D method.

Fig. 4 compares several variants of bilateral filtering with different photometric distances. Some methods achieve a greater MTF than the unfiltered image which seems incorrect. This can be explained as we use a measure that is only suited for linear methods on non-linear methods.

We have seen that bilateral filtering in the reconstruction domain gives promising results. Also projection-based filtering has shown its ability to preserve edges, however these methods should be applied carefully to avoid irregular streaking artifacts. For future work, we plan to combine 2D and 3D noise filtering in projection and reconstruction domain. Further, we plan to confirm our results by using a model-observer evaluation pipeline.

Acknowledgement. The authors gratefully acknowledge funding of the Research Training Group 1773 "Heterogeneous Image Systems" and the Erlangen Graduate School in Advanced Optical Technologies (SAOT) by the German Research Foundation (DFG).

References

1. Kachelrieß M, Watzke O, Kalender WA. Generalized multi-dimensional adaptive filtering for conventional and spiral single-slice, multi-slice, and cone-beam CT. Med Phys. 2001;28(4):475–90.
2. Zeng GL. Noise-weighted spatial domain FBP algorithm. Med Phys. 2014;41(5):051906.
3. Tomasi C, Manduchi R. Bilateral filtering for gray and color images. Proc IEEE Int Conf Comput Vis. 1998; p. 839–46.
4. Borsdorf A, Raupach R, Flohr T, et al. Wavelet based noise reduction in CT-images using correlation analysis. IEEE Trans Med Imaging. 2008;27(12):1685–703.
5. Manduca A, Yu L, Trzasko JD, et al. Projection space denoising with bilateral filtering and CT noise modeling for dose reduction in CT. Med Phys. 2009;36(11):4911–9.
6. Dirk Schäfer MG Peter van de Haar. Comparison of Gaussian and non-isotropic adaptive projection filtering for rotational 3D x-ray angiography. Fully 3D Image Reconstr Radiol Nucl Med. 2013; p. 130–3.
7. Maier A, Wigström L, Hofmann H, et al. Three-dimensional anisotropic adaptive filtering of projection data for noise reduction in cone beam CT. Med Phys. 2011;38(11):5896–909.
8. Feldkamp L, Davis L, Kress J. Practical cone-beam algorithm. J Opt Soc Am A. 1984;1(6):612–9.

The SIP-NVC-Wizard

User Guidance on Segmentation for Surgical Intervention Planning of Neurovascular Compression

D. Franz[1,2], L. Syré[1,3], D. Paulus[3], B. Bischoff[4],
T. Wittenberg[1,2], P. Hastreiter[2,4]

[1]Fraunhofer Institute for Integrated Circuits (IIS), Erlangen
[2]Computer Graphics Group, University of Erlangen-Nuremberg
[3]Active Vision Group, University of Koblenz and Landau
[4]Department of Neurosurgery, University Hospital Erlangen
daniela.franz@iis.fraunhofer.de

Abstract. Neurovascular compression syndromes (NVC) result from a compression of the entry/exit zone of cranial nerves by a vessel at the surface of the brainstem. Surgical intervention planning (SIP) for NVC enables a comprehensive spatial understanding of the patient specific anatomy. Specifically, brainstem, vessels and nerves are segmented in NVC SIP. To support segmentation for NVC SIP, we propose a wizard-based user guidance. The SIP-NVC-Wizard guides the user through the patient's individual anatomy and segmentations, and translates the parameter tuning into adequate medical terminology. We were able to show pathological nerve-vessel-contact in ten NVC cases producing results comparable to conventional NVC SIP, and performed a pilot-study to evaluate usability and functionality of the proposed wizard. With the SIP-NVC-Wizard our subjects were able to perform a NVC SIP without any knowledge in image processing. Anatomical beginners showed a steep learning curve. Time was reduced to 34 minutes compared to 1-2 hours for conventional NVC SIP.

1 Introduction

Neurovascular compression syndromes (NVC, such as trigeminal neuralgia and hemifacial spasm) result from a contact between a vessel and a cranial nerve at the nerve's entry/exit zone at the brainstem. A surgical treatment consists of a mobilisation of the blood vessel from the nerve and successive insertion of a small piece of Teflon between nerve and vessel. Preoperatively, a visualisation of the nerve-vessel-contact together with the brainstem yields a comprehensive spacial understanding of the complex anatomy in this area (Fig. 1, top). Hence, a segmentation of the anatomical structures of interest is obtained on a combination of strongly T2 weighted MR-CISS (Constructed interference in steady state) and an angiographic MR-TOF (time of flight) sequence [1, 2, 3]. The conventional approach, a semiautomatic segmentation of the structures, may take

1-2 hours for an experienced user and is a challenging task due to the complex and individual anatomy.

We propose the SIP-NVC-Wizard, a computer-assisted semiautomatic segmentation tool for NVC SIP. The SIP-NVC-Wizard uses the wizard interaction pattern [4] to guide the user through the segmentation of vessels, nerves, brainstem and surrounding CSF (cerebrospinal fluid, Fig. 1, top left). It uses the idea of divide-and-conquer to split a complex task into a series of steps, each one easy to solve. Our wizard guides users through the anatomy and translates technical image processing terms into problem-oriented medical terminology, thus closing the "semantic gap" between software and the medical expert. Tight user guidance and automatic segmentation proposals reduce the time needed for NVC SIP and enable also non-image processing experts to perform NVC SIP on their own with only the assistance of a software. The wizard considers the fact that NVC SIP is highly dependent on the anatomical expertise of the user and provides methods to edit every anatomical structure manually.

Different aspects of NVC SIP have been proposed in various publications [1, 2, 3]. An other approach that use the wizard interaction pattern for intervention planning is a wizard for the segmentation of the middle and inner ear [5]. AMIDE includes a wizard for filtering [6] and Ahmadi et al. proposed a wizard for neurosurgical planning including segmentation [7]. We use the wizard interaction pattern for guided NVC-SIP and propose new methods for the semiautomatic segmentation for the relevant structures.

2   Methods

Fig. 1 (bottom) depicts the page structure of the SIP-NVC-Wizard. After loading a MR-CISS dataset, the corresponding MR-TOF images are automatically loaded. A tutorial page shows the general interaction methods with the wizard, how to scroll through the slices, to zoom and to draw in the slices and how to set seed points. Additionally, each page provides a help window, that also describes general interaction methods and page specific tasks. The anatomical overview page asks the user to identify anatomical landmarks (CSF, brainstem, basilar artery, vertebral artery, trigeminal and facial nerves) by setting eight seed points. Afterwards, a volume of interest is computed from the points. On the next page we use a combined dataset of MR-TOF and MR-CISS to segment the CSF with volume growing and refine it with level-sets [8]. From the MR-TOF data vessels are segmented directly via thresholding. In the MRA-TOF only arteries are visible. Segmentation of the brainstem is given from the largest connected component of the inverse CSF segmentation. On the nerve candidates page, nerves are selected via seed points from a set of tubular structures under the CSF mask. Tubes are detected with a vesselness filter [9]. On the nerve/vessel refine page, the nerve segmentation and vessels from the MRI-CISS can be refined in the draw/erase mode on both masks. In the MRI-CISS small arteries and veins are visible. The draw/erase mode is available on all segmentation pages to refine the segmentation of every anatomical structure.

3 Materials

An NVC SIP expert segmented five cases of hemifacial spasm (nerve-vessel-contact on the facial nerve) and five cases of trigeminal neuralgia (nerve-vessel-contact on the trigeminal nerve) with the SIP-NVC-Wizard. Each case consists of an MR-CISS dataset (Fig. 1, top left) and a corresponding MR-TOF, each with $512 \times 512 \times 144$ voxels and a voxel size of $0.39 \times 0.39 \times 0.4mm^3$. We compared the results to conventional NVC SIP [1, 2, 3] and evaluated whether the SIP-NVC-Wizard lead to similar results showing the pathological nerve-vessel-contact. To assess the wizard's usability and functionality, we conducted a pilot-study with an expert in NVC SIP and two medical students. We observed the user and recorded their feedback. Additionally, all users answered a questionnaire assessing the usability of the wizard and how satisfied they were with the segmentations and the whole software. Possible answers had a range between 1 and 4, from "disagree" to "agree". Another part of the questionnaire refers to IsoMetrics^S for the evaluation of graphical user interfaces based on ISO 9241/10 [10]. Possible answers had a range between 1 and 5, from "disagree" to "so-so" and "agree". The pilot-study provides feedback and error-reports to improve the SIP-NVC-Wizard prior to a more comprehensive evaluation and comparison with conventional NVC SIP.

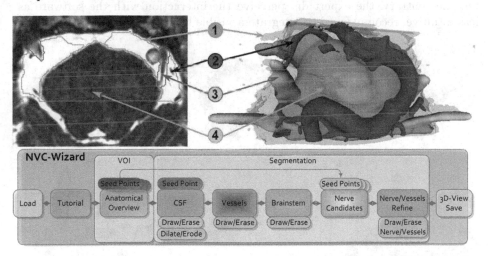

Fig. 1. Anatomical structures (top) and SIP-NCV-Wizard page structure. The anatomy is depicted in an axial slice of the MR-CISS data (left) and a 3D visualisation (right) for CSF (1), blood vessels (2), nerves (3) and brainstem (4). The image processing part of the page structure is divided into a part for setting a volume of interest (VOI) and a part for segmentation. Optional user interactions are marked in yellow, necessary user interactions are in marked red.

4   Results

We were able to visualize the pathological nerve-vessel-contact in all ten cases.
Fig. 2 demonstrates results from conventional NVC SIP and from the SIP-NVC-
Wizard. For a better evaluation, the results were both rendered with direct volume rendering (DVR) in the original planning framework (Fig. 2, left and middle
column). The right column of Fig. 2 presents results of in the SIP-NVC-Wizard
rendered with surface meshes. The NVC-SIP result show the pathological nerve-
vessel-contact (Fig. 2, pink) and are sufficiently similar to conventional results
(Fig. 2). On average, the subject took 34 minutes ($\sigma = 19$) for one SIP-NVC-
Wizard run.

Tab. 1 depicts the mean rating for criteria groups and user groups. Our observations and the feedback regarding functionality revealed a good suitability
for NVC SIP (expert) and a good learning curve with anatomy in that area
(students) that "often it is not the same as in textbooks" (quotation of a student). The expert could complete a NVC SIP with the tool and found automatic
segmentation suggestions reasonable. Regarding usability, we observed that the
students perceived the workflow as smooth and could apply the necessary user
interaction. They used the tutorial page and the help window but they would
have liked an additional labelling of the anatomic structures after segmentation.
On the contrary, the expert did perceive the interaction with the software as
less intuitive, recommended to integrate a visible brush in the draw/erase mode

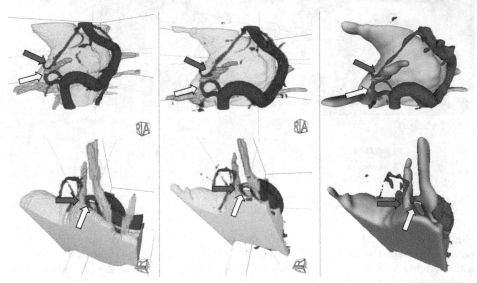

Fig. 2. Comparison of conventional and SIP-NVC-Wizard results with different 3D
visualization techniques: Original planning results rendered with DVR (left), SIP-
NVC-Wizard results rendered with DVR (middle), SIP-NVC-Wizard results rendered
with surface meshes (right). With the NVC-SIP-Wizard we were able to visualize two
nerve-vessel-contacts, one pathological (pink arrow) and one non-pathological (white
arrow), like visible in conventional NVC SIP. The visual results are sufficiently similar.

Table 1. Averaged results of the questionnaire consisting of a general part (top) and a part from IsoMetrics[S] (bottom). Note that the range is [1,4] for the top and [1,5] for the bottom.

Criterion	Expert user (n=1)	Medical students (n=2)
Usability	3 (weak agree)	3.4 (weak agree)
Satisfaction with segmentation	3 (weak agree)	3.5 (agree)
Satisfaction whole software	4 (agree)	3.8 (agree)
Suitability for the task	3.8 (weak agree)	4.7 (agree)
Self-descriptiveness	2.7 (so-so)	3.9 (weak agree)
Conformity with user expectations	3.9 (weak agree)	4.8 (agree)
Error tolerance	2.4 (weak disagree)	2.3 (weak disagree)
Suitability for learning	3.1 (so-so)	4.3 (weak agree)
Controllability	2.2 (weak disagree)	3.8 (weak agree)
Suitability for individualization	1.0 (disagree)	1.0 (disagree)

and would have liked to have a possibility to toggle linear interpolation in the volume data and the segmentation masks. All test users had difficulties with the small size of the text font and would have liked it larger. Also, we observed that the instructions on the top of the page were too detailed on some pages and not explicit enough on others.

5   Discussion

We were able to reveal the pathological nerve-vessel-contact in ten cases of NVC. The SIP-NVC-Wizard results are visually consistent with the results of a conventional NVC SIP as presented in [1, 3] (Fig. 2).

A small pilot-study showed that the SIP-NVC-Wizard is suitable for the task and consistent with user expectations, both for experts and medical students. They all could segment all structures of interest and were able to use the software intuitively. The average time of 34 minutes is distinctly smaller than 1-2 hours for conventional NVP SIP. The expert and the students gave high ratings on usability and they were satisfied with the segmentations and the whole software, though the expectations of the expert were influenced by the procedure of the conventional process. Suitability for learning got a high rating from the student users, reflecting that they could learn both software and anatomy within one run of the wizard. The medium rating of suitability from the expert did result from the fact, that he rather asked colleagues for help with the software, than using the tutorial page and help window. The parameter self-descriptiveness analyses, whether the user knows at any time what the software does. This is often achieved by clear software messages and a clear menu structure. While the students found the wizard self-descriptive, the expert gave a "so-so" rating. He would have liked shorter instructions. Suitability for individualisation and controllability was rated low, as expected for a software based on the wizard interaction pattern. The software is deliberately restricted and with tight user guidance rather than allowing for individualization. The feedback and observations showed that very few usability enhancements are necessary (brush size, font size, toggle linear interpolation) to enhance the usability. These features will be included in the next software version.

To sum up, we presented a wizard for guided neurovascular compression segmentation that leads non-image-processing experts through the complex task of NVC SIP. Automatic segmentation suggestions ease and speed up. Manual segmentation refinements are still necessary and useful due to the complex anatomy. With the SIP-NVC-Wizard both an expert in NVC SIP and non-expert medical student could perform a NVC SIP. We could reveal the relevant pathological nerve-vessel-contact in all ten cases of NVC SIP. In the future, there will be usability adaptations and a larger user study.

References

1. Hastreiter P, Naraghi R, Tomandl B, et al. 3D-visualization and registration for neurovascular compression syndrome analysis. Proc MICCAI. 2002; p. 396–403.
2. Hastreiter P, Naraghi R, Tomandl B, et al. Analysis and 3-dimensional visualization of neurovascular compression syndromes. Acad Radiol. 2003;10(12):1369–79.
3. Hastreiter P, Vega Higuera F, Tomandl B, et al. Advanced and standardized evaluation of neurovascular compression syndromes. Proc SPIE. 2004; p. 5367.
4. Tidwell J. Designing Interfaces. O'Reilly; 2007.
5. Franz D, Hofer M, Pfeifle M, et al. A wizard-based segmentation approach for cochlear implant planning. Proc BVM. 2014; p. 258–63.
6. Loening A, Sanjiv G. AMIDE: a free software tool for multimodality medical image analysis. Int J Mol Imag. 2003; p. 131–7.
7. Ahmadi SA, Pisana F, DeMomi E, et al. User friendly graphical user interface for workflow management during navigated robotic-assisted keyhole neurosurgery. Proc CARS. 2010.
8. Xu A, Wang L, Feng S, et al. Threshold-Based level set method of image segmentation. Proc Intell Netw Intell Syst. 2010; p. 703–6.
9. Sato Y, Nakajima S, Atsumi H, et al. 3D Multi-scale line filter for segmentation and visualization of curvilinear structures in medical images. Proc Joint Conf CV, VR, Robot Med Med Robot CAS. 1997; p. 213–22.
10. Gediga G, Hamborg K, Düntsch I. The IsoMetrics usability inventory: an operationalisation of ISO 9241-10. Behav Inf Technol. 1999;18:151–64.

Statistical Analysis of a Qualitative Evaluation on Feature Lines

Alexandra Baer, Kai Lawonn, Patrick Saalfeld, Bernhard Preim

Department for Simulation and Graphics, Otto-von-Guericke University Magdeburg
alexandra.baer@ovgu.de

Abstract. In this paper, we statistically analyze the results of a qualitative evaluation with 129 participants of the most commonly used feature line techniques on artificial and anatomical structures obtained from patient-specific data. For this analysis, we tested for significant differences to verify the results and the evaluation. We applied the Shapiro-Wilk test for normality, the Friedmann test to validate significant differences, and the Wilcoxon signed-rank test to compare paired samples. The results are used to give recommendations for which kind of surface which feature line technique is most appropriate.

1 Introduction

Illustrations in anatomical atlases are mostly depicted in a simplified representation to enhance essential anatomical structures. This means, only important information are illustrated to support the physician or the doctor-to-be to focus on a specific region. Traditional illustrations are hand-made which is therefore, not available on patient-specific data. Feature lines are a family of illustrative visualization techniques that can be applied on arbitrary surfaces and thus on patient-specific data. They are used to give a simplified representation of an object. For this simplification, the object is illustrated by using lines, which are placed at the most salient regions such that the object's shape can be perceived without additional shading. This abstraction of surfaces is important and has a high potential for depicting pathologies, anatomical and risk structures required for surgery planning [1] and for intraoperative visualizations [2]. Moreover, abstract illustrations of patient-specific data and therapy options support an individual patient documentation. To assess the quality of such feature lines, evaluations are important. Previous evaluations only compare a subset of the feature line methods.

This work is an extension of [3], where we qualitatively compared all different feature line techniques on three anatomical and three artificial surfaces. This first evaluation was about a ranking of the different feature line techniques according to aesthetic and realistic depiction. The participants should order the methods and rank them from place 1 to 6, with 1 being the most realistic or aesthetic technique. The rank of the feature line techniques is determined by using the Schulze method. This method is used to determine a final rank ordering, but no significance is tested. Therefore, a winner is determined, but it is not clear if this result is statistically relevant. The contribution of this paper is a statistical analysis of the feature line techniques for significant differences. For this analysis, we use different statistical tests and analyze the results on organic surfaces as they occur in biology and medicine. Afterwards, we give recommendations on what kind of surface is depicted well with which feature line technique. This guideline can be used to choose an appropriate feature line technique for an anatomical structure.

2   Materials and methods

2.1   Feature line techniques

Interrante et al. [4] introduced ridges and valley lines (RV) to illustrate salient regions. This method is curvature-based and therefore view-independent. Thus, DeCarlo et al. [5] presented a view-dependent approach: suggestive contours (SC). SC are an extension of the conventional contour definition, but fail in depicting convex structures. Therefore, Judd et al. [6] combined the advantages of RV and SC and presented apparent ridges (AR). This method uses a view-dependent curvature term and applies the RV definition to illustrate the shape. Xi et al. [7] introduced photic extremum lines (PLs). This technique determines the maximum of the variance of illumination. The user can add additional spotlights to influence the result. Kolomenkin et al. [8] presented demarcating curves (DC), a view-independent approach. This method is best suited to enhance furrows. Zhang et al. [9] introduced Laplacian lines (LL). LL extend the Laplacian-of-Gaussian for images to 3D surfaces to illustrate the shape.

2.2   Evaluation and quantitative analysis

The evaluation was conducted with 129 participants. 68 men with an average age of 30.53 years and 61 woman with an average of 30.92 years participated in this line drawing technique evaluation. The participants had a very broad spectrum of educational background. The tasks to assess the techniques' quality

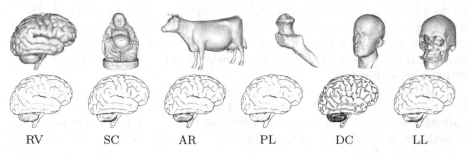

RV   SC   AR   PL   DC   LL

Fig. 1. In the first row, the different models for the evaluation are listed. In the second row, the different feature line techniques are illustrated with the brain model [3].

comprise an assessment of aesthetics, of realism and preference. For all tasks, the participants saw an original model, which was shaded using Gouraud shading. Furthermore, the feature line techniques were applied and the participants had to order them according to aesthetics and realism regarding the shaded model, see Fig. 1 for an overview of all models and techniques. The last task was about choosing a favorite technique. Six models were visualized with each of the six line drawing techniques. Three groups of 43 participants had to rate the six line drawing techniques. Each model was rated by 43 participants. The line drawing techniques are quantitatively analyzed for each model. Thus, we have 43 rank results for each model and technique. We analyzed the rating results of realism and of aesthetics in two steps; model-independent and model-dependent. Initially, the Shapiro-Wilk test was applied to analyze the normal distribution. Furthermore, we applied the Friedmann test and the non-parametric Wilcoxon signed-rank test for a pairwise comparison.

3   Results

Not normally distributed rank results were confirmed with a significant difference of $p \le .05$ for realism and of $p \le .01$ for aesthetics compared to a normal distribution. The non-parametric Friedmann test confirmed significant differences with $p \le .01$ for both assessment tasks. The Wilcoxon sign-rank test confirmed significant difference for the first analysis step (model-independent) for realism with $p \le .05$ between the techniques RV - SC, SC - LL, SC - PL and AR - LL and with $p \le .01$ between RV - AR, RV - LL, AR - PL and PL - LL. A significant difference for aesthetics with $p \le .01$ was confirmed for AR and DC pairwise compared with any other technique. In detail, the best and worst ranked technique are significantly different compared to the other techniques. All

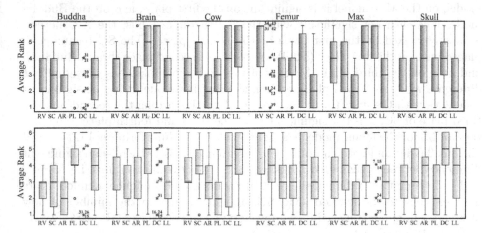

Fig. 2. The model-dependent results for realism in blue and for aesthetics in yellow visualized as boxplots. Detected outliers are displayed as an asterisk with the according sample number. Circles are potential outliers.

model-dependent results for realism and for aesthetics are illustrated in Fig. 2. The boxplots show the results for each task and model and the median result is included. The Wilcoxon sign-rank test pairwise compared the techniques for each model and task. The results are shown in Fig. 3. Each table contains the results for realism (upper blue triangular matrix) and for aesthetics (lower yellow triangular matrix) for one model. The Wilcoxon sing-rank test confirmed significant differences for realism with $p \leq .01$ between each technique pair for the Buddha and the Max model, illustrated in Fig. 3 in the upper triangular matrix with green check marks. Additionally, significant differences with $p \leq .01$ and $p \leq .05$ were confirmed for the other models and tasks, as shown in Fig. 3. A detailed result discussion follows in Sect. 4.

4   Discussion

We divide this section into the discussion of the realism and aesthetics results. Finally, we analyze the results of the preferred techniques. In the following, a statistically significant difference is in short significant or a significant difference.

4.1   Realism results

In most cases, starting from the resulting order of the feature line techniques, neighbored ranks are not significantly different. For example, regarding the result of the cow model the resulting order is: AR, PL, RV, DC, SC, LL. In this case, the statistical difference of the first place (AR) and the second place (PL) is not significant but AR compared to RV. Analyzing the first three ranks, AR, SC, and LL are dominant. In cases where AR is on the first rank (brain, Buddha, cow, Max), it is not significant with the second place only on the brain and cow model, on the Max model it is significant on the first place, and on the Buddha model it is even not significant with the fourth rank. Thus, the AR method is mostly ranked on the first place or the second place. The SC technique is placed once on the first place (skull), twice on the second place (brain, Buddha), and once on the third place (Max). On the skull model, SC has no significant difference with the second place, and on the Buddha model it has no significant difference with the first, third, and fourth place. Regarding the second and the third place of SC, it is not significant with the third and fourth place. The first rank of LL for the femur model is a significant result. Furthermore, LL is placed on rank 2 twice and once on rank 3. As mentioned, mostly there is no significant difference between neighbored ranks, but mostly between two ranks, i.e., rank 2 and 4. In summary, although the realism results are not uniquely defined, there is a tendency to the methods AR, SC, and LL. Counting the number of how often a technique was placed on a rank between 1-3, we have AR: 5, SC: 4, LL: 4, PL: 2, RV: 2, DC: 1.

4.2 Aesthetics results

The aesthetics results are similar to the realism results regarding the significance. Mostly, neighbored ranks are not statistically significant. The best result was obtained by AR. AR reaches twice the first place (Buddha, Max) with significant difference to the second rank; it reaches twice the second rank (cow, femur), whereas it has no significant difference even to the fourth rank. The LL technique reached twice the first place (brain, femur). On the brain model it has no significant difference compared to the second place, and on the femur model it has no significance even on the third place. The PL technique reached also twice the first place (cow, skull). On the cow model it is significantly better compared to the second place, and on the skull model it has no statistical significant difference to the third rank. The results for this task contain several detected outliers for the DC technique, as shown in Fig. 2 in the lower row. The Buddha, brain and Max results revealed up to seven outliers. According to the median and other DC results, we assume that the participants misunderstood rank 1 and thus ranked the technique vice versa. For this task, the techniques AR, PL, and LL were placed best. Counting the number of how often a technique was placed on a rank between 1-3, we have AR: 5, RV: 4, SC: 3, LL: 3, PL: 3, DC: 0.

4.3 Preferred techniques

The participants should also choose their favorite technique. Independent of the underlying model, we list how often which feature line technique was chosen: AR: 65, LL: 58, SC: 49, PL: 33, RV: 27, DC: 26. Here, we see a tendency to the preferred techniques AR, LL, and SC.

Buddha	RV	SC	AR	PL	DC	LL
RV		-.308	-.564	✓	✓	-.496
SC	.324		-.283	✓	✓	-.828
AR	✓	✓		✓	✓	-.496
PL	✓	✓	✓		✓	✓
DC	✓	✓	✓	✓		✓
LL	✓	✓	✓	✓	✓	

Brain	RV	SC	AR	PL	DC	LL
RV		-1.554	✓	✓	✓	-.686
SC	✓		-.471	✓	✓	-1.128
AR	.266	.192		✓	✓	✓
PL	✓	✓	✓		-.734	✓
DC	✓	✓	✓	✓		✓
LL	✓	.122	✓	✓	✓	

Cow	RV	SC	AR	PL	DC	LL
RV		✓	✓	.165	.070	✓
SC	✓		✓	✓	.388	✓
AR	.080	✓		.129	✓	✓
PL	✓	✓	✓		✓	✓
DC	.311	.264	.063	✓		✓
LL	✓	✓	✓	✓	✓	

Femur	RV	SC	AR	PL	DC	LL
RV		.083	✓	✓	✓	✓
SC	✓		✓	✓	✓	✓
AR	✓	✓		.430	.435	✓
PL	✓	✓	.350		.344	✓
DC	✓	.318	.060	.063		✓
LL	✓	✓	.372	.415	✓	

Max	RV	SC	AR	PL	DC	LL
RV		.200	✓	✓	✓	✓
SC	.099		✓	✓	✓	.075
AR	✓	✓		✓	✓	✓
PL	.134	.299	✓		.162	✓
DC	✓	✓	✓	✓		✓
LL	.325	✓	✓	✓	✓	

Skull	RV	SC	AR	PL	DC	LL
RV		✓	.096	✓	.155	✓
SC	.237		✓	✓	✓	.295
AR	.165	.378		✓	.422	✓
PL	.141	.061	✓		✓	.100
DC	✓	✓	✓	✓		✓
LL	✓	.059	.154	✓	✓	

Fig. 3. Each table contains the realism (upper blue triangular matrix) and the aesthetics (lower yellow triangular matrix) results of the Wilcoxon sign-rank for one model. A green check mark confirms a significant difference between the corresponding two techniques. If no significant difference was found, the *z-score* value is listed. If the *z-score* value is bigger than 1.96 (ignoring the minus sign), then the Wilcoxon sign-rank test confirms a significant difference with $p < .05$.

4.4 Summary

The statistical analysis showed that mostly neighbored ranks are not significantly different, but analyzing the techniques that differ from more than two ranks, the difference is mostly significant. Thus, the evaluation gives reliable results. Moreover, further evaluations can be conducted similarly, even if the results of the line techniques are visually hard to distinguish, the participants mostly agreed with the different tasks. We would strongly recommend to use one of the three different feature line techniques AR, LL, or SC for illustrating anatomical structures. In general, SC would be more appropriate as this technique uses second-order derivatives only. Compared to the other methods, which have third-order derivatives, SC is less susceptible to noisy surfaces. However, SC cannot depict convex regions and thus, surfaces with sharp edges. Sharp edges, however, rarely exist in anatomical structures. Nevertheless, in this case AR and LL are recommended. Here, the performance of AR is lower than the performance of LL. The LL method is not recommended for users without experience, as this technique needs user-defined values for calculating the Laplace operator on the surface. This can result in a trial-and-error loop where the user tests different parameters until a satisfying result is yielded. In overall, we recommend to use SC, as this is more robust against noise. For a detailed analysis of patient-specific data an extended evaluation is recommended.

References

1. Tietjen C, Isenberg T, Preim B. Combining silhouettes, surface, and volume rendering for surgery education and planning. Proc IEEE Eurograph Symp Vis. 2005; p. 303–10.
2. Ritter F, Hansen C, Dicken V, et al. Real-time illustration of vascular structures. IEEE Trans Vis Comput Graph. 2006; p. 877–84.
3. Lawonn K, Baer A, Saalfeld P, et al. Comparative evaluation of feature line techniques for shape depiction. Proc VMV. 2014; p. 31–8.
4. Interrante V, Fuchs H, Pizer S. Enhancing transparent skin surfaces with ridge and valley lines. Proc IEEE Vis. 1995; p. 52–9.
5. DeCarlo D, Finkelstein A, Rusinkiewicz S, et al. Suggestive contours for conveying shape. Proc SIGGRAPH. 2003; p. 848–55.
6. Judd T, Durand F, Adelson E. Apparent ridges for line drawing. Proc SIGGRAPH. 2007; p. 19–26.
7. Xie X, He Y, Tian F, et al. An effective illustrative visualization framework based on photic extremum lines (PELs). IEEE Trans Vis Comput Graph. 2007; p. 1328–35.
8. Kolomenkin M, Shimshoni I, Tal A. Demarcating curves for shape illustration. Proc SIGGRAPH. 2008; p. 157:1–7:9.
9. Zhang L, He Y, Xia J, et al. Real-time shape illustration ssing laplacian lines. IEEE Trans Vis Comput Graph. 2011; p. 993–1006.

Assessment of Electrode Displacement and Deformation with Respect to Pre-Operative Planning in Deep Brain Stimulation

Andreas Husch[1,2,3], Peter Gemmar[3], Jörg Lohscheller[3], Florian Bernard[1,2,3], Frank Hertel[1]

[1]Dept. of Neurosurgery, Centre Hospitalier de Luxembourg
[2]Luxembourg Centre for Systems Biomedicine (LCSB), University of Luxembourg
[3]Dept. of Computer Science, Trier University of Applied Sciences
husch.andreas@chl.lu

Abstract. The post-operative validation of deep brain stimulation electrode displacement and deformation is an important task towards improved DBS targeting. In this paper a method is proposed to align models of deep brain stimulation electrodes that are automatically extracted from post-operative CT imaging in a common coordinate system utilizing the planning data as reference. This enables the assessment of electrode displacement and deformation over the whole length of the trajectory with respect to the pre-operative planning. Accordingly, it enables the estimation of plan deviations in the surgical process as well as cross-patient statistics on electrode deformation, e.g. the bending induced by brain-shift.

1 Introduction

Deep brain stimulation (DBS) is an established therapy for movement disorders such as Parkinson's Disease (PD). It is based on the permanent implantation of electrodes in deep brain areas which are connected to a stimulation device.

The implantation of the electrodes is carried out using a stereotactic device that is fixed to the patient's head. The stereotactic device is co-registered with pre-operative medical imaging (in most centers a combination of MR and CT imaging), allowing the surgeon to plan the desired trajectory to the target on a surgical planning station. Subsequently, the computed image coordinates of the trajectory can be transferred to the mechanical system of the stereotactic device.

The accurate placement of an electrode is hampered by effects like limited mechanical accuracy of the stereotactic system, low contrast of the target structures in pre-operative MR images and the so-called brain-shift – the movement and deformation of the brain after trepanation of the skull due to loss of fluid and invasion of air. In order to compensate for those effects most centers use a stereotactic micro-drive device (MDD) to insert up to five test electrodes during surgery as detailed in Fig. 1. Intra-operative tests include micro electrode recording (MER) and test stimulations to identify the optimal placement location of the permanent stimulation electrode.

Numerous publications on DBS electrode placement discuss manual point-based approaches, i.e. considering points on the electrode trajectory in post-operative imaging and comparing them to points on the planned trajectory, often restricted to the target point as the only point evaluated [1, 2]. Lalys et al. [3] recently published an approach to automatically extract information about the implanted electrodes from post-operative CT imaging and to model them using a third-degree polynomial. Based on this, they determined a mean curvature index describing the overall bending behavior of an electrode.

The overall goal of the present paper is to enable the analysis of DBS planning vs. outcome deviations over the whole length of the electrodes, facilitating the detailed analysis of the surgical accuracy in a specific case as well as statistical evaluation of electrode behavior across multiple patients.

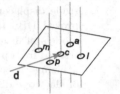

Fig. 1. Arrangement of the test electrode trajectories defined by a micro-drive device for intra-operative assessments. The electrode set is composed of a central (c), a lateral (l), a medial (m), an anterior (a) and a posterior (p) electrode. The target point (d) of the central electrode represents the original plan of the surgeon and the other four trajectories are arranged in 90° steps at a distance of 2 mm parallel to the central electrode.

2   Materials and methods

Our approach consists of three main stages – electrode segmentation, electrode modeling and electrode alignment – that are building up on each other. They are described in detail in the following subsections.

2.1   Stage 1 – Automated electrode segmentation

The electrode extraction pipeline depicted in Fig. 2 is based on the assumption that the electrodes are the only metal parts inside the brain after surgery. Therefore an initial thresholding for high intensity values (i.e. metal) is followed by the application of a convex hull brain mask to remove all metal voxels outside the brain. After these operations the m largest connected components (LCC) of voxels represent the m electrodes implanted. Finally, the LCCs are skeletonized, i.e. reduced to one point per axial slice and represented as a matrix $D = (p_1, p_2, ..., p_n)$ with $p_i \in \mathbb{R}^3$. The skeletonization is done by calculating the slice wise centroid of the LCC weighted by the image intensity values, as this has been shown to produce superior results with sub-voxel accuracy for the detection of rotational-symmetric bodies in CT [4].

The simplification to use only the convex hull of the brain instead of a detailed brain mask allows to rely solely on CT data. Therefore a post-operative thin-slice

CT volume constitutes the only input to the algorithm, which is an advantage of the proposed approach. The convex hull is sufficient for the intended usage to mask out metal (i.e. wires) outside the brain.

2.2 Stage 2 – Electrode modeling

To quantify the deviation of an implanted electrode to the pre-operative plan, the segmentation result needs to be expressed in a compact form allowing evaluations along the whole trajectory. This can be achieved by modeling the implant as a parameterized curve with restricted degrees of freedom, reflecting the fact that the possible bending of the electrode is limited by its physical properties and large oscillations between two skeleton points can be ruled out.

The goal is therefore to model the electrode in a parameterized way as a function $f : [0,1] \rightarrow \mathbb{R}^3$ with

$$f(t) = \big(f_x(t), f_y(t), f_z(t)\big)^T \quad \text{where } f_r(t) = \sum_{i=0}^{d} c_{r,i} t^i \quad \forall\, r \in \{x, y, z\} \qquad (1)$$

The parameter d for the maximum exponent of the polynomial term is defined consistently to the literature as $d = 3$ [3]. This was found to be a good trade-off between an accurate modeling of the electrode bending and the smoothness of the curve. The fitting of the model in Eq. (1) can be solved by standard linear regression as it is purely linear in the coefficients $c_{r,i}$.

To apply linear regression a mapping of a parameter t to its powers t^0, t^1, t^2, t^3 is needed. This is achieved by a mapping function $\Phi_3(\mathbf{t})$ that maps a vector $\mathbf{t} = (t_1, ..., t_n)$ to a matrix of its component wise powers from 0 to 3.

Given a matrix $D = (p_1, p_2, ..., p_n)$ of skeleton points $p_i \subset \mathbb{R}^3$ generated as described in 2.1 the desired linear regression model in its general form using a coefficient matrix $C \in \mathbb{R}^{3 \times 4}$ and applying $\Phi_3(\mathbf{t})$ is given as

$$C\Phi_3(\mathbf{t}) = D \qquad (2)$$

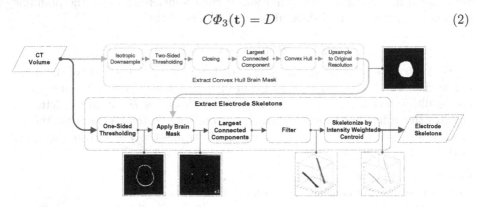

Fig. 2. Processing pipeline of the electrode segmentation including the helper pipeline to extract a convex hull brain mask.

The specific parameter vector $\mathbf{t} \in [0,1]^n$ is defined as

$$\mathbf{t} = (t_1, t_2, ..., t_n) \quad \text{with} \quad t_1 = 0, \; t_i = \frac{\sum_{j=1}^{i} \|p_j - p_{j+1}\|_2}{\sum_{j=1}^{n} \|p_j - p_{j+1}\|_2} \tag{3}$$

The vector $\mathbf{t}$ samples a path along the skeleton of the electrode from the tip to the distal part. The first point t_1 corresponds to the tip and is defined as $t_1 = 0$ and the points t_2, t_3, ... t_{n-1} reflect the distance to the tip measured in linear steps along the electrode skeleton normalized to the interval $[0,1]$.

Employing the shorthand $T = \Phi_3(\mathbf{t})$, one can write

$$CT = \begin{pmatrix} c_{x,0} & c_{x,1} & c_{x,2} & c_{x,3} \\ c_{y,0} & c_{y,1} & c_{y,2} & c_{y,3} \\ c_{z,0} & c_{z,1} & c_{z,2} & c_{z,3} \end{pmatrix} \begin{pmatrix} 1 & 1 & \cdots & 1 \\ t_1 & t_2 & \cdots & t_n \\ t_1^2 & t_2^2 & \cdots & t_n^2 \\ t_1^3 & t_2^3 & \cdots & t_n^3 \end{pmatrix} = D \tag{4}$$

for the desired third-degree polynomial model. This linear regression problem can be solved employing the normal equation, minimizing the squared error, i.e. $C = DT^T (TT^T)^{-1}$.

2.3   Stage 3 – Electrode alignment

To enable the assessment of electrode bending and plan vs. outcome deviations across patients an alignment of the electrode models is required.

Using the originally planned target point $\mathbf{d}_i$ of each electrode i to specify a common origin and defining a basis B_i that is uniquely determined by $\mathbf{d}_i$ and the fixed geometry of the surgical micro-drive device, a planning coordinate system is defined as detailed in Fig. 3.

The orthonormal vectors $\mathbf{b}_1, \mathbf{b}_2, \mathbf{b}_3$ define the basis matrix $B = (\mathbf{b}_1, \mathbf{b}_2, \mathbf{b}_3)$.

To align all electrodes i, represented by their polynomial coefficients C_i as determined in stage 2, a transformation of the coefficients C_i into the planning coordinate system is applied, resulting in the new coefficients

$$C_i^{\text{plan}} = B_i^T (C_i - (\mathbf{d}_i, \, \mathbf{0}, \, \mathbf{0}, \, \mathbf{0})) \tag{5}$$

By subtracting the destination vector $\mathbf{d}_i$ from the intercept term of the original coefficients C_i, a common origin is obtained which is followed by representing the resulting coordinates in the basis B_i by multiplying B_i^T from the left. By aligning the individual targets to a common origin and using the fact that the geometry of the micro-drive is the same for all electrodes this leads to an alignment of the electrodes in a common space.

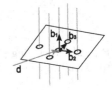

Fig. 3. Definition of the planning coordinate system. The arrangement of the five possible trajectories is fixed by the MDD. $\mathbf{b}_1$ is defined as the unit vector from the planned destination $\mathbf{d}$ to the entry point, $\mathbf{b}_2$ is the unit vector from the destination point in lateral direction of the MDD and $\mathbf{b}_3$ is the unit vector from the destination point in anterior direction of the MDD.

3   Results

All the previously introduced methods have been implemented in a MATLAB environment. The electrode segmentation and modeling was tested with 20 post-operative CT scans from two hospitals operating different types of CT scanners. The average fitting error of the skeleton points by the electrode modeling was found to be in a range of 0.125 mm with no outliers. This indicates that the third-degree curve is sufficient to accurately model the electrode bending.

Digitally readable planning data were available for six patients, five of them with bilateral electrode implantation and one with unilateral implantation leading to 11 electrodes. Fig. 4 shows the electrode models extracted from immediate post-operative CT aligned in the common planning coordinate space.

The deviations of planned electrode trajectories from the post-operative outcome are visible in the middle of Fig. 4, where traces of the electrodes in certain intervals along the planned trajectory are displayed. An increase of the variance with the distance from the planned destination can be observed. This seems consistent with the larger amount of brain-shift to be expected in upper brain areas. Calculating the mean deviation to plan error, i.e. the distance of the final electrode to the planned trajectory in millimeters along the trajectory, results in

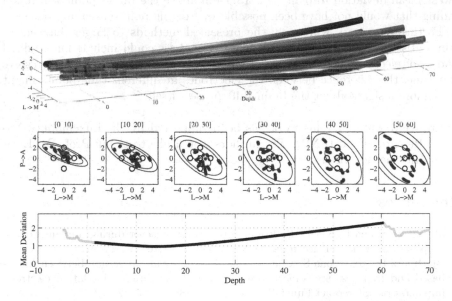

Fig. 4. Top: Electrodes aligned in the common space following stages 1 to 3. The trajectories are colored by the distance to the central plan. Middle: Block wise slicing orthogonal to the central plan. Each box shows the electrodes in lateral-medial / posterior-anterior plane in a 10 mm interval. Bottom: Mean plan deviation for the electrodes aimed at the central trajectory. The black part of the line indicates the range covered by all electrodes. Very deep areas as well as areas near to the skull are not supported by all electrodes due to different implantation depths and brain dimensions.

the curve depicted at the bottom of Fig. 4 for the electrodes aimed at the central trajectory. The error increases in upper brain areas. It is remarkable that the minimal mean plan deviation of 0.92 mm is reached about 13.5 mm above the planned destination and is slightly increasing again towards the tip.

4   Discussion

In this work, the automatic extraction of DBS electrodes from post-operative CT, their modeling utilizing linear regression to fit a parameterized polynomial curve and the transformation into a common coordinate system using the planning data and the geometry of the micro-drive device as a reference are proposed.

The novel approach of aligning electrode models into a common planning space creates a framework to analyze the behavior of DBS electrodes compared to the original planning and enables future statistical assessments of electrodes across multiple patients. This in turn allows measurements along the whole length of the electrode, i.e. the determination of deviation to plan errors for every point on the electrode instead of target point errors alone as discussed in the existing literature. The application to a relatively small dataset revealed the lowest mean deviation to plan error 13.5 mm above the target point which is a finding that would not have been possible by existing point-based approaches.

Forthcoming work will apply the presented methods to larger datasets to gain statistically reliable results. Advanced analysis could include longitudinal studies of electrode deformations. As it is known that brain-shift will resolve over time, the difference between the electrodes at different time points might allow more insights about the brain-shift process itself.

Acknowledgement. This work has been supported by the Luxembourg National Research Fund (FNR). The authors would like to thank Prof. Dr. Karl-Heinz Klösener for discussions.

References

1. Miyagi Y, Shima F, Sasaki T. Brain shift: an error factor during implantation of deep brain stimulation electrodes. J Neurosurg. 2007;107(5):989–97.
2. Bjartmarz H, Rehncrona S. Comparison of accuracy and precision between frame-based and frameless stereotactic navigation for deep brain stimulation electrode implantation. Stereotact Funct Neurosurg. 2007;85(5):235–42.
3. Lalys F, Haegelen C, D'albis T, et al. Analysis of electrode deformations in deep brain stimulation surgery. Int J Comput Assist Radiol Surg. 2014;9(1):107–17.
4. Grunert P, Mäurer J, Müller-Forell W. Accuracy of stereotactic coordinate transformation using a localisation frame and CT imaging. Neuros Rev. 1999;22(4):173–87.

Das 3D User Interface zSpace

Verwendung zur Exploration und Inspektion von Wirbeln der Halswirbelsäule

Patrick Saalfeld[1], Alexandra Baer[1], Kai Lawonn[1], Uta Preim[2], Bernhard Preim[1]

[1]OvG-Universität, Institut für Simulation und Graphik, Magdeburg, Germany
[2]Klinikum Magdeburg, Institut für Radiologie, Magdeburg, Germany
saalfeld@isg.cs.uni-magdeburg.de

Kurzfassung. Diese Arbeit untersucht die Verwendung eines stereoskopischen Monitors sowie die Stift-basierte Eingabe zur Exploration der Halswirbelsäule und Inspektion einzelner Wirbel. Die Exploration medizinischer Strukturen erleichtert das Verstehen und Erlernen anatomischer Zusammenhänge und kann somit Ärzte in der Ausbildung unterstützen. Die Stiftinteraktion basiert auf einer Metapher, welche durch eine Fokus- und Kontexttechnik unterstützt wird. Die Eignung des 3D-User Interfaces wird evaluiert sowie quantitativ und qualitativ ausgewertet.

1 Einleitung

Für das Erlernen anatomischer Zusammenhänge ist die interaktive Exploration von realistischen 3D-Modellen hilfreich [1, 2]. Diese Zusammenhänge können Eigenschaften wie die Größe einzelner Strukturen, Lokalität oder Relation zu anderen Objekten sein. Medizinstudierende und Ärzte müssen diese Eigenschaften und anatomische Zusammenhänge lernen und verstehen [1]. Eine Aufgabe von Chirurgen ist es, Bilder und Informationen der diagnostischen 2D-Bildgebung während einer Operation in die reale Welt auf den Patienten zu übertragen [3]. Hierbei liefern bspw. CT-Daten der Halswirbelsäule mit geringer Schichtdicke die Grundlage, um den Zustand des Patienten zu beurteilen [4].

Durch 3D-User Interfaces (3DUIs), also Benutzungsschnittstellen, die die *direkte* Interaktion im 3D-Raum durch Ein- und Ausgabegeräte ermöglichen, können 3D-Daten realitätsnah dargestellt werden. Dies ermöglicht die Exploration von anatomischen Zusammenhängen und erleichtert die Transferleistung, die der Chirurg beim Übertragen der 2D-Bilddaten in die Realität vollbringt. Bei der Exploration der Halswirbelsäule sollte ein 3DUI bestimmte Anforderungen erfüllen:

- Das *Ausgabegerät* sollte die Betrachtung von 3D-Objekten unterstützen. Die Wahrnehmung komplexer Strukturen, z. B. Wirbelkörper, profitiert dabei besonders von zusätzlichen Tiefenhinweisen, wie sie durch stereoskopische Displays kommuniziert werden.

– Das *Eingabegerät* sollte dem Nutzer erlauben, die 3D-Szene und einzelne 3D-Objekte flexibel und zielführend zu manipulieren. Hierzu bieten sich Eingabegeräte mit mehreren Freiheitsgraden an (Degress of Freedom, DOF). Da diese Freiheitsgrade zu einer komplizierteren Interaktion führen können, kann eine Metapher aus dem alltäglichen Leben helfen [1].
– Die *Art der Darstellung* sollte den Nutzer unterstützen, einen Gesamteindruck über die 3D-Szene zu erhalten und Strukturen von besonderer Relevanz zu erkennen. Fokus- und Kontexttechniken (F&K-Techniken) sowie illustrative Visualisierungsmethoden sind hierfür sinnvoll.

Diese Arbeit untersucht die genannten Anforderungen mit dem Ziel, Lösungen für die Exploration und Inspektion der Halswirbelsäule zu finden.

Das 3D-Puzzle von Ritter et al. [1] nutzt 3D-Visualisierungstechniken und eine Interaktionsmetapher um bspw. Medizinstudierende zu unterstützen. Auch in der vorliegenden Arbeit werden Visualisierungs- und Metapher-basierte Interaktionstechniken genutzt, um angehenden Medizinern zu ermöglichen, räumliche Strukturen und Zusammenhänge zu explorieren und zu verstehen. Ein aktueller Überblick über Anwendungen, die medizinisches Lernen in der Ausbildung und im Training unterstützen, ist in [5] zu finden. Das Potential des 3DUIs *zSpace* (www.zSpace.com) wurde für das Training einer Tympanoplastik von [6] beschrieben und wird daher in dieser Arbeit verwendet. F&K-Techniken können zusätzlich helfen, indem sie einen Überblick über die gesamten dargestellten Daten geben (Kontext) und gleichzeitig ermöglichen, Elemente im Detail zu betrachten (Fokus). Neben *räumlichen* F&K-Techniken wie Fish-Eye-Views [7], *dimensionale* Techniken wie magischen Linsen zur Betrachtung von Wirbeln [8], existieren auch Techniken, die visuelle Parameter von Objekten wie den Kontrast ändern. In dieser Arbeit wird eine solche *hinweisende* Technik verwendet.

2 Material und Methoden

In diesem Abschnitt wird ein Überblick über das verwendete Ein- und Ausgabegerät und die genutzte Interaktions- sowie F&K-Technik gegeben. Anschließend wird das Konzept der durchgeführten Evaluierung beschrieben.

Die 3D-Modelle der einzelnen Wirbel basieren auf einem CT-Datensatz mit 0,7 mm Schichtdicke im Knochen- und Weichteilkern. Aus diesem wurden die Wirbel C1 bis C7 segmentiert und in 3D-Oberflächenmodelle umgewandelt.

2.1 3DUI und F&K-Technik

Diese Arbeit verwendet das zSpace, welches einen 3D-Monitor mit Stift-basierter Interaktion durch einen 6DOF-Stylus kombiniert (Abb. 3(a)). Der hochauflösende Monitor ermöglicht die stereoskopische Betrachtung von 3D-Modellen durch eine polarisierte passive 3D-Brille. Zusätzlich wird die Position der Brille vom System getrackt (Kopf-Tracking), was die Erfassung der Position und Orientierung des Kopfes des Nutzers erlaubt (*Fishtank-VR*). Dies erlaubt dem Arzt die dargestellte Halswirbelsäule durch alleiniges Bewegen des Kopfes stereoskopisch von verschiedenen Seiten zu betrachten. Die Interaktion mit 3D-Daten ist neben herkömmlicher Mausinteraktion mit dem Stylus möglich, welcher räumlich getrackt wird. Die Ausrichtung des Stifts wird virtuell in die 3D-Szene verlängert und ermöglicht es so auf einzelne Wirbel der Halswirbelsäule zu zeigen. Diese werden, sobald markiert, rot gefärbt (Abb. 1). Zur Wirbelselektion wird ein Knopf am Stylus genutzt. Zur Inspektion einzelner Wirbel muss der Nutzer in der Lage sein, diesen zu verschieben und zu rotieren. Zur Realisierung wird folgende Metapher verwendet: Beim Drücken des Knopfes wird der Wirbel *aufgespießt*, ist somit am virtuell verlängertem Strahl befestigt und kann nun simultan verschoben und rotiert werden.

Beim Selektieren eines Wirbels wird die *Ghost Copy Technique* aus [9] verwendet. Hierbei wird der Wirbel nicht aus der Gesamtstruktur entfernt, sondern eine temporäre Kopie erstellt. Dies hat den Vorteil, dass der Kontext für den Nutzer geometrisch unverändert sichtbar bleibt, er aber dennoch den Wirbel als Kopie inspizieren kann. Als F&K-Technik wird eine hinweisende Methode umgesetzt, welche auf Tiefenschärfe basiert. Normalerweise werden vom Auge fokussierte Objekte scharf wahrgenommen – Objekte, die sich davor oder dahinter befinden, werden mit größerer Distanz zum Fokusobjekt unschärfer. Diesen Prozess kann man umkehren, um die Aufmerksamkeit des Nutzers zu lenken [10]: Lässt man die Kontextstruktur, hier die Halswirbelsäule, unschärfer erscheinen, so konzentriert sich der Nutzer automatisch auf das Fokusobjekt und kann dieses immer noch mental in den Kontext einordnen (Abb. 1). Die F&K-Technik wird angewendet, sobald der Nutzer einen Wirbel selektiert, wobei die Unschärfe der Halswirbelsäule so animiert wird, dass die Unschärfe stetig stärker wird. Nachdem der Nutzer den Wirbel inspiziert hat, kann dieser durch Drücken eines zweiten Knopfes am Stylus repositioniert werden (Abb. 2). Die zum Ende langsamer verlaufende Animation wird dabei so ausgeführt, dass sich das Objekt gleichmäßig zur ursprünglichen Stelle verschiebt und orientiert. Dabei wird der Unschärfe-Effekt der Kontextvisualisierung mit der Transformation des in-

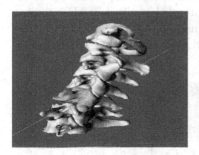
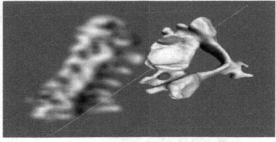

Abb. 1. Der Wirbel C5 wird mit dem Stylus markiert (links). Mit gedrücktem Knopf am Stylus kann der Wirbel inspiziert werden (rechts). Nach der Selektion wird der Kontext (Wirbelsäule) unscharf dargestellt, um die Fokusstruktur (Wirbel) hervorzuheben.

spizierten Objektes synchronisiert, sodass die Gesamtstruktur zeitgleich scharf dargestellt wird, sobald das Objekt seine Ausgangsposition erreicht hat.

2.2 Konzept der Evaluierung

Im Rahmen dieser Arbeit wurde eine strukturierte Befragung bezüglich der persönlichen Einschätzung der Visualisierung und Interaktion durchgeführt. Hierzu wurde ein Fragebogen erstellt, welcher in folgende fünf Bereiche unterteilt wurde: die *Stereovisualisierung*, das *Explorieren mittels Kopf-Tracking*, die *Stylus-Interaktion*, die *Fokus- und Kontextdarstellung* sowie die *Animation der Repositionierung*. Eine persönliche Bewertung jedes Bereiches wird mittels einer 5-Punkte Likert-Skala mit einer Einteilung von (−−, −, 0, +, ++) dokumentiert. Neben Fragen bezüglich der Explorationsunterstützung wird in jedem der fünf Bereiche die Benutzerfreundlichkeit erfragt. Die Ergebnisse werden quantitativ ausgewertet sowie mithilfe des Mittelwertes und Medians eine Tendenz der Probanden ermittelt. Weiterhin werden Äußerungen notiert sowie die Möglichkeit für individuelle schriftliche Kommentare gegeben.

3 Ergebnisse

3.1 Ablauf der Evaluierung

Allen Probanden wurde das 3D-Modell der Halswirbelsäule präsentiert. Zu Beginn erfolgte eine individuelle Exploration des Modells durch Mausinteraktion. Danach wurden die Probanden gebeten, das Modell nur durch Änderung der Kopfposition zu untersuchen. Anschließend wurden die Probanden aufgefordert mithilfe des Stylus einen Wirbelkörper zu selektieren, aus der Halswirbelsäule herauszuholen und die so gewählte Fokusstruktur separat zu inspizieren (Abb. 1). Abschließend wurde die animierte Repositionierung der Fokusstruktur in den Kontext durch die Probanden ausgelöst und betrachtet (Abb. 2). Jeder Proband erhielt einen Fragebogen, welcher *während* der Interaktion mit dem Modell ausgefüllt werden sollte. Dies ermöglichte den Probanden unmittelbar nach Ausführung der Aufgaben die Fragen zu beantworten und ggf. explizit ihre Einschätzung durch erneute Ausführung zu überprüfen.

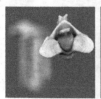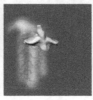

Abb. 2. Der inspizierte Wirbel wird nach Druck auf einen Stylus-Knopf mit einer Ease-out-Animation an seine ursprüngliche Stelle transformiert. Synchron dazu ändert sich die Darstellung der Kontextstruktur von unscharf zu scharf.

3.2   Auswertung der Evaluierung

Insgesamt haben neun Probanden an der Evaluierung teilgenommen. Davon waren sieben männlich und zwei weiblich im Alter von 26 bis 45 Jahren (Ø 32,3 Jahre). Während zwei Probanden keine Erfahrung mit Stiftinteraktion hatten, gaben alle Teilnehmer an, Erfahrung mit 3D-Visualisierungen und Stereovisualisierungen zu haben. Ein Proband hatte keine Erfahrungen mit medizinischen Daten; die anderen waren mit medizinischen Visualisierungen vertraut. Für die Analyse der Antworten wurde die Skalen-Einteilung mit numerischen Werten von -2 bis $+2$ gleichgesetzt, was einer üblichen Vorgehensweise in der Statistik zur Bestimmung eines Mittelwertes $\bar{x}$ entspricht. Die Stereovisualisierung wurde mit $\bar{x} = 1,44$ und einem Median von $md = 2$ bewertet, was „++" der Likert-Skala entspricht. Die Ergebnisse für das Kopf-Tracking erreichen einen Mittelwert von $\bar{x} = 1,22$ und $md = 1$, für die Animation $\bar{x} = 1,78$ und $md = 2$ und für die Unschärfe-Darstellung $\bar{x} = 1,22$ und $md = 1$. Zwei Probanden kommentierten, dass ihnen die Unschärfe der Kontextstruktur zu stark ist, wobei nur einer die Teilfrage aus dem Bereich Unschärfe, wie „angenehm die Unschärfe empfunden wird", mit „−" bewertete. Alle anderen Bewertungen entsprachen „+" (55,5%) oder „++" (33,3%). Der Stylus als Eingabegerät wurde von den Probanden mit $\bar{x} = 1,00$ und $md = 1$ bewertet. Die Beantwortung der Frage, ob eine Verschiebung mithilfe des Stylus erleichtert wird, wurde von 55,5% mit „++" und von 44,4% mit „+" bewertet. Die Rotation mit dem Stylus wurde hingegen nur einmal mit „++", dreimal mit „+", dreimal mit „0" und zweimal mit „−" bewertet. Differenzierter analysiert und auch durch Beobachtungen während der Studie bestätigt, empfinden die Probanden es leichter mithilfe des Stylus eine Struktur zu verschieben ($\bar{x} = 1,55$, $md = 2$) als diese zu rotieren ($\bar{x} = 0,33$, $md = 0$). Drei Probanden gaben an, dass ihnen die Rotation Schwierigkeiten bereitete, wobei einer anmerkte, dass ihm diese Interaktion durch Übung leichter fallen würde. Die Ergebnisse des Fragebogens sind in Abb. 3(b) zusammengefasst.

4   Diskussion

Die Evaluierung zeigt, dass die Bewertung der Probanden in allen Bereichen im Median zwischen „++" und „+" liegt. Dies ist ein Indikator dafür, dass sich das

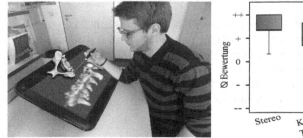
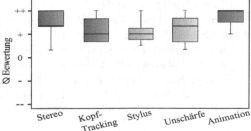

Abb. 3. Inspektion eines Wirbels mit dem zSpace (links). Die Ergebnisse der fünf abgefragten Bereiche sind als Boxplots dargestellt (rechts).

zSpace kombiniert mit der auf Unschärfe-basierenden F&K-Technik zur Exploration und Inspektion der Halswirbelsäule sowie einzelner Wirbel eignet. Auffallend ist, dass die Interaktion mit dem Stylus, im Speziellem die Rotation einzelner Wirbel, mit „+" bewertet wurde. Dies ist auf die geringe Erfahrung der Probanden mit dieser Interaktionstechnik zurückzuführen. Dies wird zum einen durch die Aussage eines Probanden bestätigt. Zum anderen konnte während der Nutzerstudie beobachtet werden, dass Probanden mit Stylus-Erfahrung weniger Interaktionsschritte benötigten, um einen Wirbel in die gewünschte Ausrichtung zu rotieren. Die vorliegende Arbeit hat ein 3DUI für das Betrachten, Verstehen und Erlernen anatomischer Zusammenhänge der Halswirbelsäule vorgestellt. Zukünftige Arbeiten können die Frage untersuchen, wie dem Nutzer verständlicher die Funktionsweise des Stylus kommuniziert werden kann. Weiterhin ist die Übertragung der beschriebenen Techniken auf andere medizinische Anwendungsgebiete wie die Exploration von Gefäßpathologien interessant.

Danksagung. Diese Arbeit wurde im Zusammenhang mit dem STIMULATE-Projekt durch das Bundesministerium für Bildung und Forschung BMBF (Förderkennzeichen 03FO16101A) gefördert. Weiterhin danken wir Dornheim Medical Images für die Bereitstellung des Dornheim Segmenters.

Literaturverzeichnis

1. Ritter F, Preim B, Deussen O, et al. Using a 3D puzzle as a metaphor for learning spatial relations. Proc Graph Interface. 2000; p. 171–8.
2. Höhne KH, Bomans M, Riemer M, et al. A volume-based anatomical atlas. IEEE Comput Graph Appl. 1992;12(4):73–8.
3. Kellermann K, Salah Z, Mönch J, et al. Improved spine surgery and intervention with virtual and interactive training cases and augmented reality visualization. Proc Digit Eng. 2011; p. 8–15.
4. Friedburg H. Bildgebende Verfahren und ihre Wertigkeit. In: Die obere Halswirbelsäule. Springer Berlin Heidelberg; 2005. p. 183–191.
5. Preim B, Botha CP. Visual Computing for Medicine: Theory, Algorithms, and Applications. Elsevier Science; 2013.
6. Baer A, Hübler A, Saalfeld P, et al. A comparative user study of a 2D and an autostereoscopic 3D display for a tympanoplastic surgery. Proc EG Vis Comput Bio Med. 2014; p. 181–90.
7. Furnas GW. Generalized Fisheye Views. Proc SIGCHI. 1986;17:16–23.
8. Bichlmeier C, Heining SM, et al MR. Virtually extended surgical drilling device: virtual mirror for navigated spine surgery. Proc MICCAI. 2007; p. 434–41.
9. Tan DS, Robertson GG, Czerwinski M. Exploring 3D navigation: combining speed-coupled flying with orbiting. Proc SIGCHI. 2001; p. 418–25.
10. Kosara R, Miksch S, Hauser H. Semantic Depth of Field. Proc IEEE Symp INFOVIS'01. 2001; p. 97–104.

Passive 3D Needle Tip Tracking in Freehand MR-Guided Interventions with Needle Model Visualization

Sebastian Schmitt[1], Christian Sobotta[1], Morwan Choli[2], Heinrich M. Overhoff[1]

[1]Medical Engineering Laboratory, Westfälische Hochschule, University of Applied Sciences, Gelsenkirchen, Germany
[2]MR:comp GmbH, Testing Services for MR Safety & Compatibility, Gelsenkirchen, Germany
sebastian.schmitt@w-hs.de

Abstract. In freehand MR-guided interventions, the monitoring of the current needle position relative to the target is crucial. In this work, a method for fast passive needle tip tracking in 3D is presented. For a true-FISP sequence, it is shown that proper k-space sub-sampling and signal processing allow for an accurate estimation of the needle tip position. A reduction in scan time is achieved by drastically reducing the number of measurements. The calculated needle tip positions are superimposed on a pre-interventional 3D planning volume in form of a needle model to ensure a continuous monitoring of the current needle tip position.

1 Introduction

Magnetic Resonance Imaging (MRI) offers an excellent soft tissue contrast without using ionizing radiation. In addition, it enables imaging of arbitrary oriented slices. Therefore, it is a well-established modality for minimally invasive diagnostic or therapeutic procedures (e.g. biopsies of suspicious lesions).

These interventional procedures can be performed (a) freehand [1] or (b) with robotic or manual needle-guidance templates [2]. In the latter cases (b) the required needle path is planned based on a pre-interventional planning volume. The needle is then pushed forward along the planned trajectory and a control scan is performed afterwards. Usually the needle position is not being controlled continuously during the procedure.

The success of freehand MR-guided needle interventions (a) depends on the determination of the needle tip position with respect to the target throughout the procedure. Thus, the visibility of the needle and the target in MR images is crucial [3]. Due to the large susceptibility artifact of the intervention needle, the biopsy of small suspicious lesions can be difficult, in the case that the signal void occludes the lesion. Therefore, it can be advantageous to automatically determine the current position of the intervention needle and superimpose a needle model on a pre-interventional 3D planning volume. The needle tracking can be performed actively (e.g. by using external measurement devices [4, 5]) or passively (image or raw data based [6, 7]). Since no external measurement devices are required, the advantages of passive needle tracking over active tracking are a drastically reduced measurement setup, and a more convenient procedure for the surgeon. Typically, passive needle tracking is performed by an image based detection of fiducial markers (paramagnetic particles) or segmentation of the needle in reconstructed images.

In [8] we developed a raw data based method for needle tip tracking in a series of 2D+t images. This method neither requires reconstruction of whole images (segmentation of the needle or marker identification) nor any modification of the intervention needle or the measurement setup (active or passive markers) and allows for a fast monitoring of the needle tip position throughout a freehand MR-guided intervention.

In this work we extend this method to the three-dimensional case. For a trueFISP (true fast imaging with steady state precession) sequence, it is shown that proper k-space sub-sampling and signal processing allow for an accurate estimation of the needle tip position in a small acquired volume. For the purpose of an appropriate visualization of the needle in the pre-interventional 3D planning volume, we developed a visualization program which among others allows for superimposition of needle models on 3D volumes.

2   Materials and methods

2.1   Materials

In 8 experiments an amagnetic biopsy needle (SOMATEX®, MR Chiba Needle 20 G, $d^{\text{needle}} = 0.95\,\text{mm}$, $l^{\text{needle}} = 150\,\text{mm}$) has been inserted into a measurement phantom filled with agar-agar and (i) a fixed melon, and (ii) a fixed piece of pork inside. For each experiment the different reference trajectories were determined by a needle holder's (NH) geometric parameters (Fig. 1).

The inclination angle $\varphi^{\text{NH}} \in \{0°, 15°, 20°, 30°\}$ and the azimuthal angle $\vartheta^{\text{NH}} \in \{0°, 90°\}$ have been varied for each experiment and the penetration depth of the needle has been increased step by step. After each step, k-space raw data have been acquired with a Siemens MAGNETOM Aera 1.5 T. In this way, a needle path $s(n)$ is imaged in a time discrete series of data volumes (3D+t) consisting of N_K parallel images $\mathbf{G}_k(n)$ with n the index of discrete time steps of data acquisition. The imaging sequence was a trueFISP sequence with a FOV of $210.0 \times 210.0 \times 25.2\,\text{mm}^3$ and a resolution of $N_I \times N_J \times N_K = 192 \times 192 \times 7$, where N_I and N_J denote the numbers of pixels per image row and column and N_K denotes the number of image slices.

2.2   Methods

The k-space (raw data) $\mathbf{K}$ represents the amplitudes and phases of the spatial wave numbers $\mathbf{k}$ of the image $\mathbf{G}$. The raw data and the image are linked via a 2D-Fourier Transform ($\mathbf{K} = \mathcal{F}\{\mathbf{G}\}$).

Localization of the needle tip in one image slice In [8] we assumed that the needle's susceptibility artifact in one image slice is stretched symmetrically to the needle axis, and that sectional views in those image slices which are orthogonal to the needle axis are contrast rich and resemble a rectangle-like grayscale value profile (Fig. 2).

It has been stated that the difference $\Delta s(n)$ of the needle feed between two time samples can be estimated from the difference image $\Delta \mathbf{G}_k(n)$ by approximating an enclosing rectangle of height $\Delta i(n)$ and width $\Delta j(n)$ located at image position $(i_0(n), j_0(n))$.

The approximation can be performed by analyzing only a fraction of the k-space data. This sub-sampled k-space consists of $N_{\text{traj}} = 5$ rows $\widetilde{\mathbf{k}}_x$ and columns $\widetilde{\mathbf{k}}_y$ of the k-space $\mathbf{K}_k$ and is denoted by $\widetilde{\mathbf{K}}_k$.

The acquired sub-k-space data $\widetilde{\mathbf{K}}_k(n)$ of the current time frame are subtracted from the data of the previous frame $(n-1)$ to get the difference data $\Delta \widetilde{\mathbf{k}}_x(n)$ and $\Delta \widetilde{\mathbf{k}}_y(n)$, respectively.

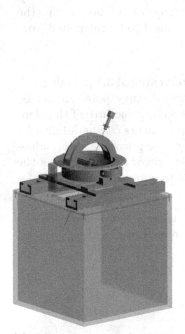
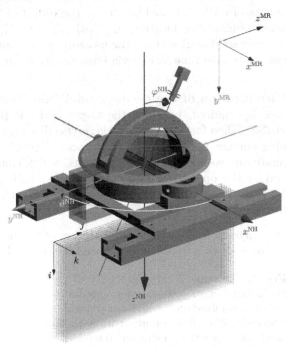

(a) Measurement phantom. The interior has been filled with agar-agar and different objects fixed inside.

(b) Needle holder. The inclination angle φ^{NH} and the azimuth angle ϑ^{NH} of the needle can be varied in the ranges $\varphi^{\text{NH}} = [-60°, 60°]$ and $\vartheta^{\text{NH}} = [0°, 360°]$. The aquired image slices are adumbrated with dotted lines. Image coordinate system i, j, k.

Fig. 1. Schematic depiction of the measurement phantom and the needle holder for $\varphi^{\text{NH}} = 30°$ and $\vartheta^{\text{NH}} = 90°$.

The parameters of the above mentioned enclosing rectangle of the needle feed in the difference image $\Delta \mathbf{G}(n)$ are determined by approximating the inverse Fourier Transforms of $\tilde{\mathbf{k}}_x(n)$ and $\tilde{\mathbf{k}}_y(n)$ by rectangle functions $\mathbf{r}(i_0, \Delta i)$ and $\mathbf{r}(j_0, \Delta j)$

$$\min_{i_0, \Delta i} \left\| \mathcal{F}^{-1}\left\{ \Delta \tilde{\mathbf{k}}_x(n) \right\} - \mathbf{r}\left(i_0, \Delta i\right) \right\|_1 \tag{1}$$

$$\min_{j_0, \Delta j} \left\| \mathcal{F}^{-1}\left\{ \Delta \tilde{\mathbf{k}}_y(n) \right\} - \mathbf{r}\left(j_0, \Delta j\right) \right\|_1 \tag{2}$$

Localization of the needle tip in parallel image slices For each image slice of index k which contains the needle artifact an enclosing rectangle can be approximated, such that all these rectangles shape a cuboid of height $\Delta i(n)$, width $\Delta j(n)$, and depth $\Delta k(n)$ centered at the position $(i_0(n), j_0(n), k_0(n))$ in the acquired volume.

The index of the slice containing the automatically determined needle tip is denoted by $k_{\mathrm{tip}}^{\mathrm{meas}}(n)$ and is equal to the center of the cuboid $(k_{\mathrm{tip}}^{\mathrm{meas}}(n) = k_0(n))$. To determine the location $(i_{\mathrm{tip}}^{\mathrm{meas}}(n), j_{\mathrm{tip}}^{\mathrm{meas}}(n), k_{\mathrm{tip}}^{\mathrm{meas}}(n))$ of the needle tip, the needle's solid angles inside the measurement volume need to be calculated from two successive time frames via trigonometric functions.

Visualization of the needle model One pre-interventional 3D planning volume is acquired, in which the target and the planned entry point should be visible. Therefore, it is desireable to visualize only crucial structures of the planning volume and to hide irrelevant ones. These requirements can be fulfilled by modifying so-called transfer functions, which change the grayscale/color values and/or the opacity of each voxel. Our visualization program, which uses the VTK library [9], provides three controlling elements to manually adjust transfer functions like

1. grayscale/color values as a function of the original grayscale/color values,
2. opacity as a function of the original grayscale/color values, and

Fig. 2. Example for the geometry of the needle artifact in sectional view (needle inserted into a fixed melon, inverted grayscale). The artifact is alligned symmetrically to the needle axis, contrast rich, and resembles a rectangle-like grayscale value profile.

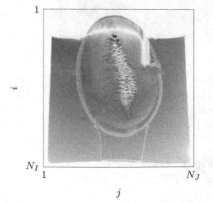

3. opacity as a function of the original grayscale/color values' gradients,

to achieve an optimal visualization result.

The needle tracking method presented here, yields the indices $(i_{\text{tip}}^{\text{meas}}(n)$, $j_{\text{tip}}^{\text{meas}}(n)$, $k_{\text{tip}}^{\text{meas}}(n))$ of the needle tip. Via the DICOM header information of the acquired image slices, the 3D coordinates $(x_{\text{tip}}^{\text{meas}}(n), y_{\text{tip}}^{\text{meas}}(n), z_{\text{tip}}^{\text{meas}}(n))$ of the needle tip at the current time frame n can be calculated. These coordinates can be used to superimpose a needle model on the pre-interventional planning volume.

3   Results

3.1   Needle tip tracking in 3D

The difference between the automatically determined positions of the needle tip $(x_{\text{tip}}^{\text{meas}}(n), y_{\text{tip}}^{\text{meas}}(n), z_{\text{tip}}^{\text{meas}}(n))$ and the reference points $(x_{\text{tip}}^{\text{ref}}(n), y_{\text{tip}}^{\text{ref}}(n), z_{\text{tip}}^{\text{ref}}(n))$ have been compared for the different datasets ((i) needle inserted into a fixed melon, (ii) needle inserted into a fixed piece of pork).

For (i) the needle tip could be determined with an error of $e_{xyz}^{\text{MR}} = 0.66 \pm 1.44$ mm, for (ii) the error was $e_{xyz}^{\text{MR}} = 0.93 \pm 1.21$ mm. The errors were roughly the same for different inclination and azimuth angles φ^{NH} and ϑ^{NH} of the needle.

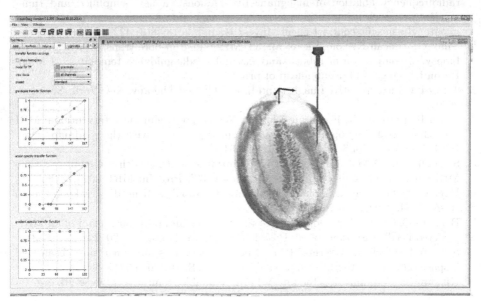

Fig. 3. Superimposition of the needle model on the 3D planning volume. The position of the needle tip and the orientation of the needle axis have been calculated automatically.

3.2 Visualization of the needle model

The needle's diameter $d^{needle} = 0.95\,\text{mm}$ and length $l^{needle} = 150\,\text{mm}$ are known previously. Therefore, it is possible to superimpose a predefined needle model on the pre-interventional planning volume, in order to monitor the current needle position (Fig. 3). The positioning of the needle model is based on the results of the needle tip tracking.

4 Discussion

The choice of a reduced sampling scheme determines the duration of image data acquisition. Therefore, with the presented method a fast passive tracking of the needle tip position is possible, which does not require the choice of specially designed instruments with an increased visibility in MR images [3]. The method is applicable under nearly real conditions, i.e. a reduced motion of the ROI. In a next step the method shall be validated for clinical data.

References

1. Fischbach F, Lohfink K, Gaffke G, et al. Magnetic resonance-guided freehand radiofrequency ablation of malignant liver lesions: a new simplified and time-efficient approach using an interactive open magnetic resonance scan platform and hepatocyte-specific contrast agent. Invest Radiol. 2013;48(6):422–8.
2. Tilak G, Tuncali K, Song SE, et al. 3T MR-guided in-bore transperineal prostate biopsy: a comparison of robotic and manual needle-guidance templates. J Magn Reson Imaging. 2014;[Epub ahead of print].
3. Jolesz FA. Intraoperative Imaging and Image-Guided Therapy. New York: Springer; 2014.
4. Viard R, Betrouni N, Rousseau J, et al. Needle positioning in interventional MRI procedure: real time optical localisation and accordance with the roadmap. Proc IEEE Eng Med Biol Soc. 2007;2007:2748–51.
5. Schaudinn A, Otto J, Linder N, et al. Clinical experience with a virtual real-time MRI navigation option for prostate biopsies at 3T. Proc Int MRI. 2014;10:29.
6. Kochavi E, Goldsher D, Azhari H. Method for rapid MRI needle tracking. Magn Reson Med. 2004;51(5):1083–7.
7. Bergeles C, Qin L, Vartholomeos P, et al. Tracking and position control of an MRI-powered needle-insertion robot. Proc IEEE Eng Med Biol Soc. 2012;2012:928–31.
8. Schmitt S, Choli M, Overhoff HM. Needle position estimation from subsampled k-space data for MRI-guided interventions. Proc SPIE. 2015;9415.
9. Kitware Inc. Visualization toolkit (VTK). Available from: http://www.vtk.org.

Evaluation verschiedener Ansätze zur 4D-4D-Registrierung kardiologischer MR-Bilddaten

Timo Kepp, Jan Ehrhardt, Heinz Handels

Institut für Medizinische Informatik, Universität zu Lübeck
timo.kepp@googlemail.com

Kurzfassung. 4D-MR-Bilddaten des Herzens ermöglichen die Bestimmung diagnostisch relevanter Funktionsparameter. Grundlage für die Berechnung kardiologischer Funktionsparameter sind Segmentierungen des linken bzw. rechten Ventrikels. Die atlasbasierte Segmentierung bietet ein automatisiertes Verfahren, dessen Grundlage nicht-lineare Registrierungsverfahren sind. Dieser Beitrag beschäftigt sich mit der räumlich-zeitlichen Registrierung von zwei 4D-Bildsequenzen, auch 4D-4D-Registrierung genannt, durch eine Multichannel-3D-Registrierung mit Trajektorienbeschränkung. Die Trajektorienbeschränkung bildet korrespondierende Bildpunkte innerhalb einer Sequenz über die Zeit ab und ermöglicht das gleichzeitige Registrieren aller Zeitpunkte zweier 4D-Bildsequenzen durch einen Multichannel-3D-Ansatz. In dieser Arbeit wurde die Multichannel-3D-Registrierung mit weiteren Registrierungsverfahren verglichen und anhand von kardiologischen Cine-MR-Bildsequenzen evaluiert. Es zeigte sich, dass die direkte 3D-Registrierung leicht bessere Ergebnisse erzielte als die Multichannel-3D-Registrierung. Darüber hinaus konnte eine erhöhte Robustheit und Konsistenz durch die Anwendung der Trajektorienbeschränkung festgestellt werden.

1 Einleitung

Kardiovaskuläre Erkrankungen gehören heutzutage zu den häufigsten Todesursachen in der westlichen Welt. Die Bestimmung relevanter Parameter wie das end-systolische und end-diastolische Volumen (ESV/EDV) spielt in der Funktionsdiagnostik des Herzens eine wichtige Rolle. Die Grundlage für die Bestimmung dieser Parameter stellen dabei Segmentierungen des linken bzw. rechten Ventrikels (LV/RV) in 4D-Bilddaten dar. Die manuelle Segmentierung von 4D-Bildsequenzen stellt eine sehr zeitaufwendige Aufgabe dar, sodass in den vergangenen Jahren verschiedene (semi-)automatische Verfahren für die Segmentierung von 4D-Bilddaten vorgestellt wurden. Da die Zeitdimension nicht als zusätzliche räumliche Dimension angesehen werden darf, ist die Erweiterung von (bestehenden) 3D-Bildverarbeitungswerkzeugen jedoch nicht trivial.

Die atlasbasierte Segmentierung ist ein automatisches Verfahren, welches die Einbringung von a priori Wissen in den Segmentierungsprozess ermöglicht. Die wesentliche Grundlage hierbei ist eine nicht-lineare Registrierung zwischen einem Atlas- und einem Patientendatensatz. Für die atlasbasierte Segmentierung von 4D-Bildsequenzen werden geeignete 4D-Registrierungsverfahren benötigt. In [1, 2, 3, 4, 5] wurden bereits Ansätze für die Angleichung und Registrierung von 4D-Bilddaten vorgeschlagen. In dieser Arbeit wird der Ansatz von Peyrat et al. verwendet, die für die 4D-4D-Registrierung eine Multichannel-3D-Registrierung mit Trajektorienbeschränkung vorgeschlagen haben [6]. Der Ansatz wurde mit zwei weiteren Registrierungsverfahren verglichen und im Gegensatz zu Peyrat et al. anhand von kardiologischen Cine-MR-Bildsequenzen evaluiert.

2   Material und Methoden

2.1   Räumlich-zeitliche Registrierung von 4D-Bilddaten

Tomographische 4D-Bilddaten $I(\boldsymbol{x}, t)$ bestehen meistens aus einer Reihe von N einzelnen 3D-Bildern $I_j(\boldsymbol{x}) = I(\boldsymbol{x}, t_j)$, die zusammen eine Bildsequenz mit $\Omega \times \tau \subset \mathbb{R}^3 \times \mathbb{R}$ darstellen. Hierbei beschreibt Ω die Bilddomäne und τ das Aufnahmeintervall mit $t_j < t_{j+1} \in \tau$. Bei der räumlich-zeitlichen Registrierung wird eine Transformation Ψ zwischen einer Referenzsequenz R und einer Targetsequenz T gesucht, die einen Bildpunkt $(\boldsymbol{x}, t)$ auf den Bildpunkt $(\boldsymbol{x}', t')$ abbildet

$$
\begin{aligned}
\Psi : \Omega_R \times \tau_R &\to \Omega_T \times \tau_T \\
\Psi(\boldsymbol{x}, t) &= (\psi_{\text{space}}(\boldsymbol{x}, t), \psi_{\text{time}}(t))
\end{aligned}
\tag{1}
$$

Die Transformation Ψ lässt sich in eine rein zeitliche Transformation ψ_{time} und eine rein räumliche Transformation ψ_{space} auftrennen, die unabhängig voneinander betrachtet werden können [6]. Dabei garantiert ψ_{time}, dass dieselben physiologischen Ereignisse, wie bspw. die Phasen des Herzzyklus, aufeinander abgebildet werden, wohingegen ψ_{space} den Punkt $\boldsymbol{x}$ zum Zeitpunkt t auf den korrespondierenden Punkt $\boldsymbol{x}'$ abbildet. Unter der Annahme, dass physiologische Ereignisse nicht ortsabhängig sind, ist ψ_{time} lediglich von t abhängig. Für die Bestimmung von ψ_{time} werden globale physiologische Parameter wie EKG oder Blutvolumenverläufe der Ventrikel verwendet. Ist ψ_{time} bekannt, werden R und T zeitlich angepasst, so dass $R_j(\boldsymbol{x})$ und $T_j(\boldsymbol{x})$ physiologisch korrespondieren. In einer diskreten Betrachtung (Abb. 1) beschreibt ψ_j durch die Entkopplung von ψ_{space} und ψ_{time} nur noch die räumliche Transformation zum Zeitpunkt t_j zwischen Referenz- und Targetsequenz, sodass $\psi_j = \psi_{j_{\text{space}}}$ gilt. Gesucht werden nun N räumliche Transformationen ψ_j. Auf der einen Seite ist es möglich jeden Zeitpunkt getrennt voneinander zu berechnen, indem eine 3D-Registrierung zwischen R_j und T_j durchführt. Hierbei wird jedoch die zeitliche Korrespondenz nicht beachtet. Auf der anderen Seite kann die Registrierung durch Trajektorien eingeschränkt werden, sodass ein gleichzeitiges Registrieren aller Zeitpunkte möglich ist, was fortführend vorgestellt wird.

2.2 Beschränkung der Registrierung durch Trajektorien

Seien $\varphi_{R_{j,k}} : \Omega_R \to \Omega_R$ und $\varphi_{T_{j,k}} : \Omega_T \to \Omega_T$ die Bewegungstransformationen zwischen den Zeitpunkten t_j und t_k innerhalb der Bildsequenz R bzw. T, d.h. $y = \varphi_{R_{j,k}}(x)$ beschreibt die Position des Punktes (x, t_j) zum Zeitpunkt t_k. Für korrespondierende Punkte $x \in R_j$ und $x' \in T_k$ ergibt sich $x' = \varphi_{T_{j,k}} \circ \psi_j(x)$ bzw. $x' = \psi_k \circ \varphi_{R_{j,k}}(x)$ (Abb. 1). Die aus dieser Beziehung entstehenden Beschränkungen werden als Trajektorienbeschränkungen (TB) bezeichnet

$$\psi_k \circ \varphi_{R_{j,k}} = \varphi_{T_{j,k}} \circ \psi_j \Leftrightarrow \psi_k = \varphi_{T_{j,k}} \circ \psi_j \circ \varphi_{R_{j,k}}^{-1} \qquad (2)$$

und koppeln ψ_j mit ψ_k und $\varphi_{R_{j,k}}$ bzw. $\varphi_{T_{j,k}}$ [6]. Sind die Bewegungstransformationen bekannt, so kann ψ_k für alle übrigen Zeitpunkte durch Gl. (2) aus einem berechneten ψ_j zum Zeitpunkt t_j rekonstruiert werden.

2.3 Multichannel-3D-Registrierung

Durch das Integrieren der Trajektorienbeschränkungen entsteht eine Kopplung zwischen allen ψ_j, sodass diese nicht mehr unabhängig von einander betrachtet werden können. Es soll nun das SSD-Distanzmaß (sum of squared differences)

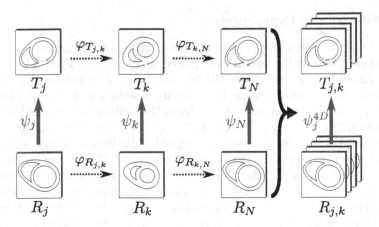

Abb. 1. Links: Zeitliche Diskretisierung der 4D-Registrierung. ψ_j beschreibt die Intersequenztransformation zum Zeitpunkt t_j und $\varphi_{R_{j,k}}$ bzw. $\varphi_{T_{j,k}}$ beschreiben die Intrasequenztransformation (Bewegungstransformationen) zwischen den Zeitpunkten t_j und t_k. Rechts: Mithilfe der Trajektorienbeschränkungen kann die 4D-Registrierung durch eine einzelne Transformation ψ_j^{4D} formuliert werden und dadurch als Multichannel-3D-Registrierung parametrisiert werden. Hierzu werden alle Zeitpunkte R_k und T_k jeweils auf den Referenzzeitpunkt registriert und transformiert ($R_{j,k}$ und $T_{j,k}$). Alle übrigen ψ_j^{4D} können anschließend über die Trajektorienbeschränkungen rekonstruiert werden.

für alle Zeitpunkte der Bildsequenzen minimiert werden. Mit Gl. (2) ergibt sich

$$
\mathcal{D}^{4D}[R_j, T_j; \psi_j^{4D}] := \int_{\Omega_j} (T_j \circ \psi_j^{4D}(\boldsymbol{x}) - R_j(\boldsymbol{x}))^2 \, d\boldsymbol{x} +
$$

$$
\sum_{k \neq j}^{N} \int_{\hat{\Omega}_k} (T_k \circ \varphi_{T_{j,k}} \circ \psi_j^{4D} \circ \varphi_{R_{j,k}}^{-1}(\boldsymbol{x}) - R_k(\boldsymbol{x}))^2 \, d\boldsymbol{x} \tag{3}
$$

Wird zusätzlich $\hat{\Omega}_k = \Omega_j = \Omega$ angenommen, vereinfacht sich (3) zu

$$
\mathcal{D}^{4D}[R_{j,k}, T_{j,k}; \psi_j^{4D}] := \frac{1}{2} \left(\int_{\Omega} \sum_{k=1}^{N} \alpha_k (T_{j,k} \circ \psi_j^{4D}(\boldsymbol{x}) - R_{j,k}(\boldsymbol{x}))^2 \right) d\boldsymbol{x} \tag{4}
$$

mit $R_{j,k} = R_k \circ \varphi_{R_{j,k}}$ und $T_{j,k} = T_k \circ \varphi_{T_{j,k}}$. Hierdurch kann die 4D-Registrierung als gleichzeitiges Abbilden mehrerer Bildpaare verstanden werden (Abb. 1), was einer Multichannel-3D-Registrierung entspricht. $\alpha_k < 0$ beschreibt den Einbezug der Volumenänderung durch die Bewegungstransformation, was einer voxelweisen Gewichtung mit $|\operatorname{Jac}(\varphi_{R_{j,k}})(\boldsymbol{x})|$ entspricht. Für den Fall $k = j$ gilt zusätzlich $R_{j,j} = R_j$ bzw. $T_{j,j} = T_j$ und $\alpha_j = 1$.

2.4 Material und Experimente

Für die Evaluation wurden 10 (von insgesamt 33) kardiologische 4D-Cine-MR-Bildsequenzen von Andreopoulus et al.(2008) verwendet [7]. Die Bilddaten wurden mit einem GE Genesis Signa MR-Scanner unter Verwendung der FIESTA-Pulssequenz aufgenommen. Jede Bildsequenz besteht aus 20 Zeitpunkten, die einen kompletten Herzzyklus abdecken. Jedes 3D-Teilbild besteht aus $256 \times 256 \times 8 - 15$ Voxeln. Das Spacing beträgt $0.93 - 1.64\,\text{mm}$ innerhalb und $6 - 13\,\text{mm}$ zwischen den Bildschichten. Zusätzlich liegen für die Bildsequenzen manuell generierte Segmentierungen vom Endo- und Epikard des LV vor. Ferner wurde der Blutpool des RV für diese Arbeit nachträglich manuell segmentiert. In einem ersten Schritt wurde eine Angleichung der Bildsequenzen durch eine zeitliche Registrierung erreicht, die anhand von Blutvolumenkurven des LV durchgeführt wurde. Des Weiteren wurden mehrere Vorverarbeitungsschritte durchlaufen, um die Bilddaten für die Evaluation vorzubereiten. Durch eine Bias-Korrektur konnten lokale Intensitätsinhomogenitäten korrigiert werden. Die relativ großen Schichtabstände wurden über ein registrierungsbasiertes Interpolationsverfahren verringert, um nahezu isotrope Voxel zu erhalten [8]. Darüber hinaus wurde Rauschen über eine anisotrope Glättung minimiert. Schließlich wurden die Grauwertprofile der Bildsequenzen über eine Histogrammangleichung angepasst [5]. Folgende Registrierungsverfahren wurden miteinander verglichen:

- *Direkte variationelle 3D-Registrierung (3D-direkt):* Bei diesem Verfahren wird zu jedem Zeitpunkt t_k die Transformation ψ_k direkt zwischen Referenz- und Targetsequenz bestimmt. Das bedeutet, dass alle ψ_k unabhängig voneinander berechnet werden.

Tabelle 1. Ergebnisse der 4D-Registrierung. Die Dice-Koeffizienten sowie symmetrischen Oberflächendistanzen $d_{\mu_{\text{sym}}}$ wurden jeweils zwischen den verformten Segmentierungen der Targetsequenz und der Referenzsequenz bestimmt. Die Werte wurden über alle Zeitpunkte und allen Patienten gemittelt.

	3D-direkt		3D-MC+TB		3D+TB	
	Dice	$d_{\mu_{\text{sym}}}$	Dice	$d_{\mu_{\text{sym}}}$	Dice	$d_{\mu_{\text{sym}}}$
Endokard	0.82	$1.99 \pm 1.20\,\text{mm}$	0.82	$1.92 \pm 0.89\,\text{mm}$	0.82	$2.04 \pm 1.19\,\text{mm}$
Epikard	0.86	$2.38 \pm 1.21\,\text{mm}$	0.86	$2.41 \pm 1.10\,\text{mm}$	0.86	$2.47 \pm 1.19\,\text{mm}$
RV	0.78	$2.53 \pm 1.25\,\text{mm}$	0.77	$2.75 \pm 1.26\,\text{mm}$	0.77	$2.81 \pm 1.35\,\text{mm}$
Mittelwert	0.82	$2.30 \pm 1.24\,\text{mm}$	0.82	$2.36 \pm 1.14\,\text{mm}$	0.82	$2.44 \pm 1.29\,\text{mm}$

– *Variationelle 3D-Registrierung mit TB (3D+TB):* Im Vergleich zu 3D-direkt wird die Intersequenztransformation zum Referenzzeitpunkt $(j = 5)$ unabhängig berechnet. Alle anderen Intersequenztransformationen werden durch $\psi_k = \varphi_{T_{j,k}} \circ \psi_j \circ \varphi_{R_{j,k}}^{-1}$ rekonstruiert, um die Trajektorienbeschränkungen zu erfüllen.
– *Multichannel-3D-Registrierung mit TB (3D-MC+TB):* Die Intersequenztransformation werden durch die Multichannel-3D-Registrierung zum Referenzzeitpunkt $(j = 5)$ berechnet. Alle übrigen Intersequenztransformationen werden wie bei 3D+TB durch $\psi_k = \varphi_{T_{j,k}} \circ \psi_j \circ \varphi_{R_{j,k}}^{-1}$ bestimmt.

Für die Berechnung der Transformationen wurden für 3D-direkt, 3D+TB und 3D-MC+TB dieselben Parametereinstellungen verwendet. Bei allen drei Verfahren wird ein Multi-Level-Verfahren mit drei Leveln verwendet, wobei die gewählte Anzahl der Iterationen 500 für das höchste, 300 für das mittlere und 150 für das niedrigste Level beträgt. Weiterhin wurde eine diffusive Regularisierung mit einem Gewichtungsfaktor $\beta = 1.5$ gewählt. Die Berechnung der Transformationen erfolgt an fünf äquidistanten Zeitpunkten $(t_1, t_5, t_9, t_{13}, t_{17})$.

3 Ergebnisse

Um die Registrierungsergebnisse miteinander vergleichen zu können, wurden die Segmentierungen der Targetsequenz mit der berechneten Transformation verformt und anschließend mit denen der Referenzsequenz verglichen. Hierbei wurde als Metrik der Dice-Koeffizient und die mittlere symmetrische Oberflächendistanz $(d_{\mu_{\text{sym}}})$ zwischen den Segmentierungen bestimmt.

Die Ergebnisse der Evaluierung sind in Tab. 1 dargestellt. Insgesamt erzielten alle drei Registrierungsverfahren gute Ergebnisse. Dabei waren 25-50% aller gemessenen Oberflächendistanzen unter 2 mm. Insgesamt erreichte 3D-direkt die besten Resultate. Die schlechtesten Resultate erzielte 3D+TB. Des Weiteren zeigt 3D-MC+TB eine erhöhte Konsistenz und Robustheit der Registrierungsergebnisse (s. Std-Abw. von $d_{\mu_{\text{sym}}}$). Des Weiteren sind alle Ergebniswerte bis auf die Dice-Koeffizienten zwischen 3D-direkt und 3D-MC+TB statistisch signifikant verschieden.

4 Diskussion

In dieser Arbeit wurde der von Peyrat et al. vorgestellte Ansatz der Multichannel-3D-Registrierung (3D-MC+TB) adaptiert und mit zwei weiteren Verfahren (3D-direkt, 3D+TB) verglichen. Hierbei zeigten alle drei Ansätze gute Registrierungsergebnisse. Des Weiteren sind die Registrierungsergebnisse im Bezug auf 3D-MC+TB mit den Ergebnissen, die Peyrat et al. in ihrer Evaluation erzielte, vergleichbar.

In ihrer Arbeit evaluierten Peyrat et al. die 3D-MC+TB anhand von fünf kardiologischen 4D-CT-Bildsequenzen. Diese weisen im Vergleich zu Cine-MR-Sequenzen deutlich homogenere Grauwertverteilungen auf, was die Registrierung solcher Bildsequenzen vereinfacht. Dennoch sind die Ergebnisse der dieser Arbeit in Bezug auf die 3D-MC+TB durchaus mit den Ergebnissen von Peyrat et al. vergleichbar. Besonders die Robustheit durch die Verwendung der Trajektorienbeschränkungen konnte bestätigt werden. Jedoch schnitt das Verfahren 3D-direkt in den Ergebnissen von Peyrat et al. [6] wesentlich schlechter ab, was in der vorliegenden Arbeit nicht bestätigt werden konnte. Des Weiteren wurde eine Verbesserung der 3D-direkt Methode durch die Verwendung der Trajektorienbeschränkungen beschrieben, durch die hier durchgeführten Experimente ebenfalls nicht reproduziert werden konnte. Darüber hinaus zeigte sich während der Evaluation, dass die Angleichung der Bildsequenzen durch die zeitliche Registrierung einen starken Einfluss auf die Rekonstruktion durch die Trajektorienbeschränkungen hat.

Literaturverzeichnis

1. Caspi Y, Irani M. Spatiotemporal alignment of sequences. IEEE Trans Pattern Anal Mach Intell. 2002;24:1409–24.
2. Lorenzo-Valdés M, Sanchez-Ortiz GI, Mohiaddin R, et al. Atlas-based segmentation and tracking of 3D cardiac MR images using non-rigid registration. Proc MICCAI. 2002; p. 642–50.
3. Perperidis D, Mohiaddin RH, Rueckert D. Spatio-temporal free-form registration of cardiac MR image sequences. Med Image Anal. 2005;9(5):441–56.
4. Durrleman S, Pennec X, Trouvé A, et al. Spatiotemporal atlas estimation for developmental delay detection in longitudinal datasets. Proc MICCAI. 2009; p. 297–304.
5. Ehrhardt J, Kepp T, Schmidt-Richberg A, et al. Joint multi-object registration and segmentation of left and right cardiac ventricles in 4D cine MRI. Proc SPIE. 2014; p. 90340M.
6. Peyrat JM, Delingette H, Sermesant M, et al. Registration of 4D cardiac CT sequences under trajectory constraints with multichannel diffeomorphic demons. IEEE Trans Med Imaging. 2010;29(7):1351–68.
7. Andreopoulos A, Tsotsos JK. Efficient and generalizable statistical models of shape and appearance for analysis of cardiac MRI. Med Image Anal. 2008;12(3):335–57.
8. Ehrhardt J, Säring D, Handels H. Structure-preserving interpolation of temporal and spatial image sequences using an optical flow-based method. Methods Inf Med. 2007;46(3):300–7.

Binary Image Inpainting with Interpolation-Enhanced Diffeomorphic Demons Registration
Application to Segmentation Defects of Proximal Femora

A. Friedberger, O. Museyko, K. Engelke

Institute of Medical Physics, University Erlangen-Nürnberg, Erlangen, Germany
andreas.friedberger@imp.uni-erlangen.de

Abstract. There is a wide range of segmentation methods for bone structures in CT images. Many of these methods are declared as automatic, but it is not guaranteed, that the resulting segmentation labels the volume of interest correctly in any case. This work presents a technique, which assists the user with the necessary corrections of the segmentation errors. The procedure must be started manually, but the following steps are fully automatic. First, a similar, correct segmentation is selected from a database, which is used to mask the defects. Then the selected segmentation is registered onto the defect one using the diffeomorphic demons algorithm. Thereby, the region inside the mask is excluded from registration but the displacement field is interpolated. The method has been implemented and tested for segmentations of the proximal femur head, but can easily be transferred to segmentations of other bone regions.

1 Introduction

In medical image processing, the segmentation of bone in CT images is a well known problem and a variety of methods exist [1]. But especially when segmenting pathological images, there is no guaranty, that the used algorithm separates the volume of interest correctly from the background. In the case of such segmentation failures, manual user interaction is necessary, which can be tedious and time consuming.

In literature, one can find some promising, semi-automatic methods proposed for correction of segmentation errors, see [2] and references therein. In contrast to those, the proposed method in this work does not need marking of the defects by the user. Started manually, this method works fully automatic. The basic idea of it was inspired by the methods proposed by Henn et al. in [3] and Lamecker and Pennec in [4]. In [3] the goal is the warping of MRI images of a brain with lesions to a brain atlas while preserving these lesions. The missing correspondence due to the lesion was resolved by masking of the affected regions and exclusion from registration. Minimization of the introduced similarity functional lead to a smooth interpolation in these regions. The method presented in this work adopts this general idea, however does not use atlas-based registration for segmentation, but rather for the repair of a given segmentation. This segmentation is represented by a binary image and is gained with the help of some other algorithms, which are extraneous to this work. Furthermore, while the interpolation in [3] arose naturally from minimizing a special similarity functional, the interpolation in this work is explicitly introduced to the registration algorithm. This equals the method in [4]. But instead of local interpolation based on the Laplace equation with inhomogeneous Dirichlet boundary conditions defined on the boundary of the mask, the method proposed in this work uses interpolation on the base of an image-wide solution of the diffusion equation.

The proposed technique is used for automatic correction of segmentation defects at the proximal femur head. However this method is quite general and can easily be applied to many other binary segmentations.

2   Materials and methods

The basic idea of the method is to substitute the defects in a segmentation by the corresponding regions of a similar shaped segmentation without defects. This substitution is obtained by means of registration. Therefore, the presented method compares the defect segmentation with a database consisting of correct segmentations of similar objects and chooses the best matching one. Then this optimum image is used to mask the defect regions. After that, the selected image is warped onto the defect segmentation by diffeomorphic demons registration. During registration, the masked defect regions are excluded, so the calculated displacement field would vanish there. To avoid this, the displacement field in the defect regions is interpolated at each iteration with the help of the diffusion equation.

2.1   Template selection and defect masking

The used template for registration (the correct segmentation) should be similar to the reference (the segmentation with defects). This avoids large deformations and yields a "predictable" displacement field. Therefore, the defect segmentation is compared with a database, consisting of several aligned, correct segmentations of similar objects. The database was created once beforehand and its alignment was done by rigid registration of all images onto one arbitrarily chosen image within the database. The measure for the comparison with the database is the absolute sum of distances.

The best matching database image (the optimum template) is used to mask the defect automatically. To this end, one takes the asymmetric difference of this image and the defect segmentation. After that, a morphological opening removes small structures, which probably do not represent defects.

2.2   The diffeomorphic demons registration with interpolation

The demons algorithm, introduced by Thirion in his seminal paper [5], calculates a displacement field s, which maximizes some similarity criterion between the reference image R and the template T if the latter is warped with it. To this end, at every iteration an update field u is computed, whereby the masked regions are excluded from registration. To avoid a vanishing field in these regions, the update field is interpolated.

The interpolation is done on the basis of the diffusion equation for some vector field d and the source vector field u (the update field)

$$\frac{\partial d}{\partial t} - \alpha \Delta d = u \tag{1}$$

Δ denotes the Laplace operator and α the diffusion constant. In three dimensions, expression (1) consists of three separate equations. These can be rewritten based on the implicit scheme with a discretization of time (time step τ)

$$(\mathbb{I} - \alpha \tau \Delta) d^{k+1} = d^k + \tau u \tag{2}$$

where d^k stands for the vector field $d(k\tau)$ at time k and $\mathbb{I}$ denotes the identity operator. The used boundary conditions are of homogeneous Neumann type. (2) can be solved by Fourier transformation [6]. Then the update field u in the masked regions is replaced with the solution of (2). This partially interpolated update field has to be combined in some way with the displacement field s. In the diffeomorphic demons algorithm, this is done through the exponential mapping $s \leftarrow s \circ \exp(u)$, which leads to a one-to-one diffeomorphic transformation [7].

After the displacement field s is joined with the update u, it is smoothed with a Gaussian kernel K_σ to constrain the deformation of the template. A high standard deviation σ of the kernel results in a more restrictive deformation, whereas a low σ leads to more relaxed deformations.

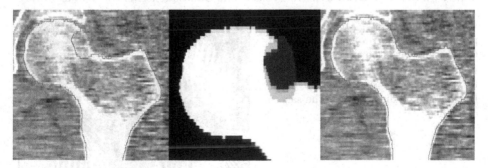

Fig. 1. The defect segmented CT image of the proximal femur (left) is converted to a binary image (middle) and the defect is automatically masked (red region). The following registration with interpolation could restore the segmentation (right).

2.3   The workflow

Given a segmentation with defects and an appropriate database, the general workflow consists of the following steps, which do not need further user interaction once started:

1. Rigid registration of the defect segmentation to the database.
2. Selection of the optimum template.
3. Masking of the defects.
4. Registration with interpolation between the optimum template and the defect segmentation.
5. Substitution of the defect segmentation by the registration result (warped template) within the masked regions.

2.4   Application to the proximal femur

The method was tested on 25 defect segmentations of proximal femora. The defects addressed in this test are "holes" in the segmentation, thus these holes have to be "filled up". The dual problem, cropping of segmentation defects, can be addressed by this method, too. Due to the opposed defect masking step, both modes can not be applied simultaneously but consecutively. The segmentations were created with the Medical Image Analysis Framework (MIAF, developed at the Institute for Medical Physics, Erlangen, Germany) from CT scans of postmenopausal women.

The method was implemented in C++, utilizing the Insight Toolkit (ITK, *www.itk.org*) and the Fastest Fourier Transform in the West (*www.fftw.org*), a C subroutine library computing discrete Fourier transforms. The database with potential templates consisted of 30 correct segmentations of different patients of the same study. The morphological opening during the defect masking step was done with radius of 2 times the voxel size. The Gaussian kernel K_σ was set to 0.01

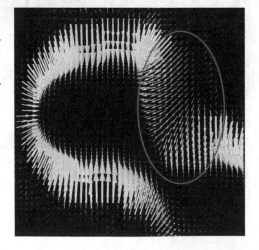

Fig. 2. The coronal MPR of the displacement field corresponding to Fig. 1. Comparing with the middle picture of Fig. 1, one can detect the smooth interpolated region. Note that only every third vector is displayed for the sake of clearness.

times the voxel size, which is low enough to allow for quasi-free deformations. The time step and the diffusion constant were chosen to be $\tau = 1$ resp. $\alpha = 3$. The computation time was about 20 s on a computer with a 3.6 GHz Quadcore processor.

3   Results

Fig. 1 left shows a coronal multiplanar reformation (MPR) of a defect segmentation of a proximal femur. Apparently, the segmentation failed in the transition zone of neck and head. This segmentation is converted to a binary image, the defect is masked automatically (red, overlaid region in Fig. 1 middle) and the registration with interpolation method restored the defect (Fig. 1 right). Fig. 2 shows one coronal MPR of the displacement field. This MPR corresponds to the one of Fig. 1. The interpolated region is indicated by the red ellipse. For the sake of clearness, only every third vector is displayed. Fig. 3 left shows a larger segmentation failure due to low bone mineral density in the affected regions. The usage of the correction method yields the blue regions in Fig. 3 right, which can be merged with the main segmentation (red). As one can see, the method did not fully restore the segmentation and additional user interaction is necessary.

The correction tool was tested on 25 defect segmentations and could reduce the overall time for user interaction from 60 min (without the tool) to 30 min (with the tool). 5 segmentations did not need further user interaction.

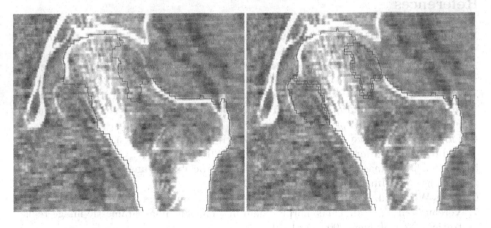

Fig. 3. The left picture shows a MPR of a segmentation with larger failure. The blue regions in the right picture are the results of the presented method. These regions do not sufficiently restore the segmentation defects. Primarily, this can be explained by the large scale of the defects.

4 Discussion

The presented method to automatically correct defects in segmentations works well for small to medium sized defects at the proximal femur (Fig. 1). It significantly reduces the user interaction time. However, with increasing defect size, the difference between the corrected image and the desired result (Fig. 3) gets bigger. This arises from local variances of the femur shape, which cannot be reproduced by the smooth, mask wide interpolation.

A way to increase performance of the method may be the use of a statistical shape model (SSM) instead of the database. With a SSM one could create a specific adjusted template for each segmentation. This, and the impact of the method on the segmentation precision will be attended in following studies.

Yet, one drawback of the method is the loss of information when binarizing the segmented CT image. But even for large defects, the results of the automatic correction are good approximations to the desired correct segmentation (Fig. 3). Thus, these results could also serve as a starting point for subsequent methods, which may further improve the obtained correction by working on the gray value image.

Although the presented method was tested on improvement of proximal femur segmentations only, the generalization to other bones, bone regions or even arbitrary binary images is quite straightforward.

References

1. Bankman IN. Handbook of Medical Imaging: Processing and Analysis. Burlington: Academic Press; 2009.
2. Kronman A, Joskowicz L. Image segmentation errors correction by mesh segmentation and deformation. Med Image Comput Comput Assist Interv. 2013;16:206–13.
3. Henn S, Hoemke L, Witsch K. A generalized image registration framework using incomplete image information - with application to lesion mapping. In: Mathematics in Industry. vol. 10. Springer; 2006. p. 3–25.
4. Lamecker H, Pennec X. Atlas to image-with-tumor registration based on demons and deformation inpainting. Proc MICCAI. 2010.
5. Thirion JP. Image matching as a diffusion process: an analogy with Maxwell's demons. Med Image Anal. 1998;2:243–60.
6. Press WH, et al. Numerical Recipes. New York: Cambridge University Press; 2007.
7. Vercauteren T, et al. Diffeomorphic demons: efficient non-parametric image registration. NeuroImage. 2009;45:61–72.

Handling Non-Corresponding Regions in Image Registration

David Drobny[1,2], Heike Carolus[2], Sven Kabus[2], Jan Modersitzki[1]

[1]Institute of Mathematics and Image Computing, University of Lübeck
[2]Philips Research, Hamburg
drobny@informatik.uni-luebeck.de

Abstract. Image registration is particularly challenging if the images to be aligned contain non-corresponding regions. Using state-of-the-art algorithms typically leads to unwanted and unrealistic deformations in these regions. There are various approaches handling this problem which improve registration results, however each with a focus on specific applications. In this note we describe a general approach which can be applied on different mono-modal registration problems. We show the effects of this approach compared to a standard registration algorithm on the basis of five 3D CT lung image pairs where synthetic tumors have been added. We show that our approach significantly reduces unwanted deformation of a non-corresponding tumor. The average volume decrease is 9% compared to 66% for the standard approach while the overall accuracy based on landmark error is retained.

1 Introduction

One of the central assumptions in image registration is that each region of one image has a corresponding region in the other one. There are several scenarios for medical images where this assumption does not hold, for example tissue resection, bone drill out, tumor growth, different filling of digestive organs, or display of medical equipment. State-of-the-art non-rigid registration algorithms, which do not explicitly handle non-corresponding regions typically estimate a deformation which either shrinks or expands an image structure to compensate for the missing correspondence. There are several approaches which cope with this problem. Most of them are specialized in certain applications, first and foremost in brain resection. Due to the specialization, assumptions can be made to simplify the problem. Either the segmentation of the missing volume [1], or certain characteristics of the non-corresponding areas (e.g. intensity range, location) [2, 3, 4] are assumed to be known. In [5] the central idea is to model the probability for each voxel to be corresponding between both images based on the residual of the images. Similar to [5] we propose an approach which makes no explicit assumption and is thus applicable to various scenarios. Following this idea, we extend an elastic registration framework [6, 7] to reduce the impact of non-corresponding regions. To demonstrate the feasibility and the advantage compared to a standard approach, we conduct experiments on lung CT data. We alter images to feature non-corresponding areas and show the superior handling of these regions by our proposed approach.

2 Materials and methods

For our experiments we use five inhale-exhale lung 3D CT image pairs provided by the DIR-lab project [8]. Each image has a size of 256×256 voxel in-slice and covering the thorax with a voxel size between (0.97×0.97) and $(1.16 \times 1.16)\,\mathrm{mm}^2$ and a slice thickness of $2.5\,\mathrm{mm}$. For each image pair 300 corresponding reference landmarks are provided. To simulate a non-corresponding structure, we altered each template image which is to be deformed by adding an ellipsoid into the lung, once centered and once peripheral. This synthetic tumor enables analysis of the registration behavior in a controlled and well understood environment.

Following [6], we use a variational framework for image registration, i.e we minimize the function

$$J[R,T,\varphi] = D[R,T,\varphi] + \alpha\, S[\varphi] \tag{1}$$

where D is the sum of squared differences (SSD) and S the elastic potential, see [6] for details. For later references we denote the implementation of [7] as the standard approach. In the following we describe how this standard approach is extended to deal with non-corresponding regions.

The probability for a region to be corresponding in the reference image R and the template image T can be evaluated for each voxel. To do so, we introduce two models. The first model M_1 assumes a relationship of the voxels of R and T which is explained by the displacement $\varphi = id + u$. The second model M_2 represents a non-correspondence of the voxels. For the model M_1 a Gaussian distribution depending on the residual $R - T(\varphi)$ is assumed [5]. With $r = R(x)$, $t = T(\varphi(x))$, we have

$$P_{M_1} = P(r,t|M_1) = e^{-\frac{(r-t)^2}{16\,\sigma^2}} \tag{2}$$

where $\sigma^2 = \mathrm{var}(R - T(\varphi))$ is the variance of the residual image.

This results in lower probabilities for larger differences between voxel intensities. The model M_2 is assumed to have a uniform distribution. Since we do not have prior knowledge about the type of non-correspondence, any value of the residual has the same probability to depict a non-correspondence. Therefore $P_{M_2} = P(r,t|M_2) = c$ is constant with $c = 0.0025$ as an exemplary value. The amount of regions without correspondence can vary highly thus it is infeasible to predict the a-priori probabilities for M_1 and M_2 without further knowledge of the image data. Because of this we assume that the a-priori probabilities for both models are equal. Utilizing the Bayes theorem we obtain the probability map P^* which, given the residual $r - t$, indicates the probability for every voxel to have a valid correspondence: $P^* = P_{M_1}/(P_{M_1} + P_{M_2})$.

To retain the ratio of data term and regularizer and thus the elasticity of the standard approach, we introduce a scaled version of the probability map as $P = 1.2 \cdot P^*/\mathrm{mean}(P^*)$.

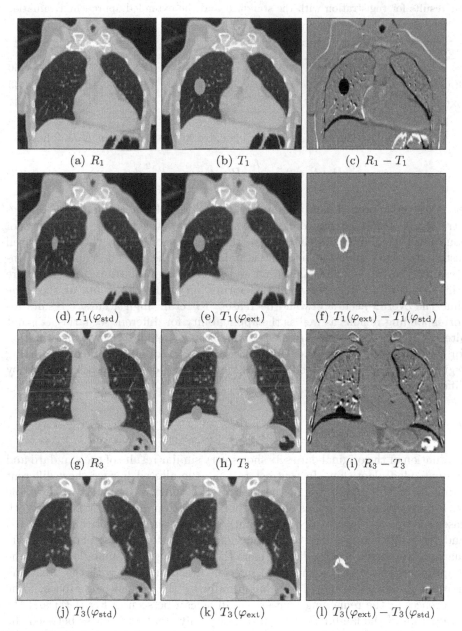

Fig. 1. Coronal view of the results of case 1 with a synthetic tumor located central in the right lung in T_1 as well as the results of case 3 with a synthetic tumor located in the diaphragm of the right lung in T_3. The reference images R (a) and (g), the template images T (b) and (h) and the residuals $R - T$ (c) and (i), the transformed templates of the reference $T(\varphi_{std})$ (d), (j) and the proposed $T(\varphi_{ext})$ (e), (k) algorithm, and the residuals of the warped template images $T(\varphi_{ext}) - T(\varphi_{std})$ (f), (l) are shown.

Table 1. Mean landmark error in mm of the unaltered images (case 1-5), showing similar results for registration with the standard and the extended approach. Evaluation is based on 300 landmarks.

Case	1	2	3	4	5	∅
No registration	3.89	4.34	6.94	9.83	7.48	6.50
Standard	1.03	1.09	1.59	1.68	1.77	1.43
Extended	1.03	1.08	1.59	1.61	1.76	1.41

P is applied to the SSD similarity measure in the data term D as follows

$$D[r,t] = 0.5 \cdot \int_{\Omega} \left[P(r,t) \cdot (r - t) \right]^2 dx \qquad (3)$$

With this modified data term and the unaltered elastic regularizer $S[\varphi]$, registration is performed according to the standard approach. The parameter α of equation (1) controls the elasticity of the registration and is chosen as a well tested standard value for both the standard and the extended approach. Increasing α in the standard algorithm and thus making the transformation more stiff, would result in less unwanted deformation of the tumor but at the same time the overall accuracy would decrease. To retain high accuracy results for corresponding regions as well as the applicability for different scenarios, α is not altered. In this way, we ensure that the algorithms yield a similar transformation for all corresponding regions. Differences in the handling of non-corresponding regions can thus be explained by effects of the proposed approach and not by different elasticity.

3   Results

Evaluation of the original data sets shows very similar results of the standard and the extended algorithm. In contrast to this, the altered images show different behavior of the algorithms in the area of the tumor. In Fig. 1 an example with central tumor as well as one with peripheral tumor are illustrated. In both cases the tumor is compressed significantly by the standard algorithm (Fig. 1 (d) and (j)) while the extended algorithm yields a transformed template with only marginal tumor shrinkage (Fig. 1 (e) and (k)). Although the tumor located at the diaphragm (Fig. 1 (h)) is moved in inferior direction along with the breathing motion, its shape is altered only marginally by the extended approach. The differences in the remaining lung are small as can be seen in Fig. 1 (f) and (l). Evaluation of the landmark error also shows only small differences between the registration algorithms (Tab. 1).

The probability map P (Fig. 2(c)) after registration mainly shows the region of the tumor as a dark blob which indicates high probability for a non-correspondence. Dark regions depict a low weighting of the data term during registration, thus the deformation of these regions is dominated by the regularizer and strong deformation of the tumor is avoided that way. This also becomes

Table 2. Volume change of the tumor relative to the baseline deformation, showing the different effect of the standard and the extended algorithm. For both algorithms, the relative volume change of each test image pair with central and peripheral tumor as well as the mean value is given.

Tumor	Case	1	2	3	4	5	Ø
Central	Standard	−71%	−72%	−61%	−56%	−70%	−66%
	Extended	− 5%	− 9%	−11%	−10%	− 8%	− 9%
Peripheral	Standard	−50%	−52%	−37%	−30%	−45%	−43%
	Extended	− 8%	− 6%	− 4%	−10%	− 8%	− 7%

apparent when looking at the determinant of the Jacobian of the displacement φ, indicating the volume change at each voxel. The standard approach (Fig. 2(a)) yields a very strong volume change in the area of the tumor while the rest of the image is very homogeneous. Our proposed approach yields only marginal aberration from a smooth deformation in the tumor area (Fig. 2(b)).

To evaluate the different effects of both algorithms quantitatively, we analyze the volume change of the tumor region. The ground-truth volume is computed with the baseline deformation, i.e. the deformation resulting from standard registration of the unaltered images. This is done to get the volume of the tumor region deformed only by the breathing motion. If registration of the altered images is not influenced by the tumor, the deformation will ideally be the same as the baseline deformation. Thus we compare the volume resulting from the registration of the altered images with the ground-truth volume. The relative tumor change for central and for peripheral tumors is shown in Tab. 2.

The standard algorithm yields an average reduction of the tumor volume of 66% (for central location) and 43% (for peripheral location) while the extended algorithm better retains the size of the tumor with an average reduction of 9% and 7%, respectively. The magnitude of the volume change depends on the

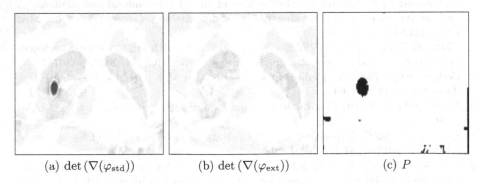

(a) $\det\left(\nabla(\varphi_{\text{std}})\right)$ (b) $\det\left(\nabla(\varphi_{\text{ext}})\right)$ (c) P

Fig. 2. Volume change of case 1 resulting from the standard algorithm (a) and the extended algorithm (b) as well as the final probability map of the extended algorithm (c). Orange and red colors in (a) and (b) denote shrinkage, while blue values denote expansion. Values close to 0 in (c) are shown dark and values close to 1 are shown bright.

tumor location. The peripheral tumors are located on the lung boundary. Since the surrounding tissue of the lung has intensities close to the tumor intensities, the volume of the tumor part located outside of the lung is less affected.

4 Discussion

In this note a standard variational registration algorithm is extended to handle non-corresponding regions. A probability map P indicating the probability of each voxel to have a valid correspondence between both images is computed and included in the data term.

The experiments show that with our proposed approach the regions without correspondences, simulated by added artificial tumors, only slightly affect the registration. We observe only a small average tumor shrinkage of 9% for central locations and 7% for peripheral locations compared to 66% and 43%,respectively, of the standard approach. For the rest of the image we observe very similar deformed template images and landmark displacements for both approaches. Thus we could show that the proposed approach is superior in regions without correspondences, while the rest of the lungs retains the high accuracy of the standard algorithm.

Note that although results are presented only for lung registration, the approach is general and can be applied in basically all areas of image registration.

References

1. Berendsen F, Kotte A, de Leeuw A, et al. Registration of structurally dissimilar images in MRI-based brachytherapy. Phys Med Biol. 2014;59(15):4033.
2. Kwon D, Niethammer M, Akbari H, et al. PORTR: pre-operative and post-recurrence brain tumor registration. IEEE Trans Med Imaging. 2014;33(3):651–67.
3. Nithiananthan S, Schafer S, Mirota DJ, et al. Extra-dimensional demons: a method for incorporating missing tissue in deformable image registration. Med Phys. 2012;39(9):5718–31.
4. Chitphakdithai N, Duncan JS. Non-rigid registration with missing correspondences in preoperative and postresection brain images. Proc MICCAI. 2010; p. 367–74.
5. Periaswamy S, Farid H. Medical image registration with partial data. Med Image Anal. 2006;10(3):452–64.
6. Modersitzki J. FAIR: Flexible algorithms for Image Registration. vol. 6. SIAM; 2009.
7. Kabus S, Lorenz C. Fast elastic image registration. Med Image Anal Clin: A Grand Challenge. 2010; p. 81–9.
8. Castillo R, Castillo E, Guerra R, et al. A framework for evaluation of deformable image registration spatial accuracy using large landmark point sets. Phys Med Biol. 2009;54(7):1849.

A Memetic Search Scheme for Robust Registration of Diffusion-Weighted MR Images

Jan Hering[1,2], Ivo Wolf[2], Tawfik Moher Alsady[1], Hans-Peter Meinzer[3], Klaus Maier-Hein[1]

[1] Junior Research Group Medical Imaging, DKFZ Heidelberg
[2] Mannheim University of Applied Sciences, Mannheim
[3] Medical and Biological Informatics, DKFZ Heidelberg
j.hering@dkfz-heidelberg.de

Abstract. Effective image-based artifact correction is an essential step in the application of higher order models in diffusion MRI. Most approaches rely on some kind of retrospective registration, which becomes increasingly challenging in the realm of high b-values and low signal-to-noise ratio (SNR), rendering standard correction schemes more and more ineffective. We propose a novel optimization scheme based on memetic search that allows for simultaneous exploitation of different signal intensity relationships between the images, leading to more robust registration results. We demonstrate the increased robustness and efficacy of our method on simulated as well as in-vivo datasets. The median TRE for an affine registration of $b = 3000\,\mathrm{s/mm^2}$ acquisitions could be reduced from $> 5\,\mathrm{mm}$ for a standard correction scheme to $< 1\,\mathrm{mm}$ using our approach. In-vivo bootstrapping experiments revealed increased precision in all tensor-derived quantities.

1 Introduction

Robust and successful head motion and artifact correction is a critical preprocessing step in diffusion tensor imaging [1] and higher-order diffusion modeling [2]. Image registration-based retrospective correction schemes are widely adopted in the community [3, 4]. At higher b-values, however, registration becomes increasingly challenging due to stronger artifacts, lower signal-to-noise ratio (SNR), and increased dependency of the signal on the gradient direction and thus larger contrast deviations between acquisitions. This renders standard correction schemes more ineffective. A pairwise registration of diffusion-weighted and non-diffusion-weighted images (Fig. 1(a)) can easily produce a remarkable amount of outliers in such a setting. In Fig. 1, the points depict acquisitions at $b_0 = 0\,\mathrm{s/mm^2}$ and $b_2 \geq b_1 \geq 0\,\mathrm{s/mm^2}$. The arrows indicate a pairwise registration of the moving (tail) and the fixed (head) image. This severely impedes advanced diffusion MRI modeling techniques that generally suffer from a higher sensitivity to noise (due to the increased number of free parameters in the models) and require longer acquisition times (potentially yielding increased head motion).

To overcome this problem, several approaches were proposed that assume a signal model, e.g. the second order diffusion tensor [5] or higher order models [6] to generate simulated reference images mimicking the contrast of the diffusion-weighted image to be corrected (Fig. 1(b)).

In theory, there are many more of such similarity relationships between different images in an acquisition that could be exploited implicitly or modeled explicitly. Instead of choosing a non-weighted or simulated image as the reference, higher b-value acquisitions can as well be registered to their already corrected "nearest neighbors" (minimal difference in the diffusion gradient direction) on a lower b-shell (Fig. 1(c)).

The hypothesis of this work is that a more consequent exploration of the intensity relations between the different images could enhance our capabilities to solve challenging registration problems during artifact correction of diffusion-weighted images. An optimal method would be able to prevent outliers and local minima by choosing the optimal combination of available registration objectives for each acquisition and at each step during the optimization process to efficiently find its way to the global optimum.

2   Materials and methods

Formally, the registration of two images I and J is an optimization over a transform space $\mathcal{T}$ with respect to a cost function C

$$\hat{T} = \arg\min_{t \in \mathcal{T}} C[I, J, t]$$

In this work, we introduce a metaheuristic memetic optimization scheme that combines local optimization methods with ideas from particle swarm optimization (PSO). The approach naturally deals with the simultaneous optimization of several cost functions or objectives at the same time. This section briefly introduces the underlying concepts.

2.1   Particle swarm optimization

Due to their capabilities in global search space exploration, evolutionary approaches have readily been applied to several intensity-based medical image registration problems [7]. Here, the optimization is directly applied to the registration scheme, e.g. by optimizing the transform parameters using PSO [8]. The

Fig. 1. Registration schemes based on signal intensity of diffusion MRI.

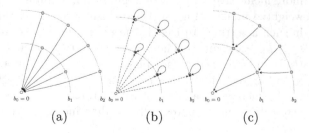

(a)   (b)   (c)

PSO technique uses a collection of particles in search space, each representing a feasible solution to the given optimization problem (in our case: a transformation). Each particle follows the swarm dynamics, which is modeled by a combination of each particle's own history and information from other particles (see [9] for a detailed description).

2.2 Memetic optimization

The main disadvantage of PSO when compared to straight local search methods is its lower performance and efficiency in computing local optima with high precision. The class of so-called memetic approaches aims at directly integrating the exploitation capabilities of local search with the exploratory power of metaheuristics like PSO. Such approaches were readily applied to image registration [10]. A memetic version of PSO iterates between two phases as depicted in Fig. 2. The local search phase is accomplished by any kind of local image registration method that is initialized by the particle's position in transform space. The second phase performs a standard PSO update [9].

2.3 Multi-objective optimization

Evolutionary approaches allow arbitrary kinds of constraints and objectives. One prominent class of techniques is formed by multi-objective PSO (MOPSO) [9]. One straight-forward approach that we also adopted here is the equally-weighted aggregation of the different objectives/cost functions [9].

2.4 Proposed approach

The proposed multi-objective memetic PSO solves the problem of affine registration of diffusion-weighted images by optimizing all previously introduced objective functions simultaneously: the unweighted objective (Fig. 1(a)), the model-based objective (Fig. 1(b)), and the nearest-neighbor objective (Fig. 1(c)). Each particle follows a specific single objective during the local search phase. The particles for the different objectives can be interpreted as different species or memes within the complete population that locally excel in different aspects of performance. The resulting positions in search space form a swarm that then undergoes the PSO update using weighted aggregation of the objectives [9] (Fig. 2).

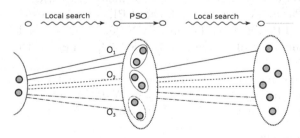

Fig. 2. Memetic search scheme for three local objectives ($O_{1,2,3}$) depicted by different line styles. The different species or memes formed by the corresponding objective's particles in the population are marked by small ellipses in the first particle set.

Fig. 3. Synthetic data: (a) full head tractogram used for the simulation in FiberFox; (b) axial view of simulated image at b=0 s/mm^2, (c) simulated image at b=3000 s/mm^2. In-vivo data: (d) acquisition at $b = 0$ s/mm^2 (e) and $b = 1000$ s/mm^2 (f) Acquisition at b=3000 s/mm^2.

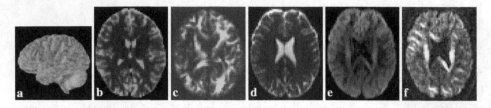

2.5   Parametrization

Several PSO parameters influence the behavior of the swarm [9]. The inertia weight ω regulates a trade-off between global and local exploration abilities. c_1 and c_2 balance individual history and the global swarm experience. Considering the powerful and PSO independent local search capabilities of the proposed memetic scheme, we chose PSO parameters that strongly favor swarm experience and global search over individual cognition and local search ($\omega = 0$, $c_1 = 0$, $c_2 = 1$). The local search was realized as regular step gradient descent using Mutual Information following a three-level resolution pyramid registration approach. The PSO update steps are placed at the different levels of the resolution pyramid. Our reference method was the same pyramidal local search method without PSO updates using the unweighted objective.

2.6   Experiments

The method was evaluated on both synthetic and in-vivo datasets (Fig. 3). Synthetic data provide a ground truth which allows a quantitative evaluation of the target registration error (TRE). The in-vivo experiments were performed using bootstrapping. We simulated a full brain dataset, 2.5 mm isotropic voxels, with one baseline ($b = 0$ s/mm^2) image and acquisitions at $b = 1000, 3000$ and 4500 s/mm^2 with 18 gradient directions each using Fiberfox[1]. We randomly added motion with up to 5 mm translation and 5 deg rotation in positive or negative direction for all three directions / axes. Rician noise with a SNR of 40 was added.

In-vivo data were acquired on a 3 T clinical scanner (Siemens Trio) with a gradient strength of 40 mT/m. Parameters were: single shot EPI, twice refocused spin echo diffusion preparation, TR/TE 8200/115 ms, FOV 250 mm, 50 axial slices, resolution $2.5 \times 2.5 \times 2.5$ mm^3. b-Values were b=0/1000/ 3000 s/mm^2 with 18/81/81 directions respectively.

In-vivo bootstrap analysis was performed by subdividing 81 gradient directions into three disjunctive subgroups of 27 directions each. A diffusion tensor was fit to the corrected data [1]. The Coefficient of Variance (CoV) among

---

[1] http://www.mitk.org/DiffusionImaging

the bootstrap samples was evaluated for the derived scalar indices: fractional anisotropy (FA), mean, axial and radial diffusivity (MD, AD and RD).

3   Results

The average TRE dropped significantly from > 5 mm for the non-weighted reference correction scheme to < 1 mm for the proposed optimization scheme ($p < 10^{-4}$, paired t-test). While this effect was particularly strong at higher b-values (Fig. 4a), the respective errors already differed significantly at the lowest shell with $b = 1000$ s/mm² ($p < 10^{-4}$). The TRE of the proposed method stayed below the voxel size of 2.5 mm for all b-values. The average TRE for the highest b-value at 4500 s/mm² was 1.5 mm.

The coefficient of variance (CoV) was significantly lower for three out of four tensor-derived scalar indices (MD, RD and FA) when applying the proposed correction scheme to the higher b-value acquisitions at b=3000 s/mm² (Fig. 4(b)). The differences only reached trend-level (not significant) for the same experiment performed at b=1000 s/mm².

The processing time on an Intel-i7 desktop PC system for the correction of in-vivo data was 19 min and 22 s on average ($\sigma^2 = 1$ min) for the standard correction and 68 min 39 s ($\sigma^2 = 9$ min) for the proposed method.

4   Discussion

We proposed a novel memetic search scheme for registration of diffusion-weighted MR datasets that significantly outperforms standard registration in synthetic and in-vivo datasets.

There are several parameters that potentially influence the performance of our method. These were set once and not touched so far during development of our approach. The number of iterations between local and global search, for example, was directly taken from the pyramidal registration scheme and thus limited to only three. This emphasized the local search phase as compared to the PSO updates. Furthermore, the number of particles and other PSO parameters were chosen very modestly and in favor of emphasizing the local

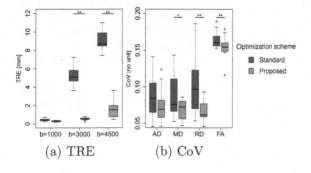

(a) TRE   (b) CoV

Fig. 4.   TRE in simulated datasets grouped by b-values (a). The proposed approach (green) outperforms the standard non-weighted reference approach (red). Coefficient of variance (CoV) in scalar indices for tensors fitted to the $b = 3000$ s/mm² shell (b). Significance levels: $p < 0.05$* and $p < 0.005$**.

search procedure. Future work will be necessary to further investigate on these choices and optimize these settings.

The in-vivo experiments at a lower b-value did not reach statistical significance. However, the proposed method showed very pronounced improvements at higher b-values ($b = 3000\,\text{s/mm}^2$ and above), which are of critical importance to a whole range of novel diffusion techniques that rely on higher-order modeling.

The computational effort of our approach increases linearly with the number of particles used. However, the particle's local search phases are independent of each other and thus highly parallelizable.

We inspected the importance of the different objective functions by evaluating the history of each particle that went through the optimization process, and could not identify one dominant objective. Interestingly, the importance of each objective differed for the different stages of the pyramid. This evidence could provide a basis for the development of more sophisticated, adaptive weighting strategies that could further improve the performance of the proposed approach.

We hope that our highly promising initial results will inspire future studies on metaheuristic optimization in diffusion MRI registration.

References

1. Basser PJ, Mattiello J, LeBihan D. MR diffusion tensor spectroscopy and imaging. Biophys J. 1994;66(1):259–67.
2. Panagiotaki E, Schneider T, Siow B, et al. Compartment models of the diffusion MR signal in brain white matter: a taxonomy and comparison. NeuroImage. 2012;59(3):2241–54.
3. Mohammadi S, Moeller HE, Kugel H, et al. Correcting eddy current and motion effects by affine whole-brain registrations: evaluation of three-dimensional distortions and comparison with slicewise correction. Magn Reson Med. 2010;64(4):1047–56.
4. Rohde GK, Barnett AS, Basser PJ, et al. Comprehensive approach for correction of motion and distortion in diffusion-weighted MRI. Magn Reson Med. 2004;51(1):103–14.
5. Bai Y, Alexander DC. Model-based registration to correct for motion between acquisitions in diffusion MR imaging. Proc ISBI. 2008; p. 947–50.
6. Ben-Amitay S, Jones DK, Assaf Y. Motion correction and registration of high b-value diffusion weighted images. Magn Reson Med. 2012;67(6):1694–702.
7. Valsecchi A, Damas S, Santamaria J. Evolutionary intensity-based medical image registration: a review. Curr Med Img Rev. 2013;9(4):283–97.
8. Li Q, Sato I. Multimodality image registration by particle swarm optimization of mutual information. Lect Notes Computer Sci. 2007; p. 1120–30.
9. Parsopoulos KE, Vrahatis MN. Multi-Objective Particles Swarm Optimization Approaches. IGI Global; 2008. p. 20–42.
10. Silva L, Bellon ORP, Boyer KL. Precision range image registration using a robust surface interpenetration measure and enhanced genetic algorithms. IEEE Trans Pattern Anal Mach Intell. 2005;27(5):762–76.

A Variational Method for Constructing Unbiased Atlas with Probabilistic Label Maps

Kanglin Chen, Alexander Derksen

Fraunhofer MEVIS Project Group Image Registration
kanglin.chen@mevis.fraunhofer.de

Abstract. We introduce a novel variational method based image registration and reconstruction to construct an average atlas with probabilistic label maps. The average atlas equipped with probabilistic label maps could be used to improve atlas based segmentation. In the experiment we validate the registration accuracy and the unbiasedness of atlas construction using clinical datasets.

1 Introduction

Average atlas is an average representative of an image database with average intensities and shapes. Nowadays it becomes an important tool in several aspects of medical image processing. In computational anatomy, it is used to study the variability between individuals and identify abnormal anatomical structures [1]. In the surface based morphometry (SBM), inter-subject averaging of cortical surface is used to perform statistical analysis of morphometric properties, such as aging and neurodegenerative diseases [2]. Besides these, average atlas is commonly used in segmentation. The transformations from datasets to atlas are computed offline, and we can transfer the segmentations of datasets to a new object by computing only one registration from the atlas to the new object. Comparing multiple atlas based segmentation, it reduces the computational time significantly [3].

There are different ways to construct an average atlas. The most simple way is to utilize stereotaxic coordinates [4]. One aligns the datasets to a template image according to the stereotaxic coordinates and then average them. This approach is straightforward, however, the registration suffers from low accuracy. More recently, a variational approach based on diffeomorphic registration has been introduced in [3]. The induced average atlas has much shaper edges than just using affine registration based on the stereotaxic coordinates. Another popular approach for constructing an average atlas is based on averaging deformation fields [5]. One computes the affine and nonlinear registrations for every image of a database to a template image, and averages deformation fields modulo affine transformations. In the end, the average warped image of the database transformed by the average deformation field yields the average atlas.

However, computing an atlas, in particular with the application for segmentation, the segmentation labels are in general not utilized in the atlas construction

Fig. 1. A volume of the PDDCA database with the segmentations- and landmarks-overlays.

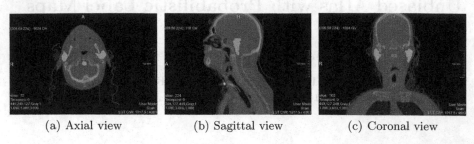

(a) Axial view   (b) Sagittal view   (c) Coronal view

process and the probabilistic label maps are computed afterwards in terms of estimated deformation fields [3]. In this work, we will introduce a novel variational method combining anatomical images and segmentations to compute the atlas. The atlas consists of an average template image and probabilistic label maps. The corresponding variational problem is based on the hyperelastic regularization for image registration and the Huber-TV regularization for image reconstruction. An alternating approach is introduced to solve the minimization problem. In the experiments, we will use 3D clinical datasets to compute the atlas. Utilizing the annotated segmentations and landmarks of the datasets, we are able to validate the accuracy of image registrations and the unbiasedness of the atlas.

2   Materials and methods

To construct the atlas, we use the public database PDDCA[1] of computational anatomy. In each dataset there exist the segmentations of brain stem, left and right parotids. In addition, the landmarks of chin, odontoid process, left and right condyloid processes are marked by triangles, crosses and dots. In Fig. 1 we visualize one dataset with the overlays. We use 27 datasets to compute the atlas with probabilistic label maps by our algorithm, which will be introduced in the following context.

We restrict our problem to 3D using the same image modality. Suppose there exist N images $\{\mathcal{I}_i\}_{i=1}^N$ with $\mathcal{I}_i : \Omega_i \to \mathbb{R}$, where Ω_i is a bounded domain of $\mathcal{I}_i$. In addition, we suppose in $\mathcal{I}_i$ there exist P binary segmentation images $\{\mathcal{S}_{i,k}\}_{k=1}^P$ with $\mathcal{S}_{i,k} : \Omega_i \to \{0,1\}$. Since we work on discrete images and segmentations, the domain Ω_i is discretized into a regular nodal grid with n_i grid points $\{x_j\}_{j=1}^{n_i}$, the acquired discrete image $I_i := \{\mathcal{I}_i(x_j)\}_{j=1}^{n_i}$ and the discrete segmentation $S_{i,k} := \{\mathcal{S}_{i,k}(x_j)\}_{j=1}^{n_i}$.

We search for an average template of anatomical images $\mathcal{T} : \Omega \to \mathbb{R}$ and P probabilistic label maps $\{\mathcal{S}_k\}_{k=1}^P$ with $\mathcal{S}_k : \Omega \to [0,1]$, where Ω is a pre-defined domain of the atlas. In the discrete setting, we discretize Ω with n nodal grid points $\{x_j\}_{j=1}^n$. Then, the discrete template is defined by $T = \{\mathcal{T}(x_j)\}_{j=1}^n$,

---

[1] http://www.imagenglab.com/pddca_18.html

and the discrete probabilistic label maps are defined by $S_k = \{\mathcal{S}_k(x_j)\}_{j=1}^n$ for $k = 1, \cdots, P$. We solve the following minimization problem to obtain the results, namely

$$
\sum_{i=1}^{N} \mathrm{hd}_i \left(\frac{1}{2} \|I_i - T \circ y_i\|_2^2 + \frac{c}{2} \sum_{k=1}^{P} \|S_{i,k} - S_k \circ y_i\|_2^2 + \mathrm{Reg}^{\mathrm{hyper}}(y_i) \right)
$$

$$
+ \lambda_T \mathrm{Reg}^{\mathrm{rec}}(T) + \lambda_S \sum_{k=1}^{P} \mathrm{Reg}^{\mathrm{rec}}(S_k) \xrightarrow{\{y_i\}_{i=1}^N, T, \{S_k\}_{k=1}^P} \min
$$

(1)

In (1) the template T is warped by with a deformation field $y_i \in \mathbb{R}^{3n_i}$, which matches I_i in the sense of the sum of squared differences (SSD) with the product of spacing hd_i. In the term involving of the probabilistic label maps, we use a parameter $c \in \mathbb{R}^+$ to emphasize the term of segmentations. In the rest domain, the registration is driven by anatomical information. To make the computation of the template image, deformation fields and probabilistic label maps possible, we set up a priori information of them using regularizations $\mathrm{Reg}^{\mathrm{hyper}}, \mathrm{Reg}^{\mathrm{rec}}$. The regularization parameters $\lambda_T, \lambda_S \in \mathbb{R}^+$ are used to balance the tradeoff between fidelity term and a priori information. The regularizations will be discussed in the following context.

A crucial ingredient for image registration is the regularization of the deformation field. In the area of atlas construction, the underlying deformation is non-linear and non-parametric. Hence, we decided to employ so called *hyperelastic regularization* [6]. A highlighted feature of hyperelastic regularization is to prevent the folding effects, since it additionally allows to control area, volume and length changes introduced by the deformation field and guarantees diffeomorphic transformations. In order to motivate the hyperelastic regularization, let us assume that $y : \Omega \to \mathbb{R}^3$ is continuously differentiable and that $y(x) = x + u(x)$. Consequently, the term $|\nabla u|_F^2$ gives a notion of the changes in length introduced by the deformation, where $|.|_F$ denotes the Frobenius norm. In addition, surface changes and volume changes can be captured by $\mathrm{cof}(\nabla y)$ and $\det(\nabla y)$. In the discrete setting, we denote the discrete Jacobian ∇u_i for the deformation field y_i. For the discrete cofactor and determinant of the deformation at a deformed voxel p^j, we write $\mathrm{surf}(p^j)$ and $\mathrm{vol}(p^j)$, $j = 1, \ldots, nc_i$, where nc_i is the number of cell-centered gridpoints of Ω_i.

Since in 3D it is desirable to control specifically the factors length, surface and volume, penalty functions are introduced yielding the *hyperelastic regularization*:

$$
\mathrm{Reg}^{\mathrm{hyper}}(y_i) := \frac{\lambda_l}{2} \sum_{j=1}^{n_i} |\nabla u_i^j|_F^2 + \lambda_s \sum_{j=1}^{nc_i} \Phi(\mathrm{surf}(p^j)) + \lambda_v \sum_{j=1}^{nc_i} \Psi\left(\mathrm{vol}(p^j)\right)
$$

(2)

Here $\lambda_l, \lambda_s, \lambda_v \in \mathbb{R}^+$ are regularization parameters and

$$
\Phi(z) := \sum_{i=1}^{3} \max\left(\sum_{j=1}^{3} z_{j,i}^2 - 1, 0\right) \text{ and } \Psi(z) := \frac{(z-1)^4}{z^2}
$$

(3)

are penalty functions yielding a well-posed registration problem. Details concerning the theory can be found in [6].

For the regularization on image reconstruction, we apply total variation based on the Huber-norm. Total variation is a standard tool to reconstruct an image from noisy data with edge preservation. In the discrete setting, the total variation of a discrete image $T \in \mathbb{R}^n$ using Huber-norm is defined as

$$\text{Reg}^{\text{rec}}(T) := \|\nabla T\|_{1,\alpha} = \text{hd} \sum_{j=1}^{n} |\nabla T_j|_\alpha \tag{4}$$

where ∇T denotes a finite difference approximation of the gradient of T and hd is the product of the spacing of the grid. The Huber-norm is defined as

$$|x|_\alpha = \begin{cases} \dfrac{|x|^2}{2\alpha} & \text{if } |x| \le \alpha \\ |x| - \dfrac{\alpha}{2} & \text{if } |x| > \alpha \end{cases} \tag{5}$$

where $\alpha > 0$ is a parameter defining the tradeoff between quadratic regularization for small values and total variation regularization for larger values. A well-known advantage of total variation regularization using Huber-norm is the reduction of the staircasing effect. The Huber-TV regularization is also applied to the probabilistic label maps construction in (1).

2.1   Optimization

The optimization of (1) is a challenging problem, since we have to simultaneously estimate the template, probabilistic label maps and deformation fields. To make the computation possible, we apply the alternating approach, which split (1) into image registration and reconstruction problems. These problems are well studied and efficient algorithms are available. For given template T and probabilistic label maps $\{S_k\}_{k=1}^{P}$, the image registration problems read

$$\frac{1}{2} \|I_i - T \circ y_i\|_2^2 + \frac{c}{2} \sum_{k=1}^{P} \|S_{i,k} - S_k \circ y_i\|_2^2 + \text{Reg}^{\text{hyper}}(y_i) \xrightarrow{y_i} \min \tag{6}$$

for $i = 1, \cdots, N$. In this work the freely available numerical implementation from FAIR [7] was used and we adjusted the implementation of the distance measure to fit our problem with multiple distance measures. For image reconstruction we consider the following problems for the fixed deformation fields $\{y_i\}_{i=1}^{N}$

$$\sum_{i=1}^{N} \frac{\text{hd}_i}{2} \|I_i - T \circ y_i\|_2^2 + \lambda_T \text{Reg}^{\text{rec}}(T) \xrightarrow{T} \min \tag{7}$$

$$\frac{c}{2} \sum_{i=1}^{N} \text{hd}_i \|S_{i,k} - S_k \circ y_i\|_2^2 + \lambda_S \text{Reg}^{\text{rec}}(S_k) \xrightarrow{S_k} \min, \quad k = 1, \cdots, P \tag{8}$$

Table 1. Average pairwise distances of landmarks chin, odontoid process (odont_P), condyloid process left (condy_PL), and condyloid process right (condy_PR) excluding self-comparisons.

	Chin	Odont_P	Condy_PL	Condy_PR
Distances (mm)	2.01	1.11	2.56	3.02

Such problems are classified into TV-l_2 denoising problems, which can be solved efficiently the Chambolle-Pock algorithm [8].

In summary, we solve (6)-(8) iteratively by incorporating a multilevel framework.

3   Results

In Fig. 2 we visualize the computed results. The template is overlayed with the probabilistic label maps of brain stem, left and right parotids. The transformed landmarks from the image spaces to the atlas space are also visualized in this figure. Regarding the registration accuracy, we consider the average distances of the landmarks. For each type of landmarks we build the pairs of all possible combinations excluding self-comparisons and compute the average distances of all pairs. The results are listed in table 1. Another important issue is to validate the unbiasedness of the atlas, and the basic idea is borrowed from [5]. Generally speaking, an unbiased point of a cluster of points is the average of the points along x-, y- and z-axis. Similarly, the average displacements of the landmarks from the image spaces to the atlas space is equal to zero for x-, y- and z-axis. The results of average displacements for each type landmarks are listed in table 2.

4   Discussion

A visual inspection of Fig. 2 shows the template and probabilistic label maps have sharp edges. The clusters of the landmarks in this figure seem to be concentrated. Combined with the average pairwise distances of the landmarks showed in table 1, we conclude that the registrations work accurately for all the datasets.

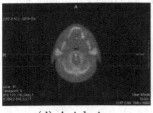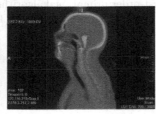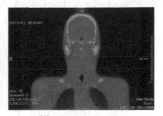

| (d) Axial view | (e) Sagittal view | (f) Coronal view |

Fig. 2. The template image and probabilistic label maps by the proposed algorithm with the landmarks-overlays. The parameter setting $c = 10, \lambda_l = \lambda_s = 1, \lambda_v = 10, \alpha = 10^{-2}, \lambda_T = 20, \lambda_S = 10^{-1}$.

Table 2. Average displacements of landmarks chin, odontoid process (odont_P), condyloid process left (condy_PL), and condyloid process right (condy_PR) according to x-, y- and z-axis.

	chin	Odont_P	Condy_PL	Condy_PR
Displacements (mm)	[0.2 -0.8 1.1]	[-0.2 -0.8 -0.7]	[-2.0 -2.4 -0.5]	[1.5 -3.0 -0.3]

Regarding the validation of unbiasedness, it is difficult to get the average displacements to be zero, since the annotated landmarks have some variability in the annotation process. However, as showed in Tab. 2, the average displacements are kept small compared to the image spacing [2.3mm, 2.5mm, 3.2mm]. Additionally, with an unknown variability of the landmarks, we consider the constructed atlas is unbiased.

In this paper, we introduced a new variational method based on the hyperelastic image registration and the Huber-TV image reconstruction to compute an unbiased atlas with probabilistic maps. Using clinical datasets, we validated the atlas has high registration accuracy and it is unbiased. In the future, we will apply this method for atlas based segmentation and the probabilistic maps could be useful to improve the segmentation.

References

1. Toga AW, Mazziotta JC. Brain Mapping: The Methods. vol. 1. Academic Press; 2002.
2. Fischl B, Sereno MI, Tootell RB, et al. High-resolution intersubject averaging and a coordinate system for the cortical surface. Hum Brain Mapp. 1999;8(4):272–84.
3. Joshi S, Davis B, Jomier M, et al. Unbiased diffeomorphic atlas construction for computational anatomy. NeuroImage. 2004;23:S151–60.
4. Evans A, Kamber M, Collins D, et al. MRI-based probabilistic atlas neuroanat. Magn Reson Scanning Epilepsy. 1994; p. 263–74.
5. Guimond A, Meunier J, Thirion JP. Average brain models: a convergence study. Comput Vis Image Underst. 2000;77(2):192–210.
6. Burger M, Modersitzki J, Ruthotto L. A hyperelastic regularization energy for image registration. SIAM J Sci Comput. 2013;35(1):132–48.
7. Modersitzki J. FAIR: Flexible Algorithms for Image Registration. SIAM; 2009.
8. Chambolle A, Pock T. A first-order primal-dual algorithm for convex problems with applications to imaging. J Math Imaging Vis. 2011;40(1):120–45.

MR-Elastographie auf dem Schreibtisch

Untersuchung der Viskoelastizität von Gewebeproben mit einem Niederfeld MR-Tomographen

Selcan Ipek-Ugay[1], Toni Drießle[2], Michael Ledwig[2], Jing Guo[3], Thomas Tolxdorff[1], Ingolf Sack[3], Jürgen Braun[1]

[1]Institut für Medizinische Informatik, Charité – Universitätsmedizin Berlin
[2]Pure Devices GmbH Würzburg, Germany
[3]Institut für Radiologie, Charité – Universitätsmedizin Berlin
selcan.ipek-ugay@charite.de

Kurzfassung. Bildgebende Verfahren gehören zu den wichtigsten Instrumenten in der medizinischen Diagnostik, während die Palpation ein wichtiges diagnostisches Werkzeug zur qualitativen Erfassung von Elastizitätsveränderungen oberflächennaher Organe ist. Die Elastographie ist die Kombination dieser beiden Techniken. Dabei wird die tastende Hand des Arztes durch niederfrequente Vibrationen und Bildaufnahme der Gewebeauslenkung mittels Ultraschall (US) oder Magnetresonanztomographie (MRT) ersetzt. Mit der Elastographie können viskoelastische Gewebeeigenschaften bestimmt und im komplexen Schermodul G* parametrisiert werden. Die Korrelation der makroskopischen, viskoelastischen Gewebeparameter und der Mikrostruktur ist für eine verbesserte Diagnostik notwendig, sie wurde allerdings bislang nur in wenigen Tierstudien adressiert. Als Lösung bieten sich systematische Untersuchungen von histopathologisch genau charakterisierten Gewebeproben an. Dies scheitert bislang einerseits an der Verfügbarkeit von Magnetresonanz-Elastographie (MRE) tauglichen Geräten, da geeignete Elastogrpahie-Techniken kommerziell noch nicht verfügbar sind. Andererseits ist der Zugang zu MR-Tomographen oftmals limitiert oder mit hohen Kosten verbunden. Im Rahmen dieser Arbeit wurde daher die Machbarkeit der MRE an einem kostengünstigen MRT-Tischgerät mit einem 0.5 Tesla Permanentmagneten untersucht. Für die MRE wurde das Gerät um eine Vibrationseinheit und eine bewegungssensitive Spin-Echo-Aufnahmetechnik erweitert. Die Auswertung erfasster Scherwellenausbreitungsmuster erlaubt die Berechnung von G* und somit die Bestimmung viskoelastischer Gewebeparameter. Die Machbarkeit des Verfahrens wurde mit Agarose- und Ultraschallgel-Proben sowie unterschiedlichen Gewebeproben (Schweineleber, Schweinemuskel und Rinderherz) durchgeführt, wobei sich eine gute Übereinstimmung mit einer Vergleichsuntersuchung an einem Hochfeld Tierscanner gezeigt hat.

1 Einleitung

Die Magnetresonanzelastographie (MRE) [1] ist ein nichtinvasives, medizinisches Bildgebungsverfahren zur Ermittlung viskoelastischer Gewebeeigenschaften für diagnostische Zwecke. Diverse Studien haben bei Leberfibrose [2], Herzerkrankungen [3], neurologischen Erkrankungen [4] und Hirntumoren [5] eine hohe Sensitivität der MRE gegenüber krankhafter Gewebeveränderungen bewiesen. Untersuchungen mittels MRE und Oszillationsrheologie als Referenzmethode haben eine hervorragende Übereinstimmung der ermittelten viskoelastischen Kenngrößen gezeigt [6]. Die hohe Sensitivität der Elastographie für pathologische Veränderungen von biologischen Weichgeweben ist auf die Empfindlichkeit des Schermoduls gegenüber Änderungen der hierarchischen Organisation mechanischer Gewebestrukturen von der zellulären bis hin zur makroskopischen Ebene zurückzuführen [7]. Versuche in Tiermodellen [8, 9, 10] sowie in vivo Studien [7] geben erste Hinweise auf eine Korrelation der MRE mit der Histologie. Die MRE wurde bisher hauptsächlich an Hochfeld-MRT Tierscannern bei 7 Tesla an Tiermodellen und Gewebeproben [11] durchgeführt. Bei Untersuchungen an einem 0.1 T System mit limitierter Gradientenstärke hat sich gezeigt, dass dies für Untersuchungen kleiner Gewebeproben aufgrund des reduzierten Signal-zu-Rausch-Verhältnisses und geringer Bewegungsempfindlichkeit nicht geeignet ist. Im Gegensatz dazu ist das hier verwendete kommerziell verfügbare MRT-Tischgerät mit einem 0.5 T Permanentmagneten ausgestattet und aufgrund des leistungsfähigen Gradientensystems sensitiv für kleine Scherwellenamplituden. Somit ist es potentiell zur MRE von Gewebeproben mit einem Volumen von ca. 1 cm^3 geeignet. Das MRT-Tischgerät zeichnet sich weiterhin durch hohe Benutzerfreundlichkeit und leicht adaptierbare Hard- und Software aus. Das Ziel dieser Arbeit ist die Untersuchung der Einsetzbarkeit des Systems für die MRE an kleinen Gewebeproben sowie die Validierung mittels Vergleichsmessungen an einem 7 T Tierscanner mit MRE-Option.

2   Material und Methoden

2.1   Probenvorbereitung

Für die Experimente wurden die Proben (Ultraschallgel, Agarose, Schweineleber, Rinderherz- und Skelettmuskel vom Schwein) in bodenseitig geschlossene Glasrohre überführt (Innendurchmesser 8 mm). Um eine Dehydrierung zu vermeiden, wurden alle Gewebeproben mit Ultraschallgel bedeckt. Bei Muskelproben mit anisotropen Gewebeeigenschaften wurde die Faserrichtung entlang der Längsachse des Probenbehältnisses ausgerichtet.

2.2   MRE-Setup und Datenakquisition

Zeitharmonische Vibrationssignale ($f=$ 500 bis 1000 Hz in 100 Hz Schritten) wurden zunächst als Wechselspannungssignale mit einem Wellengenerator (Tektronix, Beaverton, OR, USA) erzeugt und danach über einen Audioverstärker (Adam Hall, Neu-Anspach, Deutschland) an einen Lautsprecher (Visaton, Haan, Deutschland) weitergeleitet, mit dem zeitharmonische Auslenkungen induziert wurden. Diese Vibrationen wurden mit einem Karbonfaserstab und einer Klemme auf das, im Zentrum des Magneten positionierte Probenbehältnis übertragen

(Abb. 1, rote Markierung). Für die MRE-Untersuchungen der Proben wurde ein MRT-Tischgerät (Researchlab, Pure Devices GmbH, Würzburg, Deutschland) mit einem 0.5 T Permanentmagneten (MagSpec22 MHz, Pure Devices GmbH, Würzburg, Deutschland) eingesetzt. Zur Datenakquisition wurde eine, in MAT-LAB (Mathworks, Natick, MA, USA) implementierte Spin-Echo-Sequenz durch Erweiterung mit bipolaren trapezförmigen Bewegungskodiergradienten (MEG) beiderseits des refokusierenden RF-Pulses gegenüber Bewegungen sensibilisiert. Die MEG's wurden mit einer Amplitude von 250 mT/m und einer Anstiegsrate von 2000 T/m/s synchron zu den Vibrationsfrequenzen (f = 500, 600, 700, 800, 900 und 1000 Hz mit jeweils 16, 18, 22, 26, 28, und 32 Perioden) geschaltet. Die Messungen wurden über eine, mit einem Laptop verbundene Research-Konsole (drivel, Pure Devices GmbH, Würzburg, Deutschland) gesteuert. Ein Scherweellenzyklus wurde in 8 Zeitschritten mit einem Trigger-Delay von $1/(8f)$-Inkrementen relativ zum Startpunkt der MEG's abgetastet. Pro Vibrationsfrequenz wurden insgesamt 8 Phasendifferenzbilder (16 Wellenbilder mit jeweils umgekehrter Polarität der MEG's zur Elimination statischer Phasenbeiträge) erfasst. Die gesamte Messdauer war abhängig von der Repetitionszeit (TR), die zwischen 500 und 1500 ms variierte und betrug 8 bis 25 Minuten pro Vibrationsfrequenz. Weitere Bildgebungsparameter waren: Echozeit (TE): 40 ms, Matrixgröße: 64 × 64; Field of View (FOV): 15 × 15 mm^2, 3 mm Schichtdicke.

2.3 Datenauswertung

Nach zeitlicher Fourier Transformation über die phasenentfalteten Phasendifferenzbilder wurden die resultierenden komplexen Wellenbilder mit einem Bandpassfilter mit in [11] ermittelten frequenzabhängigen Grenzen gefiltert (für 500, 600, 700, 800, 900 und 1000 Hz jeweils 0.0016, 0.0016, 0.0015, 0.0014, 0.0014, 0.0014 m (untere Schwellwerte) sowie 0.0257, 0.0199, 0.0157, 0.0124, 0.0124, 0.0124 m (obere Schwellwerte)). Daraufhin wurden in den resultierenden geglätteten Wellenbildern der Proben manuell Regions of Interest (ROI's) definiert, für die nachfolgend der komplexe Schermodul G* mit Hilfe einer 2D Helmholtz-

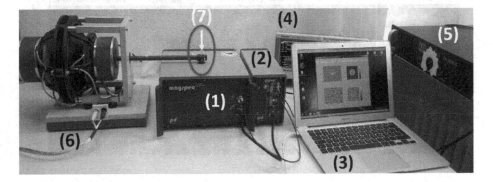

Abb. 1. Experimenteller Aufbau: (1) 0.5 T Permanentmagnet, (2) Konsole, (3) Laptop, (4) Funktionsgenerator, (5) Verstärker, (6) Lautsprecher, (7) Reagenzglas mit Probe.

Inversion [12] berechnet wurde. Ausgehend von G* wurden für alle Proben Speichermodul G' (Elastizität), Verlustmodul G" (Viskosität) sowie das Verhältnis G"/ G' berechnet.

3   Ergebnisse

Abb. 2 zeigt die Wellenbilder (Scherwellenauslenkung) aller Proben bei 500 und 1000 Hz Vibrationsfrequenz mit den zur Auswertung definierten ROI's. Individuelle Scherwellenamplituden können durch Multiplikation der links oben angegebenen Skalierungsfaktoren mit den rechts in den Farbbalken definierten Auslenkungen berechnet werden. Unterschiede erklären sich durch manuelle proben- und frequenzabhängige Anpassung der Verstärkerleistung.

Abb. 3 stellt die frequenzaufgelösten Auswerteresultate für G' und G" sowie das Verhältnis G"/G' dar. Skelettmuskulatur (Abb. 3, rote Kurve) zeigt sowohl für G' als auch für G" die höchsten Werte, gefolgt von Herzmuskelgewebe (schwarze Kurve) und dem Agarosegel-Phantom (blaue Kurve). Die Leberprobe (cyanfarbige Kurve) hat die geringsten Elastizitäts- und Viskositätswerte, die nahezu mit denen der Ultraschallgel-Probe (grüne Kurve) übereinstimmen. Die Ultraschallgel-Probe wurde zusätzlich an einem 7 T Tierscanner mit vergleichbaren Aufnahmeparametern untersucht (grüne gestrichelte Kurve).

4   Diskussion

Im Rahmen dieser Arbeit wurde die Einsetzbarkeit eines für die MRE modifizierten kommerziell verfügbaren MR-Tomographen zur Untersuchung kleiner, biologischer Gewebeproben demonstriert. Mit Hilfe der Ultraschallgel-Probe wurde eine gute Übereinstimmung viskoelastischer Kenngrößen zu einem 7 T Hochfeld-Tierscanner mit MRE-Option gefunden. Dies belegt in Übereinstimmung mit

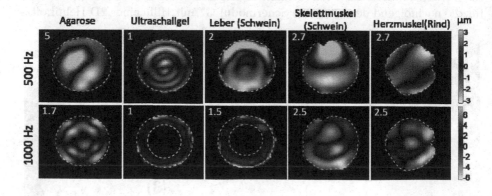

Abb. 2. Wellenbilder der Proben bei 500 Hz und 1000 Hz mit den eingezeichneten ROI's und Skalierungsfaktoren (links oben) zur Berechnung individueller Scherwellenamplituden.

früheren Arbeiten, dass mittels MRE ermittelte viskoelastische Parameter als feldunabhängig betrachtet werden können. Das Verhältnis von Speicher- und Verlustmodul steht in Übereinstimmung mit früheren Ergebnissen [11] und ist am höchsten für Proben mit niedrigem G' bei hohem G" und somit am höchsten für Lebergewebe und Ultraschallgel-Probe, gefolgt von Muskelgewebe. Für Agarosegel sind Schwankungen sichtbar, die auf schwache Dämpfung und daraus resultierender Reflexionen zurückzuführen sind. Interessanterweise sind die viskoelastischen Kenngrößen des Ultraschallgels vergleichbar zum Lebergewebe, wodurch es sich als Material für Leberphantome eignet. Die Auswerteresultate ermöglichen eine Kategorisierung der Gewebeproben anhand ihrer viskoelastischen Eigenschaften.

Bei MRE-Untersuchungen ist das Verhältnis zwischen Scherwellenamplitude und Rauschen im Phasenbild ein wichtigstes Qualitätskriterium für die Güte berechneter viskoelastischer Parameter. Dazu wurden die maximalen Phasenwerte aus der Fundamentalfrequenz (Scherwellenamplitude) mit den der höchsten Harmonischen (Phasenrauschen aus der 3. Harmonischen aufgrund der Abtastung einer Scherwellenperiode in 8 Zeitschritten) normalisiert. Für das 0.5 T MRE-Tischsystem ist das Verhältnis um einen Faktor 4.2 geringer gegenüber dem 7 T Tierscanner. Die durchgeführte Machbarkeitsstudie mit dem vorläufigen experimentellen Setup hat Limitationen, die in weiterführenden Arbeiten optimiert werden können. Beispielsweise kann die, mit langen Aufnahmezeiten verbundene Spin-Echo basierte MRE Sequenz durch Turbo-Spin-Echo Aufnahmetechniken ersetzt werden, welche eine effektivere Auslesung des k-Raums erlauben. Eine Verbesserung der MRE-Hardware kann durch Verwendung von für hochfrequente Vibrationen optimierte piezoelektrische Aktoren und einen externen Gradienten verstärker zur Erhöhung der Bewegungssensitivität erreicht werden. Schließlich können Vibrationen unterschiedlicher Frequenzen in ein Signal überlagert werden [2], wodurch in nur einer Messung die Frequenzabhängigkeit viskoelastischer Parameter ermittelt werden kann. Dies ist wichtig für die angestrebte effiziente Akquisition multifrequenter Datensätze des kompletten Wellenfeldes als Grundlage für die Verwendung neuer Inversionsverfahren zur Erzeugung hochaufgelöster Karten viskoelastischer Parameter.

Zusammengefasst wurde ein kostengünstiges MRE-System zur Analyse kleiner Gewebeproben auf Basis eines 0.5 T MR-Tischgeräts entwickelt und validiert. Das Scherwellenamplituden-Rausch-Verhältnis der MRE-Daten im Rahmen der

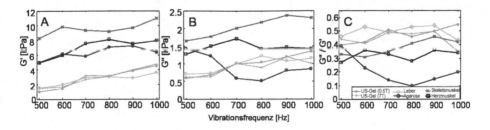

Abb. 3. Auswerteresultate für G', (B) G" und, (C) Verhältnis G"/G' für alle Proben.

vorläufigen MRE-Implementierung ist nur um einen Faktor 4.2 geringer als an einem 7 T Tierscanner. Die Tischgerät-MRE hat somit das Potential zu Untersuchungen kleiner Gewebeproben für eine systematische Analyse der Korrelation von histopathologisch gesicherter Mikrostruktur mit makroskopischen viskoelastischen Parametern.

Literaturverzeichnis

1. Muthupillai R, Lomas DJ, Rossman PJ, et al. Magnetic resonance elastography by direct visualization of propagating acoustic strain waves. Science. 1995;269:1854–7.
2. Asbach P, Klatt D, Schlosser B, et al. Viscoelasticity-based staging of hepatic fibrosis with multifrequency MR elastography. Radiology. 2010;257:80–6.
3. Elgeti T, Knebel F, Hattasch R, et al. Shear-wave amplitudes measured with cardiac MR elastography for diagnosis of diastolic dysfunction. Radiology. 2014;(131605).
4. Wuerfel J, Paul F, Beierbach B, et al. MR-elastography reveals degradation of tissue integrity in multiple sclerosis. NeuroImage. 2010;49:2520–5.
5. Simon M, Guo J, Papazoglou S, et al. Non-invasive characterization of intracranial tumors by MR-Elastography. New J Phys. 2013;15(085024).
6. Yasar TK, Royston TJ, Maginl RL. Wideband MR elastography for viscoelasticity model identification. Magn Reson Med. 2013;70:479–89.
7. Sack I, Joehrens K, Wuerfel E, et al. Structure sensitive elastography: on the viscoelastic powerlaw behavior of in vivo human tissue in health and disease. Soft Matter. 2013;9:5672–80.
8. Klein C, Hain EG, Braun J, et al. Enhanced adult neurogenesis increases brain stiffness: in vivo magnetic resonance elastography in a mouse model of dopamine depletion. PLoS One. 2014;9(0092582).
9. Freimann FB, Muller S, Streitberger KJ, et al. MRE in a murine stroke model reveals correlation of macroscopic viscoelastic properties of the brain with neuronal density. NMR Biomed. 2013;26:1534–9.
10. Klein C, Hain EG, Braun J, et al. Enhanced adult neurogenesis increases brain stiffness: in vivo magnetic resonance elastography in a mouse model of dopamine depletion. PLoS One. 2014;44:1380–6.
11. Riek K, Klatt D, Nuzha H, et al. Wide-range dynamic magnetic resonance elastography. J Biomech. 2011;44:1380–6.
12. Papazoglou S, Hamhaber U, Braun J, et al. Algebraic Helmholtz inversion in planar magnetic resonance elastography. Phys Med Biol. 2014;10(92582).

Portability of TV-Regularized Reconstruction Parameters to Varying Data Sets

Mario Amrehn[1], Andreas Maier[1,2], Frank Dennerlein[1], Joachim Hornegger[1,2]

[1]Pattern Recognition Lab, FAU Erlangen-Nürnberg
[2]Erlangen Graduate School in Advanced Optical Technologies (SAOT)
mario.amrehn@fau.de

Abstract. In C-arm computed tomography there are certain constraints due to the data acquisition process which can cause limited raw data. The reconstructed image's quality may significantly decrease depending on these constraints. To compensate for severely under-sampled projection data during reconstruction, special algorithms have to be utilized, more robust to such ill-posed problems. In the past few years it has been shown that reconstruction algorithms based on the theory of compressed sensing are able to handle incomplete data sets quite well. In this paper, the iterative iTV reconstruction method by Ludwig Ritschl et al. is analyzed regarding it's elimination capabilities of image artifacts caused by incomplete raw data with respect to the settings of it's various parameters. The evaluation of iTV and the data dependency of iterative reconstruction's parameters is conducted in two stages. First, projection data with severe angular under-sampling is acquired using an analytical phantom. Proper reconstruction parameters are selected by analyzing the reconstruction results from a set of proposed parameters. In a second step multiple phantom data sets are acquired with limited angle geometry and a small number of projections. The iTV reconstructions of these data sets are compared to short-scan FDK and SART reconstruction results, highlighting the distinct data dependence of the iTV reconstruction parameters.

1 Introduction

C-arm systems with a mounted X-ray tube and flat panel detector are very popular in medical image acquisition [1]. The C-arm device is typically rotated around the patient in a 200° radius or less. During rotation projection images are acquired and utilized for reconstructing a 3D distribution of the object's X-ray attenuation coefficients. Due to the limited projection angle of the C-arm and a small number of projections severe artifacts may show in the computed coefficients. Reconstructing from limited raw data, the very popular reconstruction method of Feldkamp-Davis-Kress (FDK) [2] does not yield optimal results. Iterative methods are designed to compensate those artifacts by iteratively alternating between backprojecting data into the reconstructed image and projecting intermediate reconstruction images back into the raw data domain. Especially a combination of iterative algorithms with insights from Compressed Sensing [3] seems to improve reconstruction results from limited raw data [4]. The problem arising from those hybrid approaches is twofold. The runtime for a final solution to emerge may significantly increase. Furthermore, the number of parameters to be set by the user may be the sum of the combined method's free variables. This introduces a high dimensional optimization space. In the following, the impact of changes to the parameter set is analyzed.

2   Materials and methods

A method to solve the inverse problem of the Radon transform is to formulate the reconstruction problem as a system of linear equations. A reconstruction is performed minimizing an objective function which may incorporate prior knowledge about the image. One unconstrained objective function for an iterative reconstruction approach is defined by the SSD measure between the original projection values and the projected current image

$$\min \|R\,f(r) - p\|_2^2 \tag{1}$$

where $f(r)$ is the value of voxel $r = (r_1, r_2, r_3)$ in the reconstructed image f. $R\,f(r)$ is the system of linear equations with X-ray transform R. p denotes the measured raw projection data.

2.1   Compressed sensing

Compressed Sensing is a signal processing technique to deal with the problem of incomplete data sets [3, 5] when reconstructing by finding solutions to underdetermined linear systems. It takes advantage of the signal's sparseness or compressibility in some domain, allowing the entire signal to be determined from relatively few measurements. This sparseness can be incorporated into a constraint. A signal is transformed by a sparsifying operator Ψ into a suitable domain for measuring it's compressibility. For a signal $f \in \mathbb{R}^n$ the transformation in an orthonormal basis is defined as $f(t) = \sum_i^n x_i \Psi_i(t)$, where x_i is the coefficient sequence of f, $x_i = \langle f, \Psi_i \rangle$ in the basis Ψ. With under-sampled data, only a subset of all n coefficients of f can be measured

$$y_k = \langle f, \phi_k \rangle, \quad k \in M \subset [1 \ldots n] \tag{2}$$

ϕ_k is the function discretizing f to samples y_k and may be a Dirac delta function shifted by k. The reconstruction is given by $\hat{f} = \Psi \hat{x}$ where $\hat{x}$ is the solution of the convex optimization

$$\min_{x_{\text{app}} \in \mathbb{R}^n} \|x_{\text{app}}\|_{\ell 1} \text{ subject to } y_k = \langle \phi_k, \Psi_{x_{\text{app}}} \rangle \quad \forall k \in M \tag{3}$$

There may be multiple solutions for $\hat{f} = \Psi x_{\text{app}}$. The one is chosen which coefficient sequence minimizes the $\ell 1$ norm, a suitable measure for the function's sparsity. This also penalizes image artifact creation during reconstruction.

2.2   Simultaneous algebraic reconstruction technique (SART)

Starting from an initial guess for the reconstructed object, SART performs a sequence of iterative grid projections and correction back-projections until the reconstruction has converged [6]. An update of the current image is performed after all rays in one projection are processed. Correction terms are computed to update the image voxel values with respect to their objective function, then combined by a weighted sum

$$f_i^{\nu+1} = f_i^\nu + \beta \cdot \sum_{k \in s(\nu)} \frac{1}{\sum_j (R^T)_{i,j}^k} (R^T)_{i,j}^k \frac{\sum_i R_{j,i}^k f_i^\nu - p_j^k}{\sum_i R_{j,i}^k}, \; \nu \in [0, N_{\text{Sub}}[\quad (4)$$

where the system matrix $R_{i,j}^k$ of the k-th projection maps f on p^k. The index i represents an image voxel r. j is a projection's element. The relaxation parameter $\beta \in]0,1]$ controls the convergence speed of the minimization. The choice of the number of subsets N_{Sub} affects the angular distance between successively used projections. All elements of f_i are processed in each sub iteration ν [4]. Iterating over all subsets ν yields one full SART-iteration f_{n+1}^{SART}. SART has many advantages over FDK, such as better noise tolerance and handling of sparse and non-uniformly distributed projection datasets. However, computation time is considerably higher [6].

2.3   Constrained total variation optimization (TV)

With incomplete data the inverse problem to (1) is under-determined causing an infinite number of possible solutions for a reconstructed image. One proposed approach utilizes an iterative reconstruction combined with Compressed Sensing by extending the cost function with a constraint from a priori knowledge. The signal $f(r)$ can be completely reconstructed with a high probability with less samples than required by the Nyquist criterion, if most entries of $\Psi f(r)$ are zero i.e. a sparsifying transformation is known. This is approximated by the $\ell 1$-norm of $\Psi f(r)$ [4, 7] as seen in (3). This yields an inequality-constraint convex optimization function as a penalized least squares approach (Tikhonov regularization)

$$\min \|\Psi f(r)\|_1 \text{ subject to } \|R f(r) - p\|_2^2 < \epsilon \quad (5)$$

minimizing the raw data cost function with the sparsity constraint at a low value. To speed up the computation, iTV [4] minimizes the raw data cost function via SART and image sparsity separately in their own domain, using the image gradient ∇ as Ψ and a Gradient Descent approach, which in each of it's M steps reduces the cost function $\|\nabla f(r)\|_1$, called the total variation

$$f_{n+1,m+1}^{TV}(r) = f_{n+1,m}^{TV}(r) + \alpha \cdot \nabla \|\nabla f_{n+1,m}^{TV}(r)\|_1 \quad (6)$$

$$\nabla \|\nabla f_{n+1,m}^{TV}(r)\|_1 \approx \frac{\left(\nabla_{xx} f_{n+1,m}^{TV} + \nabla_{yy} f_{n+1,m}^{TV} + \nabla_{zz} f_{n+1,m}^{TV}\right)}{\sqrt{\left(\nabla_x f_{n+1,m}^{TV}\right)^2 + \left(\nabla_y f_{n+1,m}^{TV}\right)^2 + \left(\nabla_z f_{n+1,m}^{TV}\right)^2 + \text{regul}^2}}$$
$$(7)$$

Table 1. Default parameters for the iTV reconstruction and it's variations.

Type	β	ω	$\lambda_{\max}$	eTV-Iterations	regul	α_{init}	GD-Iterations
Default	0.4	0.8	1.2	20	10^{-4}	0.3	25
Changes	0.8	0.4	$\{5, \infty\}$	$\{10, 30\}$	10^{-2}	0.8	10

The linear combination of the two resulting intermediate images form a full iTV iteration. An optimal parameter value $\lambda \in]0; 1]$ is determined in the raw data domain by solving the quadratic (9), since ϵ_{n+1} is known and ω is set by the user [4]

$$\epsilon_{n+1} = (1 - \omega) \cdot \|R f_{n+1}^{SART}(r) - p\|_2^2 + \omega \cdot \epsilon_n, \quad \omega \in]0; 1[\tag{8}$$

$$\|R[(1 - \lambda) f_{n+1}^{SART}(r) + \lambda f_{n+1,M}^{TV}(r)] - p\|_2^2 = \epsilon_{n+1} \tag{9}$$

$$f_{n+1} = (1 - \lambda) f_{n+1}^{SART}(r) + \lambda f_{n+1,M}^{TV}(r) \tag{10}$$

3   Results

To evaluate the portability of a parameter set for iTV, a two-pass experiment is performed. In the first stage a proper parameter set for a given reconstruction problem is evaluated. In the second stage, the parameter set is used for different reconstruction scenarios as proposed in [8]. All reconstructions were computed on projection images corrupted with Poisson distributed noise and a simulated radiation dose of $k = 10^6$ X-ray photons.

On a circular trajectory of radius 750 mm with a detector-source distance of 1200 mm, 227 projections are simulated on an angle of 170.25° with an angular increment of .75°. The detector's 800×800 pixel size is 6 mm in each dimension. The ground truth data is a $512 \times 512 \times 174$ centered version of the FORBILD head phantom with 6 mm regular hexahedron voxels. For the parameter search, a star-shaped pattern is chosen, i.e. from a default set only one parameter is altered prior to a new reconstruction run. After these ten reconstructions seen in Tab. 1 the best set is chosen by the RMSE, Pearson Correlation, MSSIM, PSNR, TV norm metrics as well as human inspection. The unambiguously best result comes from the default set plus relaxation parameter $\beta = 8$ In the second part, phantoms were reconstructed with limited angle and few projections through angular incrementation. Results for limited angle are presented in Tab. 2. Graphical results are presented in Fig. 1.

4   Discussion

The fixed set of parameters optimized for a limited angle acquisition of the FORBILD head phantom was used during reconstruction of various scenarios.

Table 2. Reconstruction results with limited angle relative to ground truth or FDK in percent. Left FORBILD head, right human head phantom.

		200°	185°	170°	155°	140°	200°	185°	170°	155°	140°
	RMSE	56.0	49.9	50.5	51.1	46.7	57.7	49.1	55.8	56.7	53.9
	PC	101.5	102.6	103.1	103.1	105.7	57.7	49.1	55.8	56.7	53.9
SART	MSSIM	96.7	89.9	100.9	113.5	124.1	99.2	108.5	118.1	122.4	134.2
	PSNR	155.7	171.8	156.0	163.6	208.7	141.5	145.2	140.5	148.4	147.3
	TVNORM	135.4	117.1	122.9	129.4	144.5	125.5	112.0	119.0	121.4	133.7
	RMSE	16.6	19.4	29.2	31.5	37.9	44.9	38.2	52.4	51.7	47.1
	PC	102.1	103.4	103.9	104.0	106.6	102.2	103.8	104.6	105.3	110.4
iTV	MSSIM	140.9	131.5	149.1	168.7	180.5	111.9	123.2	131.2	137.3	159.4
	PSNR	149.1	138.1	127.1	134.8	168.1	122.8	129.3	120.9	121.9	128.5
	TVNORM	57.2	49.9	46.1	45.8	47.8	40.8	35.6	29.4	29.8	34.2

4.1 Limited angle

For the FORBILD head phantom data and limited angle geometry, the SART and the iTV algorithm are superior to the short-scan FDK method in terms of the introduced error metrics, the RMSE in particular. The iTV reconstruction is superior to the SART method according to every metric except the Peak Signal-to-Noise Ratio causing more blurred transitions at the inner boundaries

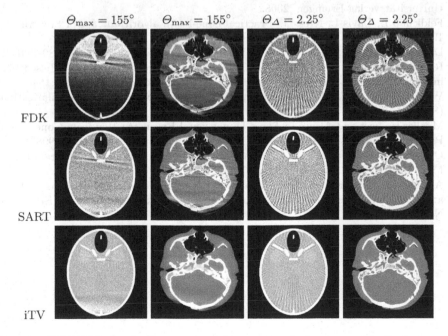

Fig. 1. FORBILD head phantom and human head phantom with limited angle ($\Theta_{max} = 155°$) and few projections ($\Theta_\Delta = 2.25°$). WC:0, WW:{200, 1000}.

of the object. The inhomogeneous regions resulting from the X-ray photon noise induced and streak artifacts are less prominent in iTV improving the perception of low contrast elements. However, the porous bone structure of the human head phantom got blurred significantly using the same set of parameters for this reconstruction.

4.2 Few projections

According to the error metrics, there is a clear hierarchy in the assessment of data quality with few projections. The RMSE of the iTV method is less than half the SART's. Elements with small changes in their attenuation coefficients are better preserved and not partially overlayed by streaks. For the FORBILD head phantom iTV performs a superior preservation of resolution. Again, more structure is lost in the human head phantom reconstruction. Altogether, iTV handles under-sampled data due to a high angular increment over a short-scan acquisition procedure quite well. However, it becomes apparent that a proper parameter set for limited angle may not be transferable to different geometries without a loss in quality.

References

1. Dennerlein F. Image Reconstruction from Fan-Beam and Cone-Beam Projections. Universitätsverlag Erlangen; 2008.
2. Feldkamp L, Davis L, Kress J. Practical cone-beam algorithm. J Opt Soc Am A. 1984;1(6):612–9.
3. Donoho DL. Compressed sensing. IEEE Trans Inf Theory. 2006;52(4):1289–306.
4. Ritschl L, Bergner F, Fleischmann C, et al. Improved total variation-based CT image reconstruction applied to clinical data. Phys Med Biol. 2011;56(6):1545.
5. Wu H, Maier A, Fahrig R, et al. Spatial-temporal total variation regularization (STTVR) for 4D-CT reconstruction. Proc SPIE. 2012; p. 83133J.
6. Mueller K. Fast and Accurate Three-Dimensional Reconstruction from Cone-Beam Projection Data Using Algebraic Methods. The Ohio State University; 1998.
7. Chambolle A. An algorithm for total variation minimization and applications. J Math Imaging Vis. 2004;20(1-2):89–97.
8. Amrehn M. Implementation and Evaluation of a Total Variation Regularized Iterative CT image Reconstruction Method. Friedrich-Alexander-University Erlangen-Nürnberg; 2014.

Projection-Based Denoising Method for Photon-Counting Energy-Resolving Detectors

Yanye Lu[1,5], Michael Manhart[1,3], Oliver Taubmann[1,4], Tobias Zobel[1],
Qiao Yang[1], Jang-hwan Choi[2], Meng Wu[2], Arnd Doerfler[3], Rebecca Fahrig[2],
Qiushi Ren[5], Joachim Hornegger[1,4], Andreas Maier[1,4]

[1]Pattern Recognition Lab, Department of Computer Science,
Friedrich-Alexander-Universität Erlangen-Nürnberg, Germany
[2]Department of Radiology, Stanford University, CA, USA
[3]Department of Neuroradiology, Universitätsklinikum Erlangen, Germany
[4]Erlangen Graduate School in Advanced Optical Technologies (SAOT), Germany
[5]Department of Biomedical Engineering, Peking University, Beijing, China
yanye.lu@fau.de

Abstract. In this paper, we present a novel projection-based novel noise reduction method for photon counting energy resolving detectors in Spectral Computed Tomography (CT) imaging. In order to denoise the projection data, a guidance image from all energy channels is computed, which employs a variant of the joint bilateral filter to denoise each energy bin individually. The method is evaluated by a simulation study of cone beam CT data. We achieve a reduction of noise in individual channels by 80% while at the same time preserving edges and structures well in the results, which indicate that the methods are applicable to clinical practice.

1 Introduction

Polychromatic X-ray sources are commonly employed for medical Computed Tomography (CT). However, most of them are processed as mono-energetic CT measurements by conventional CT detectors which can not take advantage of the energy information in the X-ray beam. In recent years, development of Spectral Computed Tomography (SCT), which plays a vital role in Quantitative Computed Tomography (QCT) [1], has been accelerated by many technologies in both hardware and software. For QCT-reconstruction, spectral input data requires multiple measurements with different spectral characteristics of each projection bin. SCT facilitates the quantitative measurement of material properties. It has broad potential for applications in the preclinical and the clinical field, allowing for visualization of bone and plaque, measurement of blood volume, or quantification of contrast agent concentrations.

Unfortunately, by splitting the acquired photons into different energy bins, each energy channel suffers from a low signal-to-noise ratio leading to noisy projection images, especially in the low energy portion of the energy spectum. Therefore an appropriate noise reduction method is required to obtain reliable image quality in clinical applications. Iterative reconstruction methods have shown superior advantages in noise reduction, but suffer from high complexity, which is a shortcoming in practical applications, especially in interventional medical image processing cases. It is worth mentioning that the noise from photon-counting energy-resolving detectors can be modeled by using Poisson statistics accurately and easily, which is a great advantage in projection based denoising processing. In light of this, besides post-processing approaches on reconstructed images, filtering in pre-processing on projection data is also presented by several studies, such as using noise adaptive filter kernels [2, 3] and edge preserving filters [4, 5].

In this paper, we present a novel contribution to bring this new technology closer to clinical practice: improved noise reduction using non-linear techniques in fluoroscopic imaging. Below we give a short review of X-ray absorption physics, then describe our denoising approach. Subsequently, simulated results are presented.

2   Materials and methods

2.1   Polychromatic X-ray absorption

Traditional X-ray detectors measure the integral of the incident X-ray spectrum at each pixel

$$I = \sum_{i=1}^{E} N_i L_i e^{-\sum_{j=1}^{M} \mu_{ij} l_j} \tag{1}$$

where E denotes the number of considered energy levels, N_i the number of emitted photons at energy level L_i, M the number of considered materials, μ_{ij} the energy and material dependent X-ray absorption, and l_j the path length in the respective material j. In this measurement, each photon is weighted with its energy, which results in a weighted sum of Poisson distributed random variables.

Photon-counting detectors are able to detect each photon individually. Thus, the integral from (1) simplifies to

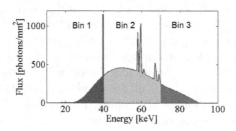

Fig. 1. Binning of a X-ray spectrum into 3 bins.

$$I = \sum_{i=1}^{E} N_i e^{-\sum_{j=1}^{M} \mu_{ij} l_j} \qquad (2)$$

In the energy-resolving case, we get more than a single measurement per pixel (Fig. 1). We differentiate the photons into $b = 1 \ldots B$ different energy channels or bins

$$I_b = \sum_{i=l_b^s}^{l_b^e} N_i e^{-\sum_{j=1}^{M} \mu_{ij} l_j} \qquad (3)$$

where l_b^s and l_b^e are the respective start and end indices of the considered energies in bin b. The energy-selective channels suffer from more noise than the measurements over the complete spectrum, because number of photons corresponding to each bin is is reduced from $I_0 = \sum_{i=0}^{E-1} N_i$ to $I_b^0 = \sum_{i=l_b^s}^{l_b^e} N_i$ and the signal-to-noise ratio in the Poisson process in proportional to $\sqrt{I^0}$ and $\sqrt{I_b^0}$, respectively.

2.2   Noise reduction with joint bilateral filtering

To obtain an image with distinct structures and reduced noise, we add the photons of all energy-selective projection images I_b to recover the projection image I covering the full energy spectrum

$$I = \sum_{b=1}^{B} I_b \qquad (4)$$

Note that this procedure is optimal in terms of weighting of the noise variances. We use I as a guidance image for a joint bilateral filter (JBF) [6] to compute energy-selective projection images I_b' with reduced noise but preserved structures

$$I_b'(x, y) = \frac{1}{c(x, y)} \sum_{i,j} g_s(x, i, y, j) g_I(x, i, y, j) I_b(x, y) \qquad (5)$$

$$c(x, y) = \sum_{i,j} g_s(x, i, y, j) g_I(x, i, y, j) \qquad (6)$$

$$g_s(x, i, y, j) = e^{-\frac{(x-i)^2 + (y-j)^2}{2\sigma_s}} \qquad (7)$$

$$g_I(x, i, y, j) = e^{-\frac{(I(x,y) - I(i,j))^2}{2\sigma_I}} \qquad (8)$$

where $g_s(x, i, y, j)$ is the spatial kernel controlled by σ_s and $g_I(x, i, y, j)$ is the range kernel controlled by σ_I and the guidance image I.

The range kernel is configured such that a certain contrast difference D is preserved

$$D = I_1 - I_2 \tag{9}$$

In case of a monochromatic angiography image, D can be defined using $I_1 = I^0 e^{-\mu^{bg} l^{bg}}$ and $I_2 = I^0 e^{-(\mu^{bg} l^{bg}) - (\mu^v l^v)}$. The X-ray absorption μ^{bg} and the path length l^{bg} correspond to the anatomic background, while μ^v and l^v define absorption and path length corresponding to a contrast agent filled vessel. Insertion into (9) yields

$$D = I_1 - I_2 = I^0 e^{-\mu^{bg} l^{bg}} - I^0 e^{-(\mu^{bg} l^{bg}) - (\mu^v l^v)} = I_1 (1 - e^{-\mu^v l^v}) = I_1 z \tag{10}$$

where the parameter z is only dependent on the vessel size and material. Note that z can be conveniently computed as $z = 1 - \frac{I_2}{I_1}$. This leads to a contour adaptive definition of the bilateral filter with $\sigma_I = \bar{I}(x, y) \cdot z$, where $\bar{I}(x, y)$ is the mean value of the guidance image in a local neighborhood.

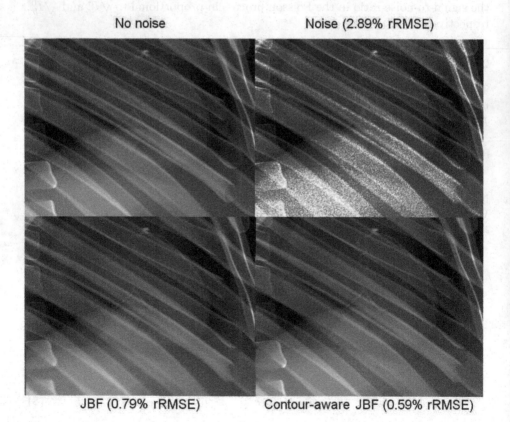

Fig. 2. Line integral images with and without noise (top row) and after restoration using JBF filtering (bottom row).

2.3   Experimental setup

We simulated a set of fluoroscopic images using an append buffer based rendering procedure [7] using XCAT [8]. An X-ray spectrum with the same half layer values as a commercially available C-arm system is used. Projection size was simulated with 620×480 pixels with a pixel size of 0.6×0.6 mm. The peak-voltage was set to 90 kV. We applied a time current product of 2.5 mAs, which is comparable to the dose setting per projection in a clinical 3D scan. The projection was centered around the heart to focus on the coronary arteries, which were filled with an iodine-based contrast medium (comparable to Ultravist 370). Energy-dependent X-ray absorption coefficients for elemental data and compounds such as bone were obtained from the NIST database [9]. All methods were implemented in the CONRAD framework [10] and will be made available as open source software.

3   Results

Fig. 2 displays the simulated images of the first energy channel with and without noise. The relative root mean square error (rRMSE) that is normalized with the maximal intensity in the noise-free image is reduced from 2.89% to 0.59%. Note that the rRMSE was only evaluated at pixels that did not suffer from photon starvation (excessive white noise) in the noisy image, while all pixels were considered for the JBF denoised images.

4   Discussion

We presented a novel approach for noise reduction of energy-resolved projection images. The idea of a contour-aware joint bilateral filtering to energy-resolving detectors is applied in this study, which could reduce noise but well preserve edges and structures. As shown in the result, denoising with JBF and contour-aware JBF is very successful, which could reduce noise by 80% while at the same time preserving edges and structures well. We will apply this method to realistic data in the future work and explore potential clinical applications.

Acknowledgement. The authors gratefully acknowledge funding of the Medical Valley national leading edge cluster, Erlangen, Germany, diagnostic imaging network, sub-project BD 16, research grant nr. 13EX1212G.

References

1. Heismann BJ, Schmidt BT, Flohr TG. Spectral computed tomography. Proc SPIE. 2012.
2. Kachelrieß M, Watzke O, Kalender WA. Generalized multi-dimensional adaptive filtering for conventional and spiral single-slice, multi-slice, and cone-beam CT. Med Phys. 2001;28(4):475–90.

3. Zeng GL, Zamyatin A. A filtered backprojection algorithm with ray-by-ray noise weighting. Med Phys. 2013;40(3):031113-1-7.
4. Manduca A, Yu L, Trzasko JD, et al. Projection space denoising with bilateral filtering and CT noise modeling for dose reduction in CT. Med Phys. 2009;36(11):4911-9.
5. Manhart M, Fahrig R, Hornegger J, et al. Guided noise reduction for spectral CT with energy-selective photon counting detectors. Proc CT Meet. 2014; p. 91-4.
6. Petschnigg G, Szeliski R, Agrawala M, et al. Digital photography with flash and no-flash image pairs. ACM Trans Graph. 2004;23(3):664-72.
7. Maier A, Hofmann HG, Schwemmer C, et al. Fast simulation of x-ray projections of spline-based surfaces using an append buffer. Phys Med Biol. 2012;57(19):6193-210.
8. Segars WP, Sturgeon G, Mendonca S, et al. 4D XCAT phantom for multimodality imaging research. Med Phys. 2010;37(9):4902-15.
9. Hubbell JH, Seltzer SM. Tables of X-ray Mass Attenuation Coefficients and Mass Energy Absorption Coefficients. National Inst. of Standards and Technology-PL, Gaithersburg, MD (United States). Ionizing Radiation Div.; 1995.
10. Maier A, Hofmann H, Berger M, et al. CONRAD: a software framework for cone-beam imaging in radiology. Med Phys. 2013;40(11):111914-1-8.

Reference Volume Generation for Subsequent 3D Reconstruction of Histological Sections

Martin Schober[1], Philipp Schlömer[1], Markus Cremer[1], Hartmut Mohlberg[1],
Anh-Minh Huynh[1], Nicole Schubert[1], Mehmet E. Kirlangic[1],
Katrin Amunts[1,2], Markus Axer[1]

[1]Institute of Neuroscience and Medicine (INM-1), Research Center Jülich, Germany
[2]C. and O. Vogt Institute for Brain Research, Heinrich Heine University Düsseldorf,
Germany
m.schober@fz-juelich.de

Abstract. Anatomical reference brains are indispensable tools in human brain mapping, enabling the integration of multimodal data or the alignment of a series of adjacent histological brain sections into an anatomically realistic space. This study describes a robust and efficient method for an automatic 3D reconstruction of blockface images taken from postmortem brains during cutting as a prerequisite for high-quality 3D reconstruction of brain sections. The refinement technique used in this registration method is applicable for a broad range of pre-registered histological stacks.

1 Introduction

High-resolution 3D models of the human brain are necessary prerequisites to understand the brain's organization at the microscopical level. This has recently been shown for 3D cytoarchitectonics [1] and for revealing the nerve fiber architecture [2] including the distribution of axons and thin fiber bundles. In order to compute 3D reconstructed stacks of histological sections, it is necessary to eliminate artifacts, which are introduced during tissue processing, e.g. cutting and mounting [3]. Blockface images, which are obtained during cutting brains, are largely undistorted and therefore represent an important reference to recover the spatial coherence of the non-linearly deformed histological sections. Blockface registration using corners of a checkerboard placed underneath a postmortem brain has been introduced by our own group in order to achieve a high-quality 3D reconstruction [4]. Here we show a robust and efficient method for the automatic 3D reconstruction of blockface images, which is based on two steps of registration.

2 Materials and methods

The presented method comprises two parts of registration: a marker-based alignment and a median-based refinement of the volume stack using 3D information.

The first part of the algorithm is based on the use of ARTag markers, which have been established in the fields of augmented reality and computer vision to trace camera positions and orientations in real-time [5]. Each marker represents an individual identifying number and encodes a triplicate of a 12-bit number in a 6x6 array of black and white pixels. Fig. 1 shows a blockface image of the left temporal lobe of a human brain placed on a pattern of ARTag markers.

The patterns of markers guarantee a robust code identification by a "majority vote"; such algorithm is important in an environment, where the markers are likely to be partially covered, e.g. by ice crystals or sectioning residues. The detection of the markers was realized by implementation of the ARToolkitPlus library [6]. The basic idea to use ARTag markers for blockface image registration is to extract the coordinates of the same markers in different blockface images and to align them to each other by means of an affine registration transformation.

However, the approach using only marker matching in the background causes perspective errors in the brain tissue due to the fact that the cutting plane of the brain and the background containing the marker pattern have decisively different distances to the camera lens. If the registration algorithm has to correct higher translations of a brain section, these perspective errors will become larger (Fig. 2). This figure demonstrates the accuracy of registration in the marker plane in contrast to the tissue plane.

These larger perspective errors appear in average in 10% of all brain sections. Therefore, in the second part of the developed algorithm the median along the depth (z-axis) of the marker-based aligned sections was calculated to eliminate these outliers caused by perspective errors. Fig. 3 shows the principle of this median calculation. Here, the sliding window radius is set to 2 pixels, the datasets

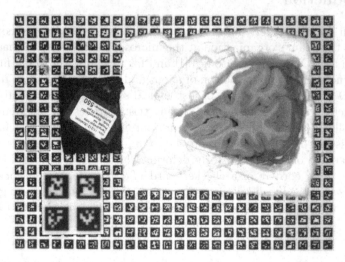

Fig. 1. Blockface image of the left temporal lobe of a human brain placed on a pattern of ARTag markers. The tissue block has been cut in coronal plane from anterior to posterior and was further processed for 3D-PLI[2]. The image size is 3272x2469 pixels with a pixel size of 66 μm x 66 μm.

Fig. 2. Two adjacent mouse brain sections registered by alignment of ARTag markers. The two upper lines show the registration error between the tissue sections while the lower line indicates the high accuracy of the marker alignment.

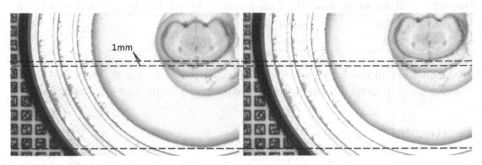

shown in this article have been processed with a radius of 5 pixels. In a next step, the marker-based aligned images were registered section-by-section onto the median volume using a translation transform estimated by the pixel-based image registration algorithm provided by the Insight Toolkit Library, ITK [7]. By using this technique there is taken advantage of 3D information in an actually 2D section-by-section registration method. This procedure has been applied to different types of blockface images acquired from both paraffin embedded and frozen brains in different types of microtomes with different camera setups. A total number of about 12,000 blockface images has been processed so far, which includes brain sections from tissue blocks and whole brains of different species (mouse, rat, vervet monkey, human). The examples shown in this study were taken from a left human temporal lobe, a left human hemisphere, a vervet mon-

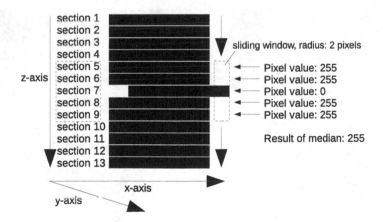

Fig. 3. Calculation of median volume: The median of pixel values is calculated within a sliding window with constant pixel radius along z-axis. In this example the pixel value in the picked xy-coordinate in section 7 is set to a pixel intensity of 255 in the new median section. This filtering is done for all xy-coordinates of each section and results in a stack of median sections.

Table 1. Averaged sum of squared intensity differences between neighboring sections of unprocessed and registered stacks. Values have been averaged for each stack.

Dataset	Hum. temp. lobe	Hum. hemisphere	Vervet Monkey brain	Mouse brain
Unprocessed	439.8	404.4	278.0	498.2
Registered	20.2	88.3	21.6	24.2

key brain and a mouse brain, which were further processed for 3D Polarized Light Imaging to map nerve fibers and their pathways in white and gray matter [2].

3   Results

The first step of the algorithm, the marker-based alignment, provided highly accurate results in the pattern plane in each of the processed datasets as visually examined by an expert. However, this accuracy can not inevitably be transferred to the sectioning plane of the brain (Fig. 2). In case of using small-scale microtomes for small tissue samples from rodent brains, for instance, the perspective errors in the cutting plane were most significant due to the close distance to the camera lens. The elimination of perspective outliers in the cutting plane using the median-based refinement improved the accuracy of results significantly. Fig. 4 indicates the importance of this refinement step.

The quality of the registration results has been evaluated by using the sum of squared intensity differences algorithm as similarity measure between neighboring sections [8]. These measures have been taken in unprocessed and in registered stacks of the four datasets mentioned before. For each stack all measured values have been averaged (Tab. 1).

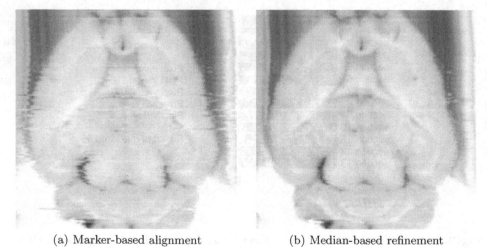

(a) Marker-based alignment   (b) Median-based refinement

Fig. 4. Orthogonal views of the registered blockface images of a mouse brain demonstrating the difference between marker-based alignment and the median-based refinement.

Furthermore, the quality of all reconstructed stacks of brain sections was approved by visual evaluation. An important criterion for a visual evaluation of the quality of registration results is the improvement of recognizability of fine structures and the smoothness of structures, e.g., the transition between white and gray matter [9]. To give an example, the Hippocampus of the human left temporal lobe in Fig. 5(a) is clearly recognizable in the registered volume in contrast to the unprocessed volume. Fig. 5 demonstrates the quality of the finally generated blockface references of a human temporal lobe and a left human hemisphere as a volume, a vervet monkey brain and a mouse brain in orthogonal views. The quality of the results is independent of the considered species, brain size and quality of datasets. Since the algorithm was parallelized, the processing time of a dataset of 1,000 sections was reduced from four hours to 15 minutes using six compute nodes of the iDataplex Cluster JuDGE (Juelich Dedicated GPU Environment) in the Juelich Supercomputing Centre of the Research Centre Juelich in Germany.

4 Discussion

We have successfully implemented a fully automated and robust method to align different kinds of blockface datasets acquired with different microtome setups using ARTag markers. It has been demonstrated that the results are highly accurate and the quality of reconstruction is reproducible. The results are independent of the considered species, the type and any characteristics of the object we want to generate a reference for. Blockfaces are not distorted by cutting processes, and therefore provide an excellent reference (i) due to their high in-plane

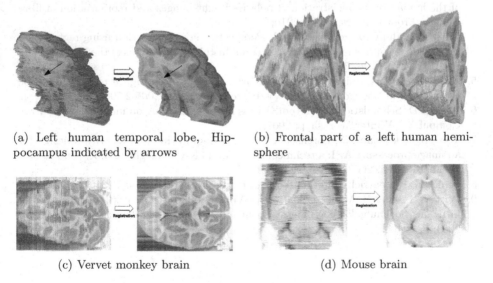

(a) Left human temporal lobe, Hippocampus indicated by arrows

(b) Frontal part of a left human hemisphere

(c) Vervet monkey brain

(d) Mouse brain

Fig. 5. Results of the registration process for various types of datasets. Unprocessed volumes are shown on the left and registered volumes on the right.

resolution and (ii) due to their correspondences to the scanned and analyzed histological sections. In this context, the blockface volume bridges the gap between MRI measurements and anatomical individual sections of the same brain sample. Blockface images reconstructed by the algorithm described in this article are used as references for histological brain sections, autoradiographic images and 3D-PLI Fibre Orientation Maps.

The last step of the registration process, the alignment to the median, can be integrated into any kind of registration workflows or methods. This technique is also applicable to pre-registered 3D-PLI Fibre Orientation Maps [2] or any kind of pre-registered histological stacks.

Acknowledgement. This study was partially supported by the National Institutes of Health under grant agreement no. R01MH 092311, by the Helmholtz Association through the Helmholtz Portfolio Theme "Supercomputing and Modeling for the Human Brain", and by the European Union Seventh Framework Programme (FP7/2007-2013) under grant agreement no. 604102 (Human Brain Project).

References

1. Amunts K, Lepage C, Borgeat L, et al. BigBrain: an ultrahigh-resolution 3D human brain model. Science. 2013;340(6139):1472–5.
2. Axer M, Amunts K, Gräßel D, et al. A novel approach to the human connectome: ultra-high resolution mapping of fiber tracts in the brain. NeuroImage. 2011;54(2):1091–101.
3. Palm C, Axer M, Gräßel D, et al. Towards ultra-high resolution fibre tract mapping of the human brain–registration of polarised light images and reorientation of fibre vectors. Front Hum Neurosci. 2010;4.
4. Eiben B, Palm C, Pietrzyk U, et al. Perspective error correction using registration for blockface volume reconstruction of serial histological sections of the human brain. Proc BVM. 2010; p. 301–5.
5. Fiala M. Artag revision 1, a fiducial marker system using digital techniques. Proc IEEE Comput Soc Conf Comput Vis Pattern Recognit. 2005;2:590–6.
6. Wagner D, Schmalstieg D. ARToolKitPlus for pose tracking on mobile devices. Proc Comput Vis Winter Workshop; 2007.
7. Yoo TS, Ackerman MJ, Lorensen WE, et al. Engineering and algorithm design for an image processing API: a technical report on ITK-the insight toolkit. Stud Health Technol Inform. 2002; p. 586–92.
8. Sonka M, Fitzpatrick JM. Handbook of medical imaging. Proc SPIE. 2000;2.
9. Wirtz S, Fischer B, Modersitzki J, et al. Vollständige Rekonstruktion eines Rattenhirns aus hochaufgelösten Bildern von histologischen Serienschnitten. Proc BVM. 2004; p. 204–8.

3D Reconstruction of Histological Rat Brain Images

Nicole Schubert[1], Mehmet E. Kirlangic[1], Martin Schober[1], Anh-Minh Huynh[1], Katrin Amunts[1,2], Karl Zilles[1,3], Markus Axer[1,2]

[1]Institute of Neuroscience and Medicine (INM-1), Research Centre Juelich
[2]C. a. O. Vogt Institute of Brain Research, Heinrich-Heine-University Düsseldorf
[3]Department of Psychiatry, Psychotherapy and Psychosomatics, RWTH University Aachen
n.schubert@fz-juelich.de

Abstract. Histology of brain sections provides the opportunity to analyse the brain structure on a microscopic level. Histological sections have to be aligned into a 3D reference volume to obtain a correct spatial localization of cell structures. This paper presents a new approach of a rigid registration method of histological sections to a blockface volume. The method and the results are validated by using synthetic data and experimental histological rat brain images. The results indicate a robust, simple and valid image registration method.

1 Introduction

Despite the progress in neuro-imaging, the microscopical analysis of brain structure is still required to understand the organisation of the brain. Therefore, histological imaging is an important modality in neuroscience to investigate cell types, structures and spatial localization of neurons. Thereby, postmortem brains were processed in a microtome and thin brain sections were prepared. This results in loss of spatial correlation between brain sections. Hence, it is necessary to re-align the sections to obtain correct 3D information of the neuronal structures across the whole brain.

Different approaches of image registration methods investigate the problem of 3D reconstruction. For instance, Palm et. al. [1] used rigid methods, whereas others applied elastic methods [2]. In [3] image registration of sectioned brains was comprehensively reviewed. A fundamental problem in 3D reconstruction is the anatomically correct alignment of the brain sections, where a "cucumber effect" can occur due to the lack of a suitable 3D reference [1].

To show the quality of the methods an accurate gold standard has to be found. This is a major challenge in image registration validation [4]. Common ways for validation are phantom studies, simulations, comparison with other registration methods or assessment by experts.

This paper presents a rigid registration approach to align histological sections into a 3D reference. A reconstructed brain volume of so called blockface images

(images of the surface of the brain block during sectioning) was used as an anatomical reference. A validation of the registration method was shown using generated test data. In addition, the results of the test data and experimental rat brains were validated with the help of three uncorrelated quality criteria and a landmark based validation. We introduce a simple, fast and robust method for reconstructing histological sections.

2 Materials and methods

2.1 Data acquisition

Whole rat brains (Fig. 1, left) were frozen and embedded in Tissue Tek® on a specimen holder in a microtome cryostat. Before sectioning a blockface image of every section was taken with a CCD camera (Fig. 1, middle), which was installed above the cryostat (2588 × 1958 pixels, 0.015 mm × 0.015 mm, RGB). The brain was serially cut in coronal sections of 0.02 mm thickness. Thus, a whole rat brain was sectioned into approximately 1500 sections. After melting the sections onto a glass slide, every third section was stained with a modified silver method to visualize important structural features of neurons [5] (Fig. 1, right). The remaining sections were used for quantitative autoradiography [6]. The resulting resolution of the histological sections in cutting direction was therefore 0.06 mm. Histological sections were digitized by using a high resolution camera system (4164 × 3120 pixels, 0.005 mm × 0.005 mm, RGB).

2.2 Reconstruction workflow

The details of the reconstruction of the blockface images were described in [7]. The marker based method provides a 3D reference without cut artefacts or spatial loss of structure. After the reconstruction the blockface volume was segmented from background (Tissue Tek®) using a 3D watershed algorithm.

The following section describes the workflow of the reconstruction of the histological sections:

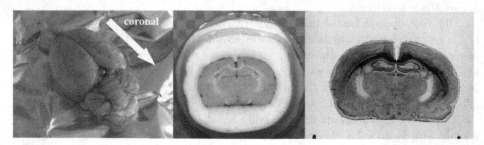

Fig. 1. Left: rat brain after removal, middle: blockface image, right: histological image.

1. In a *preprocessing step* each image was visually inspected. Completely damaged sections, for instance with huge gaps or folds, were replaced by a neighboring section without artefacts. These damaged sections were not used for a later analysis. This substitution was possible due to the fact, that the anatomical structures did not vary significantly between directly neighboring sections.
2. In the *segmentation step*, the histological tissue was separated from the background. Because of the high contrast between the tissue and the background, and the homogeneity of the background, a simple thresholding method could be used. The segmentation results were approved by an anatomical expert.
3. The reconstruction was performed by means of a *rigid registration* of a histological stack to the corresponding section of the blockface volume based on their segmentation masks. First, the centers of gravity in both images were calculated and aligned. Thereafter, a brute force optimizer systematically tested all the potential combinations of rotation angles in search for the best solution. We used sum of squared differences as the metric.
4. An optional *refinement step* was used to handle sections with loss of tissue. Here, the additional optimization of translation also considered the inner structures of the sections.

2.3   Reconstruction validation

Finding a ground truth for validation of an algorithm is a well known problem in image registration. To simulate test data, which were close to our experimental data, we used the recently published Waxholm Space atlas of the Spraque Dawley rat brain (WHS atlas) [8]. It is a volumetric atlas based on high resolution MRI, which also provides a volumetric brain mask. The high resolution of the rat atlas ($512 \times 1024 \times 512$ pixels, 0.039 mm isotropic) is comparable with our data sets. The test data were generated by reslicing the WHS brain mask in the coronal direction to simulate a coronal sectioning. Afterwards, the sectioned masks were randomly translated and rotated within specific ranges ($[-5\,\text{mm}, 5\,\text{mm}], [-90°, 90°]$), similar to our histological sections. The histological sections are smaller than the blockface images due to the freezing procedure. Hence, the test sections were shrinked about 0.03% by removing contour pixels.

2.4   Quality measures

One approach to determine the quality of the registration is to calculate the mean square error between the known transformation of the test data and the estimated transformation of the reconstructed data [9]. The known transformation is applied to a circle, on which a point is marked. The new position of the point can be calculated with the rigid transformation equation with rotation angle θ, translation values (t_x, t_y), rotation centre (c_x, c_y) and the point coordinates (x, y)

$$T_{\text{rigid}}(x, y, \theta, t_x, t_y) = \begin{pmatrix} \cos\theta & -\sin\theta \\ \sin\theta & \cos\theta \end{pmatrix} \begin{pmatrix} x - c_x \\ y - c_y \end{pmatrix} + \begin{pmatrix} t_x + c_x \\ t_y + c_y \end{pmatrix} \tag{1}$$

The estimated transformation of the registration is inverted and applied to the original circle. Now, with both transformed points the mean square error by the Euclidean distance between the two points provides measure of the quality of the registration algorithm independent of any metric or interpolation method.

Another approach is to compare the results of the registration with the help of several discrepancy measures usually used in segmentation validation. A comprehensive evaluation suggests the use of three uncorrelated measures, that cover different aspects of the segmentation: the Dice coefficient, the average surface distance and the Hausdorff distance [10]. The Dice coefficient determines the overlap of two segments, whereby 0 is the result of disjunct segments and 1 is the result of the same segments. The average surface distance determines the minimal distance in mm of one segment to the other and vice versa. This value is 0 for a perfect registration. The Hausdorff distance is defined as the maximum distance in mm of a segment to the nearest point in another segment and vice versa. A low Hausdorff distance indicates a good match. These measure values were applied to both, the test data and the experimental data.

Although, the measures enable the validation of the algorithm and the results of matching the masks, they do not prove the correctness of the inner anatomical structures. Thus, the inner structure of the tissue is needed to be compared with the help of corresponding landmarks set in blockface and histological images by an anatomical expert. The quality is determined with the Euclidean distance between the landmarks after the registration procedure.

3   Results

The registration method was applied to 10 generated test data. The reconstructed volume is quite similar to the original 3D volume (Fig. 2). The mean distance error of the transformations is 0.058 ± 0.004 mm, which indicates a very

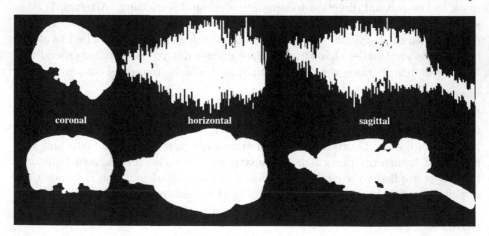

Fig. 2. Generated test data set, first row: before registration, second row: after registration.

Table 1. The validation by using landmarks results in a total mean square error (mse) of 0.213±0.091 mm. The table shows mse and standard deviation σ of selected sections.

Section	32	62	116	166	249	266	307	351	385	439
mse	0.125	0.080	0.166	0.163	0.114	0.115	0.196	0.175	0.077	0.265
σ	0.075	0.012	0.056	0.088	0.096	0.032	0.112	0.050	0.018	0.182

small registration error. Also, the discrepancy measures show satisfactory results: the Dice coefficient is 0.983 ± 0, the Hausdorff distance is 0.109 ± 0.001 mm and the average surface distance is 0.034 ± 0.003 mm.

Two histological data sets, which were experimentally obtained from rat brains, were reconstructed. In $5 - 10$ out of 500 sections per brain, we had to use the refinement step. The computing time of the parallel algorithm for the reconstruction per brain was one hour, the optional refinement step took four hours per section. The applied algorithm shows a clearly recognisable improvement of the surface smoothness (Fig. 3). The quality measures support the visual inspection. The results of the first brain are: Dice coefficient of 0.982, Hausdorff distance of 0.659 mm and average surface distance of 0.296 mm. The results of the second brain are: Dice coefficient of 0.97, Hausdorff distance of 0.408 mm and average surface distance of 0.239 mm. An expert set 130 anatomi-

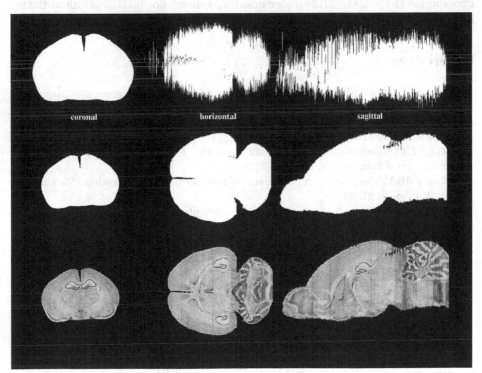

Fig. 3. Experimental data set, first row: masks before registration, second row: masks after registration, third row: histological sections after registration.

cal and evenly distributed landmarks in histological and blockface images of one brain. The mean square error distance measure of the landmark of randomly selected sections are listed in Tab. 1. These low values indicate the validity of the reconstruction results, also of the inner structures (Fig. 3, third row).

4   Discussion

We developed a simple, robust and fast method for the registration of histological brain sections to a 3D reference. The validation method based on transformation comparison, which is independent of any metric and interpolation, showed the correctness of the registration algorithm. The quality of the results were approved by uncorrelated measures as well as a landmark based validation.

As a next step, we will study nonlinear registration methods to get an idea of potential improvements of structural details.

Acknowledgement. This study was partially supported by the National Institutes of Health under grant agreement no. R01MH092311, by the Helmholtz Association through the Helmholtz Portfolio Theme "Supercomputing and Modeling for the Human Brain", and by the European Union Seventh Framework Programme (FP7/2007-2013) under grant agreement no. 604102 (Human Brain Project).

References

1. Palm C, Vieten A, Salber D, et al. Evaluation of registration strategies for multi-modality images of rat brain slices. Phys Med Biol. 2009;54(10):3269–89.
2. Gefen S, Tretiak O, Nissanov J. Elastic 3-D alignment of rat brain histological images. IEEE Trans Med Imaging. 2003;22(11):1480–9.
3. Schmitt O, Modersitzki J, Heldmann S, et al. Image registration of sectioned brains. Int J Comput Vis. 2007;73(1):5–39.
4. Maintz JBA, Viergewer MA. A survey of medical image registration. Med Image Anal. 1998;2(1):1–36.
5. Palomero-Gallagher N. Cyto and receptor architecture of area 32 in human and macaque brains. J Comp Neurol. 2013;521:3272–86.
6. Zilles K, Schleicher A, Palomero-Gallagher N, et al. Brain Mapping: The Methods. USA: Elsevier; 2002.
7. Schober M, Schloemer P, Cremer M, et al. How to generate a reference volume for subsequent 3D-reconstruction of histological sections. Proc BVM. 2015.
8. Papp EA, Leergaard TB, Calabrese E, et al. Waxholm space atlas of the sprague dawley rat brain. NeuroImage. 2014;97:374–86.
9. Pluim JPW, Maintz JBA, Viergewer MA. F-information measures in medical image registration. IEEE Trans Med Imaging. 2004;23(12):1508–16.
10. Heimann T, Thorn M, Kunert T, et al. Empirische Vergleichsmaße für die Evaluation von Segmentierungsergebnissen. Proc BVM. 2004; p. 165–70.

Joint Reconstruction of Multi-Contrast MRI for Multiple Sclerosis Lesion Segmentation

Pedro A Gómez[1,2,3], Jonathan I Sperl[3], Tim Sprenger[2,3],
Claudia Metzler-Baddeley[4], Derek K Jones[4], Philipp Saemann[5],
Michael Czisch[5], Marion I Menzel[3], Bjoern H Menze[1]

[1]Computer Science, Technische Universität München, Munich, Germany
[2]Medical Engineering, Technische Universität München, Munich, Germany
[3]GE Global Research, Munich, Germany
[4]CUBRIC, School of Psychology, Cardiff University, Cardiff, Wales, UK
[5]Max Plank Institute of Psychiatry, Munich, Germany
pedro.gomez@tum.de

Abstract. A joint reconstruction framework for multi-contrast MR images is presented and evaluated. The evaluation takes place in function of quality criteria based on reconstruction results and performance in the automatic segmentation of Multiple Sclerosis (MS) lesions. We show that joint reconstruction can effectively recover artificially corrupted images and is robust to noise.

1 Introduction

Multi-contrast MR imaging enables the quantification of metrics that provide information on tissue micro-structure. In the domain of neuroimaging, these metrics deepen our understanding of the brain in both health and disease, and could potentially assess the early onset of neurological disorders, such as Multiple Sclerosis (MS). Quantitative metrics are obtained from different MRI techniques, generating multiple contrasts and a wide-range of information regarding tissue micro-structure. Obtaining this information, however, comes at the expense of long acquisition times and low signal to noise ratios (SNR).

One possibility for overcoming the limitation of long scan times is through accelerated data acquisitions by compressed sensing (CS). In Diffusion Spectrum Imaging (DSI), acceleration by CS has been successfully demonstrated [1] and is currently being validated in clinical settings. A different approach is to use spatial context to increase data quality without further incrementing acquisition times. One of these methods, presented by Haldar et al. [2], takes advantage of structural correlations between datasets to perform a statistical joint reconstruction. This is achieved by incorporating gradient information from all contrasts into the regularization term of a maximum likelihood estimation.

In this study we evaluate the performance of joint reconstruction under different noise levels. Furthermore, we investigate the performance of this approach using a metric that evaluates the segmentation accuracy of MS lesions – i.e., the tasks the images were acquired for – rather than focusing on the common reconstruction error calculated from image intensities.

2   Materials and methods

2.1   Data acquisition

Five volunteers were scanned with a 3T GE HDx MRI system (GE Medical Systems, Milwuakee, WI) using an eight channel receive only head RF coil. MRI datasets were acquired for a HARDI protocol, a mcDESPOT [3] protocol, and a high resolution T1 weighted anatomical scan (FSPGR). The HARDI protocol consisted of 60 gradient orientations around a concentric sphere with $b = 1200$ s/mm^2 and 6 baseline images at b=0. HARDI datasets were corrected for motion using FSL's FLIRT and FNIRT [4] and both HARDI and mcDESPOT were rigidly registered to the T1 anatomical scan with FLIRT [3].

Seven MS patients were scanned with a CS-DSI acquisition protocol using a GE MR750 scanner (GE Medical Systems, Milwaukee, WI). The CS-DSI protocol comprised of 514 volumes acquired on a Cartesian grid with maximal b-value $= 3000$ s/mm^2. Additionally, high resolution T1, T2, and FLAIR contrasts were acquired. DSI volumes were co-registered to the first b=0 image, corrected for motion using FLIRT and FNIRT, and a brain mask was obtained using BET [4]. T1, T2 and FLAIR images were down-sampled to the same resolution as the DWIs and all of the volumes were once again co-registered with each other. Finally, for every patient, 11 slices were selected and lesions were manually labelled using a basic region growing algorithm on thresholding FLAIR intensity values.

2.2   Multi-constrast joint reconstruction

In a first experiment we want to evaluate whether joint reconstruction can effectively remove noise and maintain data quality in datasets of our multi-contrast sequence. To this end, we studied the reconstruction error under different noise level and optimized the necessary regularization parameters.

After data acquisition and pre-processing, volunteer datasets were artificially corrupted with homogeneous Rician noise and reconstructed using joint reconstruction. Then, or a given set of M images, the reconstructed data $\hat{\mathbf{x}}$ was obtained from the corrupted data $\mathbf{y}$ using

$$\{\hat{\mathbf{x}}^1, \hat{\mathbf{x}}^2, \ldots, \hat{\mathbf{x}}^M\} = \operatorname*{arg\,min}_{\{\mathbf{x}^1,\mathbf{x}^2,\ldots,\mathbf{x}^M\}} \sum_{m=1}^{M} \mu_m^2 \|\mathbf{F}_m\mathbf{x}^m - \mathbf{y}^m\|_2^2 + \Phi\left(\mathbf{x}^1, \mathbf{x}^2, \ldots, \mathbf{x}^M\right)$$

(1)

where $\mathbf{F}$ is the Fourier encoding operator, μ is a parameter that adjusts data consistency, and $\Phi(\cdot)$ is a regularization term. As in [2], we define the regularization term as the finite differences over all images. We have to optimize μ and Φ as a function of data quality.

2.3   Lesion segmentation

In a second experiment we evaluate the performance of a joint reconstruction for our sequence using *not* the reconstruction performance of the images, but the DICE scores of an automatic lesion segmentation algorithm. Here, we compare the DICE scores of the ground truth patient datasets with corrupted and jointly reconstructed versions of the datasets.

Random forests have already been implemented to segment MS lesions in multi-contrast MR images, achieving performance comparable to other state of the art segmentation methods [5]. We also propose the use of discriminative classifiers within a random framework to classify voxels, but, given the nature of our patient data, replace context rich features with scalar diffusion features calculated from the CS-DSI protocol.

The feature vector consists of a total of 27 features: three structural MRI intensity channels (T1, T2, and FLAIR), eight diffusion features and 16 kurtosis features. Diffusion features were estimated from the Eigenvalue decomposition of the diffusion tensor $D \in \mathbb{R}^{3 \times 3}$, while kurtosis features were estimated from projections of the fourth order kurtosis tensor $W \in \mathbb{R}^{3 \times 3 \times 3 \times 3}$ into spherical and elliptical coordinates. Both tensors were calculated by fitting the data to the diffusional kurtosis model defined in [6] and to a version of the model with a coordinate system rotated into the main directions of diffusion.

The classification task with random forests was accomplished using Matlab's (The Mathworks, Inc) Statistics Toolbox. For this work, a total of 30 trees were grown from four randomly selected datasets and the trained forest was fit to the other three patients. Every tree received a randomly subsampled dataset of voxels and lesion voxels where weighted to proportional to non-lesion voxels.

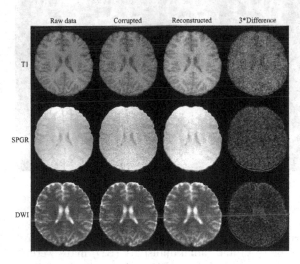

Fig. 1. Reconstructed datasets from a noisy input. Rows show, from top to bottom, three different acquisition protocols: T1, SGPR, and DWI. Columns, from left to right, display: raw data, data corrupted with $\sigma = 4\%$ homogeneous Rician noise, reconstructed data, and absolute difference between the raw data in the first column and the reconstructed data in the third column multiplied times three for better visualization.

3   Results

3.1   Optimization of joint reconstruction parameters

In the first experiment we determine regularization parameters of the joint reconstruction algorithm that are optimal for our imaging sequence. We use the high resolution volunteer data set.

Volunteer datasets were artificially corrupted with homogeneous Rician noise and reconstructed with different parameter settings. The three regularization parameters, which control for data consistency, regularization, and sensitivity of edge detection, were optimized in function of the remaining noise fraction (RNF) of the reconstructed images, and the root mean square error (RMSE) and structural similarity index (SSIM) [7] of these images to the original raw data.

Tab. 1 shows exemplary results for a given parameter set with optimized regularization parameters, and Fig. 1 provides a visual comparison of each of the reconstructed contrasts. In this example, joint reconstruction was able to remove more than 75% of the artificially added Rician noise, leading to RNF computations between 17.7 and 24.7%.

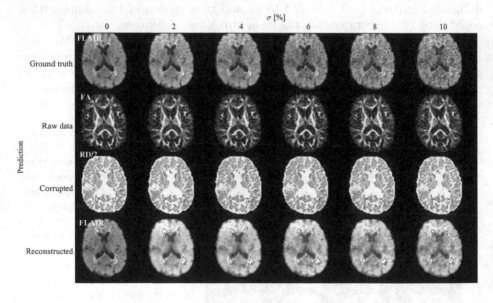

Fig. 2. Segmentation performance with respect to noise. Each row shows a different contrast, indicated in white letters, and the labeled lesions for ground truth (top row) plus predictions on raw data, corrupted data and reconstructed data (bottom three rows). Note that fractional anisotropy (FA) and radial diffusivity (RD) maps weren't directly corrupted, but estimated from corrupted data. RD is shown divided by two for better visualization.

Quality criteria	Protocol T1	MCDESPOT	DWI
$\sigma_{\hat{\mathbf{x}}}$ [%]	0.992	0.981	0.981
RNF	0.177	0.238	0.247
RMSE	0.090	0.050	0.042
SSIM	0.711	0.683	0.772

Table 1. Quality metrics estimated for different jointly reconstructed datasets. Every dataset was individually corrupted with $\sigma = 4\%$ homogeneous Rician noise and jointly reconstructed using (1).

3.2   Evaluation of MS lesion segmentation accuracy

The second experiment evaluated whether joint reconstruction can effectively remove noise without losing critical information, such as the borders between lesions and non-lesions. We evaluate the scores on the patient data set.

For five different noise levels, the following was done: homogeneous Rician noise was added to all of the images to corrupt them, images were subsequently reconstructed using joint reconstruction, two different kurtosis and diffusion models were fit to the corrupted and reconstructed datasets, and lesion segmentation was performed. The experiment was repeated over 10 iterations and a mean DICE score for every noise level was obtained. Fig. 2 shows the segmentation results of an exemplary dataset and Fig. 3 displays the general performance and robustness to noise.

As seen in Figs. 2 and 3, joint reconstruction has a significant impact on segmentation results. At low noise levels, jointly reconstructed datasets yield lower DICE scores than raw data and even noisy datasets. This is most likely do

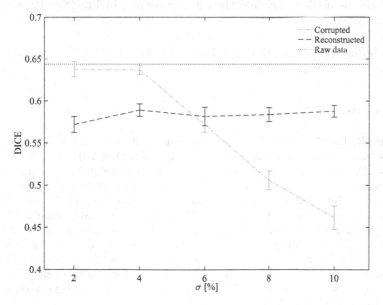

Fig. 3. DICE scores for corrupted and reconstructed datasets as a function of noise levels. Plots show mean ± standard deviation of 10 iterations and the black line indicates the average DICE score obtained from raw data.

to the fact that joint reconstruction has a smoothing effect and that, for certain parameter settings, small edge structures are ignored and blurred out. These small edge structures include the boundary between lesions and non-lesions, especially since this boundary is not completely clear or the same in the multiple contrasts. As noise levels increase, DICE scores of corrupted datasets decrease while reconstructed datasets maintain similar values.

4   Discussion

In this work, joint reconstruction was evaluated for multi-contrast MR images according to multiple criteria and the role of the method on lesion segmentation was further studied. From this analysis, it was established that joint reconstruction has a significant impact on lesion segmentation, especially at low noise levels, where over-smoothing can lead to decreased performance of the segmentation algorithm. On the other hand, joint reconstruction proved to be robust to noise, and at higher noise levels, was able to remove noise while still capturing the differences between lesions and non-lesions.

Parameter settings play a crucial role on the joint reconstruction framework. Optimizing parameters with respect to the reconstruction errors may not lead to the parameter set that is optimal for lesion segmentation. Furthermore, data quality of each particular dataset also affects the optimal parameter set. Consequently, future work will focus on developing novel, disease-specific and data-adaptive metrics that effectively discriminate between normal state and disease and that can be used to optimize the entire imaging pipeline from data acquisition to analysis.

Acknowledgement. This work was funded by the European Commission under Grant Agreement Number 605162.

References

1. Menzel MI, Tan ET, Khare K, et al. Accelerated diffusion spectrum imaging in the human brain using compressed sensing. Magn Reson Med. 2011;66:1226–33.
2. Haldar JP, Wedeen VJ, Nezamzadeh M, et al. Improved diffusion imaging through SNR-enhancing joint reconstruction. Magn Reson Med. 2013;69(1):277–89.
3. Deoni SCL, Rutt BK, Arun T, et al. Gleaning multicomponent T1 and T2 information from steady-state imaging data. Magn Reson Med. 2008;60:1372–87.
4. Jenkinson M, Beckmann CF, Behrens TEJ, et al. FSL. NeuroImage. 2012;62:782–90.
5. Geremia E, Clatz O, Menze BH, et al. Spatial decision forests for MS lesion segmentation in multi-channel magnetic resonance images. NeuroImage. 2011;57:378–90.
6. Jensen JH, Helpern JA, Ramani A, et al. Diffusional kurtosis imaging: the quantification of non-gaussian water diffusion by means of magnetic resonance imaging. Magn Reson Med. 2005;53:1432–40.
7. Wang Z, Bovik AC, Sheikh HR, et al. Image quality assessment: from error visibility to structural similarity. IEEE Trans Image Process. 2004;13:600–12.

Rekonstruktion zerebraler Gefässnetzwerke aus in-vivo μMRA mittels physiologischem Vorwissen zur lokalen Gefässgeometrie

Markus Rempfler[1,2], Matthias Schneider[2,3], Giovanna D. Ielacqua[4],
Xianghui Xiao[5], Stuart R. Stock[6], Jan Klohs[4], Gábor Székely[2],
Bjoern Andres[7], Bjoern H. Menze[1,8]

[1]Departement für Informatik, TU München
[2]Institut für Bildverarbeitung, ETH Zürich
[3]Institut für Pharmakologie und Toxikologie, Universität Zürich
[4]Institut für Biomedizinische Technik, Universität und ETH Zürich
[5]Advanced Photon Source, Argonne National Laboratory, USA
[6]Feinberg School of Medicine, Northwestern University, Chicago IL, USA
[7]Max-Planck-Institut für Informatik, Saarbrücken
[8]Institute for Advanced Studies, TU München

markurem@vision.ee.ethz.ch

Kurzfassung. In diesem Beitrag adressieren wir die Rekonstruktion zerebrovaskulärer Netzwerke mit einem Ansatz, der es erlaubt, Vorwissen über physiologisch plausible Strukturen zu berücksichtigen und gegenüber Bildinformation abzuwägen. Ausgehend von einem überkonnektierten Netzwerk wird in einer globalen Optimierung – unter Berücksichtigung von geometrischer Konstellation, globaler Konnektivität und Bildintensitäten – das plausibelste Netzwerk bestimmt. Ein statistisches Modell zur Bewertung geometrischer Beziehungen zwischen Segmenten und Bifurkationen wird anhand eines hochaufgelösten Netzwerks gelernt, welches aus einem μCT (Mikrocomputertomographie) eines zerebrovaskulären Korrosionspräparats einer Maus gewonnen wird. Die Methode wird experimentell auf in-vivo μMRA (Magnetresonanzmikroangiographie) Datensätze von Mausgehirnen angewandt und Eigenschaften der resultierenden Netzwerke im Vergleich zu Standardverfahren diskutiert.

1 Einleitung

Das Rekonstruieren von Gefässnetzwerken aus in-vivo Datensätzen ist eine herausfordernde Aufgabe: Die Netzwerke zeigen eine hohe Variabilität feiner Strukturen, die sich bei den μMRA Aufnahmen von Mäusen, welche in diesem Beitrag betrachtet werden, nahe an der unteren Auflösungsgrenze befinden.

Viele existierende Methoden zur Gefässsegmentierung basieren auf lokalen Massen der Tubularität wie [1], gefolgt von Entscheidungsalgorithmen verschiedenster Art. Die resultierenden Segmentierungen können anschliessend skeletonisiert werden, beispielsweise mittels [2], um die Netzwerkstruktur zu erhalten. Alternativ können Trackingalgorithmen, wie ausführlich reviewt in [3, 4], direkt genutzt werden um einzelne Gefässe zu extrahieren. Derartig rekonstruierte Gefässnetzwerke sind jedoch oftmals unzureichend hinsichtlich ihrer Konnektivität und verlangen nach applikationsspezifischem Postprocessing. So sind in-fill Methoden zur Korrektur fehlender lokaler Verbindungen nicht ungewöhnlich, wie beispielsweise in [5] vorgeschlagen. Lediglich in wenigen Ansätzen wird das Netzwerk als Gesamtes, unter Berücksichtigung dessen physiologischer Eigenschaften und Konnektivität, in die Rekonstruktion einbezogen: In [6] werden Annahmen über Gefässradien in eine Optimierung integriert, die sich auf Gefässbäume beschränkt. Währenddessen findet sich eine generellere Formulierung zur Rekonstruktion von kurvenförmigen Strukturen in [7]. Dabei wird ein überkonnektierter Graph erstellt um daraufhin mittels integer programming den Subgraph zu bestimmen, der die unterliegende Struktur am besten repräsentiert. Dazu wird ein Pfadklassifikator trainiert, der die lokale Kohärenz der Pfade evaluiert und diese entsprechend gewichtet.

Im diesem Beitrag verfolgen wir den Ansatz, geometrisch-physiologisches Vorwissen, das typisch für zerebrale Gefässnetzwerke ist, in eine globale Optimierung im Stil von [7] zu integrieren, wodurch es möglich wird, *Evidenz* für Gefässe im Bild mit *Prior* über deren Form und Konnektivität in einer globalen Optimierung abzuwägen. Wir präsentieren damit eine Fortsetzung der Arbeit aus [8], mit einer verfeinerten Formulierung und einer erweiterten Diskussion der Experimente.

2 Material und Methoden

2.1 Segmentierung

Um eine initiale Segmentierung der Gefässstrukturen zu erhalten, wird als erster Schritt eine Filterbank von Steerable Filter Templates (SFT) auf das Bildvolumen I angewandt, gefolgt von einem Random Forest (RF) zur Klassifikation, wie vorgeschlagen in [9]. Die resultierende Confidence Map $P(I)$ beschreibt für jedes Voxel v die Wahrscheinlichkeit $p_v \in [0, 1]$ zu einem Gefäss zu gehören und kann schliesslich durch setzen eines Thresholds bei θ in eine binäre Segmentierung überführt werden.

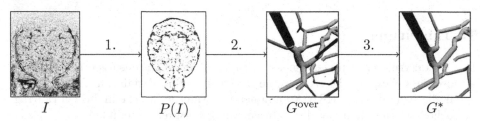

Abb. 1. Workflow: 1. Segmentierung des Bildvolumens I, 2. Konstruktion des überkonnektieren Netzwerkgraphs G^{over} aus $P(I)$, 3. Optimierung des Netzwerks: Der optimale Subgraph G^* wird unter Berücksichtigung von physiologischem Prior über die Struktur angrenzender Segmente sowie Evidenz aus I bestimmt.

Mehrfaches Anwenden verschiedener Thresholds $\{\theta_i\}$ auf $P(I)$, jeweils gefolgt von einer Skeletonisierung mittels Distance-ordered homotopic thinning (DOHT) [2] führt zu einem Set von Graphen, die anschliessend in einen *überkonnektierten* Graphen $G^{\mathrm{over}}(\{\theta_i\})$ zusammengeführt werden. Dieser bildet die Grundlage für den folgenden Optimierungsprozess, indem er verschiedene Segmente (von unterschiedlicher Wahrscheinlichkeit gemäss $P(I)$, d.h. mit unterschiedlicher Evidenz) vorschlägt, die in der finalen Rekonstruktion des Netzwerks vorkommen können.

2.2 Optimierung der Netzwerke

Ausgehend vom überkonnektierten Graphen $G^{\mathrm{over}}(\{\theta_i\})$, wird nun versucht, den Subgraph G^* zu bestimmen, der das unterliegende Gefässnetzwerk am besten repräsentiert unter Berücksichtigung von Evidenz im Bildvolumen sowie geometrisch-physiologischer Vorinformation über die Netzwerkstruktur. Wir formulieren dies als diskrete Optimierung, ähnlich wie [7], wozu für alle Segmente e_i in G^{over} eine binäre Variabel $x_i \in \{0,1\}$ eingeführt wird. Der optimale Subgraph G^* und damit das rekonstruierte Netzwerk wird schliesslich durch das Set dieser Variabeln, $X = \{x_i\}_{i=1}^{N}$, repräsentiert, wobei $x_i = 1$ bedeutet, dass die entsprechende Verbindung e_i in G^* enthalten ist. G^* ergibt sich dann durch optimieren von

$$\min \quad \alpha \sum_{x_i \in X} w_i x_i + \sum_{\substack{x_i,x_j \in X: \\ e_i,e_j \text{ adjacent}}} w_{ij} x_i x_j + \sum_{\substack{x_i,x_j,x_k \in X: \\ e_i,e_j,e_k \text{ adjacent}}} w_{ijk} x_i x_j x_k \qquad (1)$$

$$\text{s.t.} \quad \boldsymbol{A}\boldsymbol{x} \geq \boldsymbol{b} \qquad (2)$$

$$x_i \in \{0,1\} \quad \forall x_i \in X \qquad (3)$$

wobei w_i das Gewicht für einzelne Segmente ist, w_{ij} das Gewicht für zwei fortführende Segmente und w_{ijk} das Gewicht für mögliche Bifurkationen. $\alpha > 0$ ist ein Parameter, der es erlaubt, den Fokus auf dem Evidenz-Term anzupassen. Das Set von Bedingungen $\boldsymbol{A}\boldsymbol{x} \geq \boldsymbol{b}$ dient dazu, die Lösung auf konnektierte Netzwerke zu beschränken.

Wahl der Gewichte Die Kostenfunktion (1) kann als Kombination eines Evidenz-Terms, $\propto -\log P(I,G|\boldsymbol{X} = \boldsymbol{x})$, sowie eines geometrisch-physiologischen Prior-Terms, $\propto -\log P(\boldsymbol{X} = \boldsymbol{x}|\boldsymbol{\Theta})$, interpretiert werden. Entsprechend ergeben sich die folgenden zwei Arten von Gewichten für die jeweiligen Terme:

Evidenz. Die Gewichte w_i der ersten Summe von (1) erlauben es, einzelne Gefässsegmente zu bewerten und damit die Evidenz für Gefässe im Bildvolumen zu berücksichtigen. Sie sind daher wie folgt definiert:

$$w_i = -\log \frac{P(x_i = 1|I_i)}{P(x_i = 0|I_i)} = -\log \frac{p_i}{1 - p_i} \qquad (4)$$

wobei $P(x_i = 1|I_i) = p_i$ die lokale Konfidenz gemittelt entlang des Segments e_i gemäss dem RF ist.

Prior. Die zwei letzteren Summenterme gewichten jeweils aneinandergrenzende Paare von Segmenten, sowie Triplets von Segmenten, die eine mögliche Bifurkation bilden. Anders als in [8] definieren wir diese als

$$w_{ij} = -\log \frac{P(\gamma_{ij}|\text{continue}, \Theta)P(\text{continue}|\Theta)}{P(\gamma_{ij}|\text{terminate}, \Theta)P(\text{terminate}|\Theta)} \tag{5}$$

$$w_{ijk} = -\log \frac{P(\gamma_{ijk}|\text{branch}, \Theta)P(\text{branch}|\Theta)}{P(\gamma_{ijk}|\text{terminate}, \Theta)P(\text{terminate}|\Theta)} - w_{ij} - w_{ik} - w_{jk} \tag{6}$$

wo $P(\gamma_{ij}|\text{continue}, \Theta)$ die Wahrscheinlichkeit darstellt, bei einem kohärenten Paar e_i und e_j die geometrischen Features γ_{ij} zu beobachten, und analog dazu ist $P(\gamma_{ijk}|\text{branch}, \Theta)$ die Wahrscheinlichkeit bei einer Bifurkation γ_{ijk} anzutreffen. Sie werden mittels einem parametrischen Modell Θ berechnet. γ_{ij} respektive γ_{ijk} sind in diesem Fall Gefässradien und Winkel der involvierten Segmente. Durch Berücksichtigen der Priors $P(\text{continue}|\Theta)$, $P(\text{branch}|\Theta)$ und $P(\text{terminate}|\Theta)$ sowie der Annahme von $P(\gamma|\text{terminate}, \Theta) \sim$ uniform, lassen sich die Gewichte schliesslich direkt, d.h. ohne Parametertuning der zwei Divisoren, bestimmen.

2.3 Experiment

Datensätze Bei den verwendeten Datensätzen handelt es sich um vier μMRA Volumen (248 × 248 × 109 px, 60 μm isotropes Voxelspacing) sowie ein hochaufgelöstes μCT (1024 × 1024 × 1857 px, 5.8 μm isotropes Voxelspacing) eines Korrosionspräparats des vaskulären Netzwerks eines Mausgehirns.

Vorverarbeitung & Lernen des physiologischen Priors Alle Datensätze werden als erstes durch das Segmentierungsframework (Abschn.t 2.1) verarbeitet. Parameter der Filterbank und des RF werden in einer leave-one-out Crossvalidation bestimmt. Da der hochaufgelöste μCT Datensatz mit der Standardmethode (i.e. einfaches Thresholding gefolgt von DOHT) zuverlässig zu einem Gefässnetzwerk verarbeitet werden kann, führen wir an diesem eine statistische Auswertung der geometrischen Beziehungen zwischen den Gefässsegmenten durch und fitten das parametrische Modell Θ (Abschnitt 2.2).

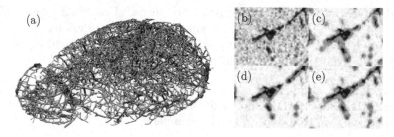

Abb. 2. Rekonstruiertes Gefässnetzwerk eines Mausgehirns resultierend aus Optimierung (a); die geschätzten Gefässdurchmesser sind entsprechend farbkodiert: (b) originaler Bildausschnitt, (c) rasterisiertes Netzwerk erzeugt durch Alternativmethode mit $\theta = 0.5$, (d) alternativmethode mit $\theta = 0.9$, (e) optimiertes Netzwerk G^*.

Rekonstruktion zerebraler Gefässnetzwerke von μMRA Bilddaten Als Kern des Experiments wird die beschriebene Methode zur Netzwerkrekonstruktion mittels diskreter Optimierung auf die vier in-vivo μMRA Datensätze angewandt um ihren Mehrwert gegenüber Standardverfahren zu ermitteln. Als Vergleichsbasis werden dazu Netzwerke mittels einfachem Thresholding und gefolgter Skeletonisierung durch DOHT (fortan als *Alternativmethode* bezeichnet) erzeugt. Zur Evaluation werden makroskopische Eigenschaften (relatives Gefässvolumen, mittlere Distanz zum nächsten Gefäss) berechnet, die über die Plausibilität der Gefässnetzwerke Auskunft geben. Ausserdem wird der Dice Score der gerasterten Netzwerke gegenüber manuellen Annotationen auf jeweils drei zentralen Slices ausgewertet.

3   Ergebnisse

Abb. 2 zeigt eine Visualisierung eines ganzen Netzwerks. Detailansichten der gerasterten Netzwerke sind als Overlay (rot) zum originalen Bildausschnitt gegeben. Quantitative Resultate in Form von makroskopischen Eigenschaften der Netzwerke, rekonstruiert mittels der vorgestellten Optimierung sowie der Alternativmethode unter verschiedener Parametrisierung, finden sich in Abb. 3.

4   Diskussion

Die diskutierte Methode zur Gefässnetzworkrekonstruktion wurde auf den in-vivo μMRA Datensätzen angewandt, wobei der physiologische Prior über plausible Konstellationen von Gefässsegmenten automatisch von dem hochaufgelösten μCT Datensatz gelernt werden konnte. Die verfeinerte Formulierung führt zu äquivalenten Resultaten verglichen mit [8], benötigt aber weniger Feintuning der Gewichte. Die Auswertung der makroskopischen Kennzahlen sowie des Dice Scores weisen darauf hin, dass sich die optimierten Netzwerke jeweils im

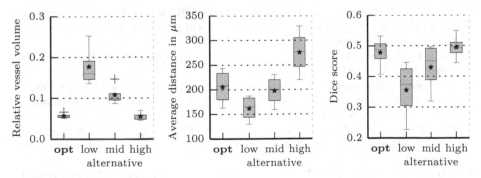

Abb. 3. Vergleich der makroskopischen Eigenschaften der Gefässnetzwerke aus der vorgestellten Methode (opt) sowie der Alternativmethode mit verschiedenen Parametrisierungen (low: $\theta = 0.2$, mid: $\theta = 0.5$, high: $\theta = 0.9$). Boxplots (median in rot, mean: $\star$) zeigen Statistiken für alle vier Datensätze.

physiologisch-plausibleren Bereich befinden, während alle Alternativen mindestens in einem Mass unplausible Werte, d.h. ein zu grosses Gefässvolumen, zu grosse Lücken oder einen wesentlich tieferen Dice Score aufweisen. Ferner adressiert die diskutierte Methode den Aspekt, dass es sich um ein verbundenes Netzwerk handelt – eine Eigenschaft die von höchster Bedeutung ist, wenn das Resultat beispielsweise für Simulationen weiterverwendet werden soll. Es wird jedoch auch deutlich, dass während der Konstruktion des Graphen G^{over}, z.B. bei Radiusschätzungen von kleinen Gefässen, noch Verbesserungspotenzial besteht (Abb. 2c-e). Für zukünftige Arbeiten wird es interessant sein, diese Konstruktion zu verfeinern, komplexere Formen des physiologischen Priors zu testen, oder die Vorhersage struktureller Information (z.B. arteriell/venös) zu integrieren.

Danksagung. This research was supported by the TU München – IAS (funded by the German Excellence Initiative and the EU 7th Framework Programme under grant agreement n 291763, the Marie Curie COFUND program of the the EU), by grants from the EMDO foundation, SNSF grant 136822, and the NCCR Co-Me supported by the SNSF. Use of the Advanced Photon Source was supported by the US Department of Energy, Office of Science, Office of Basic Energy Sciences, under Contract No. DE-AC02-06CH11357.

Literaturverzeichnis

1. Frangi AF, Niessen WJ, Vincken KL, et al. Multiscale vessel enhancement filtering. Lect Notes Computer Sci. 1998;1496:130–7.
2. Pudney C. Distance-ordered homotopic thinning: a skeletonization algorithm for 3D digital images. Computer Vis Image Understand. 1998;72(3):404–413.
3. Kirbas C, Quek F. A review of vessel extraction techniques and algorithms. ACM Compute Surv. 2004;36(2):81–121.
4. Lesage D, Angelini E, Bloch I, et al. A review of 3D vessel lumen segmentation techniques: models, features and extraction schemes. Med Image Anal. 2009;13(6):819–45.
5. Schneider M, Hirsch S, Weber B, et al. TGIF: topological Gap in-fill for correction of vascular connectivity: a generative physiological modeling approach. Lect Notes Computer Sci. 2014;8674:89–96.
6. Jiang Y, Zhuang ZW, Sinusas AJ, et al. Vessel connectivity using Murray's hypothesis. Proc MICCAI. 2011;14:528–36.
7. Türetken E, Benmansour F, Andres B, et al. Reconstructing loopy curvilinear structures using integer programming. Proc IEEE Comput Soc Conf Comput Vis Pattern Recognit. 2013; p. 1822–9.
8. Rempfler M, Schneider M, Ielacqua GD, et al. Extracting vascular networks under physiological constraints via integer programming. Lect Notes Computer Sci. 2014;8674:505–12.
9. Schneider M, Hirsch S, Weber B, et al. Joint 3D vessel segmentation and centerline extraction using oblique hough forests with steerable filters. Med Image Anal. 2015;19(1):220–49.

Reconstructing a Series of Auto-Radiographic Images in Rat Brains

Anh-Minh Huynh[1], Mehmet E. Kirlangic[1], Nicole Schubert[1], Martin Schober[1], Katrin Amunts[1,2], Karl Zilles[1,3,4], Markus Axer[1]

[1]Institute of Neuroscience and Medicine (INM-1), Research Center Juelich
[2]Cécile&Oskar Vogt Institute of Brain Research, Heinrich Heine University Düsseldorf
[3]Department of Psychiatry, Psychotherapy and Psychosomatics, RWTH Aachen
[4]JARA Jülich-Aachen Research Alliance, Translational Brain Medicine, Jülich
a.m.huynh@fz-juelich.de

Abstract. Quantitative in vitro receptor auto-radiographic studies in brains require the preparation of thin microtome sections. Due to the sectioning process, the spatial coherence is lost and needs to be recovered, if 3D analysis is envisaged. This study describes a new processing pipeline for 3D realignment of auto-radiographs of rat brain sections based on image features. Automatically extracted image features from neighboring sections are matched using their descriptors by rejecting false matches. An intermediate objective is to achieve an intra-subject reconstruction to reduce the manual effort in the next registration step. These steps are followed by a semi-automatic method which aligns already preregistered auto-radiographic stacks into a blockface reference volume to ensure anatomical correctness. The validity of the approach is illustrated by using the mean squared error between the user-defined landmarks as the quality measure.

1 Introduction

The analysis of auto-radiographic data is important to investigate the role of neurotransmitter receptors in the molecular organization of the brain [1]. Furthermore, distribution changes of the receptors and their regional densities can be an indication for neurological and psychiatric diseases. Auto-radiographic images have a high resolution and are used in Quantitative in vitro receptor auto-radiography enables the determination of neurotransmitter receptors densities in the brain. For auto-radiographic studies deep-frozen brains are sectioned into 20 micron thin sections, which are then exposed to tritium-labeled tracers which bind with high specificity to transmitter receptors. Following this step, sections are exposed to beta-sensitive film together with radioactive scales. The exposition to beta-sensitive films reveals the distribution and densities of receptors indicated by intensity of gray values.

During the sectioning process the spatial coherence between sections is lost, but the analysis of receptor distributions across the entire brain is essential.

Therefore, an accurate 3D reconstruction is required. The intra-subject reconstruction of auto-radiographic data recovers the spatial relationship. Nevertheless, for inter-subject comparisons, a common reference volume is needed to perform multimodal analysis.

Intra-subject registration of auto-radiograms was performed in [2] based on edge features. Other authors used an intensity based method by minimizing normalized cross correlation cost functions [3]. Another approach made use of a disparity analysis method which utilizes contours or image intensity to obtain a metric for the optimization in the registration process [4]. A registration based on contours and center of gravity was performed across two modalities in [5]. Due to the fact that tissue can be damaged during the sectioning process, a contour based approach is not sufficient. In addition, depending on the receptor type, corresponding images may have an extremely low signal-to-noise ratio.

Hence, a two-step registration pipeline is introduced in the present study. First a intra-subject preregistration of the auto-radiographic images is performed. Second, the preregistered stack is aligned into a 3D blockface reference volume. This approach to reconstruct auto-radiographic data can deal with a small signal-noise-ratio. Auto-radiographic images are typically noisy, which is likely to lead to feature detection in the background and causes false matching. Another issue is the signal itself. The description of the surrounding area of the detected features is too similar, so the matching of feature descriptors is ambiguous.

2   Material and methods

In this study a rat brain was frozen and sectioned using a cryostat microtome. During sectioning a blockface image was obtained for each section with a camera mounted above the cryostat. The blockface images provide an adequate anatomical reference for further analysis. The thickness of sections is $20 \mu m$. The sections were sorted into immediately following groups of three serial sections. One of them was cell body stained. After cleansing the two other sections of the natural neurotransmitters, the two other sections were immersed in buffer solutions containing known concentrations of two different radioactive tracers. Hence, the resolution in the z-direction is $60 \mu m$ (two different receptors, one cell body staining). These sections were exposed to beta-sensitive films. The resulting auto-radiographic images were digitized with a high resolution camera (4164×3120 pixels, about $5 \times 5 \mu m$ pixel resolution). In this study data of the muscarinic cholinergic receptor are used as an example for the here proposed method.

2.1   Pre-processing and pre-registration

Data should be visually inspected for artefacts and large damage beforehand. In this study damaged sections which were unusable for further analysis (e.g. histological artefacts, such as folds and tears), have been replaced by a neighboring section. This reduces possible registration errors.

The approach for a processing pipeline described here relies on image features, which are automatically extracted. Especially SIFT features and the belonging descriptors are used [6]. In comparison to intensity-based approaches, a point-based method needs less computational time, since the calculation is reduced to few points.

First, autor-adiographic images are smoothed by a median filter to remove noise in the background. With the smoothed image, a basic mask is created by threshold. Afterwards, contours are computed around each area. By the length of the contours it is possible to determine the largest components (i.e. anatomically associated areas). The final mask is generated by filling these contours.

In the next step image features are extracted from the original images. The mask indicates which features finally are extracted. The descriptors are computed on the smoothed images. To calculate the corresponding transformation of two neighboring sections, it is necessary to find matches between the two sets of features on each section. Therefore a brute-force approach helps to find matching features, this implies comparing each feature from one image with all the features from the other image. The best fit is chosen by comparing the Euclidean distances between the descriptor vectors. The surrounding area of features is too similar whereby not all feature pairs are well matched. Therefore, false matches have to be rejected. A robust estimation algorithm is used to eliminate these false matches. Therefore, the iterative method RANdom SAmple Consensus (RANSAC) is used [7]. The rigid transformation model is implemented in RANSAC as mathematical model of the observed data. To calculate the rigid transformation, at least three corresponding points are needed to solve the linear equation. This is done for every neighboring pair of sections individually. By concatenating the transformations and applying them to the auto-radiographic images, a preregistered stack is obtained.

2.2 Registration to blockface reference volume

Blockface images are captured with a camera installed above the cryostat before each section is cut. The reconstruction of the blockface images is described in [8]. The reconstructed blockface image volume is considered as the reference data set. A semi-automatic method is implemented to register the auto-radiographic volume to the reconstructed blockface volume. Assuming that the preregistered volume is consistent, meaning that all sections are realigned to each other to form a volume, there is no need to define corresponding landmarks in every fixed and moving image. It is sufficient only to define landmarks for every 30th section and to determine the corresponding transformation. All rigid transformations for sections in-between are approximated by linearly weighting their impact.

3   Results

The results are shown in Fig. 3 with views along the three principle axes: coronal, horizontal and sagittal. The physical sectioning is in coronal direction. The reconstructed blockface volume, which is used as the reference, is shown in the first row. The second row depicts the unregistered auto-radiographic data. The third row illustrates the result of the preregistration step. The last row shows the auto-radiographic volume after registration onto blockface volume. The most significant effects are labeled with arrows. The labels on the coronal plane point to structures which are suitable to set landmarks.

   Tab. 1 shows the mean squared error calculated between landmarks set by an anatomical expert. On every 30th section, five landmark pairs are set. An

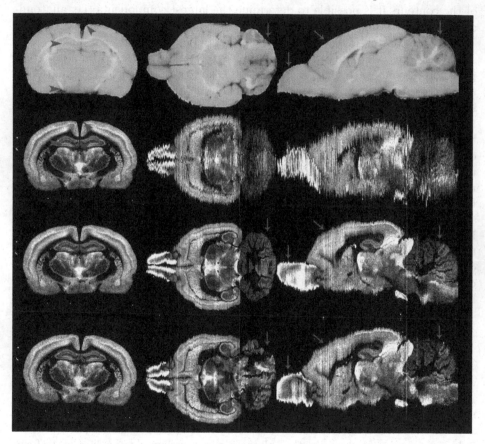

Fig. 1. Views along principle axes. The columns from left to right: coronal, horizontal, sagittal. The first row shows the reconstructed blockface volume. Second row depicts the unregistered auto-radiographic data. Third row shows the result from the preregistration. The last row depicts the registration's result of preregistered auto-radiographic volume onto blockface volume. The arrows mark the areas where the most significant differences can be seen. The brightness and contrast are adjusted to offer more details, since the original image data have by far less signal. The arrows on the coronal plane are examples of user-defined landmarks.

Table 1. Mean distances computed from user-defined landmarks set by an anatomical expert. The distances are calculated from the fixed and moving landmarks. Fixed landmarks are set in the blockface volume (Fig. 3 first row) and the moving landmarks are set in the original auto-radiography data (Fig. 3 second row).

#Section	62	92	122	152	182	212
MSE in mm	0.141	0.195	0.258	0.194	0.136	0.237
#Section	242	272	302	332	362	392
MSE in mm	0.386	0.201	0.148	0.338	0.197	0.351
#Section	422	452	482	512	542	572
MSE in mm	0.147	0.166	0.376	0.158	0.345	0.165
#Section	602	632	662	692	722	752
MSE in mm	0.259	0.386	0.206	0.255	0.309	0.218
#Section	782	812	842	872	902	932
MSE in mm	0.237	0.216	0.227	0.218	0.229	0.269
#Section	962	992	1022	1052	1082	1113
MSE in mm	0.243	0.478	0.171	0.258	0.200	0.232

example where landmarks are set, is shown in Fig. 3 (coronal plane). For each five pairs, mean distances are calculated between fixed and moving landmarks.

4   Discussion

An approach to reconstruct noisy auto-radiographic images is presented. This processing pipeline is based on image features and uses a pre-processing step.

The preprocessing step is used to enhance the reliability of automatically extracted image features. The median filter has been used, since it is convenient to purge noise in the background and it preserves contours. Furthermore, using median filtering, before the calculation of the descriptors a significant descriptor is obtained for each point. Matching these significant descriptors reduces the ratio of false matches. Remaining outliers are eliminated by a robust estimation algorithm, namely, the iterative method RANdom SAmple Consensus (RANSAC). This method is robust, even if the given set of inliers is very small. With the eliminated set of matches it has been possible to compute the rigid transformation parameters. Fig. 3 shows that the inner structures of the brain are reconstructed (third row). However, in comparison with the blockface volume (Fig. 3 first row), it is recognizable that the auto-radiographic volume is still deformed in its form. This deformation is corrected using a semi-automatic method which aligns preregistered auto-radiography to a blockface reference volume. By means of a preregistered volume it has been feasible to reduce the manual effort by setting landmarks in intervals.

The most significant effects are observed in the olfactory bulb, cerebral cortex and cerebellum (Fig. 3 third and last row, marked with arrows). The tip of the olfactory bulb is curved in caudal direction. The position of cerebellum is raised in cranial direction and the shape of cerebral cortex is flattened.

The quality of the registration is measured by the mean squared error of distances between fixed and moving landmarks (an error of 0 indicates a perfect alignment). Landmark pairs are affected by small inaccuracies, because there is no guarantee that visible anatomical landmarks in the blockface images also exist in auto-radiographic images. Examples are depicted in Fig. 3 in the coronal plane. Due to this fact, setting corresponding landmark pairs is not a simple task and can affect the error value. The registration achieves a maximum error of 0.478 mm and an overall mean value of 0.249 mm. These values reflect validity of the described approach.

Despite the possible inaccuracy of manually set landmarks, the presented processing pipeline is a practical and robust approach to reconstruct noisy autoradiographic data. As seen in the last row of Fig. 3 some registration errors still remain, since the sectioning process also causes non-linear distortions which are not examined in this study. Whether the manual effort in the second step can be avoided, if this step is substituted by a 3D registration of volumes, is the topic of further investigations.

Acknowledgement. This study was partially supported by the National Institutes of Health under grant agreement no. R01MH 092311, by the Helmholtz Association through the Helmholtz Portfolio Theme "Supercomputing and Modeling for the Human Brain", and by the European Union Seventh Framework Programme (FP7/2007-2013) under grant agreement no. 604102 (Human Brain Project).

References

1. Zilles K, Schleicher A, Palomero-Galagher N, et al. Quantitative analysis of cyto- and receptor architecture of the human brain. Brain Mapp: Methods. 2002;2:573–602.
2. Rangarajan A, Chui H, Mjolsness E, et al. A robust point-matching algorithm for autoradiograph alignment. Med Image Anal. 1996;7:379–98.
3. Ribes D, Parafita J, Charrier R, et al. A software tool for 3D reconstruction and statistical analysis of autoradiographic mouse brain sections. PloS One. 2010;5(11):e14094.
4. Zhao W, Young T, Ginsberg M. Registration and three-dimensional reconstruction of autoradiographic images by the disparity analysis method. IEEE Trans Med Imaging. 1993;12(4):782–91.
5. Nissanov J, McEachron DL. Advances in image processing for autoradiography. J Chem Neuroanat. 1991;4(5):329–42.
6. Lowe DG. Distinctive image features from scale-invariant keypoints. Int J Computer Vis. 2004;60(2):91–110.
7. Hartley R, Zisserman A. Multiple View Geometry in Computer Vision. vol. 2. Cambridge University Press; 2004.
8. Schober M, Schlömer P, Cremer M, et al. How to generate a reference volume for subsequent 3D-reconstruction of histological sections. Proc BVM. 2015; p. in press.

3D Shape Reconstruction of the Esophagus from Gastroscopic Video

Martin Prinzen, Jonas Trost, Tobias Bergen, Sebastian Nowack,
Thomas Wittenberg

Department of Image Processing and Medical Engineering,
Fraunhofer Institute for Integrated Circuits IIS Erlangen
martin.prinzen@iis.fraunhofer.de

Abstract. In gastroscopy, video endoscopic imaging is applied for the assessment of the esophagus. Video sequences which provide a narrow two dimensional insight are thereby generated. Three dimensional shape reconstructions from such video sequences offer opportunities for intuitive and enhanced visualization of the esophagus, providing additional contextual and geometrical information. Due to lack of features and the variability of the scene, the shape reconstruction bears a challenge for computer vision. In this contribution, a three dimensional reconstruction from gastroscopic video is presented by first computing a panorama image of the esophagus wall using a novel shape from shading approach followed by a 3D alignment of thereby provided 2D contours of the esophagus wall. The resulting 3D point cloud is then registered contour-wise, leading to a regular triangulation which is then texturized using the panorama image and visualized.

1 Introduction

Endoscopy is one of the most common methods for minimal invasive assessment of body cavities. Video sequences and still images are thereby acquired which are used for diagnosis and documentation. A major disadvantage of endoscopic imaging lies in the considerably constrained field of view, which only provides a narrow insight that lacks of contextual information and may affect diagnosis, treatment planning and the treatment itself.

Some methods have been presented that try to compensate the spatial view limitation by computing a panorama image of the body cavities surface from endoscopic video sequences [1, 2, 3]. A panorama reconstruction bears a challenge when dealing with the in-vivo esophagus due to its domain specific properties, such as its alterable appearance of tubular geometry and wall surface over time. This results in a deficiency of stable image features which are a key aspect in computer vision for panorama imaging solutions.

In this contribution, a three dimensional reconstruction of the esophagus is presented which builds on an approach for the computation of a panorama image from gastroscopic video. Given a gastroscopic video sequence showing a steady withdrawal of the endoscope from the esophagus, starting at the cardia and ending at the larynx, each frame contributes to the resulting panorama image, cf. Fig. 1 (right). For each frame, the approximated section of the esophagus at fixed depth is computed. This geometrical information is used in the proposed approach by executing an extension to the existing processing pipeline in a straight forward manner. In combination with the panorama image of the esophagus wall, as well as the mapping of the panorama to the unaltered original video frames, a three dimensional reconstruction offers an intuitive additional general-view of the geometrical properties of the esophagus and offers opportunities for improved documentation and enhanced context-aware diagnosis.

2   Materials and methods

The computation of a 3D reconstruction of the esophagus from a gastroscopic video sequence follows a straight forward processing pipeline (Fig. 2). Given a gastroscopic video sequence of the esophagus showing a withdrawal of the endoscope, the panorama mapping step consists of pre-processing, unwinding and concatenation of all video frames. First, the background image content is masked from the remaining 'valid' region. Next, a gray color conversion followed by a large Gauß filter is applied and a contour is unwound at a fixed intensity value using a marching squares approach. A resulting contour (one per frame), which approximately describes the esophagus wall at constant depth are then subsequently concatenated frame by frame (section by section) resulting in a panorama image of the esophagus wall. Using the contours centroid, its start point is chosen as its nearest neighbor, only regarding the x-coordinates with greater y-coordinate. Fig. 1 exemplarily shows the the processing of the panorama image by using computed contours from video frames.

All unwound contours and the panorama image state the input for the processing pipeline of the proposed 3D reconstruction method, which consists of 3D alignment of the contours followed by a contour to contour registration leading to a 3D mesh triangulation and conclusively followed by texturizing using the panorama image color information and visualization of the result.

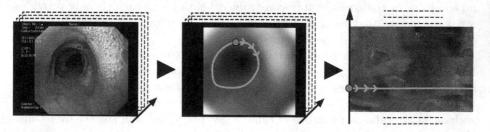

Fig. 1. Computation of a panorama image from a gastroscopic video sequence. Left: An input video frame; Center: the pre-processed and unwound frame; Right: the output panorama. The orange dot denotes the starting point of the unwound contour which is depicted as blue line.

Fig. 2. Processing pipeline for computing a 3D panorama reconstruction from gastroscopic video sequences. It is build as extension of an existing panorama mapping pipeline (unshaded), which provides the panorama image of the esophagus wall and unwound contours.

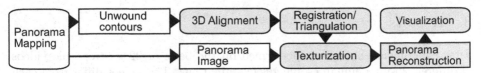

The 3D alignment of a given 2D contour and frame is achieved by subtracting the mean values for x- and y-coordinates from each point of the contour and adding a z-coordinate, which in case of frame i is set to $z = ci$ with c being a constant value for scaling. This results in retrieving a set of 3D contours, one for each frame, that are centered at their individual centroids. In order to simplify the next step of pairwise contour registration, all contours are interpolated to the same length by applying a linear interpolation.

For the registration of the given set of contours, they are treated as lines that are horizontally aligned on a regular grid. Their starting point (most left point on the grid) are set to their centroids nearest neighbor point, when regarding only its x-coordinate and using the point with greater y-coordinate. The contours are closed by copying their start points to the respective contours end. A contour to contour registration is then achieved by the triangulation of this regular grid, similar to building a vertex list used in computer graphics, describing the order of point traversal. This assignment of consecutive points of contour pairs to such a vertex list is illustrated in Fig. 3. Since contours from consecutive frames undergo little change in most cases and since the tubular geometry of the esophagus wall is commonly less concave, this approach results in a stable and steady triangulation.

The texturization step of the obtained triangulated mesh is performed using the panorama image as texture image, providing all contour points with color information. For a smooth visualization, the texture color is linearly interpolated

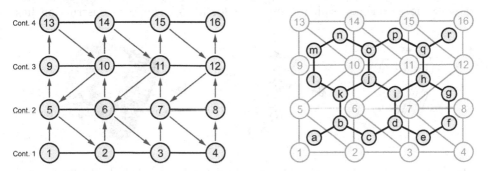

Fig. 3. Illustration of the vertex ordering (left) and its dual graph (right) of four contours of length four.

between vertices when rendering. The processing of a three dimensional esophagus reconstruction from a gastroscopic video sequence is depicted in Fig. 4.

3   Results

First experiments have been performed on the basis of 22 gastroscopic videos of different in-vivo human esophagus examinations. The videos differ from each other in terms of number of frames, image quality, esophagus wall texture and color, amount and density of contaminates, consistency of illumination, steadiness of the endoscopes movement, consistency of withdrawal speed and direction and steadiness of the patients movements. More stable video material tends to result in visually better panorama images and thus 3D reconstructions. Currently, the parameter optimization has to be applied empirically and case-related. Some qualitative results are shown in Fig. 5.

An approach for the quantitative evaluation of the presented method bears several challenges. For the matter of measuring robustness, completeness and accuracy, the main difficulty lies in the missing ground truth information of actual and measurable in-vivo esophagus geometry, as well as esophagus wall texture. A first evaluation environment has been build, consisting of a rigid esophagus model using a pipe and a series of printed textures as interchangeable wall texture. A series of video sequences has been acquired by slowly withdrawing the endoscope as smooth and centered as possible. The obtained video sequences have been processed by the proposed method and the resulting 3D reconstructed models were visually examined. The findings contributed to a set of possible adjustments and improvements for upcoming implementations, described in the following discussion.

4   Discussion

Based on an existing processing pipeline for the computation of panorama images of the esophagus wall, an approach for its 3D shape reconstruction has

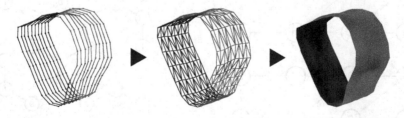

Fig. 4. 3D reconstruction of an esophagus segment. Left: 3D aligned contours of equal length; Center: a registration of contours that results in a triangle mesh; Right: the texturized panorama reconstruction.

been presented in this contribution. Next to panorama images, 3D visualizations of the esophagus enable an intuitive additional general-view of the tubular geometry which provides an enriched contextual information and may provide opportunities for

- an enhanced documentation of the esophagus,
- improved context-aware diagnosis, and
- new educational possibilities.

On the basis of first promising experiments, a series of possible improvements are pointed out. Up to date, parameters are chosen case-related, since they depend on the quality and properties of a given input video. These parameters might be set automatically or adaptively, if applicable, by using plausibility tests or assert auxiliary conditions to the algorithms outcomes.

The geometric accuracy of the reconstructed esophagus depends highly on the smoothing of the masked input frame. The stronger the frame has been smoothed, the more stable the 3D shape reconstruction performs but geometric

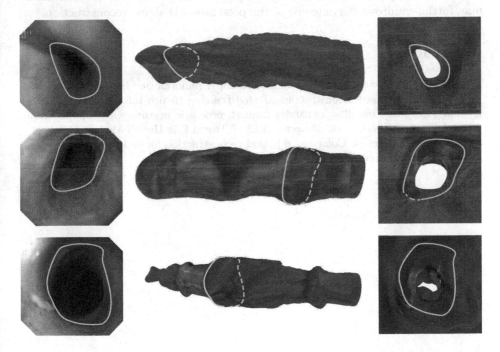

Fig. 5. 3D shape reconstructions from three different gastroscopic video sequences. Left: an input video frame with its unwound contour; Center: the 3D reconstructed model of the esophagus; Right: a view inside the related part of the 3D shape model. The blue line marks the unwound contour at this frame which approximately follows the geometry of the esophagus wall at constant depth. Approximated geometric features, such as constrictions, are preserved (top). Texture information, such as mucous congestion are re-attached to the model (bottom).

details get lost. A constraint on the overall geometry of the esophagus by applying a mathematical tube-model can hereby allow for a more stable 3D shape retrieval whilst preserving geometric details.

The illumination intensity of the endoscope may change over time due to its optional integrated and automated control feature to protect from overexposure. Using a constant intensity value b for the unwinding of a contour of a given frame, this leads to contours of varying extent over time, although the esophagus spatial extent may remain constant (compare bottom example in Fig. 5). An intensity normalization can hereby adaptively adjust the unwinding value b resulting in robust spatial extent of contours and thus of 3D shape reconstructions.

The swallowing reflex may cause a collapse of the contour up to zero spatial extent. In this case, a registration of such virtually non-existent contour fails and the triangulated mesh breaks. The detection of the swallowing reflex as well as contours of poor quality can help to automatically discard contours that are unusable for registration and triangulation.

Since the contributed method builds on a preceding processing pipeline for panorama mapping of the esophagus, improvements of the preceding methods may further improve the outcome of the presented 3D shape reconstruction.

References

1. Ishii T, et al. Novel points of view for endoscopy: panoramized intraluminal opened image and 3D shape reconstruction. J Med Imaging Health Inf. 2011;1(1):13–20.
2. Ishii T, et al. Urine flow dynamics through prostatic urethra with tubular organ modeling using endoscopic imagery. IEEE J Transl Eng Health Med. 2014;2:1–9.
3. Tokgozoglu HN, et al. Color-based hybrid reconstruction for endoscopy. IEEE Conf Comput Vis Pattern Recognit Workshops. 2012; p. 8–15.

Computerunterstützte Planung von Bonebridge Operationen

M. Scherbinsky[1], G. J. Lexow[1], Th. S. Rau[1], B. Preim[2], O. Majdani[1]

[1]Medizinische Hochschule Hannover, Klinik für Hals-Nasen-Ohrenheilkunde,
Hannover, Deutschland
[2]Institut für Simulation und Graphik, Otto-von-Guericke-Universität Magdeburg
Lexow.Jakob@mh-hannover.de

Kurzfassung. Zur Unterstützung der präoperativen Planung zur Platzierung eines Hörimplantats am Schädelknochen eines Patienten mit Hörschädigung wurde ein Prototyp einer Planungssoftware basierend auf präoperativen DVT-Daten entwickelt. Die Umsetzung erfolgte mittels eines VTK-Widgets, das Manipulationen der Implantatlage sowohl in zweidimensionalen Schnittansichten als auch in einer dreidimensionalen Darstellung des Schädelknochens erlaubt. Zusätzlich wurde auch die Biegung des Implantats berücksichtigt. Dabei lag der Fokus auf einfacher Anwendbarkeit und der Umsetzung geeigneter Manipulationstechniken mittels eines 2D-Eingabegerätes.

1 Einleitung

Bei Patienten mit einer diagnostizierten Schädigung der natürlichen Schallweiterleitung zum Innenohr wird ein Knochenleitungsimplantatsystem, z.B. die Bonebridge (MED-EL, Innsbruck, Österreich), eingesetzt. Eine Bonebridge überbrückt die geschädigte Schallübertragung, von Außen- und Mittelohr zum Innenohr. Ein externer Empfänger auf der Haut nimmt dazu Schallwellen aus der Umgebung auf und überträgt sie elektromagnetisch auf das Implantat, das Vibrationen im Knochen erzeugt und so den Schall zum Innenohr weiterleitet. Abb. 1 zeigt den Aufbau des Hörimplantats und eine skizzenhafte Platzierung. Der kritische Teil des Implantats ist der Transducer für die Vibrationserzeugung, der für eine gute Übertragung in den Knochen des Mastoids implantiert wird. Aus dem klinischen Alltag sind Mediziner mit 2D-Schnittansichten topografischer Bilddaten sehr gut vertraut. Diese Darstellungen liefern den Medizinern den Ist-Zustand der individuellen anatomischen Strukturen eines Patienten. Die Größe und Form der relevanten Strukturen, insbesondere der Risikostrukturen und deren Lage, können zur Planung des operativen Eingriffs herangezogen werden. Kritische Strukturen für die Bonebridge-Implantation sind der Sinus sigmoideus und die Dura. Gegenwärtig basiert die Planung der Implantatposition relativ zu diesen Strukturen einzig auf der räumlichen Vorstellung des Chirurgen. Das ist insbesondere bei untypischer Anatomie (z. B. durch krankhafte Veränderung des Felsenbeins oder vorhergehende Operationen) eine schwierige Aufgabe. Mit

Blick auf die umfangreichen Formen von Computerunterstützung in der HNO [1] ist es naheliegend, auch diese Aufgabe durch die Verwendung einer geeigneten Planungssoftware zu vereinfachen.

In einer solchen Software muss der Anwender virtuell die Lage des Implantats relativ zum Schädelknochen in allen drei Dimensionen ausrichten können. Dammann et al. [2] beschreiben eine Methode zur Simulation eines chirurgischen Eingriffs zur Bestimmung einer geeigneten Position und der Vorbereitung eines Implantatbetts. Die einzelnen Objekte können mit einer konventionellen 2D- oder 3D-Maus beliebig transformiert werden. Zur präoperativen Planung einer geeigneten Position eines BoneBridge-Implantats verwenden Wimmer et al. [3] eine farbcodierte Darstellung der Knochendicke. Darüberhinaus werden Methoden zum Ausrichten des Implantats nicht weiter beschrieben. Während des operativen Eingriffs hat der Chirurg Zugriff auf die Planungsdaten. Ein Software-Tool zur Platzierung einer BoneBridge haben Ramm et al. umgesetzt [4] . Während der Ausrichtung der BC-FMT am Schädelknochen bekommt der Benutzer ein visuelles Feedback zur Eignung der gewählten Position durch die farbliche Codierung der Knochendichte, der Entfernung der Risikostrukturen und das Hinzufügen von Warnhinweisen zur Eignung der Platzierung der BC-FMT. Die meisten Benutzer, so auch Mediziner, favorisieren traditionelle 2D-Eingabegeräte. Zur Manipulation der 3D-Objekte müssen dem medizinischen Anwender geeignete Interaktionstechniken zur Verfügung gestellt werden. Eine gute Basis zur Umsetzung geeigneter Manipulationstechniken bieten 3D-Widgets. Ein Widget zur Rotation, Translation und Skalierung von Objekten mit Hilfe der 2D-Maus haben Conner et al. umgesetzt [5]. Handles werden dabei zur eingeschränkten Interaktion entlang einer Achse oder um eine Achse eingesetzt. Ziel dieser Arbeit war die Umsetzung eines Prototypen eines Widgets zur Manipulation der räumlichen Lage von Objekten. Das Widget sollte den Medizinern in vertrauten 2D-Ansichten und in einer 3D-Ansicht zur Verfügung gestellt werden.

Abb. 1. Skizzenhafte Platzierung des Implantats am Schädelknochen. Zur Platzierung des Implantats muss die Beschaffenheit des Schädels des Patienten berücksichtigt werden. Eine Bonebridge besteht aus 1. Transducer (Bone Conduction-Floating Mass Transducer - BC-FMT), 2. Demodulator und 3. Spule: Der BC-FMT hat einen Durchmesser von 15,8 mm und benötigt für die Einbettung eine Tiefe von 8,7 mm. Die Verbindung zwischen dem Transducer und dem Demodulator ist beweglich. Die Bewegung beschränkt sich auf ±90° in horizontaler Ebene und -30° in vertikaler Ebene.

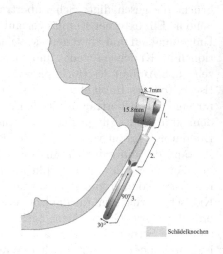

2 Material und Methoden

Die Programmierung der Anwendung erfolgte in der Programmiersprache C++ unter Verwendung der Open-Source-Libraries Qt (Version 4.8.4, qt-project.org) und VTK (Version 5.10.0, vtk.org). Bilddaten eines digitalen Volumentomographen (DVT) dienen als Ausgangspunkt für den Workflow dieser Computerunterstützung. Diese werden in den standardisierten 2D-Ansichten (sagittal, coronal und axial) und in einer 3D-Ansicht visualisiert. In der 3D-Ansicht wird der Knochen mithilfe eines schwellenwertbasierten Segmentierungsalgorithmus visualisiert. Zur Planung einer geeigneten Position des Implantats wird ein geometrisches Modell des Implantats als CAD-Objekt im STL-Format verwendet. Dieses Modell wird sowohl in den 2D-Ansichten (Umriss in Schichtebene) als auch in einer 3D-Ansicht (Oberflächenmodell) dargestellt. Zur Platzierung des Implantats wird dem Chirurgen ein Widget zur Verfügung gestellt, das an das Implantat gebunden ist. Die Realisierung des Widgets erfolgt in Anlehnung an in VTK umgesetzte Widgets, das heißt das Verhalten und die Geometrie des Objektes werden getrennt voneinander gesteuert. Das Widget dient zur Ausführung von 2D- und 3D-Transformationen zur Platzierung eines Hörimplantats. Es kann sowohl innerhalb der im medizinischen Bereich üblicherweise verwendeten 2D-Schichtansichten (sagittal, coronal und axial) als auch im 3D-Raum benutzt werden und erlaubt das Verschieben (Translate), Rotieren (Rotate) und das Verbiegen des Implantats (Bend):

2.1 Translate

Zum Verschieben des Implantats werden die Koordinatenachsen im Zentrum des BC-FMT eingeblendet. Mit der Darstellung der Koordinatenachsen kann der Chirurg das Implantat mittels einer 2D-Maus frei im Raum bewegen. Die Selektion einer Achse beschränkt sich auf das Verschieben des Implantats entlang dieser Achse. Die Verschiebung des Implantats entspricht der Translation eines Punktes p um den Verschiebevektor v. Der Verschiebevektor wird aus den aktuellen 2D-Mauspositionen (x, y) berechnet.

2.2 Rotate

Zur Darstellung des Dreh-Modus wird zusätzlich zu den Koordinatenachsen die Drehrichtung abgebildet. Diese entsprechen der Drehung des Implantats um einen Rotationswinkel und die zugehörige Rotationsachse, die sich aus der Bewegungsrichtung der Maus ergibt. Rotationen können mathematisch durch orthonormale Matrizen oder durch Quaternionen dargestellt werden. Quaternionen wurden verwendet, da sich diese einfach normieren lassen und numerische Probleme vermieden werden können.

2.3 Bend

Das Verbindungsstück zwischen Transducer und Demodulator ist in horizontaler und vertikaler Ebene beweglich und somit auf die Rotation des Transducers beschränkt. Die Manipulationstechnik Bend soll diese Bewegungen umsetzen. Der Knickpunkt wird im Mittelpunkt der Verbindung des Transducers mit dem Demodulator platziert. Die Manipulation der Handles ist auf das Verbiegen des Implantats um ±90° in horizontaler Ebene und -30° in vertikaler Ebene beschränkt. Die Manipulation des Implantats erfolgt im lokalen Koordinatensystem.

3   Ergebnisse

Ein Prototyp einer Software zur präoperativen Planung von Bonebridge-Operationen wurde programmiert. Zur Umsetzung geeigneter Manipulationstechniken wurde ein Widget für die präoperative Platzierung des Hörimplantats mittels eines 2D-Eingabegeräts entwickelt. Radiologische Bilddaten des Patientenschädels werden aus dem DICOM-Dateien und das Implantat als CAD-Objekt aus dem STL-Format geladen. Beide Objekte stehen dem Chirurgen sowohl in den üblicherweise verwendeten 2D-Schichtansichten (sagittal, coronal und axial) als auch einer 3D-Ansicht zur Verfügung. Die 2D-Ansichten können vom Chirurgen zur Beurteilung der Abstände zu kritischen Strukturen wie dem Sinus sigmoideus und der Dura genutzt werden. Zur Platzierung des Implantats stehen unterschiedliche Interaktionsmöglichkeiten zur Verfügung. Der Chirurg kann mit der gesamten Szene interagieren, die sich aus dem segmentierten Schädel des Patienten und dem 3D-Modell des Implantats zusammensetzt. Der Betrachter erhält einen globalen Überblick über die Szene sowie über die Stellung der Objekte zueinander. Die Selektion des Implantats und die damit verbundene Aktivierung des 3D-Widgets, zur Manipulation des Implantats, legt den Fokus für weitere Interaktionen auf das Implantat. Das 3D-Widget stellt dem Chirurgen Handles zur Verfügung, mittels derer er zwischen den einzelnen Techniken wählen kann:

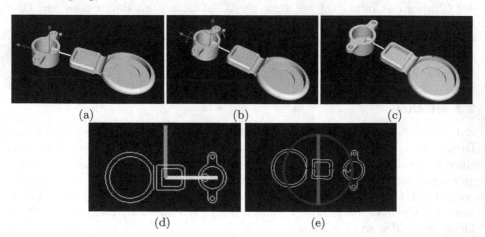

(a)   (b)   (c)

(d)   (e)

Abb. 2. Darstellung der Handles des 3D-Widgets als (a) Koordinatenachsen zum Verschieben und als gebogene Pfeile zum (b) Rotieren und (c) Verbiegen des Implantats. Die Anpassung der Handles in den 2D-Ansichten (d) zum Verschieben und (d) zum Rotieren.

- *Translate* dient der Bewegung des Implantats im Raum. Die eingeblendeten Koordinatenachsen (siehe Abb. 2 a) dienen dabei als Handles. Durch die Selektion einer einzelnen Achse wird diese farblich hervorgehoben und das Verschieben des Implantats auf diese Achse beschränkt. In den 2D-Ansichten werden schichtspezifische Handles eingeblendet (siehe Abb. 2 d).
- *Rotate* dient der Veränderung der Orientierung des Implantats. Als Handles werden in der 3D-Ansicht Pfeil-Darstellungen um den Drehpunkt platziert (siehe Abb. 2 b). Diese zeigen die Drehung um die entsprechende Achse an. In den 2D-Ansichten werden Orbits als Handles um den Drehpunkt platziert (siehe Abb. 2 e). Die Selektion eines Handles hebt diesen farblich hervor und beschränkt die Rotation um dessen Achse.
- *Bend* (Verbiegen des Implantats) beschränkt sich auf die horizontale ($\pm 90°$) und vertikale Ebene (-30°). Die Handles werden als Pfeil-Darstellungen an der Spule des Implantats platziert (siehe Abb. 2 c).

Translate und Rotate können sowohl innerhalb der 2D-Ansichten als auch in der 3D-Ansicht ausgeführt werden, wobei die Transformationen in den jeweiligen Ansichten in Echtzeit angepasst werden. Die Darstellung des 3D-Widgets wird innerhalb der 2D-Ansichten angepasst. Bend ist nur auf den 3D-Raum beschränkt.

4 Diskussion

Das vorgestellte Programm bietet eine einfache und intuitive Möglichkeit zur Planung der Implantatlage bei einer Bonebridge-Implantation. In ihrer operativen Praxis sind es Chirurgen gewohnt, innerhalb komplexer 3D-Strukturen zu interagieren. Somit bilden, neben traditionellen 2D-Schichtansichten, 3D-Visualisierungen, auf Grund ihrer besseren Abbildung der Realität, eine optimale Möglichkeit zur Planung operativer Eingriffe. Demgegenüber lassen sich in den Schichtansichten Abstände zu Risikostrukturen besser erkennen, worin der Vorteil der kombinierten Lösung liegt. Ein alternatives Software-Tool zur Planung einer Bonebridge-Implantation haben Ramm et al. [4] umgesetzt. Während der Ausrichtung der BC-FMT am Schädelknochen bekommt der Benutzer ein visuelles Feedback zur Eignung der gewählten Position auf Basis der Abstände zu autosegmentierten Risikostrukturen. Das erfordert eine höhere Rechenleistung als der hier vorgestellte Ansatz. Auch findet die Position der Spule keine Berücksichtigung, was insbesondere für das kosmetische Ergebnis der Operation nachteilig ist, da die Spule die Position des externen Teils des Implantats bedingt. Ein Verfahren zur automatisierten Berechnung der Knochendicke wurde von Lexow et al. entwickelt [6]. Dies ist eine sinnvolle Ergänzung zu der hier vorgestellten Software, um die initiale Positionierung zu erleichtern. Das hier vorgestellte Widget bietet die zeitgleiche Verwaltung der Geometrie des Hörimplantats und der umgesetzten Manipulationstechniken zur Ausrichtung des Implantats. Bei der Umsetzung der Manipulationstechniken wurde insbesondere auch das Verbiegen des Implantats berücksichtigt, um eine realitätsnahe Computerunterstützung zu gewährleisten. Die Nutzung eines Widgets bietet eine multifunktionale Anpassung notwendiger Interaktionstechniken und eine Erweiterung weiterer Handles. Kontextbezogenes Ein- und Ausblenden gewünschter Handles gewährleistet eine vereinfachte Anpassung des Widgets an weitere Objekte zur Platzierung sowohl im 3D-Raum als auch innerhalb der 2D-Ansichten. Zur präzisen Ausrichtung des Objektes durch den Anwender ist mittels der Handles, orientierend an den Achsen, eine sehr genaue Platzierung des Objektes möglich. Zur weiteren Verbesserung des Planungsprozesses wäre ein visuelles Feedback für den Chirurgen hilfreich, im Kontext der Bestimmung einer geeigneten Position für das Implantat. Weitere Untersuchungen sind zur vereinfachten Übertragung der Planungsdaten auf den Patienten geplant.

Literaturverzeichnis

1. Preim B, Botha CP. Visual Computing for Medicine, Second Edition: Theory, Algorithms, and Applications (The Morgan Kaufmann Series in Computer Graphics). 2nd ed. Morgan Kaufmann; 2013.
2. Dammann F, Bode A, Schwaderer E, et al. Computer-aided surgical planning for implantation of hearing aids based on CT data in a VR environment. Radiographics. 2001.
3. Wimmer W, Guignard J, Gerber N, et al. A preoperative planning method for Bonebridge implantations using surface distance maps. Int J Comput Assist Radiol Surg. 2013.
4. Ramm H, Morillo OSV, Todt I, et al. Visual support for positioning hearing implants. Proc CURAC. 2013; p. 116–20.
5. Conner BD, Snibbe SS, Herndon KP, et al. Three-dimensional widgets. Proc Symp Interact 3D Graph. 1992; p. 183–8.
6. Lexow GJ, Rau TS, Eckardt F, et al. Automatisierte Bestimmung der Schädelknochendicke in CT- und DVT-Bilddaten. Proc CURAC. 2012.

Real Time Medical Instrument Detection and Tracking in Microsurgery

Mohamed Alsheakhali[1], Mehmet Yigitsoy[1], Abouzar Eslami[2], Nassir Navab[1]

[1]Technichal University of Munich, Munich, Germany
[2]Carl Zeiss Meditec AG, Munich, Germany
alsheakh@in.tum.de.de

Abstract. The detection of surgical instruments in real time is one of the most challenging problems in retinal microsurgery operations. The instrument's deformable shape, the presence of its shadow, and the illumination variations are the main contributors for such challenge. A new approach for the detection of the tip of the surgical tool is proposed, which can handle the shape deformation, and the presence of the its shadow or the presence of blood vessels. The approach starts by segmenting the tool-like objects using the L*a*b color model. One of these segments is selected as the target tool based on tool's shaft model. The probabilistic Hough transform was used to get the structural information which can guide us to optimize the best possible candidates' locations to fit the tool model. The detected tool tip and its slope are propagated between the frames in the images sequence. Experimental results demonstrate the high accuracy of this technique in addition to achieve the real time requirements.

1 Introduction

Instrument Detection and tracking in retinal microscopic surgery is a crucial part for the minimal invasive procedures due to the limited sight conditions and indirect access to retinal tissues during the operation which requires further assistance to reduce the damage during the surgery. On one hand, artificial markers have been used for detection and tracking [1] which requires working on specific and predefined color information. On the other hand, depending only on the geometry of the tool [2] definitely requires a large database for the tool with different orientations and scales, which might work on an eye phantom but not in intra-operative surgery.

Allan et al. [3] learns a random forest on color information extracted from a set of color spaces which is considered to be expensive and not applicable in real time operations. Different methods [4, 5] were proposed to detect the tool tip based on learning a classifier on a large training datasets.

Herein, a new approach is proposed to detect and track the tool tip in microscopic images in real time surgery in a more precise fashion. We define the tool tip position as a point on the tool centerline where it touches the retinal tissues (Fig. 1(a) as point A). The L*a*b transform [6] is used mainly for the

segmentation process as shown in Fig. 1, because it highlights the perceptual
uniformity of the tool which is characterized as a textureless object. In general,
the structural information is considered to reduce the search space and to localize the potential tool segments in real time. Once the tool segment is detected in
a frame, the tool centerline and the tool tip are extracted and propagated to the
next frame to make the detection and tracking much more faster and accurate.

2 Methodology

2.1 Tool segmentation

As observed in a previous work [7], one dataset was taken into consideration for
validation. In this work, one more challenging dataset was included. In both
cases, the tool is included in a small range of the lowest intensity values of the
a* channel within the retina region. Applying a thresholding function on the a*
channel gives the results shown in Fig. 2(a) , where most of the tool pixels are
preserved in addition to some parts of the background which can be removed
easliy by subtracting a thresholded L* channel from the image in Fig. 2(a) to
produce the refined a* channel as shown in Fig. 2(b).

2.2 Tool edges detection

The refined a* channel gives an image with many segmented objects. A prior
information in different ways to give preference for some segments against others
can be incorporated. Many of these segments could be discarded if they are not
aligned with strong edges, or even if they aligned with bended edges, this is why

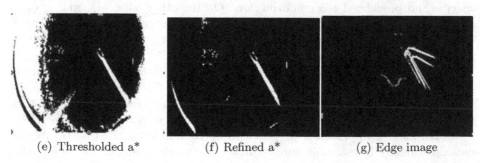

(e) Thresholded a*   (f) Refined a*   (g) Edge image

Fig. 2. Tool shaft component extraction (originals from [7]).

we structural information with the refined a* channel needs to be included. The gradient of the green channel is used to get structural information, and after thresholding, it gives the output shown in Fig. 2(c). The thresholding is important to eliminate the contribution of the background and other eye components in the edges image. From the edge image in Fig. 2(c) and the refined a* channel in Fig. 2(b), the tool object could be defined without resorting to the intensity values by just applying the propabilistic hough transform to detect the lines in the edges image as shown in Fig. 3(a). The strongest 150 linear segments were extracted and superimposed on the refined a* channel as shown in Fig. 3(b). At each line, a tool model as shown in Fig. 3(c) is fit to find the tool edge line. The model consists of two areas, where all white pixels in one area are given positive weight while the white pixels in second area are given a negative weight. The selected tool edge line is the one which maximizes the cost function F given by

$$F = w_1 * \sum_{p \in A_1} X(p) + w_2 * \sum_{p \in A_2} X(p) \tag{1}$$

where w_1 , and w_2 are the weights given to the white pixels p of the refined a* image (X) located in A_1 and A_2, respectively. If the value of w_1 is positive and w_2 is negative, then (1) detects the right side of the tool shaft. The negative value of w_2 is chosen to penalize the existence of the white pixels on the right side of the hough lines. The yellow line in Fig. 3(b) is the detected line based on (1), and the white segment aligned to it is considered the tool object.

2.3   Tool tip and centerline detection

The tool centerline can be detected if the detected left and right tool edges were parallel. Unfortunately, in most cases they are not parallel due to the tool's fast motion, image blurring, and the large illumination changes which influence the quality of the a* channel. Hence, it yields a distorted non-parallel edges. To overcome this problem and to find the tool centerline, it is better to rely on the tool object aligned to the detected tool edge line. The centers of masses for a bunch of lines perpendicular to that line are computed which produce m

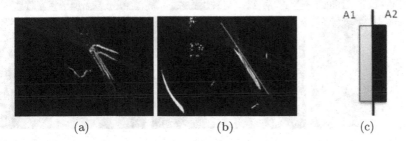

(a)   (b)   (c)

Fig. 3. (a) The detected Hough lines in the Edge image. (b) The same Hough lines obtained from the edges image and superimpsoed on the refined a* channel.(c) The tool model where the mid-line should lay on each Hough line. (Original images were taken from [7]).

candidate points. The tool centerline is found by fitting a line to these m points using RANSAC. The center of mass (X_L, Y_L) for each line is calculated based on (2)

$$X_L = \frac{1}{n} * \sum_{i=1}^{n} x_i, \quad Y_L = \frac{1}{n} * \sum_{i=1}^{n} y_i \qquad (2)$$

where n is the number of white pixels along one line L orthogonal to the tool edge line at point p. x_i and y_i are the coordinates of these pixels. The resultant line forms a signal where the transition from the foreground to the background is the tool tip position in case of using a vitrectomy tool, but if the tool has a forceps-like shape then the transition point is the joint point and further processing is required to find the tool tip position. The processing in this case is to start from the detected joint point and find the connected components around the centerline on both sides. The farthest point in the connected component from the joint point is kept, and the projection of this point perpendicularly on the centerline is the tool tip position.

2.4   Tool tip tracking

Once the tool centerline and the tool tip are detected in the current frame, these information is propagated to the next frame. Therefore, there is no need to process the entire frame each time. Assuming the tool tip position P_t and the tool slope S_t have been detected at frame t, then the search for the candidate hough lines at frame t+1 is limited to the lines within a rectangular box centered at P_t. These candidates lines are filtered out again to get rid of the ones which

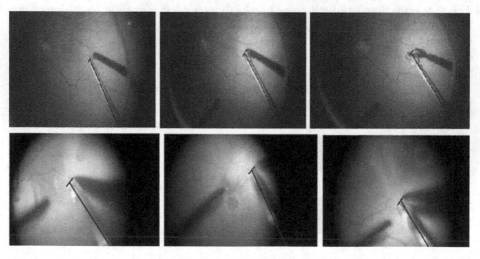

Fig. 4. Random samples from different datasets with different conditions. The first top row is from the first dataset where the red component is prominent and the tool is evenly illuminated. The second bottom row is from the second dataset where the green component is prominent, and the tool is unevenly illuminated.

have a large slope difference from the tool slope detected at the previous frame based on

$$|S_{i(t+1)} - S_t| < \epsilon \qquad (3)$$

where $S_i(t+1)$ is the i-th candidate line at frame t+1, and ϵ is a small value chosen empirically to be around 0.2.

3   Experiments and results

This algorithm was implemented using C++ and OpenCV installed on a machine with Core-I7, 2.8GHz CPU, and it runs at 23 fps.

3.1   Retinal microscopic datasets

Two microscopic datasets for real human eye surgery have been used in order to validate the technique, where 400 (1080X1920) images have been manually annotated for each dataset. The annotation includes the tool tip position, and one point on the centerline of the shaft to calculate the tool slope. The images were resized to one fifth of their original size during processing, while the validation and visualization both consider the original size. Fig. 4 shows the detected tool tip and centerline for samples from both datasets.

3.2   Datasets evaluation

The model width is 7 pixels on each side and the height is 140 pixels. The weights w_1 and w_2 in (1) were chosen to be 1 and -5 respectively. The tracking box has the size of 20x80 pixels. As an augmentation to our previously reported study [7], for quantitative validation and analysis of this approach, the percentage of the images where the tool tip is correctly detected as a function of the accuracy threshold was calculated. For each accuracy threshold (T1), we consider the percentage of the images in which the detected tool tip is at distance less than or equal to T1 pixels from the actual position based on the ground truth. This threshold varied from 5 to 50 pixels. From Fig. 5(a), it can be noticed that the tool tip positions have been correctly detected in 90 percent of the images within

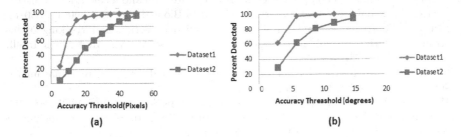

Fig. 5. Tool tip and centerline detection accuracy measurments.

a threshold of only 20 pixels for the first dataset, which shows the high accuracy in detection, and for the second dataset, the detection error is higher due to the large illumination variations and the unevenlly illuminated parts of the tool, in addition to the nature of the images which is blurred in comparison with the first dataset.

Fig. 5(b) shows the accuracy of our method in detecting the centerline of the tool. Another accuracy threshold (T2) has been defined as the angular difference in degrees between the actual slope measured based on the ground truth and the detected slope of the tool. The results show that in 90 percent of the images, centerlines were detected with angular error smaller than 6 degrees for the first dataset, and 12 degrees for the second dataset.

4   Conclusion

Herein, we presented a new real time approach for the detection and tracking of the medical tool in retinal microsurgery operations. The approach detects the tool tip position with high accuracy without using any learning techniques or prior information about the color or the geometry of the tool. The results showed the efficiency of using this approach to handle cases that contain not only the tool but also blood vessels, tool shadow, and light sources. The approach also works well regardless of blurring effects, and small lightning changes. However, the quality of the a* channel has an impact on the accuracy of the approach, and the accuracy gets lower as the tool gets darker. As a future work, a more robust technique to the occlusions, darkness along the tool, and the severe illumination changes to be achieved.

References

1. Tonet O, Thoranaghatte RU, Megali G, et al. Tracking endoscopic instruments without a localizer: a shape-analysis-based approach. Comput Aided Surg. 2007;12(1):35–42.
2. Baek YM, Tanaka S, Harada K, et al. Robust visual tracking of robotic forceps under a microscope using kinematic data fusion. IEEE Trans Mechatronics. 2014;19(1):278–88.
3. Allan M, Ourselin S, Thompson S, et al. Toward detection and localization of instruments in minimally invasive surgery. IEEE Trans Biomed Eng. 2013;60(4):1050–8.
4. Sznitman R, Richa R, Taylor RH, et al. Unified detection and tracking of instruments during retinal microsurgery. IEEE Trans Pattern Anal Mach Intell. 2013;35(5):1263–73.
5. Sznitman R, Ali K, Richa R, et al. Data-driven visual tracking in retinal microsurgery. Proc MICCAI. 2012; p. 568–75.
6. Hunter RS. Photoelectric color difference meter. J Opt Soc Am. 1958;48(12):985–93.
7. Alsheakhali M, Yigitsoy M, Eslami A, et al. Surgical tool detection and tracking in retinal microsurgery. Proc SPIE. 2015; p. accepted.

Enabling Endovascular Treatment of Type A Dissections
Measurement Scheme for Aortic Surface Lengths

Cosmin Adrian Morariu[1], Tobias Terheiden[1], Daniel Sebastian Dohle[2],
Konstantinos Tsagakis[2], Josef Pauli[1]

[1]Intelligent Systems Group, Faculty of Engineering, University of Duisburg-Essen
[2]Department of Thoracic and Cardiovascular Surgery, Universitätsklinikum Essen
adrian.morariu@uni-due.de

Abstract. Our goal is to provide a means of enabling minimally invasive therapy within the ascending aorta as a standard clinical procedure in case of aortic dissections. Exact knowledge of the inner and outer surface lengths of the ascending aorta (AA) is essential for producing patient-specific stent-grafts in order to avoid interference with any of the branch vessels connected to the AA. This contribution introduces a genuine approach to quantifying these key parameters. Furthermore, we employ an unique and precise result validation, namely by comparing the accuracy of the inner and outer curvature lengths, determined within a cadaveric CT dataset, with manual measurements performed by a vascular surgeon on the body donor's excised aorta. Our validated scheme is also being applied under identical circumstances on three patient datasets in pursuance of assessing the variability pertaining to human aortic pathological morphology.

1 Introduction

Even if treated promptly, aortic dissections reveal desolate long-term survival rates related to open surgical repair, which implies cardiopulmonary bypass and hypothermic circulatory arrest [1]. Unfortunately, it still represents nowadays the most viable intervention modality with regard to Type A dissections, which affect the ascending aorta (AA) [2]. In contrary to the descending vessel's part, the AA and aortic arch possess a more complex vascular anatomy. Hence, exact knowledge of the inner and outer surface lengths of the AA would be required for endovascular therapy due to the proximity of the coronary ostia, respectively of the supraaortic branches to both landing zones of the stent-graft.

On application level, contributions [3] and [4] noticed the crucial importance of the inner/outer aortic lengths regarding endoluminal repair. The authors demonstrate that these lengths may significantly deviate from the corresponding length along the centerline. Thus, only aortic centerline measurement is highly insufficient for planning the stent's landing zone. In [3] the inner/outer lengths are computed based on three parameters: cross-sectional aortic radius, the radius of curvature of the aortic arch and the length along the centerline.

However, especially in cases of severe pathologies such as aortic dissections, neither the cross-sectional aortic radius, nor the radius of curvature of the arch may be assumed as being constant. Consequently, we contrive a precise measurement scheme and we additionally validate the determined lengths within a cadaveric CT dataset, by comparing them with measurements performed by a vascular surgeon on the body donor's excised aorta.

2 Materials and methods

This contribution unveils an universal method capable to determine both crucial lengths along the 3D aortic mesh for any arbitrary vessel segment. The aortic mesh, together with an aortic centerline, originate from the aortic segmentation described in [5]. The measurement is performed within a sectional plane defined by three input points specified by the clinician in axial slices in order to define the desired segment. Coronal and sagittal views provide further guidance if required. In case of type A dissections the desired outer length extends from above the heart, distal to the right coronary artery (RCA), to the first supraaortic branch, the truncus brachiocephalicus (TB). The corresponding inner length starts distally to the left coronary artery (LCA), to reach the point on the opposite side to the TB. This point, denoted as TBi due to its position on the inner side of the aortic model, across the TB, will be computed automatically, since a manual placement would be difficult and error prone. For this reason we seek a plane E_{TB}, orthogonal to the aortic centerline and in immediate vicinity of the point TB. Fig. 1 (a) and (b) depict the position of RCA, LCA and TB within a CTA dataset.

For determining the sought plane E_{TB} we consider a set $P = (p_1, ..., p_n)$ of n centerline points in proximity to TB and extract n MPRs of size $m \times m$ orthogonal to the spline, each plane containing one of these points. In order to accomplish this goal, we compute

$$d_i = (x_{di}, y_{di}, z_{di}) = \frac{p_{i+1} - p_{i-1}}{\|p_{i+1} - p_{i-1}\|} \tag{1}$$

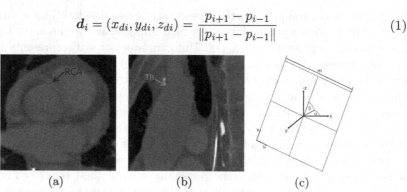

(a)	(b)	(c)

Fig. 1. Right (RCA) und left (LCA) coronary artery within an axial slice (a). Starting point of the TB within a sagittal view (b). Angles α and β characterize the extraction of an MPR plane in uv coordinate sytem and from the 3D volume in xyz-coordinate system (c).

representing the normalized orientation vector of the spline curve at location p_i. Extraction angles α_i and β_i for the multi-planar reformatted (MPR) plane having p_i as center are calculated by

$$\alpha_i = \operatorname{atan}\left(\frac{x_{di}}{y_{di}}\right), \text{ respectively } \beta_i = \operatorname{atan}\left(\frac{-\frac{y_{di}}{|y_{di}|}\sqrt{x_{di}^2 + y_{di}^2}}{z_{di}}\right) \qquad (2)$$

The uv-coordinate sytem of the MPR lies at first within the xy-plane and gets rotated around the z-axis by α_i. Rotation by β_i describes a subsequent rotation of the MPR around the new u-axis (Fig. 1(c)). 2D/3D mapping of intensity values is achieved by

$$\mathcal{M}(u,v) = I(x_{uv}, y_{uv}, z_{uv}) \qquad (3)$$

for the MPR $\mathcal{M}(u,v)$ with spline point $P = (p_x, p_y, p_z)$ as 3D center of the quadratic ROI. When extracting the ROI has to be taken into consideration that the slice spacing of some CT datasets (up to 6 mm) is much coarser than the axial within-slice resolution (ca. 0,6 mm). This aspect correlated with the varying mean intensity distribution of axial slices during the CT slice acquisition process determines the extraction of MPR – slices $\mathcal{M}(u,v)$ from the 3D input subvolume $V(x,y,z)$ by introducing a stretch-factor λ in cranio-caudal direction

$$\lambda = \frac{\sqrt{(vxsz_x \cdot \cos\alpha)^2 + (vxsz_y \cdot \sin\alpha)^2}}{1 + |\sin\beta| \cdot (vxsz_z - 1)}$$
$$= \frac{vxsz_x}{1 + |\sin\beta| \cdot (vxsz_z - 1)} \qquad (4)$$

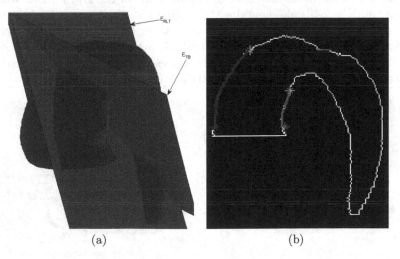

(a)	(b)

Fig. 2. Intersection of the planes E_{RLT}, E_{TB} with the aortic mesh yields the point TBi (a), which is the rightmost, yellow point in (b). The white contours represent the intersection of E_{RLT} and the aortic mesh. In blue – measured outer length. In red – determined inner length along the aortic curvature.

with $vxsz_{x/y/z}$ the voxel sizes in x, y and z-direction, respectively. Please note that for all our datasets $vxsz_x = vxsz_y$. Using λ we calculate

$$x_{uv} = p_x + \cos(\beta) \cos(\alpha) \ (v - m/2) - \sin(\alpha)(u - m/2)$$

$$y_{uv} = p_y + \cos(\beta) \sin(\alpha) \ (v - m/2) + \cos(\alpha)(u - m/2) \tag{5}$$

$$z_{uv} = p_z + \lambda \sin(\beta)(v - m/2)$$

for $\forall u, v$ and for $0 \le u < m - 1$, respectively $0 \le v < m - 1$.

Correction by λ of the scaling in z-direction causes staircase-like image artifacts. Linear interpolation of the intensities in z-direction rectifies this issue. Therefore, we alter equation 3 to

$$
\begin{aligned}
\mathcal{M}(u, v) = &(\lceil z_{uv} \rceil - z_{u,v}) \ I(x_{uv}, y_{uv}, \lfloor z_{uv} \rfloor) \\
&+ (z_{uv} - \lfloor z_{uv} \rfloor) \ I(x_{uv}, y_{uv}, \lceil z_{uv} \rceil)
\end{aligned} \tag{6}
$$

The rounding up or down of z_{uv} returns the indices $\lceil z_{uv} \rceil$ and $\lfloor z_{uv} \rfloor$ of the two axial slices between which the intensities have to be interpolated. For this purpose, we perform a z_{uv}-dependent blending of the intensities $I(x_{uv}, y_{uv}, \lfloor z_{uv} \rfloor)$ and $I(x_{uv}, y_{uv}, \lceil z_{uv} \rceil)$.

Finally, after extracting all MPRs $\mathcal{M}_i(u, v)$, with $i \in \{1, ..., n\}$, passing through the closest n spline points, plane E_{TB} will be selected based on the shortest distance between TB and each of the n MPRs. The line of intersection between the plane E_{RLT}, defined by the initial points TB, LCA and RCA, and the calculated plane E_{TB} penetrates the inner side of the aortic mesh through the quested point TBi. Fig. 2(a) illustrates the planes E_{RLT}, E_{TB} and the aortic mesh for one of the datasets. Since the intersection of the E_{RLT} plane with the aortic mesh (Fig. 2(b)) also contains the desired inner/outer contour lengths, we perform the measurement within the E_{RLT} plane. Due to the fact that we cannot assume that the points RCA, LCA and TB have been placed exactly on the aortic boundary, we compute at first the corresponding points on the contours of intersection between E_{RLT} and the 3D aortic mesh.

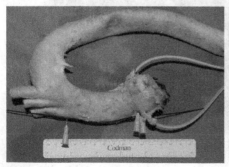 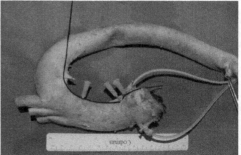

Fig. 3. Manually measuring the outer, respectively the inner contour length of an excised aorta belonging to a body donor.

3   Results

In order to guarantee the accuracy of our quantification method for the curvature lengths, a vascular surgeon performed manual measurements on the excised aorta belonging to a human body donor (Fig. 3), which we weigh against our measurements within the cadaveric CT dataset in Tab. 1. Our quantification result deviates for the outer length by only 0.51 mm from the native measurement and for the inner length by 3.4 mm. The cadaveric CTA dataset possesses a within-slice resolution of 0.92 mm and a slice spacing of 1.5 mm. Fig. 4 (a) depicts an MPR of the plane E_{RLT}, including all 4 points used for the measurement, as well as the measured inner and outer lengths of the AA. Due to the fact that the aorta pertaining to the cadaveric CT dataset contained fully thrombosed blood and also air, it has been manually marked on axial slices by a vascular surgeon. Hence, segmentation by a 3D region growing generated an unbiased 3D mesh prior to the quantification step.

Fig. 4 (b), (c) and (d) illustrate the quantification results for 3 patient CTA datasets. Within these datasets, the aorta has been segmented using the approach proposed by [5]. A further technique for extracting dissected aortas has been proposed in [6]. Tab. 1 also summarizes the results for the inner/outer curvature lengths of the patients, all of them being diagnosed with aortic dissection. Obviously, an extremely severe pathology such as aortic dissection leads to highly variable morphological characteristics of the patient's anatomy. The ratio between outer in inner curvature length significantly differs from one patient to another (ratio 1.49 in patient 1 compared to 2.18 / 2.26 in the other patients, Tab. 1). Furthermore, patients who underwent prior cardiovascular procedures often reveal a major deflection of the aortic morphology in comparison to the preinterventional stage.

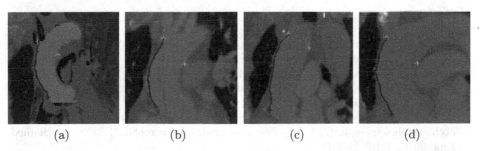

(a)   (b)   (c)   (d)

Fig. 4. MPR slices containing ROIs of E_{RLT} together with the measured inner and outer contour lengths of the AA for a) the cadaveric CT dataset, respectively b), c) and d) for 3 patient datasets. Due to the fact that the aorta pertaining to the cadaveric CT dataset contained fully thrombosed blood and also air, it has been manually marked on axial slices by a vascular surgeon.

Table 1. Inner/outer curvature lengths of the AA using our proposed method within a cadaveric CTA dataset compared to the manual measurement performed by the vascular surgeon on the body donor's excised aorta. Additionally, the results after quantifying the corresponding lengths within 3 patient CTAs.

	Outer (RCA→TB)	Inner (LCA→TBi)	Ratio O/I
Excised aorta (manual)	80 mm	54 mm	1.48
Cadaveric CTA dataset	80.51 mm	50.60 mm	1.59
Patient 1	102.94 mm	68.88 mm	1.49
Patient 2	86.12 mm	39.43 mm	2.18
Patient 3	97.71 mm	43.23 mm	2.26

4 Discussion

This contribution demonstrates that only morphological characteristics obtained from each patient's CTA dataset are able to guarantee the conformability of the stent-graft in regard to the various Type A dissection phenotypes. The validation against ground truth of the 3D contour lengths quantification method, represents a significant and, to the best of our knowledge, also unique step towards custom-designed stent-grafts according to individual CTA data. In contrast to previous approaches, we contrived a scheme, which allows us to precisely measure the surface lengths, without assuming neither constant aortic radii, nor a constant curvature of the aortic arch. For profoundly understanding the development of aortic pathologies in time, including different perioperative stages, further research has to be conducted towards quantification of anatomical changes in follow-up patient datasets.

References

1. Wendt D, Thielmann M, Melzer A, et al. The past, present and future of minimally invasive therapy in endovascular interventions: a review and speculative outlook. Minim Invasive Ther Allied Technol. 2013;22(4):242–53.
2. Zimpfer D, Schima H, Czerny M, et al. Experimental stent-graft treatment of ascending aortic dissection. Ann Thorac Surg. 2008;85(2):470–3.
3. Wörz S, von Tengg-Kobligk H, Henninger V, et al. 3D quantification of the aortic arch morphology in 3D CTA data for endovascular aortic repair. IEEE Trans Biomed Eng. 2010;57(10):2359–68.
4. Kaladji A, Spear R, Hertault A, et al. Centerline is not as accurate as outer curvature length to estimate thoracic endograft length. Eur J Vasc Endovasc Surg. 2013;46(1):82–6.
5. Morariu CA, Terheiden T, Dohle DS, et al. Graph-based and variational minimization of statistical cost functionals for 3D segmentation of aortic dissections. In: Pattern Recognit. Springer; 2014. p. 511–22.
6. Morariu CA, Dohle DS, Terheiden T, et al. Polar-based aortic segmentation in 3D CTA dissection data using a piecewise constant curvature model. Proc BVM. 2014; p. 390–5.

Outliers in 3D Point Clouds Applied to Efficient Image-Guided Localization

Ekaterina Sirazitdinova[1], Stephan M. Jonas[1], Deyvid Kochanov[1], Jan Lensen[2],
Richard Houben[2], Hans Slijp[2], Thomas M. Deserno[1]

[1]Institut für Medizinische Informatik, RWTH Aachen
[2]Applied Biomedical Systems, Maastricht, Netherlands
ekaterina.sirazitdinova@rwth-aachen.de

Abstract. In this work, the tasks of improving positioning efficiency and minimization of space requirements in image-based navigation are explored. We proved the assumption that it is possible to reduce image-matching time and to increase storage capacities by removing outliers from 3D models used for localization, by applying three outlier removal methods to our datasets and observing the localization associated with the resulting models.

1 Introduction

Nowadays, medical imaging processing is not limited to radiography or MRI but novel imaging modalities are presented including optical imaging technologies. For instance, photography is a prominent modality in wound documentation and skin lesion quantization. Furthermore, photography has been applied in other fields supporting patient. For instance, we are developing a guidance system for visually impaired and blind people that is based on optical imaging [1]. The aim is to locate a blind or visually impaired user in outdoor environments. Using structure from motion (SfM), 3D reconstructions of given tracks are created and stored in a database in the form of sparse point clouds. With a client-side App, query images are acquired and matched with the model to retrieve the precise location and orientation of the camera. High computational costs of the matching process and limited storage capacity cause the necessity of compressing 3D point clouds without loss of localization performance. It is likely that positioning accuracy can be maintained after removing outliers from 3D data.

According to the definition of Grubbs [2], an outlying observation, or outlier, is "one that appears to deviate markedly from other members of the sample in which it occurs". Outliers in a 3D point cloud may be of different nature. Firstly, they may result from errors occurring during the reconstruction process, such as inherent inaccuracies in feature detection, false matching, and errors in estimation of fundamental and projection matrices. Second, non-static environment objects (e.g., cars, chairs and tables of street cafes, advertisings, market stalls) create reconstruction noise.

In this paper, we analyse outlier removal in generated 3D point clouds for pedestrian navigation. Our hypothesis states that it is possible to maintain positioning accuracy while reducing the number of outliers in a reconstructed 3D model.

2   Materials and methods

2.1   Outlier removal

We implemented outlier removal approaches of Sotoodeh [3] and Wang et al. [4].

The *density-based* approach of Sotoodeh [3] is outlier detection algorithm based on local outlier factor (LOF) [5] applied to laser point clouds. LOF is depending on the local density of the neighborhood of an object being observed. The neighborhood is defined by the distance to the k-th nearest neighbor.

The *connectivity-based* method of Wang et al. [4] is a 2-step pipeline for outlier filtering. The authors detect sparse outliers applying a scheme based on the relative density deviation of the local neighborhood and the average local neighborhood, providing a scoring strategy that includes a normalization to become independent from the specific data distribution. To remove further small dense outliers, a clustering method is used. While the density-based method runs in a linear time, the second part of the connectivity-based approach, performed by agglomerative hierarchical clustering, has the run-time complexity of $O(n^3)$.

To asses the potential of computational speedup, a *distance-based* method of outlier detection in 3D point clouds was proposed. Our approach is based on the assumption that points belonging to building wall structures are normally distributed. Thus, we apply a double-threshold scheme: firstly, we reduce the impact of infrequent points in the model, the relative distances from which to the other points in the model are comparatively big. After eliminating such points, we estimate the second filtering factor based on the global mean over mean distances of each point's neighborhood.

2.2   Dataset

Evaluation was performed on a dataset recorded at the downtown of Maastricht, the Netherlands. The dataset results from 7 walks with a recording device (iPhone 5 with acquisition application running on it) attached with a chest mount utility to the body of the person acquiring images. Within a walk an image was sequentially acquired every second. A total of 3291 images were recorded. All recordings differ in date, time and weather condition.

The route passes by several landmarks. The main characteristics of the location are a large number of pedestrians, high vehicle traffic, narrow streets and houses located close to the road.

Processing with VisualSFM [6] resulted in a dataset consisting of 17 separate models. Each model represents a reconstructed set of building walls or a single wall as a sparse 3D point cloud. The models contain from 200 to 12792 points.

2.3   Preparation of test models

To evaluate our initial hypothesis, we selected as a reference a model from our dataset allowing for the best automatic alignment to the real world coordinates. We aligned all models to the OpenStreetMap [7] inspired by the approaches of Strecha et al. [8] and Untzelmann et al. [9]. The selected model contains 11650 points and 374 cameras.

This model was then reconstructed again by 10-fold cross-validation: all images used in the reference model were randomly partitioned into 10 subsamples of equal size. For each new reconstruction, a newly selected single subsample containing 10% of original images was used as test data, the remaining 90% of images were used to reconstruct a model.

2.4   Testing process

To test the hypothesis, the following sequence of steps was applied to 8 test reconstructions:

1. Align each model to the map to estimate their scaling factors relatively to the real world coordinate system.
2. Align the test reconstruction to the reference reconstruction. For that, we apply the estimated scaling parameters to the test and the reference models. Roughly estimate translation between the models by calculating the difference between the models' centroids.
3. Refine translation and rotation by applying the Iterative Closest Point (ICP) algorithm [10].
4. Estimate a position of each test image not used for the reconstruction like it was described in [1].
5. Use the corresponding positions of the reconstructed images from the reference model to estimate the localization error of each image. The error is calculated as the distance between the estimated position and the reference position in 2D (as we localize the user in 2D, the z-component is omitted).
6. Apply the three outlier removal methods to the aligned test reconstruction. Repeat the two previous steps with the resulting models.

2.5   Performance measures

We evaluate the performance of localization distinguishing between efficiency and quality indicators.

Efficiency indicators refer to performance in terms of time and space and estimate matching time T_m (in seconds) and model size S_m (in KB) accordingly. In order to show the changes in performance caused by the application of a certain outlier removal method, we introduce the parameters for changes in matching time ΔT_{m0j} and space requirements ΔS_{m0j}, defined as

$$\Delta T_{m0j} = \frac{T_{m0} - T_{mj}}{T_{m0}} \times 100\% \tag{1}$$

$$\Delta S_{m0j} = \frac{S_{m0} - S_{mj}}{S_{m0}} \times 100\% \qquad (2)$$

where $j = 1, ..., 4$ corresponds to a model in a test case. A *test case* contains four models: one model before outlier removal and three after different outlier removal methods applied.

Quality indicators, i.e. matching rate R and matching error E, describe localisation performance associated with a certain model.

Let n be a total number of test images associated with a certain tested model. Given a test image contained in the reference model, an image is considered as *matched* if it is possible to reconstruct its position p in the tested model. Accordingly, n_m is the total number of matched images in the model. A match is considered as a *correct* match if the positioning error, estimated as a distance between a reconstructed position p and its corresponding position p_0 in the reference model, is less than a threshold τ

$$\|p_0 - p\| < \tau \qquad (3)$$

where we set $\tau = 1.6$ m (2-3 human steps).

The number of correct matches n_c is estimated as

$$n_c = \sum_{i=1}^{n_m} [\|p_{0i} - p_i\| < \tau] \qquad (4)$$

The matching rate R is then calculated as the ratio of the number of correct matches n_c and the total number of images n

$$R = \frac{n_c}{n} \times 100\% \qquad (5)$$

The matching error E is the average value of all positioning errors of the correct matches

$$E = \frac{\sum_{i=1}^{n_m} \|p_{0i} - p_i\| \left(\|p_{0i} - p_i\| < \tau \right)}{n_c} \qquad (6)$$

Finally, we estimate the weighted error E_w as

$$E_w = wE \qquad (7)$$

where w is the corresponding weighting coefficient of a certain model. For each j-th model in a test case, where $j = 1, ..., 4$, the coefficient w_j is calculated as follows

$$w_j = 1 - \frac{R_j - \min\{R_1, ..., R_4\}}{100\%} \qquad (8)$$

The ICP alignment of a test model to the reference model might contain an error up to 1 m. Thus, the absolute values of localization measurements might

Table 1. Results.

	Outliers removed	Benefit in computational time	Benefit in storage requirments	Loss in the accuracy of localization
	P_r	ΔT_{m0j}	ΔS_{m0j}	ΔE_{w0j} (cm)
Density-based	33.3%	31.1%	28.97%	8
Connectivity-based	20.4%	17.6%	19.24%	4
Distance-based	10.2%	8.8%	10.1%	1

not be precise. However, as we always use the same alignment within a test case, estimation of relative errors is possible. Thus, our final quality indicator is

$$\Delta E_{w0j} = E_{w0} - E_{wj} \qquad (9)$$

where E_{w0} is the weighed localization error associated with the reference model, and E_{wj} $(j = 1, ..., 3)$ are the corresponding weighed errors in localization using the models after the outlier removal methods applied.

We apply Student's t-test to the entire sample of positioning errors to see whether the changes in positioning performance are significant or not.

3 Results

We achieved the following performance: on average, the density-based method classified the biggest number of points (33.3% of the initial number) as outliers, while the smallest result was obtained by the distance-based method (10.2%) (Tab. 1).

In all cases the reduction of outliers leads to significant improvement in matching time T_m and has a positive impact on model's size S_m, comparing to the performance associated with a model before outlier removal. The benefits in matching time ΔT_{m0j} and storage requirements ΔS_{m0j} are proportional to the number of points P_r removed from the model (Tab. 1).

In the worst case, the probability to locate an image with a precision up to 1.6 m was 70%. The absolute error values were below 0.56 m for all of the cases. The average localization error resulted as the lowest (0.51 m) for our outlier removal method. At the same time, the relative weighted localization error tended to increase for the methods classifying a greater number of points as outliers. The Student's t-test resulted in the probabilities of 0.28, 0.2, 0.39 for the distance-based, the connectivity-based, and for the density-based approaches, respectively.

4 Discussion

The results have shown that image-based localization achieves a significantly higher positioning precision than the one reached by modern consumer-level

GPS sensors (34 m [11]). Average error of localization is 0.56 m including the biggest detected loss in quality of 8 cm after outlier removal. Furthermore, this value additionally accumulates an error gained in the process of alignment to the reference model, which we are unable to extract from the final result. Comparing our results to the average GPS error of 34 m, we consider the loss in quality of 8 cm as reliable and acceptable. The Student's t-test confirms our conjecture classifying those losses as insignificant. Together with the fact that the conducted experiment has shown obvious benefits of outlier removal in terms of matching time and space requirements, it makes us believe that our initial hypothesis holds.

References

1. Kochanov D, Jonas S, Hamadeh N, et al. Urban positioning using smartphone-based imaging. Proc BVM. 2014; p. 186–191.
2. Grubbs FE. Procedures for detecting outlying observations in samples. Technometrics. 1969;11(1):1–21.
3. Sotoodeh S. Outlier detection in laser scanner point clouds. In: International Archives of Photogrammetry, Remote Sensing and Spatial Information Sciences XXXVI-5; 2006. p. 297–302.
4. Wang J, Xu K, Liu L, et al. Consolidation of low-quality point clouds from outdoor scenes. Comput Graph Forum. 2013;32(5):207–10.
5. Breunig MM, Kriegel HP, Ng RT, et al. LOF: identifying density-based local outliers. Proc ACM SIGMOD. 2000; p. 93–104.
6. Wu C. Towards linear-time incremental structure from motion. Proc 3DV. 2013; p. 127–134.
7. OpenStreetMap. OpenStreetMap contributors; 2014. [Online; accessed 2014 Jul 21]. Available from: https://www.openstreetmap.org/.
8. Strecha C, Pylvänäinen T, Fua P. Dynamic and scalable large scale image reconstruction. Proc IEEE CVPR. 2010; p. 406–413.
9. Untzelmann O, Sattler T, Middelberg S, et al. A scalable collaborative online system for city reconstruction. Proc IEEE ICCVW. 2013; p. 644–651.
10. Zhang Z. Iterative point matching for registration of free-form curves and surfaces. Int J Comput Vision. 1994 Oct;13(2):119–152.
11. Modsching M, Kramer R, ten Hagen K. Field trial on GPS accuracy in a medium size city: the influence of built-up. Proc 3rd Workshop on Positioning, Navigation and Communication. 2006; p. 209–218.

Iterative Algorithms to Generate Large Scale Mosaic Images

Lorenzo Toso[1], Stephan Allgeier[2], Franz Eberle[1], Susanne Maier[2],
Klaus-Martin Reichert[1], Bernd Köhler[1]

[1]Institute for Applied Computer Science
[2]Institute for Applied Computer Science/Automation
Karlsruhe Institute of Technology (KIT), Germany
lorenzo.toso@kit.edu

Abstract. The process of creating mosaic images from non-linear registration image sequences consists of various complex subtasks. The two most time consuming and hardware resource intensive operations are the image registration process and the solution of an equation system in order to determine image positions in the mosaic. This work presents methods that allow quick calculation of image positions while reducing the necessary hardware resources. A novel graph-based method to determine promising image pairs for the registration process was developed, resulting in a reduction of runtime by 87.5%.

1 Introduction

The corneal subbasal nerve plexus (SNP) of the human eye is the most densely innervated region of the human body. It provides an opportunity for in vivo and non-invasive analysis of the nerve structure. Efron [1] describes that the analysis of the SNP can be used to assess and diagnose neuropathy. High resolution images are required to visualize thin nerve structures of the SNP. Today such images can be obtained through confocal laser scanning microscopy (CLSM) [2]. Even though the image quality of CLSM is adequate, the field of view of a single CLSM image of about $0.16\,\text{mm}^2$ is insufficient for a reliable diagnosis. One way to increase the assessed area of the SNP is to create mosaic images from sequentially recorded single images. To increase the field of view of the mosaic image we have previously proposed an automated scheme by which images are recorded while moving the patients eyes in a spiral form using an on-screen fixation target [3].

The two most time intensive subtasks of the mosaicking process are the image registration and global positioning. The image registration process performs a series of image registrations to calculate relative offsets between images. It is necessary to perform non-linear registrations due to distortions of images induced by the guiding process and also by unconscious eye movements during recording [4]. The currently employed strategy to register images, called step strategy, performs a predefined set of registrations. Initially all images are registered to their close neighbors. Afterwards images are skipped with a predefined step size creating registrations between different spiral windings [5].

Purpose of the global image positioning process is to calculate global coordinates of single images from detected relative offsets [4]. This is the most time consuming task of the mosaicking process. From the calculated offsets a system of linear equations (SLE) is generated. It needs to be solved in order to obtain the global coordinates of all images. Currently the solution is computed using the Gaussian elimination algorithm, which requires two copies of the stored matrices in the main memory and therefore causes big hardware requirements.

Using the step strategy together with the Gaussian elimination algorithm, a series containing 2500 single images requires a processing time of about six hours (2x Intel® Xeon® E5-2630 CPU; 8x 8GB DDR3 RAM). To reduce the processing time and the hardware requirements, we developed the iterative method presented in this work.

2   Materials and methods

The following methods use known mathematical procedures which have been adapted to our application as well as specially developed algorithms to reduce the processing time and hardware requirements of the mosaicking process.

2.1   Efficient calculation of global coordinates

Since the system matrix of the SLE is very sparsely populated (approximately 98% unpopulated depending on image and registration count), the memory usage can be reduced by a special data structure optimized to store sparse matrices. Sparse matrices generally do not provide constant access time to random elements, but allow an efficient computation of multiplications. This allows to use more efficient algorithms for the solution of the SLE. We have successfully tested the Jacobi-Iteration [6] and the more advanced conjugate gradient (CG) method [7]. They can provide a quick approximation of the global coordinates, which can be used to improve the registration process.

2.2   Position based image registration

The previously used step strategy tends to perform too many registrations in the center of the mosaic image, while registering too few image pairs between different spiral windings. This can cause a badly distributed net of registrations which can in turn induce image artifacts such as duplicate nerve fibers in outward areas of the mosaic (Fig. 3). Based on iterative algorithms to calculate global image coordinates, it is possible to develop a more efficient strategy for the image registration.

The position-based strategy (PBS) tries to only register adjacent images that overlap according to their approximate position. Therefore the global positioning does not start after the registration process, but is done concurrently. In order to build up a well distributed net of registrations, a graph of successful image registrations is created. Only images that have a predefined minimal distance in the registration graph are candidates for a registration. They are registered if they overlap according to their approximate position. This causes a reduction of registrations in the center of the mosaic where many images overlap, while enforcing registrations in outward areas where fewer images overlap. Distances in the registration graph are computed using the Breadth-First-Search algorithm [7]. The effect of this strategy is illustrated in Fig. 3. Positions of unregistered images are extrapolated from previous image positions, assuming constant eye movement.

3   Results

All presented methods were tested on 28 image sequences of 25 study subjects acquired within two image recording sessions. The sizes of the image sequences range from 167 to 2555 single images.

Fig. 1 shows that a shift to a data structure specialized to contain sparse matrices reduces the required memory by a factor of 10^3. Therefore the memory requirements of an image sequence of 2500 images could be reduced from approximately 12 Gigabytes to less than 11 Megabytes.

The approximation of global coordinates through iterative algorithms produced very similar results compared to the solution of the Gaussian elimination algorithm. Only rare cases showed quality reductions of the resulting mosaic images due to divergence of adjacent images caused by too sparsely populated matrices. For example the time to solve the SLE of an image sequence of 2500 images can be reduced from 5.5 hours to approximately 9 seconds.

The iterative calculation of global image positions allow to implement the PBS as a new image registration strategy. Based on approximate and extrapolated image positions it is possible to reduce the number of necessary registrations by an average of 39.2% and the calculation time by 22.4% over all image

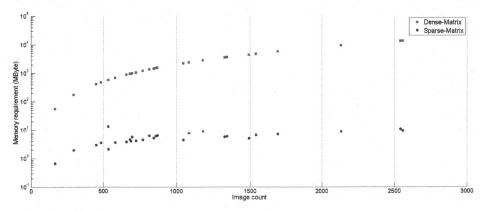

Fig. 1. Comparison of memory requirements for the SLE system matrix using different matrix data structures.

sequences. A comparison of calculation times for the two registration strategies is shown in Fig. 2.

4   Discussion

The usage of a data container for sparse matrices, reduces the required memory allowing it to be stored in the main memory without the need to swap parts of the matrix to hard disk. Therefore a significant increase in speed was obtained, even though a sparse matrix does not allow constant access time to single elements.

Global coordinates that were calculated using the Gaussian elimination algorithm show the overall best and most reliable results. The CG method produces only slightly worse results in terms of positioning. Occasionally occurring quality reductions which have not been observed by solving the SLE using the Gaussian elimination are traced back to the SLE being too sparsely populated. In few other cases the mosaic images were compressed in their Y-coordinate by about 5% causing an almost indiscernible distortion. In most cases however, the CG method produced exact results 1000 times faster than the Gaussian elimination algorithm and is therefore definitely the more suitable algorithm. In addition the usage of iterative algorithms allows output of intermediate results, which can be used to improve the registration process. The CG method produced better and faster results throughout all tested series compared to the Jacobi-Iteration and is therefore the preferable method for any further developments.

Mosaic images which were created using the PBS show less artifacts compared to images that were created using the previously used step strategy. Especially the number of registrations across different spiral windings could be

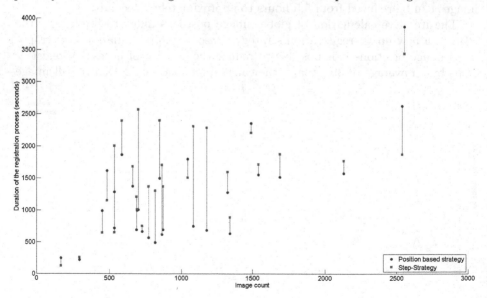

Fig. 2. Duration of the registration process using different strategies.

improved. In addition, the registration density in inner windings is lowered, which enables quicker processing times, without reducing the image quality due to a high amount of overlapping images. Overall the PBS needs significantly less image registrations by creating a much more equally distributed net of image registrations. Fig. 3 shows a comparison between the two graphs of successful registrations of the different registration strategies. Each line represents a successful registration. The magnified area shows an example of image artifacts that could be reduced using PBS.

Even though the number of performed registrations is lower using the PBS, the time needed for registering all images of an image sequence only marginally differs or is partially increased. This can be traced back to the following rea-

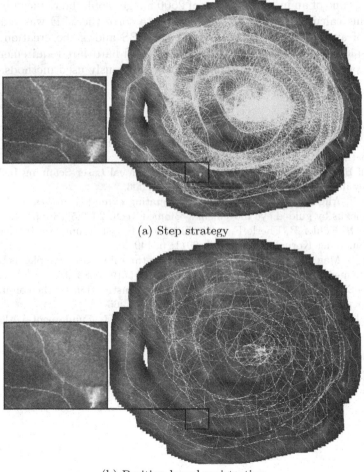

(a) Step strategy

(b) Position-based registration

Fig. 3. Mosaic images with the registration graphs of the step strategy (a) and the position-based strategy (b); the magnified image areas illustrate the reduction of image artifacts using the position-based strategy.

son: Compared to the step strategy the PBS needs to perform a Breadth-First-Search [7] in the registration graph in order to determine valid image registration candidates. Therefore the image registration can only take place after the search being finished.

Since images are only registered with others that have already been processed, the PBS does not require all images to be available at the start of the process. It is therefore possible to start the registration process while not all images have yet been recorded.

Compared to the former available step strategy, the proposed set of algorithms shows some significant advances. While the calculation time for the image registration could only be reduced marginally in the mean, the time needed for global image positioning process can be reduced significantly. The overall processing time of an image sequence of 2500 images could be reduced by 87.5%. During this calculation the memory needed to solve the SLE was reduced by a factor of approximately 1000. Overall the PBS allows the creation of large scale mosaic images in a shorter time with reduced hardware requirement, while increasing the image quality compared to the previously used methods.

References

1. Efron N. The Glenn A. Fry award lecture 2010: ophthalmic markers of diabetic neuropathy. Optom Vis Sci. 2011;88(6):661–83.
2. Guthoff RF, Baudouin C, Stave J. Atlas of Confocal Laser Scanning In-Vivo Microscopy in Ophthalmology. Berlin: Springer; 2006.
3. Köhler B, Allgeier S, Eberle F, et al. Generating extended images of the corneal nerve plexus by guided eye movements. Biomed Tech. 2012;57(Suppl 1).
4. Allgeier S, Köhler B, Eberle F, et al. Elastische Registrierung von In-vivo-CLSM-Aufnahmen der Kornea. Proc BVM. 2011; p. 149–53.
5. Allgeier S, Maier S, Mikut R, et al. Mosaicking the subbasal nerve plexus by guided eye movements. Invest Ophthalmol Vis Sci. 2014;55(9):6082–9.
6. Kawata S, Nalcioglu O. Constrained iterative reconstruction by the conjugate gradient method. IEEE Trans Med Imaging. 1985;4(2):65–71.
7. Knuth DE. Art of Computer Programming, Volume 1: Fundamental Algorithms. 3rd ed. Reading: Addison-Wesley; 1997.

Variational Registration
A Flexible Open-Source ITK Toolbox for Nonrigid Image Registration

Jan Ehrhardt[1], Alexander Schmidt-Richberg[2], René Werner[3], Heinz Handels[1]

[1]Institute of Medical Informatics, University of Lübeck, Germany
[2]Biomedical Image Analysis Group, Imperial College London, UK
[3]Department of Computational Neuroscience, University Medical Center Hamburg-Eppendorf, Germany
ehrhardt@imi.uni-luebeck.de

Abstract. In this article, we present the flexible open-source toolbox "VariationalRegistration" for non-parametric variational image registration, realized as a module in the Insight segmentation and registration toolkit. The toolbox is designed to test, evaluate and systematically compare the effects of different building blocks of variational registration approaches, i.e. the distance/similarity measure, the regularization method and the transformation model. In its current state, the framework includes implementations of different similarity measures and regularization methods, as well as displacement-based and diffeomorphic transformation models. The implementation of further components is possible and encouraged. The implemented algorithms were applied to different registration problems and extensively tested using publicly accessible image data bases. This paper presents a quantitative evaluation for inter-patient registration using 3D brain MR images of the LONI image data base. The results demonstrate that the implemented variational registration scheme is competitive with other state-of-the-art approaches for non-rigid image registration.

1 Introduction

Image registration is a crucial aspect of many applications in medical image computing. During the past years, a wide variety of approaches for non-linear registration has been proposed and successfully applied for diverse registration tasks. Examples for applications of non-linear registration algorithms are the estimation of organ deformations due to respiratory or cardiac motion [1], the co-registration of images acquired from different subjects for atlas construction or statistical analyses [2], or atlas-based segmentation methods [3].

Due to the diversity and number of existing registration approaches, it is a bewildering task to choose an appropriate registration method for a given application. A number of multi-institutional studies and challenges have taken place to give an overview of the field and to evaluate and compare different

algorithms for specific registration tasks, for example in respiratory motion estimation [4, 5] or inter-patient registration for neurological applications [2]. These
studies have a competitive design and each registration algorithm is treated as
a complete pipeline. In this setting, a systematical investigation of the effects
of separate building blocks of the registration problem (distance measure, regularization, transformation space, etc.) is not possible and the influence of these
components is hardly to divide from the impact of implementation details (discretization details, stop criterion, pre- and post-processing).

In this paper, we present a flexible open-source toolbox for non-parametric
variational image registration named *VariationalRegistration*. The toolbox is implemented as a module in the Insight segmentation and registration toolkit (ITK)
and freely available with ITK version 4.6 and higher. The aim of this toolbox is
to provide a framework to systematically investigate and compare the building
blocks of registration algorithms in a variational setting. The implementation
design allows to combine and modify different components like distance measure,
regularization, stop criterion or transformation model, and new components can
easily be implemented.

The initial motivation for the development of the toolbox was a comparison
and evaluation study for lung motion estimation in thoracic 4D CT images [1].
Therefore, state-of-the-art algorithms for variational registration were implemented in the toolbox and extensively tested using publicly accessible image
data bases[1]. The results of this study show that the implemented algorithms
perform similar to other state-of-the-art methods. In contrast to [1], this paper describes implementation concepts of the toolbox, and we present results
for *inter*-patient registration of 40 brain 3D MR images used to construct the
LONI Probabilistic Brain Atlas (LPBA40) [6]. We evaluate different distance
measures, regularization methods and transformation models and compare our
results to other state-of-the-art registration algorithms.

2   Methods and materials

2.1   Variational formulation of the image registration problem

Without going into detail, this section is to shortly summarize the variational
registration setting. Given a fixed image $F : \Omega \to \mathbb{R}$ ($\Omega \subset \mathbb{R}^d$) and a moving
image $M : \Omega \to \mathbb{R}$, registration is the process of finding a (plausible) spatial
transformation $\varphi : \Omega \to \Omega$ that maps points from F to corresponding points in
M. We compute φ by minimizing an energy functional

$$\mathcal{J}[\varphi] = \mathcal{D}[F, M \circ \varphi] + \alpha \mathcal{S}[\varphi] \to \min \tag{1}$$

Thus, the main building blocks of the functional $\mathcal{J}$ can be summarized as being
the distance measure $\mathcal{D}$, the regularization term $\mathcal{S}$, and the transformation model
of φ. In our non-parametric variational setting, φ is represented by a dense

---

[1] www.dir-lab.com and www.creatis.insa-lyon.fr/rio/popi-model

Algorithmus 1 Diffeomorphic variational registration

Set $\boldsymbol{v}^{(0)} = 0$ or to an initial field, $\boldsymbol{\varphi}^{(0)} = \exp(\boldsymbol{v}^{(0)})$ and $k = 0$
repeat
    Compute the force field $\boldsymbol{f}[F, M \circ \boldsymbol{\varphi}^{(k)}]$
    Let $\boldsymbol{v}^{(k)} \leftarrow \boldsymbol{v}^{(k)} + \tau \boldsymbol{f}$
    Regularize the velocity field using $\boldsymbol{v}^{(k+1)} = (Id - \tau \mathcal{A})^{-1} \boldsymbol{v}^{(k)}$
    Calculate the corresponding transformation $\boldsymbol{\varphi}^{(k+1)} = \exp(\boldsymbol{v}^{(k+1)})$
    Let $k \leftarrow k + 1$
until $k \geq K_{\max}$ or another stop criterion is fulfilled

vector field, i.e. by a *displacement* field $\boldsymbol{u}$, with $\boldsymbol{\varphi}(\boldsymbol{x}) = \boldsymbol{x} + \boldsymbol{u}(\boldsymbol{x})$, in the small deformation setting or by a (static) *velocity* field $\boldsymbol{v}$, with $\boldsymbol{\varphi}(\boldsymbol{x}) = \exp(\boldsymbol{v})(\boldsymbol{x})$, to represent diffeomorphic transformations. To minimize (1), the Euler-Lagrange equations are analytically derived, resulting in partial differential equations that are solved by gradient descent. This optimize-than-discretize approach results in an iterative scheme (here for the small displacement setting)

$$\boldsymbol{u}^{(k+1)} = (Id - \tau \mathcal{A})^{-1} \left(\boldsymbol{u}^{(k)} + \tau \boldsymbol{f}[F, M \circ \boldsymbol{\varphi}^{(k)}] \right) \tag{2}$$

where $\boldsymbol{f}$ denotes a force field that is related to the derivative of the distance measure $\mathcal{D}[F, M \circ \boldsymbol{\varphi}]$ and $\mathcal{A}$ is a linear partial differential operator, which can be deduced from the derivative of $\mathcal{S}$ [7]) The resulting registration algorithm for the diffeomorphic setting is summarized in Alg. 1.

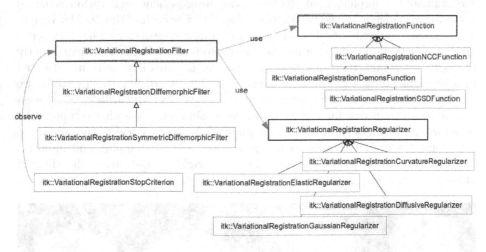

Fig. 1. Extraction from the class diagram of the toolbox *VariationalRegistration*. The overall registration algorithm is implemented in the class **VariationalRegistrationFilter** and its child classes for (symmetric) diffeomorphic registration. The force field (related to the distance measure) is computed in child classes of **VariationalRegistrationFunction** and the regularization step is done in classes derived from **VariationalRegistrationRegularizer**.

2.2   Implementation

VariationalRegistration is implemented in C++ and realized as part of ITK's finite difference solver hierarchy. A part of the class diagram is shown in Fig. 1. Further classes provide different stop criteria or handle multi-resolution schemes, for example. Within this framework, force term and regularizer remain exchangeable and additional terms can be easily integrated.

The following distance measures (i.e. its derivatives) are implemented in the current version of the toolbox: sum of squared differences (SSD), demons-based or normalized SSD (NSSD), and normalized cross correlation (NCC). The implementation of further force terms like NMI or NGF is subject of future work.

The regularization step in (2) requires to solve a linear equation system with a very large number of unknowns. We provide efficient FFT-based solving strategies for curvature and elastic regularization and a diffusive regularization based on additive operator splitting. Further, a Gaussian regularization is implemented that smooths a dense vector field with a Gaussian kernel similar to the demons registration approach. All regularizers and distance measures are multi-threaded; however, efficiency was not the main design goal of this toolbox but generalization and clarity of the source code. More implementation details can be found in [8].

2.3   Comparison and evaluation based on public data sets

We evaluate the implemented algorithms for inter-patient registration using 40 brain 3D MR images of the LPBA40 data set [6]. For each of the 3D MR images a label image containing 56 segmented structures is available. The data set is publicly available and the results therefore reproducible. Further, we can directly compare our results to 14 image registration algorithms that were investigated in a previous study performed by Klein et al. [2]. According to this study, we perform pairwise registration and compute Jaccard overlap coefficients between the labeled structures for the quantitative evaluation. We also compute the standard deviation of the Jacobian to quantify the smoothness of the computed transformations. Before non-linear registration, a skull stripping and intensity bias correction was applied and all images were rigidly registered to the MNI152 atlas space [6]. Fig. 2 shows an example image and the associated labels. To

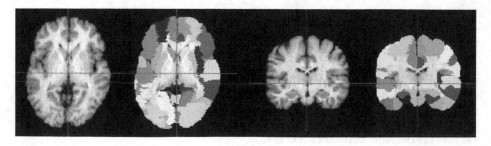

Fig. 2. An example image of the LPBA40 data set with labels used for the evaluation.

Table 1. Jaccard coefficents and standard deviations of the jacobian (σ_{Jacobian}) for twelve combinations of distance measure and regularization approach. The values are averaged over all image pairs (Jaccard coefficents and σ_{Jacobian}) and all labels (Jaccard coefficents). Registration parameters are shown in brackets.

	NCC		SSD		NSSD	
	Jaccard	σ_{Jacobian}	Jaccard	σ_{Jacobian}	Jaccard	σ_{Jacobian}
Curvature	55.9	0.55	53.6	0.44	50.8	0.58
	($\tau = 40, \alpha = 1.0$)		($\tau = 2.5e^{-6}, \alpha = 1.0$)		($\tau = 1.0, \alpha = 5.0$)	
Elastic	55.4	0.39	55.3	0.27	54.2	0.30
	($\tau = 30, \lambda = \mu = 0.1$)		($\tau = 2.5e^{-6}, \lambda = \mu = 0.1$)		($\tau = 1.0, \lambda = \mu = 0.5$)	
Diffusive	56.1	0.58	54.2	0.37	53.5	0.47
	($\tau = 30, \alpha = 0.1$)		($\tau = 2.5e^{-6}, \alpha = 0.2$)		($\tau = 1.0, \alpha = 1.0$)	
Gaussian	55.3	0.57	53.6	0.44	53.4	0.52
	($\tau = 40, \sigma^2 = 0.5$)		($\tau = 1.0e^{-5}, \sigma^2 = 1.25$)		($\tau = 1.0, \sigma^2 = 1.5$)	

analyze the influence of the building blocks of the registration algorithm each of the image pairs (in total 780) was registered with each combination of distance measure, regularizer and transformation space ($3 \times 4 \times 3 = 36$ combinations).

3   Results

Five randomly selected patient images were used to determine suitable registration parameters. We used 3 multi-resolution levels and a maximum of 300 iterations per level, other parameters are given in Tab. 1 (see [1] for explanations). Computation times largely depended on the exact algorithm configuration and vary between 5 and 40 minutes on a Quad Core PC.

Tab. 1 shows the Jaccard overlap coefficients and standard deviations of the Jacobian averaged over all labels and image pairs for the twelve combinations of regularizers and distance measures. Only results of the non-diffeomorphic transformation model are presented here due to space limitations. NCC-based

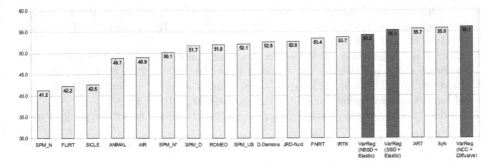

Fig. 3. Jaccard overlap (over 56 regions) for 17 registration algorithms for the LPBA40 data set. VarReg denotes algorithms from the *VariationalRegistration* toolbox, the 14 remaining algorithms were tested in [2].

registration has significant higher Jaccard values compared to SSD- and NSSD-based registration (paired t-test, $p < 0.0001$). Fig. 3 shows a comparison of the best performing algorithm for each of the three distance measures together with the 14 registration algorithms analyzed in [2].

4   Discussion and conclusion

We presented a flexible open-source toolbox for non-parametric variational image registration that is publicly available with ITK. The code design of the toolbox allows to easily combine and systematically investigate the building blocks of variational registration algorithms, as well as to implement new components. Based on publicly available data sets, the toolbox was applied for intra-patient (see [1]) and inter-patient registration and an accuracy comparable to state-of-the-art algorithms has been proven.

Analyzing the results of the inter-patient registration of MR images shows that the NCC distance measure provides the best results, however, SSD and NSSD perform surprisingly well. The elastic regularizer generates smooth displacement fields while preserving a high registration accuracy. NSSD does not perform well with curvature regularization, whereas NCC with curvature regularization combines high accuracy and smooth transformations.

References

1. Werner R, Schmidt-Richberg A, Handels H, et al. Estimation of lung motion fields in 4D CT data by variational non-linear intensity-based registration: a comparison and evaluation study. Phys Med Biol. 2014;59(15):4247–60.
2. Klein A, Andersson J, Ardekani BA, et al. Evaluation of 14 nonlinear deformation algorithms applied to human brain MRI registration. NeuroImage. 2009;46:786–802.
3. van Rikxoort EM, Isgum I, Arzhaeva Y, et al. Adaptive local multi-atlas segmentation: application to the heart and the caudate nucleus. Med Image Anal. 2010;14(1):39–49.
4. Murphy K, van Ginneken B, Reinhardt J, et al. Evaluation of registration methods on thoracic CT: the EMPIRE10 challenge. IEEE Trans Med Imaging. 2011;30(11):1901–20.
5. Brock KK, Consortium DRA. Results of a multi-institution deformable registration accuracy study (MIDRAS). Int J Radiat Oncol Biol Phys. 2010;76(2):583–96.
6. Shattuck DW, Mirza M, Adisetiyo V, et al. Construction of a 3D probabilistic atlas of human cortical structures. NeuroImage. 2008;39(3):1064–80.
7. Modersitzki J. Numerical Methods for Image Registration. Oxford University Press; 2003.
8. Schmidt-Richberg A, Werner R, Handels H, et al. A flexible variational registration framework. Insight J. 2014.

Joint Registration and Parameter Estimation of T1 Relaxation Times Using Variable Flip Angles

Constantin Heck[1], Martin Benning[1], Jan Modersitzki[1]

MIC, University of Lübeck
heck@mic.uni-luebeck.de

Abstract. Accurate and fast estimation of T1 relaxation times is a crucial ingredient for many applications in magnetic resonance imaging [1]. A fast way for T1 estimation is a model-based reconstruction from data obtained with variable flip angles as proposed in [2]. However, this technique requires multiple measurements thus patient movement can degrade the results. In this work we introduce a novel model which combines registration and T1 estimation. A discretization of the new approach is given, including a tailored optimization algorithm. The novel method is compared to conventional reconstruction techniques on 2D software phantom data. With the new method it was possible to improve the relative error in T1 maps from 0.4253 to 0.4049 using the novel algorithm.

1 Introduction

T1 estimation is a crucial step in pre-processing data obtained e.g. from dynamically contrast enhanced magnetic resonance imaging [1]. Common methods to determine T1 relaxation times are often based on inversion and saturation recovery sequences [3]. However, in clinical practice these sequences often are not fast enough [3, 4]. An alternative, faster approach proposed in [2] employs multiple measurements with spoiled gradient echo sequences with different flip angles. T1 maps can then be reconstructed using a model fit. Results from [4] indicate that this approach is capable to produce accurate measurements with significantly reduced imaging times.

Since the described method is based on multiple MR measurements, patient movement during the different acquisitions can yield degraded reconstruction results. Image registration may hence be a key factor to improve T1 estimation. However, for given images obtained with different flip-angles, co-registration is a challenging task because image contrast decreases significantly with higher flip-angles (Fig. 1). Since registration and parameter estimation are linked problems, a joint approach could be a remedy for this problem. In other applications [5], these joint approaches have shown to be capable of improving results with respect to deformation as well as parameter errors.

In this work, we present a novel model to combine registration and T1 estimation for data obtained with the variable flip-angle technique. A possible discretization of the proposed method is introduced, including a tailored optimization exploiting the specific structure of the objective function. In order to verify the new approach, we test it on phantom 2D datasets which are degraded by affine deformations as well as noise. These datasets are created using the XCAT phantom [6], realistic T1 values for multiple tissue types as well as an MR-specific modeling of noise. The results are compared to the ones from the conventional reconstruction technique [2]. Since we expect in real world applications 3D data as well as small, nonlinear deformations, this work is intended to be a first, ground laying evaluation of the proposed method. Possible future extensions will be discussed in Section 4. We begin by introducing the proposed model.

2   Materials and methods

Let $S := (S^1, \ldots, S^k) \in \mathbb{R}^{n,k}$ be a series of 2D MR images obtained at flip-angles $\alpha = (\alpha_1, \ldots, \alpha_k)$ with $\alpha_i \in (0, \pi)$. In order to reconstruct a T1 map from this series, it is necessary to establish a relationship between the signal intensities and the T1 values first. Following [2, 4], we want to outline the model used in this contribution:

2.1   Model equation for variable flip angles

Following [2, 4], the signal equation for spoiled gradient echo sequences in dependency of the flip-angle $\alpha \in [0, \pi]$ at a single voxel at location $i \in \{1, \ldots, n\}$ is given by

$$s_i^\alpha = \sin(\alpha) \frac{m_i(1 - e^{TR/T1_i})}{1 - \cos(\alpha)e^{-TR/T1_i}} \tag{1}$$

Here s_i^α is the signal intensity at a specific voxel $i \in \{1, \ldots, n\}$, α is the flip-angle, TR is the repetition-time and the steady-state magnetization m_i is given by the expression $m_i := g\rho_i e^{-TE/T2_i}$. Here ρ_i describes the proton density at voxel i, g the scanner system gain, TE the echo-time and $T2_i$ the transverse relaxation time. $T1_i$ is the voxel-specific longitudinal relaxation constant to be determined.

Substituting $\eta_i := e^{-TR/T1_i}$ and $\nu_i := m_i(1 - e^{-TR/T1_i})$ in (1) and makes it possible to reformulate the signal equation in the following way [2, 4]

$$0 = s_i^\alpha \cos(\alpha)\eta_i + \sin(\alpha)\nu_i - s_i^\alpha \tag{2}$$

Note that η_i and ν_i depend only on tissue parameters and are independent of the flip-angle. Hence we can formulate (2) for multiple measurements $s_i := (s_i^1, \ldots, s_i^k)^\top$ of the same voxel obtained at flip angles $\alpha_1, \ldots, \alpha_k$ in the following way: $0 = v_i \eta_i + w_i \nu_i - s_i$ where $v_i := (s_i^1 \cos(\alpha_1), \ldots, s_i^k \cos(\alpha_k))^\top$ and $w_i := (\sin(\alpha_1), \ldots, \sin(\alpha_k))^\top$. For an accurately motion corrected dataset, this equation is supposed to be fulfilled for every voxel.

We now introduce the variables for multiple locations in the following way: An image obtained at flip-angle α_j will be denoted by $S^j := (s_1^j, \ldots, s_n^j)^\top \in \mathbb{R}^n$. Furthermore we define the voxel-wise parameter maps $e := (\eta_1, \ldots, \eta_n)^\top \in \mathbb{R}^n$ as well as $n := (\nu_1, \ldots, \nu_n)^\top \in \mathbb{R}^n$. Hence the extension to multiple locations can be expressed as $0 = Ve + Wn - \tilde{S}$. Here V and W are block-diagonal matrices with vectors $v_1, \ldots, v_n$ and $w_1, \ldots, w_n$ on the diagonal. Note that the difference between S and $\tilde{S}$ lies in the sorting: S is sorted image-first whereas $\tilde{S}$ is sorted voxel-first. The model used in this contribution can therefore be expressed as

$$M(S, e, n, \alpha) := Ve + Wn - \tilde{S} \tag{3}$$

If signals with zero intensities s_i are present it follows from (1) that $\nu_i = 0$. Thus in this case the parameter estimation is ill posed with respect to η_i and regularization of e is crucial. Having determined η_i it is possible to obtain $T1_i$ by resubstituting $T1_i = -TR/\log(\eta_i)$. Since the change to logarithmic scale can introduce large outliers, we will force a stronger regularity of e than of n.

2.2   Objective function and optimization

We will now assume that S is degraded by affine deformations as well as noise. The idea of the proposed method is to improve the parameter estimation problem by adding the deformation parameters as additional unknowns. For k affine deformations with parameters $u := (u_1, \ldots, u_k) \in \mathbb{R}^{6,k}$ we will denote the transformed dataset by $S(u) := (S^1(u_1), \ldots, S^k(u_k))$.

For estimates (u, e, n) of the true deformations and model parameters, we define similar to [7] the following energy functional, which is to be minimized

$$\mathcal{J}(u, e, n) := h_d \left(\gamma \sum_{i=1}^{k-1} \|S^{i+1}(u_{i+1}) - S^i(u_i)\|^2 \right.$$
$$\left. + \frac{1}{2} \|M(S(u), e, n, \alpha)\|^2 + \frac{\beta_1}{2} \|\Delta_d e\|^2 + \frac{\beta_2}{2} \|\nabla_d n\|^2 \right) \tag{4}$$

Here $M(S, e, n, \alpha)$ is the physical model introduced in Section 2.1, h_d denotes the voxel volume, $\gamma, \beta_1, \beta_2 \in \mathbb{R}^+$ are regularization parameters and Δ_d and ∇_d denote forward-difference discretizations of laplace and gradient operator respectively. Note that as explained in Section 2.1 the higher order regularization on e is crucial. We will now introduce a reduced version of $\mathcal{J}$ and a suitable optimization strategy.

Since the model M depends linearly on the variables e and n it is possible to exploit the specific structure of (4) to speed up the optimization [2, 4, 8]. We will now introduce a reduced version of the functional $\mathcal{J}(u, e, n)$, which depends only on the deformation u. Given transformation parameters u, we choose optimal model variables e_u and n_u in the following sense: $0 = \frac{\partial \mathcal{J}}{\partial e}(u, e_u, n_u) = \frac{\partial \mathcal{J}}{\partial n}(u, e_u, n_u)$. These variables (e_u, n_u) can be determined as the solution of the following $2n \times 2n$ linear system

$$(V^\top V + \beta_1 \Delta_d^\top \Delta_d)e_u + \qquad\qquad V^\top W n_u = V^\top \tilde{S}$$
$$W^\top V e_u + (W^\top W + \beta_2 \nabla_d^\top \nabla_d)n_u = W^\top \tilde{S}$$

Choosing the optimal variables (e_u, n_u) for a given deformation u in the above fashion yields the following reduced objective function

$$\mathcal{J}_{\mathrm{red}}(u) := \mathcal{J}(u, e_u, n_u)$$

The optimization of $\mathcal{J}_{\mathrm{red}}(u)$ is carried out using a Gauss-Newton framework with a multilevel strategy from coarse to fine. A direct calculation using the optimality condition shows that the gradient necessary for the Gauss-Newton optimization is given by

$$\nabla \mathcal{J}_{\mathrm{red}}(u) = \frac{\partial \mathcal{J}}{\partial u}(u, e_u, n_u)$$

2.3   Evaluation

The proposed method was verified on phantom data. We used the XCAT phantom [6] to obtain ground truth data of an axial 2D scan of a human body with voxel size $1.8\,\mathrm{mm}^3$, matrix size 256×256 and $TR = 2.51\,\mathrm{ms}$. Flip angles $\alpha := (5°, 8°, 15°, 25°)$ were chosen to simulate signals the following areas using (1): Kidney (medulla/cortex/pelvis), spleen, liver, bone marrow, fat and air. T1 values for these structures were taken from [9]. Since no data for the steady-state magnetization m was at hand, we used the constant value $m = 1500$ for all tissue types as previously proposed in [4], although this value varies with the tissue. The static phantom was then perturbed by small affine deformations, yielding a dataset S_{def} (Fig. 1). Finally Riccian noise, as expected in MR data [10], was created by adding white Gaussian noise to the real and imaginary part of the Fourier-transformed data. We created multiple noise and motion corrupted datasets at various Signal to noise ratios, defined as $\mathrm{SNR} := \mu(S_{\mathrm{def}})/\mu(S - S_{def})$ where μ denotes the mean value of the respective signals. We have compared the proposed algorithm to two conventional approaches to recover T1 maps. These consist of registration and subsequent parameter estimation. For the registration two different algorithms were used, namely a *sequential registration* ($S^{i+1} \to S^i$, implementation from FAIR [7]) and a *joint registration* (minimize $\mathcal{I}(u) := \sum_{i=1}^{k-1} h_d/2 \| S^{i+1}(u_{i+1}) - S^i(u_i) \|^2$). The latter registration was chosen to investigate possible advantages introduced by the coupling of registration parameters in (4). For the subsequent parameter estimation, parameter maps (e, n) were calculated by minimizing the functional $\mathcal{P}(e, n) := 1/2(\| M(S(u_{\mathrm{opt}}), e, n, \alpha) \|^2 + \beta_1 \| \Delta_d e \|^2 + \beta_2 \| \nabla_d n \|^2)$ where u_{opt} denotes the optimized deformation parameters. The regularization terms were included to allow a fair comparison. Following the parameter estimation, T1 was reconstructed from e by calculating $T1_i = -TR/\log(e_i)$. Since changing to logarithmic scale can introduce large outliers, the relative error in T1 ($\mathrm{reT1} := \| T1^{\mathrm{rec}} - T1^{\mathrm{true}} \|_2 / \| T1^{\mathrm{true}} \|_2$) was calculated only on areas with constant T1 (Fig. 1).

Table 1. Results for various SNRs. For the initial deformation meanDE=8.7644 and maxDE=9.6766 with respect to the identity-transformation. Deformation errors are expressed in pixels.

SNR	Minimize (4) meanDE	maxDE	reT1	Sequential meanDE	maxDE	reT1	Joint meanDE	maxDE	reT1
∞	0.2781	0.3149	0.0076	0.1961	0.2256	0.0029	0.2467	0.2552	0.0039
10.66	1.2221	2.0685	0.3045	0.3412	0.4710	0.3108	0.3963	0.5262	0.2848
5.38	2.1583	2.8197	0.3692	1.2774	1.6124	0.4062	2.0694	3.0644	0.3836
4.80	2.7574	3.2040	0.4049	2.1415	2.3348	0.4381	2.1336	3.4063	0.4253

3   Results

We experimentally determined parameters $\beta_1 = 10^5$, $\beta_2 = 10^{-1}$ and $\gamma = 1$ for all experiments including noise. For the experiment without noise we chose $\beta_1 = \beta_2 = 10^{-3}$. Errors are given in maximal deformation error (maxDE), meaning the maximal error of all four deformations with respect to the mean deformation, as well as mean deformation error (meanDE), describing the mean error of the four deformations with respect to the mean deformation. Both errors are expressed in pixels. Results for various SNRs are displayed in Tab. 1. It can be seen, that the parameter error in T1 profits from the joint approach. Relative errors in T1 are reduced slightly from 0.4253 to 0.4049. However, improved reconstruction was possible regardless of larger deformation errors. Reasons for this behavior are subject to current investigations

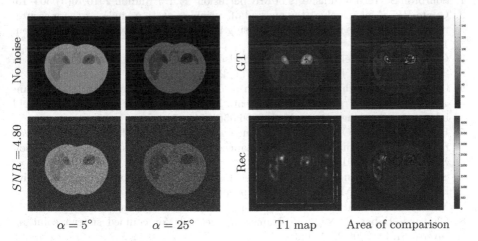

Fig. 1. Phantom data and reconstruction results. Left images: Ground-truth signals and noisy signals for minimal and maximal flip-angles $\alpha_1 = 5°$ and $\alpha_4 = 25°$. Right images: Ground-truth (GT) and Reconstructed (Rec) T1 maps for SNR=4.80 as well as the area of comparison to calculate the relative error.

4 Discussion

In this contribution we have introduced a novel method for joint registration and parameter estimation for T1 reconstruction. A discretization as well as a tailored optimization were introduced. Furthermore, a specific software phantom was used to evaluate the proposed method. It can be observed, that the inclusion of the model is capable of stabilizing the parameter estimation especially at low SNR-levels. Where at high SNR straight-forward registration methods seem to have still a small advantage, they fail to capture parameters in the presence of severe noise in a stable manner. However, evaluation of T1 times is complicated, since the change to logarithmic scale can introduce large outliers. In future work, several extensions of the proposed method will be considered: Direct regularization of T1 instead of $\eta := e^{-TR/T1}$ could stabilize parameter estimation. In order to further cope with the differences in image-contrast, an edge based distance measure could be introduced in (4). Also, as already mentioned in Sec. 1 we are planning to extend the proposed method from 2D to 3D and the deformation model from affine to nonlinear. To conclude the model driven registration approach has been shown to be capable of improving T1 estimation. The proposed concept could also be extended to many applications, as e.g. registration of DCE-MRI images similar to [5].

References

1. Sourbron S. Technical aspects of MR perfusion. Eur J Radiol. 2010;76(3):304–13.
2. Gupta RK. A new look at the method of variable nutation angle for the measurement of spin-lattice relaxation times using fourier transform NMR. J Magn Reson. 1977;25(1):231–5.
3. Crawley AP, Henkelman RM. A comparison of one-shot and recovery methods in T1 imaging. Magn Reson Med. 1988;7(1):23–34.
4. Cheng HLM, Wright GA. Rapid high-resolutionT1 mapping by variable flip angles: accurate and precise measurements in the presence of radiofrequency field inhomogeneity. Magn Reson Med. 2006;55(3):566–74.
5. Buonaccorsi GA, O'Connor JP, Caunce A, et al. Tracer kinetic model–driven registration for dynamic contrast-enhanced MRI time-series data. Magn Reson Med. 2007;58(5):1010–9.
6. Segars W, Sturgeon G, Mendonca S, et al. 4D XCAT phantom for multimodality imaging research. Med Phys. 2010;37(9):4902–15.
7. Modersitzki J. FAIR: Flexible Algorithms for Image Registration. SIAM; 2009.
8. Chung J, Haber E, Nagy J. Numerical methods for coupled super-resolution. Inverse Probl. 2006;22(4):1261–72.
9. de Bazelaire CMJ, Duhamel GD, Rofsky NM, et al. MR imaging relaxation times of abdominal and pelvic tissues measured in Vivo at 3.0T: preliminary results. Radiology. 2004;230(3):652–9.
10. Henkelman RM. Measurement of signal intensities in the presence of noise in MR images. Med Phys. 1985;12(2):232–3.

Respiratory Motion Compensation for C-Arm CT Liver Imaging

Aline Sindel[1], Marco Bögel[1,2], Andreas Maier[1,2], Rebecca Fahrig[3],
Joachim Hornegger[1,2], Arnd Dörfler[4]

[1]Pattern Recognition Lab, FAU Erlangen-Nürnberg
[2]Erlangen Graduate School in Advanced Optical Technologies (SAOT), FAU
Erlangen-Nürnberg
[3]Stanford, Department of Radiology, Stanford University, Palo Alto, CA, USA
[4]Department of Neuroradiology, Universitätsklinikum Erlangen, Erlangen, Germany
aline.sindel@fau.de

Abstract. In C-arm CT 3D liver imaging, breathing leads to motion
artifacts due to the relatively long acquisition time. Often, even with
breath-holding residual respiratory motion can be observed. These artifacts manifest in blurring and interfere clinical investigations such as liver
tissue imaging. For 3D medical image reconstruction a respiratory motion estimation and compensation is required. In this work, the motion
was estimated by tracking the motion of the diaphragm and of a vessel
bifurcation. The motion signals were integrated into a Thin-Plate-Spline
that was used for intra-scan motion compensated reconstruction. This
approach was applied to clinical C-arm CT data of the liver and showed
improved image quality. Reduced artifacts allow a more precise visual
depiction of the liver tissue for liver imaging.

1 Introduction

C-arm CT systems have enabled CT-like 3D imaging in the interventional suite
and are heavily used in many fields, e.g. angiography, cardiology, etc. Tissue
imaging of the liver supports the diagnosis of liver diseases that are indicated by
a disturbed blood flow and supports cancer treatment.

Liver imaging is a challenging task for C-arm CT systems. Due to the relatively long acquisition time of $5 - 10$ seconds, liver motion and deformation is
caused by breathing. This leads to artifacts which can be reduced by breath-
holding. Often, even with breath-holding residual respiratory motion can be
observed. Therefore, a respiratory motion compensation is required [1].

One approach to estimate motion is to use external devices, e.g. respiration
belts. However, additional equipment is required and has to be synchronized to
the X-ray image acquisition. Another approach is to extract the motion signal
directly from the acquired C-arm CT data in a projection-based respiratory
motion estimation. A promising approach is using the diaphragm motion, which
can be automatically detected [2] and has a high correlation with the respiratory
motion [3]. Schäfer et al. did first motion compensated reconstructions for liver

C-arm CT in an animal study [1]. The diaphragm based signal is an assumption of liver motion and fits particularly well for the upper parts of the liver in cranial-caudal direction [4]. In this work, we propose to estimate a more complex motion vector field using the tracked motion of a vessel bifurcation and the diaphragm, in order to get a better motion estimate within the liver.

2   Materials and methods

In this section, we will discuss two approaches for liver motion estimation and compensation. The main movement direction of the liver is cranial-caudal with around $5 - 25$ mm, but the movement in the other directions is also not negligibly small. The motion in the anterior-posterior direction varies between $1 - 12$ mm and between $1 - 3$ mm in the left-right direction [3]. Thus, we consider all three displacement directions for motion compensated reconstruction. First, we estimate the liver motion by tracking a vessel bifurcation and the diaphragm in the projection images. The resulting motion signals are then used in our main approach to interpolate a 4-D motion vector field. The other approach uses a single 3D motion signal. Our motion compensated reconstruction is a voxel-driven algorithm based on Schäfer et al. [5] and is implemented in the Software Framework CONRAD [6].

2.1   Motion signal estimation

For the upper part of the liver, the diaphragm is very suitable as a surrogate because it is clearly identifiable in the projection images and the cranial-caudal movement is well correlated with the liver movement. However, for tissue imaging a compensation of the inner structure is especially necessary. For this purpose, we tracked a vessel bifurcation that is located within the liver throughout the projection image series.

Finally, we use a rectified motion corrected triangulation algorithm to determine a 3D position for each projection based on motion corrected point correspondences in orthogonal projection image pairs and hence compute the corresponding motion of the 3D positions. The motion signal consists of the displacements of the triangulated 3D points with respect to a reference point, e.g. the first 3D position [2, 7].

Diaphragm 3D motion signal We acquire a 3D motion signal at the diaphragm top by tracking the contour of the diaphragm in the projection images. Therefore, the images are preprocessed by a gaussian low-pass filter and the Canny edge detector. The contour is tracked using a parabolic function $v = au^2 + bu + c$, where u and v are the detector coordinates. Using a triangulation algorithm, a 3D motion vector is computed [2, 7]. A plot of the motion signal is provided in Fig. 1.

Vessel 3D motion signal In order to get an estimate for internal liver motion, we manually tracked a vessel located in the center of the liver. A plot of the resulting motion signal is provided in Fig. 1. For manual tracking we require a distinctive position of the vessel, which is visible in all projections, e.g. slightly above a vessel branching. Due to the elongated shape of a vessel, we obtain precise information about the displacement in the x and y direction.

2.2   Motion compensation using a rigid motion model

For this method we assume that all parts of the liver are moving in the same direction and in the same speed. With this limitation we can describe the motion of the liver between the projections by only one 3D motion signal. Furthermore, we will not deal with compression or deformation of the liver in this method, but we assume a uniform voxel shift.

Our motion compensated reconstruction is based on Schäfer et al., in which all voxels are shifted corresponding to their current motion signal, i.e. during the backrojection process the value of the detector pixel corresponding to the shifted voxel is backprojected to the original voxel [5].

Since we refer to only one motion signal in this reconstruction method, we have a constant shift of all voxels for each projection, but the scale and direction of the shift depends on each individual projection. We use the vessel 3D motion signal to determine the displacement between the projections. As an internal part of the liver, the vessel represents the liver motion and is best suitable for this approach.

2.3   Motion compensation using a non-rigid motion model

In this method we assume a more complex motion model. We expect a stronger motion in the upper parts because these parts are directly affected by breath-

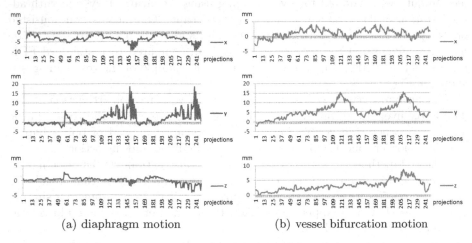

(a) diaphragm motion   (b) vessel bifurcation motion

Fig. 1. Comparison of 3D motion signals: (a) diaphragm motion, (b) vessel bifurcation motion.

ing and a decline of motion amplitude in z-direction towards the liver bottom. In order to estimate such a non-rigid motion we use a 4-D motion vector field. Therefore, we build a series of 3D Thin-Plate-Spline (TPS) consisting of the following control points: (i) 3D diaphragm signal, (ii) 3D vessel signal, (iii) boundary points. In this case boundary points refer to points located outside of the volume where we set motion to zero. Thus, the TPS algorithm is more flexible to handle rigid objects as ribs and spine.

For each projection we create a 3D motion vector field that consists of the displacement vectors determined by the TPS Interpolation. The displacement vector $\mathbf{d}(\mathbf{x})$ of an arbitrary voxel $\mathbf{x} \in \mathbb{R}^3$ is defined as

$$\mathbf{d}(\mathbf{x}) = \mathbf{A}\mathbf{x} + \mathbf{b} + \sum_{i=1}^{n} \mathbf{G}(\mathbf{x} - \mathbf{p}_i)\mathbf{c}_i \qquad (1)$$

where $\mathbf{p}_i$ are the control points and $\mathbf{G}$ is the transformation's kernel matrix to measure the euclidean distance to the control points, with the weighting coefficients $\mathbf{c}_i$. $\mathbf{A} \in \mathbb{R}^{3 \times 3}$ and $\mathbf{b} \in \mathbb{R}^3$ specify an additional affine transformation to regulate higher deviations of the spline to the control points [8]. The control points are set for each motion vector field estimation depending on the projection specific motion signals.

We use a voxel-based motion compensated backprojection as described above for the reconstruction, but in this case the voxels are shifted according to their motion vector field entries. The TPS-coefficients are estimated prior to reconstruction. The TPS is then evaluated during the backprojection on the GPU.

3   Results

We used clinical data to evaluate our motion compensation methods. The projection data was acquired for liver imaging using a C-arm CT system with administration of contrast agent and as native scans. One acquisition consisted of 248 projections with 640×480 pixels and a resolution of $0.616 \frac{mm}{pixel}$. The motion compensated reconstructions have been compared to a standard FDK reconstruction of the same projection data. An example of the result images is shown in Fig. 2.

The uncompensated reconstructions showed several motion artifacts (Fig. 2a). The whole liver tissue was blurred. This was obvious to see at the vessels in the axial view, where the vessels were half circle shaped instead of point-shaped. The liver borders and the diaphragm showed doubling and distortion.

The first method for motion compensated reconstruction (rigid motion model) indicated a great improvement (Fig. 2b). Using a single 3D motion signal of a vessel bifurcation located in the liver center, the liver tissue appeared sharper and the vessels were mapped point-like. However, there was some blurring at the upper border of the liver.

The second motion compensated reconstruction method (non-rigid motion model) combined the 3D motion signals of diaphragm and vessel in a TPS. These reconstructions further reduced motion artifacts (Fig. 2c). Additionally, they offered considerably higher image quality at the liver top and in the surrounding tissue. The vessel contour was more distinct with less streak artifacts in contrast to the first method.

We evaluated the image quality of the different reconstruction results by a survey with four experts that have scored the images on a scale from 1 to 5 (best: 5). We used four different slices of a contrast injected scan and four of a scan with residual contrast agent. The results are given as mean $\pm$ standard deviation. The compensated reconstruction images had a higher score (3.6 ± 0.51 for TPS and 3.2 ± 0.54 for one signal compensation) than the uncompensated ones (1.1 ± 0.18). In total the TPS compensation was valued best, in 6 out of 8 cases it scored better than the compensation with a single signal.

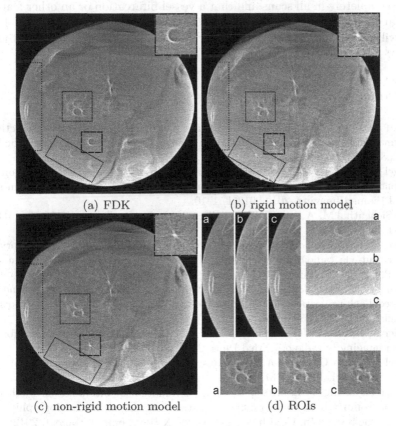

(a) FDK   (b) rigid motion model

(c) non-rigid motion model   (d) ROIs

Fig. 2. Comparison of uncompensated and motion compensated reconstruction (with contrast agent): (a) uncompensated reconstruction (FDK), (b) motion compensated reconstruction using a vessel 3D signal, (c) motion compensated reconstruction using a 4-D motion vector field. An enlarged version of the tracked vessel is to see in the top right corner. (d) These ROIs highlight the vessels in the surroundings and the ribs.

4 Discussion

We presented an algorithm to compensate respiratory motion in C-arm CT liver imaging. As shown in the result section, we observed a great improvement in image quality for liver tissue images using the motion compensated reconstruction methods. We were able to handle the artifact of distorted vessels and achieved a sharper liver border. The motion compensated reconstruction methods enable the visualization of small structures in liver tissue. We observed good results using a single tracked vessel and the diaphragm top. However, the TPS is a more flexible algorithm. More than one vessel could be used as control points and a segmented surface of the liver could contribute further control points to the TPS. For successful motion compensation it is important that the diaphragm top is visible completely in all scans and that a vessel bifurcation or an other feature is detectable in all images. So far, the vessel tracking was done manually. Future work will be looking into automatic tracking of image features in the projection images.

References

1. Schäfer D, Lin M, Rao PP, et al. Breathing motion compensated reconstruction for c-arm cone beam CT imaging: initial experience based on animal data. Proc SPIE. 2012;8313:83131D–83131D–6.
2. Bögel M, Hofmann HG, Hornegger J, et al. Respiratory motion compensation using diaphragm tracking for cone-beam c-arm CT: a simulation and a phantom study. Int J Biomed Imaging. 2013;2013(1):1–10.
3. von Siebenthal M. Analysis and modelling of respiratory liver motion using 4DMRI. ETH Zurich; 2008.
4. Balter JM, Dawson LA, Kazanjian S, et al. Determination of ventilatory liver movement via radiogrphic evaluation of diaphragm position. Int J Radiat Oncol Bio Phys. 2001;51(1):267–70.
5. Schäfer D, Borgert J, Rasche V, et al. Motion-compensated and gated cone beam filtered back-projection for 3-D rotational x-ray angiography. IEEE Trans Med Imaging. 2006;25(7):898–906.
6. Maier A, Hofmann HG, Berger M, et al. CONRAD: a software framework for cone-beam imaging in radiology. Med Phys. 2013;40(11):111914–1–8.
7. Bögel M, Riess C, Maier A, et al. Respiratory motion estimation using a 3D diaphragm model. Proc BVM. 2014; p. 240–5.
8. Müller K, Zheng Y, Lauritsch G, et al. Evaluation of interpolation methods for motion compensated tomographic reconstruction for cardiac angiographic C-arm data. Proc Second Int Conf Image Formation X-Ray Comput Tomogr. 2012; p. 5–8.

Detecting Respiratory Artifacts from Video Data

Sven-Thomas Antoni[1], Robert Plagge[1], Robert Dürichen[2],
Alexander Schlaefer[1]

[1]Institute of Medical Technology, Hamburg University of Technology
[2]Institute for Robotics and Cognitive Systems, University of Lübeck
antoni@tuhh.de

Abstract. Detecting artifacts in signals is an important problem in a wide number of research areas. In robotic radiotherapy motion prediction is used to overcome latencies in the setup, with robustness effected by the occurrence of artifacts. For motion prediction the detection and especially the definition of artifacts can be challenging. We study the detection of artifacts like, e.g., coughing, sneezing or yawning. Manual detection can be time consuming. To assist manual annotation, we introduce a method based on kernel density estimation to detect intervals of artifacts on video data. We evaluate our method on a small set of test subjects. With 86 intervals of artifacts found by our method we are able to identify all 70 intervals derived from manual detection. Our results indicate a more exact choice of intervals and the identification of subtle artifacts like swallowing, that where missed in the manual detection.

1 Introduction

The detection of anomalies or artifacts in signals is an important problem in a wide number of research areas and applications [1]. Usually an artifact refers to an unexpected pattern in data. This makes artifact detection particularly challenging for problems where a clear expectation is hard to define, e.g., for medical applications like respiratory motion prediction.

Typically, respiratory motion prediction is used in systems for motion compensation in order to overcome latencies in the setup [2, 3]. While regular motion like breathing is reliably predicted by modern algorithms, deviations from the regular pattern can pose problems [4]. Examples of such deviations include coughing, sneezing, yawning and other biological reflexes as well as, e.g., talking. Usually reflexes occur suddenly and can result in large prediction errors. We are interested in a better understanding of artifacts and in developing methods for early detection.

Motion prediction is typically based on learning a weight vector that relates the unknown future value to the signal history [3]. While this increases accuracy, it is also vulnerable towards learning unwanted patterns, e.g., from reflexes compared to regular breathing.

To gain insight in respiratory motion artifacts, we study multivariate signals from a volunteer study [3]. In the study subjects were asked to generate artifacts. While it is easy for a person to detect and classify artifacts in video images, the detection is tedious. We present an approach to analyze video images, which allows an automatic yet comprehensible anomaly detection in a controlled environment. We especially focus on artifacts that a person would notice.

A number of methods for anomaly detection have been studied in the context of, e.g., machine learning, statistics or information theory [1]. Our approach is based on kernel density estimation (KDE) which has been used to define the regular components of a signal [5, 6]. For respiratory motion it is challenging to distinguish between regular components and artifacts. Hence, we use KDE to identify artifacts and our results indicate that the proposed approach is reliable and compares favorably with manual artifact detection. It is important to note, that our current algorithm does not aim for an artifact detection on-the-fly or in a clinical environment but is supposed to assist in the manual annotation and classification of artifacts in video data from a controlled experimental setup.

2 Materials and methods

2.1 Extracting motion information from video images

Artifacts are expected to show locally higher motion in the data. We use video data $(V_k)_{k=1}^{n_f}$, with n_f the number of frames $V_k = ((v_k)_{ij})_{i,j=1}^{n_i, n_j}$, $k \in 1, \ldots, n_f$ and n_i and n_j the numbers of pixels. On the frames we define $R \subset R^2$ a region of interest (ROI) and $I^d \subset [1, n_j - d]$ an interval of interest, on which we focus. ROI and interval of interest are connected spaces. The motion between video frames V_k and V_{k+d} is estimated using the squared differences

$$D_{ijk}^d = ((v_{k+d})_{ij} - (v_k)_{ij})^2, \quad k \in I^d, (i,j) \in R \tag{1}$$

We consider different values for the difference d to limit the impact of other, non-breathing related artifacts and choose $d = 4$ for our experiments.

2.2 Detecting areas with regular motion

Motion in areas that move regularly, e.g., due to breathing or swallowing, does not carry much information. As we are mostly interested in abrupt, singular changes like coughing or yawning, we expect motion in typically static regions to be an indicator of artifacts. Hence, we mask the parts of the ROI that contain regular motion for our purpose, else events like blinking could be detected being artifacts. We introduce weights $w_{ij}, (i,j) \in R$ to suppress areas of the video which we found to show recurring motion on a connected calibration set $C \subset I$.

To identify regions of large mean motion we developed a two-phase algorithm. In the first phase we search an initial area of large mean motion for every frame. Using the overall maximum of the frame is not suited for this task, as it is not necessary in an area of large mean motion. Starting with the whole ROI we use a quad-tree based greedy search to identify regions of large mean motion determined over the sum of squared differences (1). The search terminates when the algorithm reaches a leaf.

In the second phase the subset of the ROI determined by the search algorithm is used to initialize a segmentation in order to identify the connected area of large mean motion. The segmentation $S_k = ((s_k)_{ij})_{(i,j) \in R}$, $k \in C$ is calculated using a fast marching method [7] with threshold $\phi \in [0,1]$. In Fig. 1(a) we show the result after segmentation of the quad-tree search compared to segmentation starting at the overall maximum. The area of large motion, i.e., $(s_k)_{ij} = 1$, is used to calculate the weights

$$w_{ij} = \left| \frac{s_{ij}}{\max_{i,j} s_{ij}} - 1 \right|^{\alpha}, \quad (i,j) \in R \tag{2}$$

with an attenuation parameter $\alpha \geq 0$ controlling the amount of attenuation and

$$s_{ij} = \# \{ (s_k)_{ij} \colon (s_k)_{ij} = 1, \quad k \in C \} \tag{3}$$

We chose to introduce the parameter α in order to allow higher attenuation.

We consider $\alpha \in \{0, 1, 5, 10, 20, 30, 50, \infty\}$ and $\phi \in \{0.01, 0, 05, 0.1, 0.5, 0.9, 0.99\}$ resulting in $\alpha - 20$ and $\phi = 0.01$ as our parameter choice, with $\alpha = 20$ attenuating blinking and breathing for all subjects and $\phi = 0.01$ segmenting only small areas of large motion.

2.3 Calculating the time series of motion in the ROI

Using the weights w_{ij} we calculate the time series using a frame-wise weighted sum of squared differences over the ROI

$$t_k^d = \sum_{(i,j) \in R} D_{ijk}^d \cdot w_{ij}, \quad k \in I \tag{4}$$

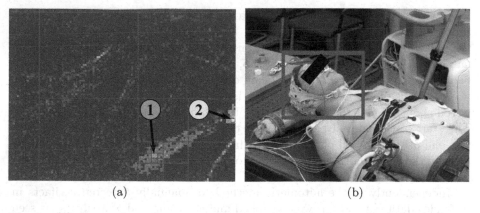

(a)   (b)

Fig. 1. (a) Comparison of segmentations starting with the result of the quad-tree search (1) or the overall maximum (2). The red lines denote the calculated boundaries of areas of the quad-tree. (b) One frame of the available video data displaying the general setup. The red box denotes the ROI.

With t_k^d being of wide range we choose to apply the common logarithm to (4) and define $L^d = (l_k^d)_{k \in I}$ with $l_k^d = \log_{10} t_k^d$, $k \in I$.

2.4 Detecting artifacts using KDE

We introduce the Gaussian kernel density estimator

$$\hat{f}(x;t) = \frac{1}{N} \sum_{i=1}^{N} K(x, X_i; t), \quad x \in \mathbb{R} \tag{5}$$

a statistical method to estimate the unknown continuous probability density function (PDF) f. Here, $X_1, \ldots, X_N$ are N independent realizations of f and $K(x, X_i; t)$ is a Gaussian kernel with location X_i and scale $\sqrt{t}$. The KDE (5) is evaluated on a discrete grid dependent on the bandwidth of the KDE. For further informations on kernel density estimators, their bandwidth and on solving (5) we refer to Botev et al. [8].

In order to detect artifacts, we calculate $\bar{l}^d$, the arithmetic mean of L^d over I and define $a^d = \{i : l_i^d > \bar{l}^d\}$, a set containing only the indexes of values greater than the mean. We assume the density of elements of a^d to be higher in an area containing an artifact compared to one without an artifact and therefore search for areas of high density in a^d. Hence, we apply (5) to a^d. The resulting estimated PDF $\hat{p}^d$ has high probability at areas of high density of elements in a^d and low probability elsewhere. We distinguish between both cases using a threshold $\theta \in \mathbb{R}$. We found $\theta = \bar{p}^d$, the arithmetic mean of $\hat{p}^d$, to yield good results. Smaller values of θ result in too wide intervals for artifacts and higher choices in too small intervals.

2.5 Validation data

We evaluate our algorithm on video data for 8 subjects (7 male / 1 female) from the multivariate data set of Dürichen et al. [3]. In Fig. 1(b) we show a frame of the video data and a ROI around the subjects head. For better comparison we name our subjects f1, m3, m4, m5, m6, m7, m8 and m9 according to [2]. We had to neglect m6 due to his face being obscured most of the time.

The focus of the experimental data is on breathing artifacts. Every session lasted about 3.5 min with 75 s of normal breathing followed by random artifacts. The start of the normal breathing and the end of the last artifact define start and end of the interval of interest I. The calibration set C is defined from the start to the end of normal breathing. More details on setup and data is given in Dürichen et al. [2].

Independently to the automatic method we manually detected artifacts in the video data. The videos were watched and start and end of artifacts, as seen by the person, were saved at full seconds.

Subject	n_{man}	n_{meth}	$n_{man-meth}$	$n_{meth-man}$
f1	10	12	0	2
m3	10	15	0	5
m4	9	11	0	2
m5	10	14	1	5
m7	12	15	0	3
m8	10	10	0	0
m9	9	9	0	0

Table 1. Comparison between manual and automatic detection per subject. n_{man}: number of manually detected artifacts; n_{meth}: number of artifacts found by our method; $n_{man-meth}$: number of manually annotated artifacts not found by our method; $n_{meth-man}$: number of artifacts found by our method, that were not manually detected.

3   Results

In the manual annotation of the data we identified intervals for 70 artifacts. Our method detects 86 artifacts using $\alpha = 20$, $\phi = 0.01$, $d = 4$ and $\theta = \bar{p}^d$;.

For an artifact to be marked as found by our method and through manual annotation, either its interval needed to be a subset of the reference interval or the distance between the limits of the intervals had to be smaller than the discretization of the KDE as set by its bandwidth.

In Tab. 1 we give the results of the manual annotations per subject and compare to the artifacts found by our method. In Fig. 2 we show results of our analysis for subject m5.

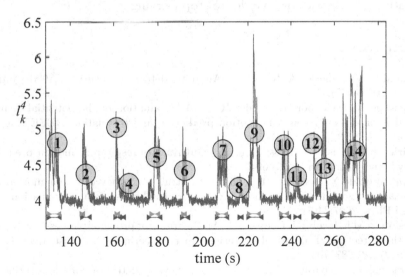

Fig. 2. Comparison of the time series L^4 on $I \setminus C$ (blue line) between the manual annotated (green bars) intervals and those found by our method (red bars) for the analyzed part of subject m5. The numbers 1 to 14 mark the intervals of artifacts as detected by our method.

4   Discussion

To summarize our approach, we consider the results for subject m5, which show the largest difference between manual and automatic detection. Due to start and end only saved at full seconds and inaccuracies in the manual detection of motion the green bars in Fig. 2 do not always align with the signal. We manually identified 10 artifacts of which 9 were marked as found. The ninth annotated interval $[250\,\text{s}, 257\,\text{s}]$ was not properly found by our method. The artifact was a long yawn, resulting in very little motion in between $251.80\,\text{s}$ and $252.68\,\text{s}$. Hence, our method separated the artifact into two artifacts 12 and 13. We found the remaining artifacts 4, 8 and 11 to be swallowing. Artifact 14 showed a remarkably longer interval than the corresponding annotated artifact, caused by motion in the background of the patient's head. An analysis of the video data of the other subjects resulted in similar explanations for all other deviations. Neither finding two artifacts instead of one nor finding additional artifacts poses a problem as our method should be used for preselection in manual assessment and classification.

Overall, our method found every manually detected artifact; with automatic detection being more reliable when it comes to subtle artifacts like swallowing. Future tasks include the determination of artifact features to distinguish between different types and research into fast artifact detection. This could lead to important improvements in motion prediction, especially by early detection of non-predictable patterns in order to stop learning.

References

1. Chandola V, Banerjee A, Kumar V. Anomaly detection: a survey. ACM Compute Surv. 2009;41(3):15.
2. Dürichen R, Davenport L, Bruder R, et al. Evaluation of the potential of multi-modal sensors for respiratory motion prediction and correlation. IEEE Eng Med Biol Mag. 2013; p. 5678 – 81.
3. Dürichen R, Wissel T, Ernst F, et al. Multivariate respiratory motion prediction. Phys Med Biol. 2014;59(20):6043.
4. Seppenwoolde Y, Berbeco RI, Nishioka S, et al. Accuracy of tumor motion compensation algorithm from a robotic respiratory tracking system: a simulation study. Med Phys. 2007;34(7):2774–84.
5. Desforges MJ, Jacob PJ, Cooper JE. Applications of probability density estimation to the detection of abnormal conditions in engineering. Proc Inst Mech Eng C. 1998;212(8):687–703.
6. Tarassenko L, Hayton P, Cerneaz N, et al. Novelty detection for the identification of masses in mammograms. Proc Inst Eng Tech. 1995; p. 442–7.
7. Sethian JA. Level set methods and fast marching methods evolving interfaces in computational geometry, fluid mechanics, computer vision, and materials science. 2nd ed. Cambridge [u.a.]: Cambridge Univ. Press; 2005.
8. Botev ZI, Grotowski JF, Kroese DP. Kernel density estimation via diffusion. Ann Stat. 2010;38(5):2916–57.

Korrektur geometrischer Verzeichnungen zur Kalibrierung von optischen Kohärenztomographiesystemen

Jenny Stritzel[1], Jesús Díaz-Díaz[2], Maik Rahlves[1], Omid Majdani[3],
Tobias Ortmaier[2], Eduard Reithmeier[4], Bernhard Roth[1]

[1]Hannoversches Zentrum für Optische Technologien, Leibniz Universität Hannover
[2]Institut für Mechatronische Systeme, Leibniz Universität Hannover
[3]Klinik für Hals-, Nasen-, Ohrenheilkunde, Medizinische Hochschule Hannover
[4]Institut für Mess- und Regelungstechnik, Leibniz Universität Hannover
jenny.stritzel@hot.uni-hannover.de

Kurzfassung. Die Optische Kohärenztomographie (OCT) ist ein etabliertes volumetrisches Bildgebungsverfahren, das insbesondere in der Ophthalmologie und Dermatologie angewandt wird. Die vorliegende Arbeit stellt eine neuartige Methode zur Kalibrierung von OCT Systemen vor, die auf Messungen einer selbst angefertigten 3D Referenzstruktur und anschließender landmarkenbasierter Registrierung beruht. Hierdurch sollen geometrische Verzeichnungen korrigiert werden, die insbesondere fehlerhafte Tiefeninformationen liefern. Mit Hilfe unserer Kalibriermethode kann der systematische Fehler um mehr als eine Größenordnung reduziert werden, sodass als Ergebnis quantitative Bildinformationen gewonnen werden können. Dieses Verfahren soll die Rekonstruktion und Interpretation von OCT-Bildern im Hinblick auf medizinische Anwendungen verbessern.

1 Einleitung

In der Medizin wurden über die Jahre zahlreiche neue bildgebende Verfahren erforscht und weiterentwickelt. So wurde 1991 die Optische Kohärenztomographie etabliert [1]. Hier wird das kurzkohärente Licht gemessen, das von der Probe reflektiert und zurückgestreut wird. Die typische Auflösung eines OCT liegt im unteren Mikrometerbereich und die Messungen sind sehr empfindlich gegenüber Brechungsindexunterschieden innerhalb einer Probe. Weiterhin sind die Messungen nicht-invasiv und kontaktlos. Man erhält nicht nur Informationen von der Probenoberfläche, sondern auch 3D Tiefeninformationen. Im Allgemeinen können in Weichgeweben einige Quadratmillimeter in lateraler Ebene (x-y-Ebene) bis in eine Tiefe (z-Richtung) von ungefähr 2 mm gemessen werden. Die Eindringtiefe ist jedoch stark abhängig vom zu untersuchenden Gewebe und vom OCT-System selbst. In stark streuenden Medien ist sie beispielsweise viel geringer als in weniger stark streuenden Medien. Daher wird das OCT besonders gerne für sehr kleine Strukturen eingesetzt, die sich nahe der Oberfläche befinden, wie zum Beispiel in biologischem Gewebe. Dazu kommt die Echtzeitfähigkeit von OCT-Systemen, die sie zu einem sehr wichtigen bildgebenden Werkzeug für die dreidimensionale in vivo Bildgebung macht, beispielsweise für die Ophthalmologie oder Dermatologie. Dies sind zumeist qualitative Anwendungen, wobei auch immer mehr quantitative Anwendungen in den Vordergrund rücken. Hierfür benötigt man zusätzliche Korrektur- und Kalibrierverfahren, die etwaige Verzeichnungen in den Bildern korrigieren.

In der Literatur [2, 3, 4, 5] wird zwischen drei Arten von Bildverzeichnungen unterschieden: die geometrischen und spektralen Verzeichnungen, sowie die, die durch Brechungsindexunterschiede innerhalb der Probe entstehen. Hier werden im Weiteren aber nur die geometrischen Verzeichnungen betrachtet. Diese werden durch nicht-telezentrische optische Strahlen mit fehlerhaften Tiefeninformationen verursacht. Ortiz et al. beschäftigen sich beispielsweise in ihren Arbeiten [3, 4] mit der 3D Korrektur von geometrischen Verzeichnungen, unter anderem angewandt beim vorderen Augensegment. Zum Einen werden geometrische Verzeichnungen durch die Architektur des Scansystems und zum Anderen durch Position und Ausrichtung der Linse in Relation zu den Spiegeln und dem Scanner beeinflusst. Daraus resultieren gekrümmte Strukturen im OCT-Bild, die in der Realität planar sind. Die Art der Krümmung hängt von der Scanspiegelkonfiguration des Scankopfes und den Linseneigenschaften ab. In jedem Fall wird aber die optische Weglänge verändert, sodass man ein OCT-Bild mit inkorrekter Probengeometrie erhält.

Die reale Probengeometrie soll mit Hilfe unserer Kalibriermethode wiederhergestellt werden, sodass man im weiteren Verlauf reale Tiefeninformationen bekommt. Die Kalibrierung beruht auf den Messungen einer selbst anfertigten 3D Referenzstruktur. Zwar gibt es bereits andere Referenzstrukturen, wie das Phantomdesign von Lee et al. [6], bei der Gitterstrukturen in Quarzglas gelasert wurden, die bei der Korrektur von Artefakten und Verzerrungen helfen sollen. Allerdings gibt es bisher keine allgemein etablierte Standardkalibriermethode für OCT-Systeme.

2 Material und Methoden

Da geometrische Verzeichnungen zu einem Fehler von mehreren 100 μm führen können, müssen insbesondere für genaue quantitative Anwendungen diese Fehler vorab korrigiert werden. Diese Arbeit stellt ein neuartiges Verfahren zur Korrektur dieses Fehlers vor. Hierfür wird eine selbst angefertigte, wohldefinierte 3D Referenzstruktur mit dem OCT vermessen. Mit Hilfe der bekannten Positionen und Ausrichtungen der auf der Struktur befindlichen Landmarken kann eine Korrektur mit linearen und nicht-linearen Transformationen vorgenommen werden. Im Weiteren werden die Referenzstruktur und die Kalibriermethode vorgestellt.

2.1 3D Referenzstruktur

Die Idee eine landmarkenbasierte Kalibrierung für OCT-Systeme zu entwickeln, die sich auf Messungen einer Referenzstruktur stützt, geht auf Arbeiten von

Ritter et al. [5] zurück. Hier wurde eine landmarkenbasierte Kalibrierstrategie für Rastersondenmikroskope und Laser Scanning Mikroskopie entwickelt.

Die von uns entwickelte 3D Referenzstruktur ist 10×10 mm^2 groß und besteht aus vier Siliziumschichten mit einem Brechungsindex von 3.5 bei einer Wellenlänge von 1300 nm, die 5×5 inverse Pyramidenstrukturen bilden (Abb. 1). Aufgrund der hohen Reflektivität der Siliziumoberfläche wurde zusätzlich eine circa 100 nm dicke Schicht Siliziumoxid aufgebracht, die die Reflektivität auf 3% reduziert. Als Landmarkendesign wurden kreisförmige Aussparungen in den vier Schichten gewählt. Diese 40×40 äquidistanten Landmarken erstrecken sich über die komplette Referenzstruktur und haben einen Durchmesser von 100 μm, was der 10-fachen Auflösung des OCT in der Strahltaille entspricht.

In Kooperation mit dem Institut für Mikroproduktionstechnik der Leibniz Universität Hannover wurde die Methode des Reaktiven Ionentiefenätzens (Bosch Prozess) benutzt, um die Referenzstruktur aus vier 500 μm $\pm$ 25 μm dicken Standardsiliziumwafern herzustellen, sodass die Struktur eine Gesamtdicke von ungefähr 2 mm hat. Die vier Schichten wurden unter dem Mikroskop mit Hilfe der Lokalisierungsmarker positioniert und verklebt. Danach wurde die komplette 3D Referenzstruktur mit einem Koordinatenmessgerät mit Hilfe der Markerlöcher vermessen, um etwaige Fehlausrichtungen zu bestimmen. Zum Schluss wurden OCT-Messungen der Referenzstruktur vorgenommen, um dann die Landmarken mittels eines auf Template Matching und Kreuzkorrelationen basierenden Algorithmus zu detektieren und so die Referenzdaten zu erhalten, die maßgeblich für die Kalibrierung sind.

2.2 Kalibriermethode

Zur Kalibrierung des OCT und somit der Korrektur von geometrischen Verzeichnungen wird eine landmarkenbasierte Registrierung verwendet. Mit Hilfe der Komposition von linearen und nicht-linearen Transformationen

$$\mathbf{x} = (x, y, z) \in \mathbf{X}_M \in \mathbb{R}^{1600 \times 3}, \ f_T : \ \mathbb{R}^3 \to \mathbb{R}^3, \ f_T(\mathbf{x}) = (T_{\text{lin}} \circ T_{\text{nicht}}) \cdot \mathbf{x} \quad (1)$$

sollen die Messdaten $\mathbf{X}_M$ möglichst gut in die Referenzdaten überführt werden.

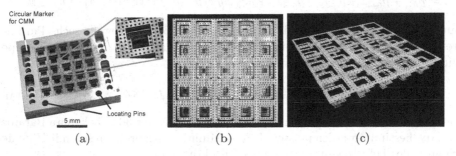

(a)   (b)   (c)

Abb. 1. 3D Referenzstruktur mit 5×5 inversen Pyramidenstrukturen und 40×40 Landmarken. (a) Bild des Standards inklusive der Lokalisierungsmarker und der Markerlöcher für das Koordinatenmessgerät (b) OCT-Bild von oben (c) OCT-Bild schräg von oben.

Abb. 2. Ausschnitt eines Volumenscans der Referenzstruktur mit einem Koordinatensystem, das die nicht-linearen Transformationsparameter, die Winkel θ, ϕ und den Tiefenversatz δ, zeigt.

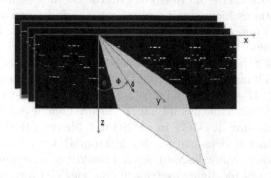

Lineare Transformationen sind Translation, Rotation, Scherung und Skalierung. Translation und Rotation sind linear extrinsische Parameter und werden benötigt, um die relative Position der Mess- und Referenzdaten zueinander mit $f_{R,t}(\mathbf{x}) = R \cdot x + t$ zu bestimmen, wobei R die Rotationsmatrix und t der Translationsvektor sind. Die Rotation wird durch die drei Eulerwinkel α, β und γ definiert. Die Translation beinhaltet ebenfalls drei Parameter, t_x, t_y und t_z. Scherung dagegen wird durch fehlende Orthogonalität der beiden Scanspiegel im OCT zueinander bzw. zur optischen Achse verursacht. Hier gibt es für jede Ebene einen Scherparameter, s_{xy}, s_{xz} und s_{yz}. Skalierung besitzt ebenfalls drei Parameter, c_x, c_y und c_z und wird verursacht durch eine unkalibrierte Scanschrittweite der beiden Scanspiegel. Scherung und Skalierung sind linear intrinsische Parameter.

Die nicht-linearen Transformationen beinhalten zwei Fehlerwinkel θ und ϕ, sowie einen Tiefenversatz δ, die für jeden A-Scan bezüglich der Referenzebene ($z = 0$) berechnet werden müssen. θ beschreibt die Abweichung vom idealen telezentrischen Strahl in x-Richtung und ϕ die Abweichung in y-Richtung. Der Tiefenversatz δ beschreibt den Fehler in z-Richtung (Abb. 2). Für alle drei Größen werden quadratische Funktionen

$$z = p_{n,1} + p_{n,2}x + p_{n,3}y + p_{n,4}x^2 + p_{n,5}xy + p_{n,6}y^2, \text{ with } \{\theta, \phi, \delta\} \in p_n \in \mathbb{R}^6 \quad (2)$$

angenommen. Daher besteht jede dieser drei Größen aus jeweils sechs Parametern, was insgesamt 18 nicht-lineare intrinsische Parameter ergibt. Die Komposition aller aufgezeigten Transformationen

$$f_T(\mathbf{x}) = (f_{R,t} \circ f_{\text{nicht}} \circ f_C \circ f_S)(\mathbf{x}) \quad (3)$$

bestimmt den gesamten Kalibrierprozess und beinhaltet 30 unbekannte Parameter, die bestimmt werden müssen. Dieses Minimierungsproblem soll mit Hilfe der Summe der Fehlerquadrate (SSE) als Gütekriterium

$$\min_{\mathbf{p}^* \in \mathcal{P}} \left\{ \mathcal{F} := SSE_{\mathbf{p}^*}(f_T(\mathbf{X}_M), \mathbf{X}_R) = \sum_{i \in \mathcal{I}} \|f_T(\mathbf{x}_{M,i}) - \mathbf{x}_{R,i}\|_2^2 \right\} \quad (4)$$

mit den Messdaten $\mathbf{x}_{M,i} \in \mathbf{X}_M$, den Referenzdaten $\mathbf{x}_{R,i} \in \mathbf{X}_R$ sowie dem Vektor $\mathbf{p}^*$, der alle idealen Kalibrierparameter enthält, gelöst werden. Da (4) hochgradig nicht-linear ist, gibt es keine analytische Lösung und erfordert eine anspruchsvollere Optimierungsmethode zur Berechnung der Parameter. Wir wenden die Sequential Quadratic Programming (SQP) Methode an, mit der die Parameter $\mathbf{p}^*$ berechnet werden. Dies ist ein häufig verwendetes und relativ einfach zu implementierendes Verfahren, das das nicht-lineare Problem durch ein leichter zu lösendes quadratisches Problem (2) ersetzt.

3 Ergebnisse

Für die geometrische Kalibrierung wurde die 3D Referenzstruktur mit einem Spectral Domain OCT Bildgebungssystem von Thorlabs (TELESTO-II mit dem Objektiv LSM03) bei einer Wellenlänge von 1300 nm ± 85 nm vermessen. Das Field-of-View beträgt $10 \times 10 \times 3.5$ mm^3 und kann die gesamte Struktur mit den 5×5 inversen Pyramidenstrukturen und 1600 Landmarken bei einer lateralen (axialen) Auflösung von 13 μm (5.5 μm) abbilden.

Wie man in Abb. 3 erkennen kann, zeigen die Messdaten eine in Realität nicht vorhandene Krümmung der planaren Referenzstruktur. Die Krümmungen in der x-z- und der y-z-Ebene sind gegenläufig, sodass eine Art Sattel entsteht. Diese Verzeichnung ist sehr massiv und muss für quantitative Anwendungen zuerst korrigiert werden. Der maximale absolute Fehler liegt in x-Richtung bei 78 μm, in y-Richtung bei 94 μm und in z-Richtung sogar bei 247 μm, was nochmal

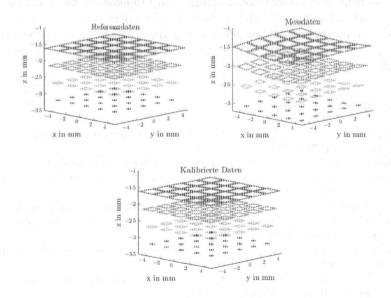

Abb. 3. Messung der 3D Referenzstruktur mit einem kommerziellen OCT, die mit Hilfe von geeigneten Transformationen in die Referenzdaten überführt werden soll. Nach Anwendung unserer Methode entstanden die kalibrierten Daten.

verdeutlicht, dass insbesondere die Tiefeninformationen verfälscht werden. Dies wird zudem deutlich an der Standardabweichung, die bei 48 μm bzw. 69 μm in x- und y-Richtung liegt und in z-Richtung mit 310 μm deutlich größer ist.

Nach der Kalibrierung kann man die Daten mit bloßem Auge nicht mehr von den Referenzdaten unterscheiden und die Referenzstruktur ist wieder sichtbar planar. Dies wird auch beim verbleibenden Fehler deutlich. Im Durchschnitt liegt der absolute Fehler in x-Richtung nach Kalibrierung bei 6 μm, in y-Richtung bei 8 μm und in z-Richtung nur noch bei 1 μm. Somit wurde insbesondere der Fehler in der Tiefe stark reduziert.

4   Diskussion

In dieser Arbeit wurde eine neuartige Methode zur Korrektur von geometrischen Verzeichnung für die Kalibrierung von OCT-Systemen beschrieben. Die Methode beruht auf den Messungen einer selbst angefertigten 3D Referenzstruktur und anschließender landmarkenbasierter Registrierung. Auf der Referenzstruktur befinden sich 1600 Markerlöcher, deren Zentrum als Landmarken dienen. Diese werden detektiert und anschließend mit geeigneten linearen und nicht-linearen Transformationsparametern an die Referenzdaten angepasst, um insbesondere die verfälschten Tiefeninformationen wiederherzustellen. Im Experiment konnte gezeigt werden, dass der geometrische Fehler nicht nur stark reduziert werden konnte, sondern auch, dass der Fehler nach Kalibrierung kleiner als die Auflösung des OCT-Systems ist, sowohl in lateraler als auch in axialer Richtung. Dies ermöglicht eine bessere Lokalisierung von Objekten in OCT-Bildern, was für viele Anwendungen sehr wichtig ist. Die Kalibriermethode kann auf andere OCT-Systeme angewandt werden, solange die Art des geometrischen Fehlers dieselbe ist. Unsere Resultate können die Rekonstruktion und Interpretation von OCT-Bildern für medizinische Anwendungen verbessern.

Literaturverzeichnis

1. Huang D, Swanson EA, Lin CP, et al. Optical coherence tomography. Science. 1991;254(5035):1178–1181.
2. Westphal V, Rollins A, Radhakrishnan S, et al. Correction of geometric and refractive image distortions in optical coherence tomography applying fermats principle. Opt Express. 2002;10(9):397–404.
3. Ortiz S, Siedlecki D, Grulkowski J, et al. Optical distortion correction in optical coherence tomography for qualitative ocular anterior segment by three-dimensional imaging. Opt Express. 2010;18(3):2782–96.
4. Ortiz S, Siedlecki D, Remon L, et al. Optical coherence tomography for qualitative surface topography. Appl Opt. 2009;48(35):6708–15.
5. Ritter M, Dziomba T, Kranzmann A, et al. A landmark-based 3D calibration strategy for SPM. Meas Sci Technol. 2007;19(12).
6. Lee G, Rasakanthan J, Woolliams P, et al. Fabrication of high quality optical coherence tomography (OCT) calibration artefacts using femtosecond inscription. Proc SPIE. 2012;8427(84271).

Automatic Single-Cell Segmentation and Tracking of Bacterial Cells in Fluorescence Microscopy Images

Vaja Liluashvili[1], Jan-Philip Bergeest[1], Nathalie Harder[1], Marika Ziesack[2],
Alper Mutlu[2], Ilka B. Bischofs[2], Karl Rohr[1]

[1]University of Heidelberg, BioQuant, IPMB, and DKFZ Heidelberg, Dept.
Bioinformatics and Functional Genomics, Biomedical Computer Vision Group
[2]Center for Molecular Biology (ZMBH) and BioQuant, University of Heidelberg,
Germany
vaj1989@gmail.com

Abstract. Automatic single-cell image analysis allows gaining deeper
insights into biological processes. We present an approach for single-cell
segmentation and tracking of bacterial cells in time-lapse microscopy
image data. For cell segmentation we use linear feature detection and
a probability map combined with schemes for cell splitting. For cell
tracking we propose an approach based on the maximal overlapping area
between cells, which is robust regarding cell rotation and accurately detects cell divisions. Our approach was successfully applied to segment
and track cells in time-lapse images of the life cycle of Bacillus subtilis.
We also quantitatively evaluated the performance of the segmentation
and tracking approaches.

1 Introduction

The bacteria of genus Bacillus, including the species Bacillus subtilis, are able to
form dormant endospores, which can survive long periods of starvation and are
resistant not only against high temperature, UV radiation, and desiccation, but
also against antibiotics. The initiation of sporulation and germination are highly
regulated processes, however, the exact mechanisms that are responsible for a
heterogeneous differentiation dynamics in isogenic populations are not yet fully
understood. Using bacterial life cycle assays in combination with quantitative
fluorescence time-lapse microscopy allows investigating bacterial cell dynamics
at each stage of the life cycle. Although the study of bacterial colonies can
provide significant insights, single-cell image analysis comprising segmentation
and tracking is necessary for a deeper understanding of the dynamic processes.

In previous work, only few approaches for segmentation and tracking of bacterial cells or rod-like structures were introduced. The segmentation approaches
are based on thresholding [1], watershed transformation [2], or level sets [3].
Thresholding-based approaches usually have problems with low contrast images and touching objects. The watershed transformation can separate merged

cells, but particularly for non-circular cells, the approach often results in over-segmentation. Level set approaches can well represent the shape of the cells, but usually a good initialisation is needed and typically these approaches cannot deal well with merged cells in low contrast images. In [4] a cell segmentation approach based on level sets and the Hessian matrix was described, however, touching cells can only be separated if they exhibit a boundary concavity at touching points, which is not always the case. In [5, 6] two segmentation approaches for rod-shaped cells were developed which are based on the detection of linear features and a probability map. These approaches yield good results, however, adjoining cells are not well separated. In [7] tracking is performed based on the minimal distance between bacterial cells in successive frames. This approach works well for relatively slow cell motion and small cell rotation, but it cannot handle cell division cases. In [8] a Gaussian mixture model was used for tracking of bacterial cells which assumes a random walk of the cells without considering cell-cell interaction. The model can handle cell division, however, it is assumed that the centroids of the daughter cells move along the major axis of the mother cell.

In this contribution, we present an approach for single-cell analysis of B. subtilis in time-lapse microscopy data. The image data contains low contrast and densely growing cells with a high division rate and large cell movement between successive frames. We developed two different segmentation methods, which are based on linear feature detection [5] and a probability map [6], and extended these approaches by incorporating a scheme for splitting highly curved segmented cells as well as by exploiting information from tracking. Our tracking approach is based on the maximal overlapping area of segmented cells in subsequent images and allows accurate detection of cell divisions. The approach is robust with respect to cell rotation, and can also handle large movements, as long as the cells in successive frames overlap. Our approach is fully automatic and was successfully applied to dynamic image data of the B. subtilis life cycle.

2   Materials and methods

We developed two segmentation approaches combined with a tracking approach for single-cell analysis of time-lapse microscopy images of the B. subtilis life cycle. The life cycle comprises the germination of the dormant endospores, the vegetative growth phase, and the sporulation (Fig. 1).

2.1   Single-cell segmentation

To segment single cells, first, the bacterial colony images are enhanced by adaptive histogram equalisation [9]. This leads to a homogenization of similar intensities, enhancing the contrast between intra and extracellular regions. Then, to determine an initial segmentation of the single cells, contours are detected using the Marr-Hildreth edge detector [5, 6]. Since the cells grow very densely, edge detection based segmentation is not sufficient to correctly separate adjoining cells. To separate touching cells we use linear feature detection [5] and a probability map [6]. Linear feature detection takes into account that bacterial cells are separated by regional minima, which are arranged along a line. The linear features are detected by local minima detection within search windows in multiple directions. Alternatively, a probability map is used [6]. This approach computes the probability of a separation along the initially segmented cell by taking into account the cell diameter and the contrast. The larger the diameter and the contrast, the higher is the splitting probability. The probabilities for the diameter and the contrast are multiplied, and cells are separated at positions, where the probability values exceed a certain threshold.

In addition, we detect segmented cells which do not have the typical straight elongated form. Such cases of highly curved segmented cells occur when after cell division the daughter cells have different orientations and low contrast, which results in an under-segmentation. In our approach we detect points with high directional changes along the skeleton of a cell and use these points for splitting. This significantly improves the segmentation result.

To further improve the segmentation we incorporated information from tracking (see below). We exploit the fact that the bacterial cells do not fuse in successive frames and assume that the increase of cell size over time is similar. In our approach, we identify fusion cases based on the tracking approach and split them using the same size ratio as for the corresponding cells in the previous frame.

In addition, we use a postprocessing step to improve the shape of the segmented cells. We apply morphological dilatation with a square structuring element at each position of the cell skeleton except at the end points, where a half-octagonal structuring element is used. An example of a segmentation result is shown in Fig. 2 (middle). There, segmented cells are visualized by different colors.

2.2 Single-cell tracking

Our tracking approach is based on the maximal overlap of cells at subsequent time points $t-1$ and t. Using the maximal overlap, an association matrix is generated. Based on this matrix, three major association cases can be distinguished:

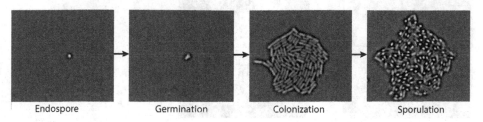

| Endospore | Germination | Colonization | Sporulation |

Fig. 1. Original images of the life cycle of B. subtilis bacteria. Red arrows point at generated spores (bright spots).

normal, division, and merging. In the normal case there exists a one-to-one correspondence between a cell in two subsequent images I_{t-1} and I_t. The division case occurs if a cell in I_{t-1} is associated with two or more cells in I_t. On the other hand, if two or more cells from I_{t-1} are associated with a cell in I_t, merging has occurred and will be corrected by our segmentation correction procedure. In cases where a cell in I_t has no association in I_{t-1}, distance-based tracking is performed. In this case, an association between a cell in I_{t-1} and a cell in I_t is generated if their centres of mass have minimal distance, but the distance should not exceed a certain threshold. If distance-based tracking cannot find an association then the segmented cell in I_t is considered an over-segmentation and is discarded. Fig. 2 (right) shows an example of a tracking result for a subset of the tracked cells.

3   Results

Our approach was applied to 49 2D+t image datasets ($[100 - 500] \times [100 - 300]$ pixels, 16 bit) with $45 - 70$ frames and $20 - 30$ minutes time intervals. The images were recorded using the DeltaVision Elite Imaging System (Applied Precision, Issaquah, USA). We performed a quantitative evaluation based on manually generated ground truth. The ground truth was determined by an expert. For the segmentation approaches we computed the object-based sensitivity and the positive predictive value (PPV), and the pixel-based Jaccard coefficient

$$\text{Sensitivity} = \frac{TP}{TP + FN}, \qquad \text{PPV} = \frac{TP}{TP + FP}, \qquad J(A,B) = \frac{|A \cap B|}{|A \cup B|} \quad (1)$$

where TP denotes true positives, FN are the false negatives, and FP denotes the false positives. $J(A,B)$ is the Jaccard coefficient for the segmented objects A and B. The tracking approach was quantified using the Jaccard coefficient. In this case, A represents the ground truth associations between cells in two successive frames and B denotes the automatically determined associations. Thus, the Jaccard index for the tracking is the quotient between the number of correctly identified associations at a time point, and the union of associations

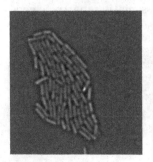 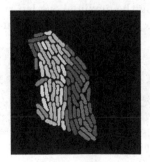 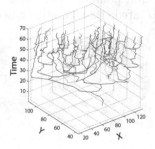

Fig. 2. (Left) Original image, (middle) segmented cells visualized by different colors, (right) tracking result (subset of trajectories).

determined by manual and automatic tracking. In following, we denote our approach based on linear feature detection by Approach1 and our approach based on a probability map by Approach2. The corresponding previous segmentation approaches [5, 6] are denoted by Previous1 and Previous2, respectively. Since the image quality decreases significantly after bacterial sporulation (Fig. 1), we investigated the performance separately for time points before and after sporulation. It turned out that before sporulation the PPV values are very high (above 0.97) for all approaches (Fig. 3, left). The performance values for the sensitivity for our approaches are better compared to the previous approaches (0.94 vs. 0.90, and 0.90 vs. 0.86). The Jaccard coefficients for our approaches are considerably higher compared to the previous approaches (0.75 vs. 0.50, and 0.74 vs. 0.48). After sporulation, the PPV values remained high for all approaches (above 0.86). For the sensitivity, our approaches yielded a considerable improvement (0.80 vs. 0.69, and 0.69 vs. 0.60). For the Jaccard coefficient we found that our approaches showed better results compared to the previous approaches also after sporulation (0.70 vs. 0.55, and 0.69 vs. 0.52)

We also investigated the performance of our tracking approach. Since the segmentation has a strong influence on the tracking result, we analysed the tracking performance when applied to both ground truth segmentation and automatic segmentation results. We found that the Jaccard coefficient was very high when tracking was applied to the ground truth segmentation (0.93 before sporulation and 0.98 after sporulation). Using automatic segmentation results, we obtained for our two approaches performance values of 0.75 and 0.75 (before sporulation) as well as 0.71 and 0.61 (after sporulation). This is a considerable improvement compared to the previous approaches with 0.64 and 0.63 (before sporulation) as well as 0.62 and 0.50 (after sporulation).

4   Discussion

We developed an approach for automatic single-cell segmentation and tracking of B. subtilis bacteria, and performed a quantitative performance evaluation. We found that our segmentation approaches yielded a considerable improvement

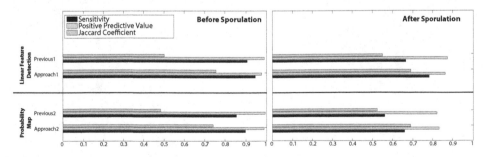

Fig. 3. (Left) Segmentation results before sporulation, (right) segmentation results after sporulation.

compared to previous approaches. We also analysed the performance of our tracking approach and found that it produced quite good results.

Acknowledgement. This work was in part supported by the European Research Council by ERC-StG ComMots 260860 and the Deutsche Forschungsgemeinschaft (Emmy Noether Program BI1213/3-1,2 and SPP1617: BE5098/1-1).

References

1. Obara B, Roberts M, Armitage J, et al. Bacterial cell identification in differential interference contrast microscopy images. BMC Bioinformatics. 2013;14(134).
2. Battenberg E, Bischofs-Pfeifer I. A System for Automatic Cell Segmentation of Bacterial Microscopy Images. Technical Report, UC Berkeley; 2006.
3. Schmitter D, Wachowicz P, Sage D, et al. A 2D/3D image analysis system to track fluorescently labeled structures in rod-shaped cells: application to measure spindle pole asymmetry during mitosis. Cell Div. 2013;8(6):1–13.
4. Liu X, Harvey CW, Wang H, et al. Detecting and tracking motion of myxococcus xanthus bacteria in swarms. Lect Notes Computer Sci. 2012;7510:373–80.
5. Vallotton P, Sun C, Wang D, et al. Segmentation and tracking individual pseudomonas aeruginosa bacteria in dense populations of motile cells. Proc ICIVC. 2009; p. 221–5.
6. Vallotton P, Turnbull L, Whitchurch C, et al. Segmentation of dense 2D bacilli populations. Proc Int Conf on Digit Image Comp: Tech and Appl, Sydney, NSW. 2010; p. 82–6.
7. Zhang HP, Be'er A, Florin EL, et al. Collective motion and density fluctuations in bacterial colonies. Proc Natl Acad Sci, USA. 2010;107(31):13626–30.
8. Juand RR, Levchenko A, Burlina P. Tracking cell motion using GM-PHD. Proc ISBI. 2009; p. 1154–7.
9. Zuiderveld K. Contrast limited adaptive histograph equalization. In: Graphic Gems IV. Academic Press Professional, San Diego; 1994. p. 474–85.

Multimodal Image Registration in Digital Pathology Using Cell Nuclei Densities

Nick Weiss[1,2], Johannes Lotz[1,2], Jan Modersitzki[1,2]

[1]Fraunhofer MEVIS, Project Group Image Registration, Lübeck
[2]Institute of Mathematics and Image Computing, Universität zu Lübeck
nick.weiss@mevis.fraunhofer.de

Abstract. 3D reconstruction and digital double staining offer pathologists many new insights into tissue structure and metabolism. Key to these applications is the precise registration of histological slide images, that is challenging in several ways. One major challenge are differently stained slides, that highlight different parts of the tissue. In this paper we introduce a new registration method to face this multimodality. It abstracts the image information to cell nuclei densities. By minimizing the distance of these densities an affine transformation is determined that restores the lost spatial correspondences. The proposed density based registration is evaluated using consecutive histological slides. It is compared to a Mutual Information based registration and shown to be more accurate and robust.

1 Introduction

In histology registration, the two prevailing applications in clinical research are 3D reconstruction and digital double staining. In 3D reconstruction, ultra thin serial sections are cut from a fixed tissue block. These sections are stained in several steps and finally digitally scanned. During this process, the sections are exposed to various deformations. Image registration is used to reestablish the spatial correspondence between the neighboring slides in order to reconstruct the original 3D object. Different approaches have been presented to solve the reconstruction problem based on image registration [1, 2].

The other application, digital double staining, has attracted less attention but still has a lot of potential. Often multiple staining chemicals are used on one tissue slide in order to discriminate different tissue properties. However, multiple chemical staining is often difficult due to the mutual reaction of the different stains. Image registration can be used to avoid the chemical double staining. In this case, different stains on consecutive slices of the tissue are applied independently. A subsequent multimodal image registration is then used to combine the information from both scans, yielding similar information to the chemical double staining. In this application, the ability of the registration to cope with different stains is fundamental.

Some solutions have been proposed to abstract the tissue information from the actual staining in the registration of histological images. Braumann et al. [3]

propose a method that automatically segments tissue regions in two different stains based on a clustering of statistical properties of pixels and their neighborhood. Lotz et al. [2] use the Normalized Gradient Fields distance measure to perform the elastic registration of image stacks with four different stains. It measures the distance of two images in terms of alignment of image gradients which works well as long as similar structures are visible in both images. Schwier et al. [4] use an automatic detection of liver vessels in the tissue to compute a rigid transformation that best maps the detected vessels onto each other. For a patch based registration, Song et al. [5] use an unsupervised content classification algorithm to learn similarity of different stains based on their color.

In this paper we propose to abstract the image information solely based on the automatically detected position of the nuclei in the tissue. However, there is not necessarily a one-to-one correspondence between nuclei in neighboring tissue slices and furthermore, not all nuclei will be detected by an automatic algorithm. We model this uncertainty by constructing a density function of the known nucleus positions and by assessing image similarity based on the difference of these density functions. As this paper focuses on the aspect of multimodality and only briefly sketches the proposed mathematical model, the reader is referred to [6] for a comprehensive discussion.

2   Materials and methods

Although the proposed method relies on a given set of nuclei positions, the work presented in this paper does not focus on nuclei detection. Therefore it is mentioned beforehand that we chose an algorithm provided by Homeyer et al. [7] for this task.

In this section we describe the three essential parts of our method: the density estimation, a distance measure that is adapted to densities and the final density registration process.

2.1   Density estimation

Given the coordinates of each cell nucleus center $X_1, ..., X_n \in \mathbb{R}^2$ within one slide the continuous density $\hat{\rho} : \mathbb{R}^2 \to \mathbb{R}$ is estimated using the Parzen window method

$$\hat{\rho}(x) = \frac{1}{nh^2} \sum_{i=1}^{n} b\left(\frac{x - X_i}{h}\right) \tag{1}$$

with a smoothing parameter h and a Gaussian basis function $b(x) = \frac{1}{2\pi} e^{-\frac{x^T x}{2}}$ as it is proposed in [8].

One could argue that such an estimation is unnecessary as the true density, given the nuclei positions, is already known. It is a sum of shifted Dirac functions ($h \to 0$ in (1)) describing the probability of finding nuclei as a certain event only at their actual positions. Considering the uncertainty of the real nuclei positions due to the automatic detection, this interpretation is far too limited. Some nuclei will be overlooked and nuclei centers will be determined with a small uncertainty. Furthermore, as we want to compare densities of neighboring slides, we cannot guarantee that a nucleus is visible at the same spot in adjacent slides due to its restricted spatial extent and orientation. Therefore an appropriate smoothing parameter h has to be chosen to represent the missing correspondences and further uncertainties.

In two perfectly aligned images, the respective nuclei positions can be seen as samples of the same unknown density, which we want to estimate.

2.2   Distance measure

We evaluate the similarity of two neighboring slices that are represented by density functions $\hat{\rho}^R$ and $\hat{\rho}^T$ by computing the Sum of Squared Differences (SSD)

$$\mathcal{D}^{\rho}_{\text{SSD}}[\hat{\rho}^R, \hat{\rho}^T] = \frac{1}{2} \int_{\mathbb{R}^2} (\hat{\rho}^R(x) - \hat{\rho}^T(x))^2 \mathrm{d}x \qquad (2)$$

The expansion of (2) unveils that the SSD is actually a sum of differently weighted Cross Correlations (CC)

$$\mathcal{D}^{\rho}_{\text{SDD}}[\hat{\rho}^R, \hat{\rho}^T] = \frac{1}{2}\mathcal{D}^{\rho}_{\text{CC}}[\hat{\rho}^R, \hat{\rho}^R] - \mathcal{D}^{\rho}_{\text{CC}}[\hat{\rho}^T, \hat{\rho}^R] + \frac{1}{2}\mathcal{D}^{\rho}_{\text{CC}}[\hat{\rho}^T, \hat{\rho}^T] \qquad (3)$$

with the CC defined as $\mathcal{D}^{\rho}_{\text{CC}}[\hat{\rho}^R, \hat{\rho}^T] = \int_{\mathbb{R}^2} \hat{\rho}^R(x)\hat{\rho}^T(x)\mathrm{d}x$. Following a detailed derivation, which can be found in [6] and is based on an idea published in [9], an analytical solution for the $\mathcal{D}^{\rho}_{\text{CC}}$ is given by

$$\int_{\mathbb{R}^2} \hat{\rho}^R(x)\hat{\rho}^T(x)\mathrm{d}x = \frac{1}{4\pi nmh^2} \sum_{i,j} e^{-\frac{\|X_j^T - X_i^R\|^2}{4h^2}} \qquad (4)$$

with nuclei positions $X_1^R, ..., X_n^R \in \mathbb{R}^2$ of the reference slide and the respective template nuclei positions $X_1^T, ..., X_m^T \in \mathbb{R}^2$. Hence, given the equations (3) and (4), the SSD between two densities, estimated as described in 2.1, can be calculated exactly.

Using the analytical solution one always has to iterate over all combinations of cell nuclei positions. In one histological slide there can be more than 500,000 nuclei, resulting in billions of combinations. In these cases, we discretize the integral in (2) on a regular grid, applying the midpoint rule. The accuracy of a discretized SSD then depends on the smoothing parameter h. On the other side a discretization can be chosen according to a desired accuracy and h. This way the densities only have to be estimated at certain grid points within a region of interest (normally defined by the image domain). Depending on h, m and n either the analytical or the discretized approach is more practicable.

2.3   Density registration

We aim to find a transformation $\varphi : \mathbb{R}^2 \mapsto \mathbb{R}^2$ that minimizes the distance between the two densities and aligns the neighboring slide images. The transformation maps from a reference coordinate frame, defined on the reference density

$\hat{\rho}^R$ onto the coordinate frame of the template density $\hat{\rho}^T$. We focus on the case of affine registration, where the deformation $\varphi(x) = Ax + b$, $A \in \mathbb{R}^{2\times2}$, $b \in \mathbb{R}^2$ is parametrized by a transformation matrix A and a translation vector b. Following the variational approach, established by, e.g., [10], the registration problem

$$\mathcal{D}^\rho_{SSD}[\hat{\rho}^R, \hat{\rho}^T \circ \varphi] \xrightarrow[A,b]{} \min \qquad (5)$$

is solved by optimizing the distance measure (2) with respect to the transformation parameters using a Gauss-Newton scheme [10].

2.4 Evaluation

The proposed density registration method was implemented in Julia and is based on a freely available image registration framework[1].

In order to evaluate our algorithm on clinically relevant samples, we applied the registration method to a stack of four slides of human lung tumor generated within the LungSys2 consortium[2]. The surgically resected material was fixed, sectioned with a slice thickness of 2 μm, and immunohistochemically stained alternately with four different stains (CD31, HE, Factor VIII, KL-1).

Similar to the evaluation in [2] we rate our registration qualitatively by visual inspection and quantitatively by measuring the alignment of manual annotations in the image. For the quantification two corresponding structures, represented by a set of discrete points, are segmented in all four slides and their distance in neighboring slides is determined by the Hausdorff distance h_d.

Furthermore these results are compared to the outcomes of a multimodal image registration based on the commonly used Mutual Information (MI) distance measure. Both registration methods rely on a multilevel or multiscale approach for faster convergence and the avoidance of local minima [10]. For the density registration different smoothing parameters h from coarse ($h = 2.0$) to fine ($h = 0.05$) are used. For the discretized approach with $h = 0.05$ we chose 1024×1024 as an appropriate grid size. The finest image level used by the MI based registration is 1860×1424.

3   Results

The Hausdorff distance between the two corresponding, annotated structures in all three slide pairs was reduced from an initial h_d greater than 1 mm to a mean h_d of 20.76 μm using the proposed density based method. In comparison the image registation with the MI distance measure reached a mean distance of 35.41 μm. This way our method presents a 41% improvement over the well established MI registration. All alignment errors are shown in Tab. 1.

The visual inspection is exemplary displayed for two slides in Fig. 1. Especially the checkerboard overlay of a specific section of the registered slides shows

---

[1] https://github.com/FraunhoferMEVIS/ImageRegistration
[2] LungSys2 is funded by the German Ministry of Education and Research.

Table 1. Alignment errors h_d (in μm) of two annotated structures after registration with either the proposed density based or the commonly used Mutual Information (MI) based multimodal distance measure. Three slide pairs were annotated.

Structure	Registered Slides	h_d (Density)	h_d (MI)
1	$1 \to 2$	39.34	55.48
2	$1 \to 2$	17.24	39.07
1	$2 \to 3$	19.13	32.57
2	$2 \to 3$	20.78	46.34
1	$3 \to 4$	17.37	24.48
2	$3 \to 4$	10.85	14.52
Mean ($\pm$ Standard Deviation)		20.76 ± 9.69	35.41 ± 14.83

a good fitting of corresponding areas. Further the small Hausdorff distance is visually confirmed by a great overlap of the annotated structures.

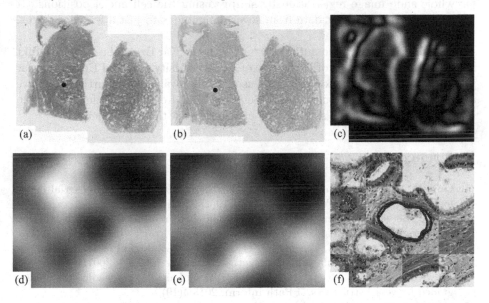

Fig. 1. Two differently stained, adjacent slides are displayed in (a) and (b). Their local differences in terms of the estimated nuclei densities ($h = 0.5$) are shown in (c). The locations of the annotated structures within the whole slides are implied by differently colored dots (● : structure 1, ● : structure 2). The estimated densities ($h = 0.05$) around structure 1 are shown in detail for slide (a) in (d) and for slide (b) in (e) after registration. The registration in this area is further evaluated by a checkerboard overlay in (f) and the mapping of structure 1 for both slides (● : (b), ● : (a)).

4   Discussion

The proposed method is able to register differently stained serial sections with an affine transformation model and outperforms the established mutual information based registration. As a proof of concept, this has been demonstrated on four sections.

Although the affine registration already aligns corresponding structures in two given sections closely, it is not able to capture elastic deformation behavior, that all slides, to some extent, have undergone during their preparation process. As shown in [2] these changes can be adjusted using a non-parametric, elastic deformation model. Extending the proposed method with such a model is currently in progress [6]. First tentative experiments have shown that the cell nuclei positions provide information, that is dense enough to determine a plausible deformation field.

Moreover this method has the potential to be a fast and memory efficient tool for whole slide image registration by simply using the cell nuclei positions. It reduces the relevant input data from several gigabytes to just a few megabytes.

Acknowledgement. The authors want to thank Kai Breuhahn and Benedikt Müller from the Institute of Pathology of the University Hospital Heidelberg for providing the histology example data used in the evaluation. Furthermore, we are grateful to André Homeyer and Henning Kost from Fraunhofer MEVIS in Bremen for providing the software we used to detect the cell nuclei.

References

1. Ourselin S, Roche A, Subsol G. Reconstructing a 3D structure from serial histological sections. Image Vis Comput. 2001;19(1):25–31.
2. Lotz J, Berger J, Müller B, et al. Zooming in: high resolution 3D reconstruction of differently stained histological whole slide images. Proc SPIE. 2014;9041:1–7.
3. Braumann U, Scherf N, Einenkel J, et al. Large histological serial sections for computational tissue volume reconstruction. Methods Inf Med. 2007;46(5).
4. Schwier M, Hahn H, Dirsch O, et al. Registration of histological whole slide images guided by vessel structures. J Path Inform. 2013;4(10).
5. Song Y, Treanor D, Bulpitt A, et al. 3D reconstruction of multiple stained histology images. J Path Inform. 2013;4(7).
6. Lotz J, Weiss N, Modersitzki J. Efficient whole slide image registration based on nuclei densities; 2015. In preperation.
7. Homeyer A, Schenk A, Arlt J, et al. Practical quantification of necrosis in histological whole-slide images. Comput Med Imag Grap. 2013;37(4):313–22.
8. Silverman B. Density Estimation. CRC Press; 1986.
9. Tsin Y, Kanade T. A correlation-based approach to robust point set registration. Eur Conf Computer Vis. 2004;3023:558–69.
10. Modersitzki J. FAIR: Flexible Algorithms for Image Registration. SIAM; 2009.

Räumliche Darstellung und Analyse von Nanopartikelverteilungen in vitalen Alveolarmakrophagen in vitro mit der Dunkelfeldmikroskopie

Dominic Swarat[1], Christian Arens[1], Martin Wiemann[2], Hans-Gerd Lipinski[1]

[1]Biomedical Imaging Group, Fachbereich Informatik, Fachhochschule Dortmund
[2]Institute for Lung Health (IBE R&D gGmbH), Münster
swarat@gmx.de

Kurzfassung. Die räumliche Wechselwirkung von Nanopartikeln mit vitalen alveolären Makrophagen wurde mit der Dunkelfeldmikroskopie, kombiniert mit einer piezogesteuerten Verschiebung der z-Achse und einer Triggerung der Kamerabilder, untersucht. Damit gelang eine räumliche Rekonstruktion von unfixierten motilen Makrophagen bei gleichzeitiger Darstellung der räumlichen und zeitlichen Verteilung der aufgenommenen Nanopartikel. Die räumliche Darstellung der Nanopartikelverteilungen ermöglicht neue Erkenntnisse zur Biokinetik von Nanopartikeln.

1 Einleitung

Die Nanotoxikologie untersucht aktuell, in wieweit Nanomaterialen gesundheitsschädlich sind und welche Wechselwirkungen überhaupt zwischen Zellsystemen und nanostrukturierten Materialen bestehen. Ein relevantes *in vitro*-Zellmodell für die Untersuchung solcher Wechselwirkungen stellen alveoläre Makrophagen dar. Allerdings zeigen diese Zellen – im Gegensatz zu ihrer meist sphäroiden Gestalt *in vivo* – flache, teils ausgedehnte Anheftungsstrukturen (Pseudopodien), die schnell verändert werden und die zur Fortbewegung dienen. Für die mikroskopischen Untersuchungen der Wechselwirkungen zwischen Zellen und Nanopartikeln wurde bereits erfolgreich ein Dunkelfeldmikroskop eingesetzt [1]. Auf Grund der Lichtstreuung an Zell- bzw. Membrangrenzen sowie an geeigneten Nanopartikeln, liefert das Gerät scharfe Bilder von der Morphologie der beteiligten Zellen, zusammen mit anheftenden oder aufgenommenen Nanopartikeln. Da diese Partikel jedoch deutlich kleiner als die Wellenlänge des sichtbaren Lichts sind, kann man die Partikel nicht direkt beobachten, sondern nur ihr Beugungsmuster. Das gilt sowohl für frei bewegliche Partikel als auch für solche Partikel, die innerhalb der Zelle in Vesikel aufgenommen wurden. Auf diese Weise kann das biokinetische Verhalten der Partikel (Transport im Cytoplasma, an Membranen oder in Vesikeln) grundsätzlich analysiert werden. Das Beleuchtungsverfahren des CytoViva Dunkelfeld-Kondensors erzeugt starken Kontrastunterschiede, die beim Durchfahren des Präparats in z-Richtung die Nutzung räumlicher Informationen möglich erscheinen lassen. Eigene Untersuchungen haben bereits gezeigt, dass die Aufnahme vom Bildstapeln (z-stack) fixierter Zellen möglich ist und eine räumliche Rekonstruktion der Zelle erlaubt [2]. Im Rahmen dieser Arbeit soll daher untersucht werden, ob neben der Darstellung der Zellmorphologie auch die räumliche und zeitliche Verteilung der Nanopartikel in vitalen Makrophagen rekonstruiert werden kann. Zudem soll auch überprüft werden, ob durch eine räumliche Rekonstruktion eine verbesserte Differenzierung des Systems „Makrophage – inkorporierte Nanopartikel" technisch möglich ist und biologisch/toxikologisch hilfreich sein kann.

2 Material und Methoden

Alveoläre Makrophagen (AM) der Rattenlunge (NR8383) wurden in F12K-Medium (angereichert mit Penicillin/Streptomycin, Glutamin und 15% fetales Kälberserum) auf einem Objektträger ausgesät und für 24 h anheften lassen. Im Anschluss an diese Vorpräparation wurden die Zellen für 30 min in F12-K Medium überführt, das AlOOH-Nanopartikel enthielt (180 μg/ml, Größe ca. 50 nm). Dabei wurden die Zellen invers inkubiert, um zu verhindern dass Nanopartikel-Agglomerate auf sie herab sedimentierten. Der Objektträger mit den vitalen AM wurde aus dem Bad genommen, gewaschen, mit einem Deckglas versehen und schließlich in einem aufrechten Dunkelfeld-Mikroskop (DFM) analysiert. Das verwendete optische System bestand aus einem Olympus Bx51 Mikroskop, das mit einem CytoViva^{TM}Dunkelfeldkondensor und einem Irisobjektiv (100x, Ölimmersion) ausgestattet war. Die im Mikroskop erzeugten Bilder wurden mit einer 12bit-Digitalkamera (PCO Pixelfly VGA) aufgezeichnet. Die Partikelgröße wurde vorab mit Hilfe eines geeigneten Gerätes (Nanosight^{TM}) und modifizierter statistischer Verfahren bestimmt [3]. Das Bildfeld betrug dabei ca. $62x46\,\mu m^2$, die korrespondierende Bildmatrix maß $650x480$ px^2. Für die räumliche Rekonstruktion der Zellen wurde ein z-Stapel mit Hilfe eines Piezo gesteuerten Systems (30DV50 / Piezojena) erzeugt. Registriert wurde überwiegend ab einer Höhe $h = 40\,\mu$m oberhalb des Objektträgers (relative Höhe $h = 0$) in Schritten von 300 nm abwärts bis zu $h = 0$, um auf diese Weise auch die obere Region der Zelle noch komplett registrieren zu können. Dieses obere Zellareal fand sich im Allgemeinen bei $h \approx 20 \mu m$, so dass der z-Stack mit den Zellbilddaten etwa 45 - 60 Bilder umfasste. Die Belichtungs- bzw. Registrierungszeit pro Schicht betrug 65 ms, die gesamte Registrierung eines z-Stapels weniger als 10 s. Parallel zu den AM-Bildregistrierungen wurde die Point-Spread-Function (PSF) des Systems experimentell, mit Hilfe von 30 nm große sphärischen Goldpartikeln, bestimmt [4].

Nach Zwischenspeicherung der Bilddaten wurde „off-line" eine Bildanalyse durchgeführt. Zunächst erfolgte eine Verbesserung der Bildauflösung durch eine 3D-Deconvolution anhand der empirisch ermittelten räumlichen PSF (Richardson-Lucy Algorithmus). Die so erzeugten Bilddaten wurden zwischengespeichert und dann einer top-down durchgeführten konventionellen Bildanalyse unterzogen. Nach erfolgter Bildkontrasterhöhung, mit Hilfe des EnhancedLocalContrast-Filters (Fenstergröße 75 px), wurden mittels LevelSetSegmentation Routine bzw.

Triple-Threshold Verfahren (jeweils ein Schwellwert für die Objekte „Zellmembranbereich", „Zellkernbereich" und mit NP gefüllte Vesikel) sowohl die entsprechenden Objektflächen als auch deren Konturen für jede Schicht des Bildstapels als Binärobjekte ermittelt werden [5]. Da die Konturen, insbesondere die des nach außen begrenzenden Zellmembranbereichs, sehr komplex sind, wurden diese Bereiche mit Hilfe von Fourier-Deskriptoren (FD) bearbeitet. Durch Verringerung der Anzahl der FD-Koeffizienten im höherfrequenten Bereich, ließ sich eine Konturglättung erzielen, die insbesondere die Erfassung der Orientierung der Zelle in der Ebene ermöglichte. Vitale Makrophagen haben die Eigenschaft, ihre äußere Form relativ rasch zu verändern. Zudem bewegen sie sich im Raum, wobei ihre Bewegungen eher zufällig sind und in eine Rotations- sowie in eine Translationsbewegung zerlegt, getrennt analysiert und letztlich korrigiert werden können.

Diese Korrektur wird erforderlich, wenn eine Spontanbewegung während (i) des Erzeugens des z-Stapels oder (ii) der Langzeitbeobachtung eines AM-stacks auftritt. Eine Rotation lässt sich durch die Anwendung der Radon- Transformation (RT) identifizieren. Hierzu werden für je zwei zeitlich versetzt aufgezeichnete Zellkonturen zunächst die RT-Spektren generiert, die dann einer Kreuzkorrelation, mit dem Ziel des Auffindens des „wahrscheinlichsten Rotationswinkels" unterzogen. Translationen lassen sich durch zeitliche Verschiebungen von Referenzpunkten (mit Hilfe der Lage von Zellschwerpunktkoordinaten) ermitteln. Sind Rotationswinkel und Verschiebung der Referenzkoordinaten bekannt, kann ein Bewegungsartefakt aus den Beobachtungsdaten weitgehend eliminiert werden. Ein biologisch wichtiger Kontrollwert, mit dem die Genauigkeit der Bildanalyse überprüft werden kann, ist das AM-Zellvolumen. Für jedes Bild im z-Stapel wurde zunächst die Objektfläche von Zelle, Zellkernareal und Vesikelbereich (gefüllt mit NP), mit Hilfe der bekannten Gaußschen Flächenmethode, bestimmt. Um den Volumenanteil zu ermitteln, wurde die Fläche schließlich mit der zugehörigen Schichtdicke multipliziert. Das Volumen der gesamten Zelle konnte dann mit den z.B. aus der Literatur bekannten Daten für AM verglichen werden. Um die räumlich orientierten Zellstrukturen auch visualisieren zu können, wurde ein konventionelles Raytracing-Verfahren bzw. ein Oberflächenvisualisierungsverfahren (Marching Cube) implementiert.

3   Ergebnisse

Es wurden beispielhaft 50 nm AlOOH-NP für die Beladung der AM verwendet. Die Generierung der 2D-Szene der AM („axiales Schichtbild") umfasst, ausgehend vom kontrastverstärkten Originalbild, die Gesamtzellkontur, das Zellkernareal und die Lage der mit NP beladenen Vesikel in der jeweiligen Bildebene. Daraus wurde für jedes der drei Objekte ein binärer Bilddatenstack erzeugt. Die Abb. 1 zeigt, ausgehend von der ausgewählten Zellebene (Abb. 1a), eine 3D-Rekonstruktion der mit NP beladenen Makrophagen. Eine Aufsicht auf eine volumenorientierte (transparente) 3D-Rekonstruktion nach der Raycasting-Methode zeigt Abb. 1(b). Der Zellkörper ist in grüner Farbe, das Zellkernareal in roter und die Verteilung der NP sind in blauer Farbe dargestellt. In Abb. 1(c) sind isoliert die mit NP beladenen Vesikel (blau) sowie der Zellkern (rot) als eine Oberflächenrekonstruktion (MarchingCube-Methode) visualisiert, während Abb. 1(d) eine Oberflächenrekonstruktion des gesamten AM darstellt. Mit dem Oberflächenmodell des AM lässt sich auch das Volumen der Zelle ermitteln. Sein

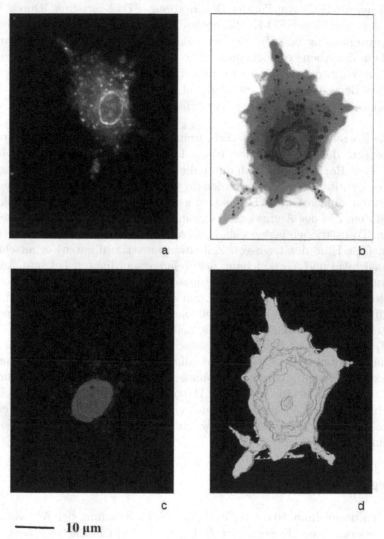

Abb. 1. 3D-Rekonstruktion eines mit NP beladenen vitalen Makrophagen. Dargestellt sind eine ausgewählte Zellschicht aus einem generierten Zellbildstapel (a), die Aufsicht auf eine aus dem Stapel mit dem Ray-Casting-Verfahren transparent dargestellte Zelle (b), die räumliche Lagebeziehung zwischen Zellkernareal und NP-beladenen Vesikeln als Oberflächenmodell mit Marching-Cube-Verfahren (c) sowie eine Oberflächenrekonstruktion der kompletten Zelle Marching-Cube-Verfahren (d).

numerischer Wert weicht praktisch nicht vom Volumenwert ab, der mit der oben beschriebenen Flächen-Höhenmethode nach Gauß bestimmt werden konnte (relative Abweichung $< 5\%$). Die ermittelten Volumenwerte lagen typischerweise bei etwa 1200 μm^3 und stimmten mit bekannten Literaturwerten gut überein [6]. Die Abb. 2(a) und (b) zeigen die Verteilung von NP innerhalb der Zelle zu verschiedenen Zeiten. Eine Registrierung nach etwa 20 min weist auf eine eher randständige Verteilung der NP innerhalb der Zelle hin (Abb. 2(a)). Nach etwa 60 min beobachtet man hingegen, dass weite Zellbereiche von den mit NP beladenen Vesikeln erfasst werden. Eine systematische Untersuchung des Quotienten von Vesikelvolumen (mit geladenen NP) V und dem Gesamtzellvolumen V_0 ergab einen mit der Zeit t sigmoidal zunehmenden Verlauf (Abb. 2(d)) bis maximal etwa 70% des Gesamtzellvolumens, während zu Beginn typischerweise nur etwa 20-30% des Gesamtzellvolumens erreicht wurde. Offenbar lässt sich hieraus ableiten, dass typische zeitliche Verteilungsmuster von NP innerhalb der Zelle darstellbar und damit analysierbar sind. Um zu testen, inwieweit eine räumliche Vermessung der Makrophagen im Hinblick auf die Verteilung der mit NP gefüllten Vesikel überhaupt sinnvoll ist, wurde zunächst von jedem der $N_0 = 37$ registrierten AM der Quotient von kleinster ($A_{\min}$) und größter ($A_{\max}$) Fläche innerhalb des jeweiligen z-stacks bestimmt, welche die mit NP gefüllten Vesikel innerhalb der Zelle repräsentiert. Der Wert dieses Quotienten ($0 < \frac{A_{\min}}{A_{\max}} \leq 1$) wurde in fünf gleichgroße Intervalle geteilt und gegen die relative Anzahl $\frac{N}{N_0}$ der zu den Intervallen gehörenden Werte abgetragen (Abb. 2(c)). Man erkennt, dass im Beispiel (das für einen Zeitpunkt von $t = 40$ min nach Messungsbeginn ausgewählt wurde) offenbar die überwiegende Zahl im Bereich von $0 < \frac{A_{\min}}{A_{\max}} \leq 0.6$ liegt. Daraus ist zu schließen, dass es innerhalb einer Zelle zu einem großen Unterschied der von den NP eingenommenen Flächen kommt, was auf eine differenzierte räumliche Verteilung der NP innerhalb der Zelle hindeutet.

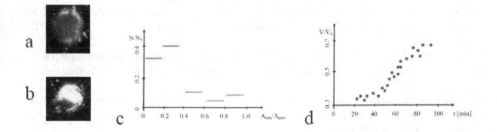

Abb. 2. Ausbreitungszustand der mit NP beladenen Vesikel in einer 2D-rekonstruierten Makrophage. Zustand der Vesikelverteilung nach 20 min (a) und nach 60 min (b) Beobachtungszeit. Verteilung der Anzahl der im Intervall Amin/Amax gefundenen mit NP beladenen Vesikelbereiche, beobachtet 40 min nach Beginn des Experiments (c). Verteilung des von Vesikeln eingenommenen Zellvolumens V in Bezug zum Gesamtvolumen der Zelle V_0 in Abhängigkeit von der Zeit t (d).

4 Diskussion

Die exemplarisch vorgestellten Untersuchungsergebnisse haben gezeigt, dass eine räumliche Rekonstruktion von lebenden Makrophagen bei Anwesenheit von Nanopartikeln *in vitro*, bis hin zu Volumenberechnungen des Vesikelkompartiments möglich ist. Zeitliche Veränderungen der NP-Verteilung innerhalb der Zelle waren detektierbar. Auch Bewegungsartefakte konnten weitgehend eliminiert werden. Insgesamt konnte auf dieser Basis eine räumliche und zeitliche Rekonstruktion der beteiligten zellulären Systeme erfolgreich durchgeführt werden. Die Dunkelfeldmikroskopie ermöglicht die gleichzeitige Visualisierung von nicht-fluoreszenzmarkierten Nanopartikeln in ebenfalls ungefärbten Zellen. Wesentliche Zellbestandteile und Kompartimente (äußere Membran, Kernhülle, Endosomen und Vesikel) lassen sich zusammen mit Nanopartikeln abbilden [1]. Beobachtungen und Analysen des dynamischen Partikelverhaltens können so unabhängig von Farbstoffeinflüssen durchgeführt werden. Da die verwendeten NR8383 Makrophagen, bei einer Höhe von bis zu 20 μm, eine vergleichsweise dicke optische Schicht mit eher ungünstigen optischen Streuungseigenschaften darstellen, lässt sich die Methodik leicht auf die Vielzahl der adhärent wachsenden und meist viel flacheren Zelltypen übertragen und stellt somit ein brauchbares Instrumentarium für die nanotoxikologische Zellforschung dar.

Danksagung. Die Arbeit wurde mit Mitteln des Bundesministeriums für Bildung und Forschung (BMBF / FKZ 17NT026) gefördert.

Literaturverzeichnis

1. Xiao L, Qiao YX, He Y, et al. Three dimensional orientational imaging of nanoparticles with darkfield microscopy. Anal Chem. 2010;82:5268–74.
2. Swarat D, Wiemann M, Lipinski HG. Three-dimensional characteristics of alveolar macrophages in vitro observed by dark field microscopy. Proc SPIE. 2014;9129:91292N–1–12.
3. Wagner T, Lipinski HG, Wiemann M. Dark field nanoparticle tracking analysis for size characterization of plasmonic and non-plasmonic particles. J Nanopart Res. 2014;16(5):1–10.
4. Cole RW, Jinadasa T, Brown CM. Measuring and interpreting point spread functions to determine confocal microscope resolution and ensure quality control. Nat Protoc. 2011;6:1929–41.
5. Sethian JA. LevelSet methods and fast marching methods. Cambridge Press, 2nd ed.; 1999.
6. Krombach F, Muenzing S, Allmeling AM, et al. Cell size of alveolar macrophage: an interspecies comparison. Environ Health Perspt. 1997;105:1261–3.

2D Plot Visualization of Aortic Vortex Flow in Cardiac 4D PC-MRI Data

Benjamin Köhler[1], Monique Meuschke[1], Uta Preim[2], Katharina Fischbach[3], Matthias Gutberlet[4], Bernhard Preim[1]

[1]Dept. of Computer Graphics and Simulation, OvG University, Magdeburg, Germany
[2]Dept. of Diagnostic Radiology, Hospital Olvenstedt, Magdeburg, Germany
[3]Dept. of Radiology and Nuclear Medicine, University Hospital, Magdeburg, Germany
[4]Dept. of Diagnostics and Interventional Radiology, Heart Center, Leipzig, Germany
ben.koehler@isg.cs.uni-magdeburg.de

Abstract. Aortic vortex flow is a strong indicator for various cardiovascular diseases. The correlation of pathologies like bicuspid aortic valves to the occurrence of such flow patterns at specific spatio-temporal positions during the cardiac cycle is of great interest to medical researchers. Dataset analysis is performed manually with common flow visualization techniques such as particle animations. For larger patient studies this is time-consuming and quickly becomes tedious. In this paper, we present a two-dimensional plot visualization of the aorta that facilitates the assessment of occurring vortex behavior at one glance. For this purpose, we explain a mapping of the 4D flow data to circular 2D plots and describe the visualization of the employed λ_2-vortex criterion. A grid view allows the simultaneous investigation and comparison of multiple datasets. After a short familiarization with the plots our collaborating cardiologists and radiologists were able distinguish between patient and healthy volunteer datasets with ease.

1 Introduction

Four-dimensional phase-contrast magnetic resonance imaging (4D PC-MRI) made great advances in the last decade [1, 2]. It enables the non-invasive acquisition of time-resolved, three-dimensional information about the intravascular hemodynamics. The gained insight supports diagnosis and severity assessment of different cardiovascular diseases (CVD). Vortex flow in the great mediastinal vessels such as the aorta is presumed to be a strong indication of several pathologies. Therefore, studies with homogeneous patient groups are performed to quantify the probability of vortex occurrence in specific vessel sections during the cardiac cycle.

Common pathline visualizations [3] of the highly complex 4D PC-MRI datasets allow qualitative analysis. Köhler et al. [4] adapted the line predicates technique to semi-automatically filter vortex flow. Such methods are essential to make 4D PC-MRI viable for the clinical routine. Nevertheless, when the pathlines are displayed all at once by ignoring their temporal component, heavy visual clutter remains. Particle animations alleviate this problem, but increase the required evaluation time per dataset.

Different works established simplified visualizations of the cardiovascular morphology. Cerqueira et al. [5] proposed the nowadays widely used 2D Bull's Eye Plot (BEP) of the left ventricle that is based on a standardized segmentation. The plot is simple, unambiguous and thus a convincing reduction of the 3D information. Angelelli et al. [6] introduced a straightening of tubular structures and applied it to the aorta in order to enhance flow analysis with reference to the main flow direction, which usually is the centerline. Yet, when the whole cardiac cycle is to be analyzed, numerous such visualizations with different temporal positions are required.

In this work, we introduce a circular 2D plot that is adaptable to various flow characteristics. We focus on vortex flow due to the strong correlation to cardiovascular pathologies. The plot provides detailed information about the temporal position and approximates the corresponding vessel section. A grid view of different datasets enables the fast assessment of vortex behavior in a user-defined database. A scalar parameter controls the plots' sensitivity towards vortex flow. The possibility to set already analyzed datasets as references enhances the classification of new cases. After a brief training our collaborating cardiologists and radiologists were able to reliably find pathologic cases in the grid view.

1.1 Medical background

The aorta is the largest artery of the body with a vessel diameter of about $2 - 3$ cm. Oxygenated blood comes from the left ventricle (LV), passes the aortic valve (AV) and is then supplied to the body. Systole denotes the phase of LV contraction, when the AV is opened. During diastole, when the LV is relaxed, the AV is closed and prevents retrograde flow. A pathologic dilation of the aorta is called ectasia. If the vessel diameter is above 1.5 the original size, it is referred to as aneurysm. The altered morphology promotes the formation of vortex flow in the corresponding vessel section. The AV normally consists of three leaflets. In bicuspid aortic valve (BAV) patients two of them adhere. Hope et al. [7] detected systolic vortex flow in the ascending aorta, the vessel section directly behind the valve, in 75 % of their BAV patients. For furthers details about the relation between vortex flow and cardiovascular pathologies we refer to [4].

2   Material and methods

In the following, the 4D PC-MRI dataset acquisition and preprocessing pipeline are described. We proceed with a detailed explanation of the 4D data to 2D plot projection, the employed λ_2-vortex measure and grid view as solution to one of its drawbacks.

2.1 Data acquisition and preprocessing

The 4D PC-MRI data were acquired using a 3 T Magnetom Verio (Siemens Healthcare, Erlangen, Germany) with a maximum expected velocity (V_{ENC}) of 1.5 m/s per dimension. A dataset contains each three (x-, y- and z-dimension) time-resolved flow and magnitude images that describe the flow direction and strength (i.e. the velocity), respectively. All temporal positions together represent one full heartbeat. The spatio-temporal resolution is 1.77 mm × 1.77 mm in a 132 × 192 grid with 3.5 mm distance between the 15 to 23 slices and about 50 ms between the 14 to 21 time steps. Artifact reduction in the flow images was performed using eddy current correction and phase unwrapping [8]. A maximum intensity projection over time (tMIP) of the magnitude images is calculated as basis for the graph cut-assisted segmentation.[1] The resulting three-dimensional binary vessel mask is postprocessed using morphological closing and opening. A surface mesh is obtained via marching cubes, subsequently low-pass filtered as well as reduced and then used to extract a centerline.[2] The GPU is utilized to integrate pathlines using an adaptive step size Runge-Kutta-4 scheme with quadrilinear interpolation of the flow velocity vectors and to calculate the λ_2-criterion for the line predicate-based vortex extraction [4]. It is ensured that each voxel in every temporal position is visited at least once.

2.2 Aortic vortex plot

Mapping Intravascular positions $x = (x, y, z, t)$ in the 4D PC-MRI dataset consist of a three-dimensional spatial and a one-dimensional temporal component. The circular plot visualization, however, offers merely an angle ϕ and a distance d to the center as degrees of freedom.

Medical research papers, which correlate the presence of vortex flow patterns to specific pathologies, have two central questions: *When* (during the cardiac cycle) does the vortex occur and in *what vessel section*? We decided to map a vortex' temporal position to the plot's angle as an analogy to a clock and due to the cyclic nature of the data. The first time step is located 12 o'clock, the direction is clockwise. Now there is only the center distance d left to map the spatial position. The idea is to employ the centerline for this purpose. The projection p of a spatial position in the vessel onto the centerline is determined and used to obtain $d \in [0, 1]$ as $\sqrt{\text{length (centerline until } p)} \ / \ \text{length (centerline)}$. Thus, the plot center corresponds to the approximate aortic valve location, where the centerline starts. Increasing d encode positions in the aortic arch and descending aorta. The square root is used to ensure that inner and outer parts of the plot are represented with equally large areas. Fig. 1 depicts the mapping.

---

[1] GridGraph_3D_26C (GridCut library)

[2] vtkMarchingCubes,   vtkWindowedSincPolyDataFilter,   vtkQuadricDecimation (VTK library) and vmtkcenterlines (VMTK library)

Fig. 1. Mapping intravascular positions to the plot. The temporal position corresponds to the angle – analogous to a clock. The first time step is at 12 o'clock, the direction is clockwise. The distance from the plot center encodes the position on the centerline. Central areas (blue, green) present vessel sections near the aortic valve, whereas increasing distances (yellow) show the descending aorta.

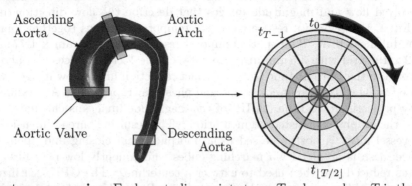

Vortex processing Each centerline point stores T values, where T is the number of time steps in the dataset. These buckets are used to accumulate a quantitative measure, in our case the λ_2-criterion since it is well suited for vortex extraction in the cardiac 4D PC-MRI context [4]. As a preprocessing the centerline is equidistantly resampled in 0.5 mm steps via cubic spline interpolation[3] in order to have the same distances in different datasets and a sufficient amount of buckets. Since the employed Runge-Kutta-4 integration uses adaptive step sizes, the vortex representing pathlines are resampled as well in the same manner. Afterwards, every point of each pathlines is processed. The closest spatio-temporal projection onto the centerline is determined and the λ_2-value of the pathline vertex is split among the two neighboring centerline buckets weighted by their inverse distance to the projection. After evaluating all pathlines the mean λ_2-value is calculated for each bucket. A binomial smoothing of the accumulated values is performed as postprocessing. Vortices are present where $\lambda_2 < 0$. The smaller λ_2 is, the stronger is the vortex flow. Unfortunately, the criterion has no fixed minimum, which negatively affects the comparability between different datasets. As a remedy, we let the user define a minimum λ_2-value as parameter α within 0 and the minimal occurring λ_2-value. The closer α is to 0, the more sensitive the visualization is towards vortex flow. The parameter is used to scale as well as clamp the λ_2-values to $[0, 1]$. The scaled values are then mapped to an arbitrary color scale. We employ the rainbow scale since this a common choice in the clinical context.

Dataset comparison A grid view is provided to enable the efficient comparison of multiple datasets. The sensitivity parameters α is used globally for all plots. The user has the option to choose known cases as reference plots in addition to the actual cases that are selected for evaluation.

---

[3] spline1dbuildcubic (ALGLIB library)

3   Results

We used 14 datasets for the evaluation: Five healthy volunteers, two patients
with an ectatic ascending aorta and seven BAV patients. Each patient has
prominent systolic vortex flow in the ascending aorta. The computation time
per case is between 2 and 5 s on an Intel i7-3930K depending on the amount of
pathlines. Fig. 2(a) shows one of the patients with a dilated ascending aorta
and depicts the relation between occurring vortex flow and the resulting plot.
Fig. 2(b) shows the proposed grid view with all datasets. The two larger plots
on the left represent healthy volunteers that were selected as references. The
sensitivity parameter α was interactively adjusted so that these two plots merely
indicate the slight physiologic helix in the aortic arch during systole. In an
informal evaluation our collaborating radiologists and cardiologists were easily
able to spot the remaining three healthy volunteers without pathologic vortex
flow.

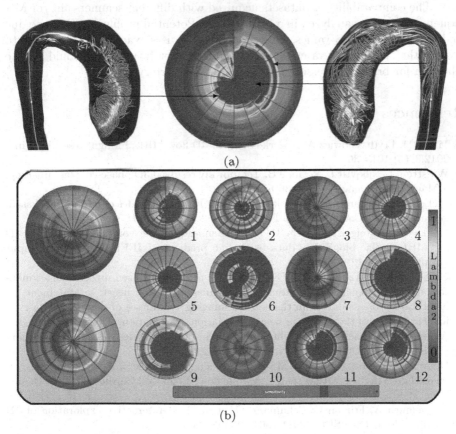

(a)

(b)

Fig. 2. (a) Diastolic (left) and systolic vortex flow (right) and the resulting vortex plot
of a patient with an ectatic ascending aorta. (b) Two healthy volunteers are shown as
larger reference plots on the left. Three more healthy volunteers (3, 7, 10) are among
two patients with an ectatic ascending aorta (1, 11) and seven BAV patients.

4   Discussion

We presented a two-dimensional circular plot visualization of aortic vortex flow. Domain experts were able to quickly assess whether or not pathologic vortices are present in a dataset and could estimate their positions and temporal extents. Presenting the temporal position based on a clock analogy was considered as intuitive, whereas the mapping of spatial positions using the centerline required a short briefing. A possible application of our method is to get a quick overview of datasets in larger studies. Tasks such as counting the BAV patients with systolic vortex flow in the ascending aorta can be performed comfortably. In addition, our method could support the clinical report generation and serve as a summary of a patient's vortex flow behavior. Our method provides no information about a vortex' wall closeness, which might be interesting due to the association with high shear forces [9]. However, a visualization or integration of other measures in the plot derived from arbitrary flow properties or line predicates is conceivable. The comparability of datasets acquired with different scanners and/or MR sequences has to be analyzed in a future work. Potential problems may arise due to differently scaled λ_2-values. Our proposed plot uses exactly one centerline to project the spatial intravascular positions. Another future topic could be the adaption for branching vessels like the pulmonary artery.

References

1. Markl M, Frydrychowicz A, Kozerke S, et al. 4D flow MRI. J Magn Reson Imaging. 2012;36(5):1015–36.
2. Wigström L, Sjöqvist L, Wranne B. Temporally resolved 3D phase-contrast imaging. J Magn Reson Imaging. 1996;36(5):800–3.
3. McLoughlin T, Laramee RS, Peikert R, et al. Over two decades of integration-based, geometric flow. Comput Graph Forum. 2010;29(6):1807–29.
4. Köhler B, Gasteiger R, Preim U, et al. Semi-automatic vortex extraction in 4D PC-MRI cardiac blood flow data using line predicates. IEEE Trans Vis Comput Graph. 2013;19(12):2773–82.
5. Cerqueira MD, Weissman NJ, Dilsizian V, et al. Standardized myocardial segmentation and nomenclature for tomographic imaging of the heart: a statement for healthcare professionals from the cardiac imaging committee of the council on clinical cardiology of the american heart association. Circulation. 2002;105(4):539–42.
6. Angelelli P, Hauser H. Straightening tubular flow for side-by-side visualization. IEEE Trans Vis Comput Graph. 2011;17(12):2063–70.
7. Hope MD, Wrenn J, Sigovan M, et al. Imaging biomarkers of aortic disease: increased growth rates with eccentric systolic flow. J Am Coll Cardiol. 2012;60(4):356–7.
8. Hennemuth A, Friman O, Schumann C, et al. Fast interactive exploration of 4D mri flow data. Proc SPIE. 2011;7964:79640E–11.
9. Castro MA, Olivares MCA, Putman CM, et al. Intracranial aneurysm wall motion and wall shear stress from 4D computerized tomographic angiography images. Proc SPIE. 2013;8672:867220–8.

Automatisierung von Vorverarbeitungsschritten für medizinische Bilddaten mit semantischen Technologien

Patrick Philipp[1], Maria Maleshkova[1], Michael Götz[1], Christian Weber[2],
Benedikt Kämpgen[1], Sascha Zelzer[2], Klaus Maier-Hein[2], Miriam Klauß[3],
Achim Rettinger[1]

[1]Institut AIFB, Karlsruher Institut für Technologie
[2]Abteilung für Medizinische und Biologische Informatik, DKFZ Heidelberg
[3]Diagnostische und Interventionelle Radiologie, Universität Heidelberg
patrick.philipp@kit.edu

Kurzfassung. Medizinische Interpretationsverfahren können Ärzte in
ihrem täglichen Arbeitsablauf unterstützen, indem Arbeitsschritte im
Bereich der Bildvorverarbeitung oder -analyse automatisiert werden. Um
dies zu ermöglichen, werden Systeme benötigt, die eigenständig Arbeitsprozesse erstellen und ausführen können. Wir stellen in dieser Arbeit unser
Framework anhand des Tumor Progression Mapping (TPM) vor. Es ermöglicht Algorithmen semantisch zu beschreiben und sie automatisch
datengetrieben ausführen zu lassen. Wir verwenden dazu Konzepte aus
dem Semantic Web: Das Resource Description Framework (RDF) ermöglicht uns Algorithmen mit Semantik anzureichern. Anschließend be-
nutzen wir Linked Data Prinzipien, um eine semantische Architektur zu
entwickeln. Wir stellen die Algorithmen als selbstbeschreibende semantische Web Services bereit und führen sie automatisch datengetrieben aus.
Wir zeigen anhand dem Tumor Progression Mapping, dass diese deklarative Architektur automatisch verschiedene Arbeitsprozesse erstellen und
ausführen kann.

1 Einleitung

Entwicklungen im Bereich der automatischen medizinischen Bildverarbeitung
erlauben es auf vielfältige Art und Weise Ärzte im klinischen Alltag zu unterstützen. Dies geschieht beispielsweise durch Entwicklung ausgereifter Analyse-
methoden von radiologischen Bildern, die in der Lage sind Läsionen automatisch
zu klassifizieren oder deren Volumen zu bestimmen.

Eine große Hürde bei der Translation solcher Verfahren in die Klinik stellt
hierbei oft die Integration in den Arbeitsablauf der Ärtze dar, weshalb in der
Praxis bevorzugt die Methoden zum Einsatz kommen, die in bereits bestehen-
de Systeme integriert sind. Ein Beispiel hierfür ist die Auswertung von ROIs
direkt am PACS, da hierbei die Repräsentation der Daten und nötigen Vorverarbeitungsschritte für den Radiologen vollkommen transparent sind. Ziel unserer

Arbeit ist es eine Framework zu schaffen, das es erlaubt Algorithmen in den klinischen Alltag so zu integrieren, dass alle Aspekte der Vorverarbeitung sowie die Kombination der Algorithmen die zur Verwendung eines Analyseverfahrens notwendig sind automatisch ablaufen können. Ebenso sollen Vorbedingungen für diese Algorithmen automatisch geprüft und aufgelöst werden.

Um diese Herausforderungen anzugehen, werden etablierte Technologien des Semantic Web in den Kontext der medizinischen Bildverarbeitung übertragen. Durch das Resource Description Framework (RDF) und Linked Data ist es möglich, Daten und Algorithmen in einer einheitlichen Form zu beschreiben, die es ermöglicht aufeinander aufbauende Verarbeitungsschritte automatisch zuzuordnen und auszuführen.

Wir demonstrieren das System beispielhaft am Tumor Progression Mapping (TPM). Es dient dazu die zeitliche Progression von Hirntumoren in einer für Radiologen intuitiven Weise zu visualisieren.

Taverna [1] ist ein verwandter Ansatz, in dem Programme als Prozesse in verteilten Laufzeitumgebungen per Drag and Drop zusammengestellt und ausgeführt werden können. Bei Semantic Workflows [2] handelt es sich um ein weiteres Framework, das ermöglicht automatische Arbeitsprozesse in heterogenen Umgebungen zu erstellen. Es werden generische semantische Beschreibungen eingesetzt, die auch Bedingungen bezüglich des Ausführbarkeit von Algorithmen beinhalten. Eine letzter Ansatz entwickelt ein Domänenmodell mit der Web Ontology Lanuage (OWL) [3]. Services werden anhand dieses Modells beschrieben und konkrete Workflows basierend auf den Metadaten instanziiert.

2 Material und Methoden

Als Fallbeispiel wird hier die Follow-up Befundung von Glioblastomen (primäre Hirntumore) behandelt. Hierbei fallen sehr viele Bilddaten unterschiedlicher Modalitäten (T1 prä & post Kontrastmittelgabe, T2 FLAIR) im zeitlichen Verlauf an. Für die radiologische Befundung ist es von Interesse, wie sich der Tumor seit der letzten OP entwickelt hat. Da Glioblastoma sehr irregulär wachsen, erfolgt die Bewertung erfolgt meist visuell durch Vergleichen der Aufnahmen in verschiedenen Schichten und zu verschiedenen Zeitpunkt. Da die Aufnahmen zu verschiedenen Zeitpunkten nicht registriert sind, ist dies eine zeitraubende und komplexe Angelegenheit. Tumor Progression Mapping ist eine Möglichkeit dem Radiologen zeitliche Veränderungen in einer übersichtlichen und intuitiven Weise zu präsentieren. Jedoch erfordern diese einige Vorverarbeitungsschritte.

Zunächst werden Bilddaten aus einem Bildarchiv (PACS) abgerufen und zur Weiterverarbeitung in ein einheitliches Format gebracht (NRRD) mit dem nachfolgende Programme umgehen können. Danach wird eine Maske für Gehirnregion erstellt (Brain Mask Generation), sodass die folgenden Schritte nur auf Gehirndaten gemacht werden und nicht von Knochen und externen Bildartefakten beeinflusst werden. Dann werden alle Bilder eines Patienten räumlich registriert (Batched Folder Registration). Im Normalisierungsschritt werden die Intensitätswerte der MR Aufnahmen angepasst, sodass gleiche Gewebetypen ähnlich

Abb. 1. Szenario: Tumor Progression Mapping.

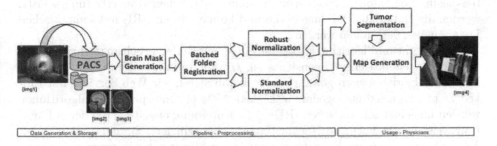

Werte erhalten. Bei diesem Schritt kann auf eventuell vorhandene Annotationen zurückgegriffen werden, um die Normalisieren robuster zu gestalten.

Nachdem die Bilder nun in einer normalisierten und registrierten Form bereitstehen, können TPM erstellt werden. Optional kann der Tumor zusätzlich noch automatisch segmentiert und in den Karten eingezeichnet werden. Abb. 1 illustriert diesen Prozess. Der gesamte Prozess dauert je nach Datenmenge 5-15 Minuten.

Die Anforderungen an die Vorverarbeitungsschritte sind:

1. Ausführbarkeit auf allen Arbeitsstationen
2. Regelmäßige Ausführung in festlegbaren Intervallen.
3. Automatische Ausführung von (neuen-) Vorverarbeitungsalgorithmen, die in einem zentralen Register aufgeführt werden.
4. Daten-getriebene Wahl von passenden Vorverarbeitungsalgorithmen, sodass verschiedene Pfade innerhalb des TPM ermöglicht werden.

2.1 Architektur

Die Basis zur automatischen Ausführung der Vorverarbeitungsschritte ist eine semantische Wissensbasis, die alle dafür nötigen Informationen enthält. Das Wissen wird kollaborativ von verschiedenen Benutzern und Systemen generiert, und durch die Benutzung der Wissensbasis erweitert. Es wird mit RDF modelliert und als Linked Data publiziert. RDF ermöglicht die semantische Annotierung von Rohdaten, um diese maschinenlesbar anzubieten. Informationen werden als Triple in Subjekt – Prädikat – Objekt Form dargestellt. Linked Data Prinzipien empfehlen, dass die mit RDF modellierten Daten mit Web Technologien verfügbar gemacht und mit anderen semantischen Datenquellen vernetzt werden.

Die semantische Wissensbasis besteht aus zwei Hauptkomponenten – einem Semantic MediaWiki (SMW), dem Surgipedia und dem Datenspeicher XNAT [1]. Surgipedia dient als zentrales Werkzeug, um Datenquellen semantisch zu beschreiben und miteinander in Beziehung zu setzen. Taxonomien ergeben sich aus Klassenzuordnungen der Rohdaten, die essentiell für die Auffindung von passenden Interpretationsalgorithmen sind; beispielsweise gibt es eine Hierarchie von Bildtypen. Es werden hierzu passende Ontologien wiederverwendet und

---

[1] http://www.xnat.org/

erweitert. XNAT ermöglicht die strukturierte Ablage von Dateien und patientenspezifischen Informationen. Durch einen zusätzlichen Konvertierungsschritt, werden die Daten als RDF angeboten und können durch URIs mit semantischen Datenquellen verbunden werden.

Interpretationsalgorithmen, wie die einzelnen Bilderverbeitungsschritte, greifen auf die semantische Wissensbasis zu. Um die Interoperabilität und Portabilität der Algorithmen zu gewährleisten, kombinieren wir Web Services mit Linked Data und erhalten sogenannte Linked APIs [4]. Interpretationsalgorithmen werden mit einer semantischen (RDF-) Beschreibung erweitert, die deren Funktionsweise, sowie Vor- und Nachbedingungen spezifiziert. Sie muss alle nötigen Metainformationen zur Klassifzierung und Ausführung des Interpretationsalgorithmus beinhalten. Die Algorithmen werden anschließ in medizinischen Linked APIs überführt; sie sind plattformunabhängig und ermöglichen Kommunikation über HTTP Methoden in RDF. Die RDF Beschreibung der Ein- und Ausgabe des Vorverarbeitungsschritts Brain Mask Generation ist in Abb. 2 zu finden. Es müssen ein Eingabebild der Klasse Headscan, sowie zwei Bilder der Klassen BrainAtlasImage und BrainAtlasMask entsprechender Formate vorhanden sein. Die Ausgabe ist eingeschränkt auf zwei Bilder der Klassen BrainImage und BrainMask.

Der Aufruf der resultierenden medizinischen Linked APIs muss passende Informationen gemäß der gesamten Vorbedingung beinhalten.

2.2   Regelbasierte Ausführung

Wir verwenden den regelbasierten Ausführungsformalismus Linked Data-Fu [5] wieder, um *medizinische Linked APIs* automatisch zu aufzurufen. Sie ermöglicht es datengetriebene Regeln zu erstellen, die eindeutig festlegen, wann eine medizinische Linked API ausgeführt wird. In unserem Szenario sollen die entwickelten medizinische Linked APIs genau dann ausgeführt werden, wenn deren Vorbedingungen für einen Patienten erfüllt sind. Wir haben eine Abstraktionsebene entwickelt, die Regeln automatisch aus den semantischen Beschreibungen erstellt, um Arbeitsabläufe deklarativ abzubilden. Die gesamte Architektur ist in ref2306-architektur visualisiert.

3   Ergebnisse

Die vorgeschlagene Architektur wurde erfolgreich implementiert; die Vorverarbeitungsalgorithmen werden automatisch gefunden und ausgeführt. Die ge-

```
              PREFIX rdf:        <http://www.w3.org/1999/02/22-rdf-syntax-ns#>
              PREFIX dc:         <http://purl.org/dc/elements/1.1/>
              PREFIX sp:         <http://surgipedia.sfb 25.de/wiki/Special:URIResolver/>

?inputImage       rdf:type      sp:Category-3AHeadscan.        ?brainImage    rdf:type    sp:Category-3ABrainImage.
?inputImage       dc:format     "image/nrrd".                  ?brainImage    dc:format   "image/nrrd".

?brainAtlasImage  rdf:type      sp:Category-3ABrainAtlasImage. ?brainMask     rdf:type    sp:Category-3ABrainMask.
?brainAtlasImage  dc:format     "image/mha".                   ?brainMask     dc:format   "image/nrrd".

?brainAtlasMask   rdf:type      sp:Category-3ABrainAtlasMask.
?brainAtlasMask   dc:format     "image/mha".
```

Abb. 2. Vor- und Nachbedingung von Brain Mask Generation Schritt.

Abb. 3. Wissensbasis, medzinische Linked APIs und regelbasierte Ausführung.

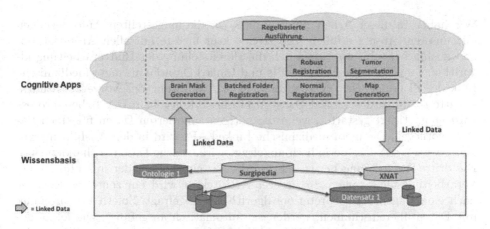

schieht datengetrieben, sodass sich verschiedene Pfade ergeben (Abb. 1). Die einzelnen Algorithmen wurden in medizinische Linked APIs überführt. Der Ausführungsformalismus Linked Data-Fu wurde in eine meta medizinische Linked API uberführt, um die Regeln periodisch mit dem annotierten Datenbestand der Patienten abzugleichen. Die Vorverarbeitungsalgorithmen wurden mit MITK [2] entwickelt. Sie lagen als Kommanozeilenprogramme mit XML Beschreibungen für Ein- und Ausgabeparameter vor. Eine beispielhafte RDF Beschreibung der Eingabe finden Sie in Abb. 2.

Die Korrektheit resultierenden medizinische Linked APIs für eine repräsentative Teilmenge der Tumor Progression Mapping Schritte haben wir bereits gezeigt [6]. Wir erweitern das Szenario hier mit datengetriebenen Entscheidungen.

Das Experiment zur Evaluierung der Pipeline führt medizinische Linked APIs automatisch aus, deren Vorbedingungen durch vorhandene Bilddaten eines jeweiligen Patienten erfüllt sind und speichert die Ergebnisse strukturiert auf der XNAT Plattform. Die medizinische Linked APIs aus Abb. 1 wurden registriert, indem die Vorbedingungen als Regeln modelliert wurden. Wenn somit für einen Patienten alle Triple von Abb. 2 vorhanden sind, wird der Brain Mask Generation Schritt ausgeführt. Die Konzepte für die jeweiligen Eingabe- und Ausgabebilder wurden in Kooperation mit Domänenexperten modelliert. Die Vor- und Nachbedingungen garantieren einen korrekten Arbeitsprozess.

Die meta medizinische Linked API für Linked Data-Fu iteriert jede 5 Minuten über alle Patienten, um medizinische Linked APIs auszuführen. Je nach vorliegendem Datenbestand, wurde der korrekte Arbeitsprozess nach spätestsens 5 Minuten angestoßen und lief durchschnittlich innerhalb 12 Minuten komplett durch.

---

[2] http://mitk.org/wiki/MITK

4   Diskussion

Wir haben in dieser Arbeit gezeigt, dass wir die aufgestellten Anforderungen mit unserem Ansatz erfüllen. Die Architektur musste auf allen Arbeitsstationen ausführbar sein, was wir durch die Bereitstellung der Bildverarbeitungsalgorithmen medizinische Linked APIs und Linked Data-Fu als meta medizinische Linked API ermöglichen. Die automatische Ausführung der Vorverarbeitungsschritte ist durch das Linked Data-Fu Framework gegeben. Der Arbeitsprozess wird auomatisiert gestartet, wenn die nötigen annotierten Daten für einen Patient vorliegen. Die meta medizinische Linked API wird in den Ausführungszustand versetzt, sodass periodisch abgefragt wird, welche Daten vorhanden sind. Die dritte Anforderung bezog sich auf die Erweiterbarkeit der auszuführenden Verarbeitungsalgorithmen. In unserer Architektur wird ein zentrales Register nach eingetragenen Interpretationsalgorithmen abgefragt. Sofern Beschreibung mit Daten übereinstimmen, werden sie automatisch ausgeführt. Die letzte gestellte Anforderung war, dass verschiedene Pfade eines komplexen Arbeitsprozesses abgebildet werden können. Dies ist durch die datengetriebene deklarative Modellierung der einzelnen Vorverarbeitungsalgorithmen gegeben, da deren Vor- und Nachbedingungen erfüllt werden müssen.

Danksagung. Diese Arbeit wurde mit Unterstützung der Deutschen Förschungsgemeinschaft (DFG) innerhalb der Projekte I01, S01, I04 und R01 des SFB/TRR 125 Cognition-Guided Surgeryëntwickelt.

Literaturverzeichnis

1. Oinn T, Greenwood M, Addis M, et al. Taverna: lessons in creating a workflow environment for the life sciences: research articles. Concurr Comput: Pract Exper. 2006;18(10):1067–100.
2. Gil Y, González-Calero PA, Kim J, et al. A semantic framework for automatic generation of computational workflows using distributed data and component catalogues. J Exp Theo AI. 2011;23(4):389–467.
3. Wood I, Vandervalk B, McCarthy L, et al. OWL-DL domain-models as abstract workflows. Proc ISoLA. 2012; p. 56–66.
4. Speiser S, Harth A. Integrating linked data and services with linked data services. In: The Semantic Web: Research and Applications. Springer; 2011. p. 170–184.
5. Stadtmüller S, Speiser S, Harth A, et al. Data-Fu: a language and an interpreter for interaction with read/write linked data. Proc Int WWW Conf. 2013; p. 1225–36.
6. Gemmeke P, Maleshkova M, Philipp P, et al. Using linked data and web APIs for automating the pre-processing of medical images. COLD (ISWC). 2014.

Towards Standardized Wound Imaging
Self-Calibrating Consumer Hardware Based on Lattice Detection on Color Reference Cards

Abin Jose[1], Daniel Haak[1], Stephan M. Jonas[1], Vincent Brandenburg[2], Thomas M. Deserno[1]

[1]Department of Medical Informatics, Uniklinik RWTH Aachen, Germany
[2]Department of Nephrology, Uniklinik RWTH Aachen, Germany
abin.jose@rwth-aachen.de

Abstract. Photographic documentation in medicine is of increasing importance. Efficient methods are required to properly register and calibrate the images. Usually, a standard reference card with special color pattern is placed in the aperature of the image. Localization and extraction of such cards is a critical step. In this paper, we adopt an iterative lattice detection algorithm developed for outdoor images. Once the lattice is extracted, crossing points of the color fields are used for perspective geometric transform while the color plates guide the color calibration process. Our method is tested on 37 images collected within the German Calciphylaxis Registry. At least, 28 out of the 35 possible grid points have been extracted in all the non-standardizes photographs, with at most two false positive detections. The lowest F-measure was above 80%. Hence, ruler and other calibration devices become obsolete and wound imaging can be performed with low-cost hardware, too.

1 Introduction

Photographic documentation is a crucial process in medical imaging. Expensive high-quality hardware and time-consuming calibration steps are required usually for quantitative photographic documentation. Calibration of images is cruical under different illumination, time, and aperture, in particular, if different hardware is used for image capturing. Any attempt to quantify the progression of the disease needs geometric as well as color calibration and therefore, as per clinical protocol it is not performed yet [1].

In a previous work [2], a color reference card and a ruler was used for color and geometric calibration, respectively. Detection of the color card was carried out by finding the scale invariant feature transform (SIFT) [3] point correspondences to a standard card image. The accuracy was dependent on precise SIFT point location and relied heavily on the SIFT parameters, which needed to be adjusted manually for different images.

A probability map computation in red white black yellow (RWBY) color space for quantitatively assessing chronic wound images was proposed by Fauzi et al [4]. This method also relies on a white label card for measurement calibration. Thus, the color card extraction is the most critical step and the success of effective photographic documentation thus depends on the robustness of the calibration card detection step. It was done making use of a reference pattern, which was printed on a white paper and placed near the wound. Manual localization and automatic delineation of images was required for color calibration. Due to corrugation and paper bending, this pattern does not support any geometric reference. However, correction of the geometric distortion is essential for assessing quantitatively the spread of a disease.

In this paper, we introduce a combined color and geometry calibration by automatic detection of a color reference card. Preliminary results of this approach have been published already in [5].

2   Materials and methods

2.1   Imaging equipment and color card

The main imaging equipment used were smart phone integrated cameras. The color card used was from CameraTrax, USA. It is a 2 × 3 inches card with 24 color plates. It consists of 24 squared color plates and covers the entire red green blue (RGB) color space. There are 35 corner points which can be used for correcting the geometric distortion. For calibration, the card is placed in the region of interest (ROI), which is usually a skin lesion or wound that needs to be monitored over a period of time to document the progress of the desease over the time.

2.2   Image processing

Park et al. have used a mean-shift belief propagation algorithm for automatically detecting deformed lattices in real world images [6]. Such lattices usually occur in man-made structures such as buildings, fences, and so on. Park's algorithmis adapted to medical images since our reference color card also contains a lattice structure. This structure becomes more prominent when we take the gradient of image after Gaussian smoothing. The main advantage of Park's approach is its robustness, which is attributed to an iterative growth of the deformed lattice interleaved with thin-plate spline (TPS) warping [6].

2.3   Calibration of geometry

Once we have detect the corner points of the color plate's lattice, the perspective transform matrix relating the distorted card as captured to the reference card's image is estimated. At least four pairs of corner points are required to find the perspective transform. We apply the least squares approach if the number of point correspondences exceeds this threshold.

The relationship between n world and image plane coordinates, (X, Y) and (x, y), respectively, is given as

$$
\begin{bmatrix}
x_1 & y_1 & 1 & 0 & 0 & 0 & -X_1x_1 & -X_1y_1 \\
0 & 0 & 0 & x_1 & y_1 & 1 & -Y_1x_1 & -Y_1y_1 \\
x_2 & y_2 & 1 & 0 & 0 & 0 & -X_2x_2 & -X_2y_2 \\
0 & 0 & 0 & x_2 & y_2 & 1 & -Y_2x_2 & -Y_2y_2 \\
.. & .. & .. & .. & .. & .. & .. & .. \\
.. & .. & .. & .. & .. & .. & .. & .. \\
x_n & y_n & 1 & 0 & 0 & 0 & -X_nx_n & -X_ny_n \\
0 & 0 & 0 & x_n & y_n & 1 & -Y_nx_n & -Y_ny_n
\end{bmatrix}
\begin{bmatrix} a \\ b \\ c \\ d \\ e \\ f \\ g \\ h \end{bmatrix}
=
\begin{bmatrix} X_1 \\ Y_1 \\ X_2 \\ Y_2 \\ .. \\ .. \\ X_n \\ Y_n \end{bmatrix}
\tag{1}
$$

where the eight parameters are denoted by $a, b, \ldots h$.

2.4 Calibration of color

The color calibration is based on averaging the 24 colors within the color plates of the color cards, as described previously [5]. In red, green, blue (RGB) color space, each color is represented by a triple (r,g,b) and (r',g',b') in source and target image, respectively. Assuming an affine three-dimensional (3D) transform in RGB color space, a set of 12 parameters is estimated, again using a least squares approach.

2.5 Evaluation study

The approach was tested on 37 photographs collected from the German Calcyphylaxis Registry [7]. We define precision p as the ratio of the number of correct lattice points detected to the total number of lattice points detected in experiment. Recall r is defined as the ratio of number of correct lattice points to the total number of lattice points in an image. The F-measure is calculated as

$$
F = \frac{2pr}{p + r}
\tag{2}
$$

3 Results

3.1 Image processing

The iterative card detection process is visualizes in Fig. 1. The candidate corner points detected is shown in panel (a). It is obtained by the Karhunen Loewe transform (KLT) corner detector on a gradient image after applying Gaussian smoothing. Panels (b) to (d) show the intermediate results during the iteration process. In Fig. 1 Panel (e), the detected lattice image is superimposed on the actual image. We could observe that the corner points are stable with respect to their exact location. The results of lattice detection algorithm are depicted in Fig. 2.

3.2   Calibration of geometry

In all cases, geometric calibration is based on a high number of corresponding pairs of reference points. Applying an inverse geometric transform is visualized in Fig. 2.

3.3   Evaluation

The recall r assesses the robustness of the geometric transform. At least, 24 out of the 35 available point correspondences have been detected correctly in all the images. With respect to just 4 required points, the least squares approach yielded reliable transform parameters. In average of all 37 images, $\bar{r} = 0.89$.

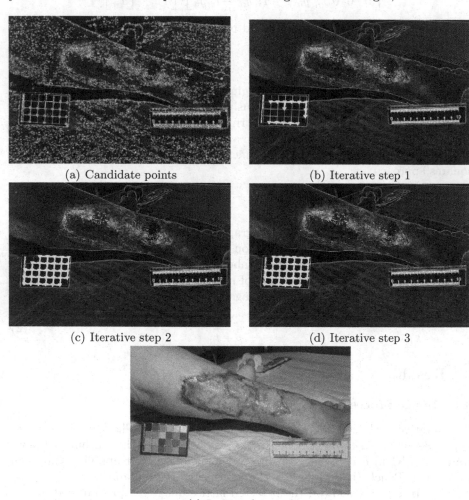

(a) Candidate points   (b) Iterative step 1

(c) Iterative step 2   (d) Iterative step 3

(e) Lattice detected

Fig. 1. Results of lattice detection.

The precision p determines the exactness of the geometric calibration. At most 2 dis-located point pairs have been detected, which do not contribute to the least squares estimation. In average of all 37 images, $\bar{p} = 0.97$.

The average F-measure on all images yields $\bar{F} = 0.93$. Hence, geometric as well as color registration is considered sufficiently accurate.

4   Discussion

A novel lattice detection algorithm approach is successfully adapted to medical domain from real world application. The approach helped in proper detection and extraction of the color card that is applied to photographic wound imaging. The method is more robust and automated compared to the previous SIFT-based algorithm. On all our images that have been acquired with low-cost hardware, a robust and fully automatic processing was possible. In future, we will perform calibrated measures of wounds with respect to their size and color. The method is applicable for other wounds of different size, such as burning lesions, if two reference cards are placed on both sides of the lesion. Robustness might also increase by moving the black and brown color plates into the middle of the card away from the black boundary.

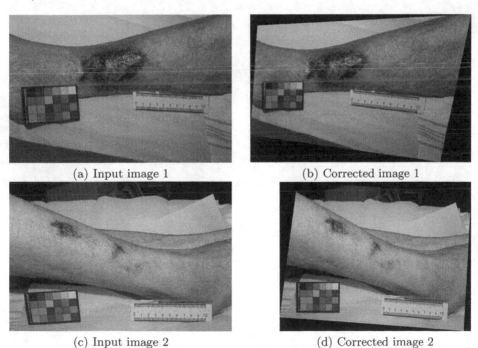

(a) Input image 1   (b) Corrected image 1

(c) Input image 2   (d) Corrected image 2

Fig. 2. Results of perspective correction. After correction, the color cards appear perfectly rectangular and appropriately aligned to the horizontal and vertical axes.

References

1. Alvarez OM, Berg WT, Chukwu EE, et al. Digital photo planimetry for wound measurement and quantitative wound assessment. Wound Care Ther. 2012;1:16–7.
2. Deserno TM, Sárándi I, Jose A, et al. Towards quantitative assessment of calciphylaxis. Proc SPIE. 2014;9035:90353C–8.
3. Lowe DG. Distinctive image features from scale-invariant keypoints. Int J Comput Vis. 2004;60(2):91–110.
4. MFA Fauzi IK, Catignani K, Gordillo G, et al. Segmentation and automated measurement of chronic wound images: probability map approach. Proc BVM. 2014;9035:1–8.
5. Jose A, Haak D, Jonas S, et al. Standardized photographic documentation using low-cost consumer hardware and automatic calibration. Proc SPIE. 2015;9414.
6. Park M, Brocklehurst K, Collins R, et al. Deformed lattice detection in real-world images using mean-shift belief propagation. IEEE Trans Pattern Anal Mach Intell. 2009;31(10):1804–16.
7. Deserno TM, Haak D, Brandenburg V, et al. Integrated image data and medical record management for rare disease registries.A general framework and its instantiation to the German calciphylaxis registry. J Digit Imaging. 2014;27(3):1–14.

Implementing a Web-Based Architecture for DICOM Data Capture in Clinical Trials

Daniel Haak, Charles E. Page, Thomas M. Deserno

Department of Medical Informatics, Uniklinik RWTH Aachen
dhaak@mi.rwth-aachen.de

Abstract. Medical imaging plays an important role in clinical trials providing qualitative and quantitative findings. Patient's data in studies is captured in electronic case report forms (eCRFs) instead of paper-based CRFs, which are provided by electronic data capture systems (EDCS). However, EDCS insufficiently support integration of image data into patient's eCRF. Neither interfacing with picture archiving and communication systems (PACS), nor managing of digital imaging and communications in medicine (DICOM) data in eCRFs is possible. Hence, manual detours for image data in study's data capture workflow increase error-proneness, latency, and costs. In this work, a completely web-based system architecture is implemented interconnecting EDCS and PACS. Our approach utilizes the open source projects OpenClinica, DCM4CHEE, and Weasis as EDCS, PACS, and DICOM web viewer, respectively. In the optimized workflow, user interaction completely takes place in the eCRF. DICOM data storage and retrieval is performed by middleware components hidden from the user, ensuring data consistency and security by identifier synchronization and de-identification, respectively. This shortens paths for image data capture in the workflow, reduces errors, and saves time and costs. Beside this, valuable data for further research is centrally and anonymously stored in a research PACS.

1 Introduction

Nowadays, medical imaging plays an important role in controlled clinical trials, performed in the process of developing novel drugs and medical devices. Image-based surrogate endpoints support qualitative and quantitative findings in clinical trials providing eligibility, efficacy, and security [1]. Nowadays, captured patient's data in such trials is stored and managed in electronic data capture systems (EDCS), which provide electronic case report forms (eCRFs) instead of the traditional paper-based CRFs. Automatic evaluation of data by range checks reveals errors directly during data entry improving data quality, saving time and costs.

OpenClinica is one of the world's most popular EDCS [2, 3]. This web-based application offers rich functionality for data storage and management. Since its release in 1993, digital imaging and communications in medicine (DICOM) [4] has established as the leading standard for storage and exchange of image data in medical applications. Picture archiving and communication systems (PACS) are used for DICOM-based storage and communication of medical image data and metadata in hospitals for patient care, as well as for research purposes. However, EDCS such as OpenClinica lack in support of DICOM, neither integration of DICOM image data into eCRFs, nor communication between EDCS and PACS is possible.

A first step in connecting EDCS and PACS has been performed by van Herk et al. [5]. A PACS is queried from the eCRF for DICOM objects using the hospital's patient identifier. After de-identification, the DICOM objects are made accessible via the web access to DICOM objects (WADO) protocol [6], and linked to the eCRF. After this, eCRF and image data is transferred to a research server. However, in this solution, the DICOM objects must be available already in the PACS for eCRF integration.

In our previous work, various architectures for EDCS and PACS connecting system have been analyzed [7]. Based on these architectures, a criteria catalog of 30 requirements has been built and 25 DICOM viewer software projects evaluated in concerns of their suitability for the presented architectures. An optimal architecture has been determined [8], in which DICOM data is integrated into the eCRF together with usual patient's data, it is then transferred to an PACS, back-linked with the eCRF and visualized in a web-based DICOM viewer. DCM4CHEE[1] and Weasis[2] have been proposed as appropriate PACS and DICOM web viewer for this architecture, respectively.

In this work, a final and workflow-optimized architecture for integration of DICOM images into the electronic data capture process of clinical trials is presented.

2   Material and methods

2.1   Architecture

The architecture for a system connecting EDCS and PACS (Fig. 1) consists on client side of (i) OpenClinica client component; (ii) OC-Big, an OpenClinica extension for integration of binary large objects (BLOBs) and (iii) Weasis, a web-based DICOM viewer. The server side includes (iv) OpenClinica server component; (v) DCM4CHEE PACS and (vi) Weasis PACS connector.

2.2   Components

OpenClinica (Community Edition, Version 3.4) is an open source EDCS and clinical data management system. The web application allows design of studies with user-defined eCRFs and is used for data capture in multi-site clinical trials. OpenClinica follows industry standards and is approved by regulatory authorities such as the Food and Drug Administration (FDA). As usual for web applications,

---

[1] http://www.dcm4che.org/
[2] http://sourceforge.net/projects/dcm4che/files/Weasis/

Fig. 1. Architecture for EDCS and PACS connection and communication flows for data and DICOM.

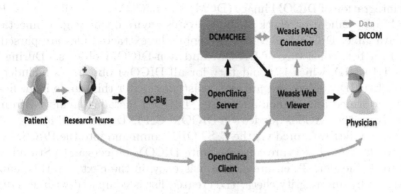

OpenClinica consists of a server and a client component. OC-Big[3] is an extension for OpenClinica developed at our department [9]. The open source plug-in allows context-based integration of BLOBs into OpenClinica's eCRF.

DCM4CHEE (Version 2.17.2) is an open source DICOM Clinical Data Manager system consisting of an archive and image manager, and a PACS. The software is designed in a modular structure and provides various communication interfaces (e.g. for DICOM or HL7 communication).

Weasis (Version 2.0.2) is a open source web-based DICOM viewer, which is developed in Java. Weasis provides a wide range of image viewing tools (e.g. for measurements) and can be easily connected to PACS via WADO. Weasis PACS connector (Version 4.0) is an add-on for Weasis and allows invocation of the web viewer from a web context via the Java Network Launch Protocol (JNLP).

2.3 Workflow

Our system architecture is composed of two communication workflows through our architecture for storage and retrieval of PACS data (Fig. 2, top & bottom, respectively) which are triggered by user actions in the eCRF.

2.4 Storage

Typical patients data is stored as usual inside the eCRF on the OpenClinica client. For storage of patient's DICOM data, OC-Big [9] is used. Here, DICOM data, such as DICOM image (DCM) and binary image (JPG) data, document data (PDF) or compressed archives (ZIP, TAR, GZIP), can be selected for transfer. In addition, an OpenClinica identifier (OC-ID) is generated and additionally sent with the data. The OC-ID is constructed by patient and study identifiers in OpenClinica (OIDs), which are extracted from the selected eCRF. After successful transfer and reception of DICOM data by the OC-Big's server component,

---

[3] https://code.google.com/p/oc-big/

large binary object (BLOB) data is extracted and stored on server's file system. In the next step, the PHP script invokes a Linux shell (bash) script for PACS integration of DICOM image (DCM) and DICOM convertible (JPG, PDF) data. After a validation check of the system's environment (e.g. connection to PACS available, DICOM converter present), the extracted files are parsed and added to a list, consisting of DICOM and non-DICOM objects. During this, the StudyInsUID, which is mandatory for all DICOM objects, is included and all StudyInsUID validated regarding consistency. After this, an de-identification step is performed and all non-mandatory DICOM metadata removed from the header. Now, the PACS is queried via DICOM C_FIND command for the OC-ID and all listed files are stored via the C_STORE command into the PACS. During this, non-DICOM objects are converted into DICOM objects and a StudyInsUID added to the header. To ensure data consistency, in the next step this mapping is validated by an integrity check: the created list is compared with all DICOM objects which are mapped to the OC-ID identifier in the PACS. If this succeeds, a Weasis URL including the OC-ID is generated and stored into the eCRF by OC-Big.

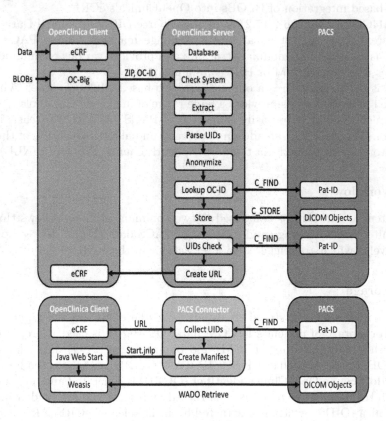

Fig. 2. Workflow of our implementation and involved components for DICOM data storage (top) and retrieval (bottom).

2.5   Retrieval

For retrieval of integrated DICOM data, a click on the Weasis URL embedded in the eCRF starts communication with the Weasis PACS connector. The connector analyzes the URL and fetches all DICOM UIDs from the PACS via C_FIND. Based on these UIDs a manifest of all DICOM objects listed in the PACS is created, written in a XML structure and encapsulated into a JNLP file, which is sent back to OpenClinica's client. Here, the execution of the JNLP file triggers the invocation of the Weasis web viewer via Java Web Start. Weasis now iteratively gathers all DICOM objects by their UIDs from the PACS via WADO and visualizes them in the web interface.

3   Results

Our resulting workflow is depicted in Fig. 3. For storage of DICOM objects in the eCRF, the data entry person (e.g. a research nurse) opens the eCRF of the patient in OpenClinica as usual and invokes OC-Big by a click on a button embedded in the eCRF (Step 1). In OC-Big, the user selects DICOM files from

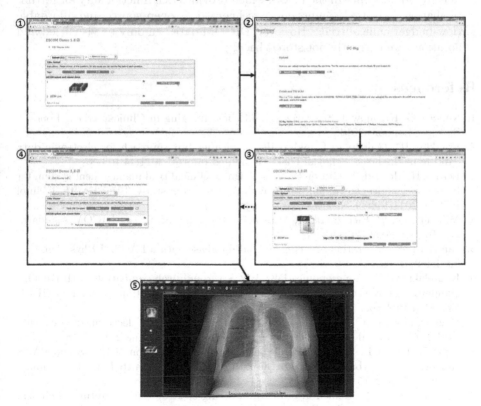

Fig. 3. Final workflow for study nurses using our implementation for DICOM data integration into EDCS.

the local file systems and starts the transfer (Step 2). After successful transfer of the DICOM data, a reference to the DICOM data is stored in the eCRF (Step 3). For retrieval of the DICOM objects, a button click in the eCRF starts Weasis web viewer (Step 4). After this, patient's DICOM data is available in Weasis for viewing or image interaction (e.g. measurements) (Step 5).

4   Discussion

In this work, a final architecture and implementation based on results of previous work for connection of EDCS and PACS has been presented. The architectures consist of multiple communicating components, whereof only two components (OpenClinica and Weasis DICOM viewer) are visible to the user. Both components are shared through web and accessible via modern web browsers, hence DICOM data can be stored and retrieved from everywhere (where an internet connection is available). Also hidden from the user, DICOM data objects and their metadata is automatically de-identified and synchronized and therefore, data consistency and security ensured, respectively. Nonetheless, all integrated data is stored only once in the PACS, which provides rich functionality for further data sharing. All used components are licensed as open source and affordable for low-budget clinical trials. However, DICOM data can only be visualized and annotations are currently not stored back, yet.

References

1. Miller CG, Krasnow J, Schwartz LH. Medical Imaging in Clinical Trials. London: Springer London; 2014.
2. Franklin JD, Guidry A, Brinkley JF. A partnership approach for electronic data capture in small-scale clinical trials. J Biomed Inform. 2011;44:103–8.
3. Leroux H, McBride S, Gibson S. On selecting a clinical trial management system for large scale, multi-centre, multi-modal clinical research study. Stud Health Technol Inform. 2011;168:89–95.
4. Mildenberger P, Eichelberg M, Martin E. Introduction to the DICOM standard. Eur Radiol. 2002;12(4):920–7.
5. van Herk M. Integration of a clinical trial database with a PACS. J Phys Conf Ser. 2014;489:012099.
6. Koutelakis GV, Lymperopoulos DK. PACS through web compatible with DICOM standard and WADO service: advantages and implementation. Conf Proc IEEE Eng Med Biol Soc. 2006;1:2601–5.
7. Haak D, Deserno TM. Integration of DICOM images into the electronic data capture workflow of clinical trials. Accepted on SPIE Medical Imaging 2015. 2015.
8. Haak D, Page CE, Deserno TM. Workflow-based integration of EDCS and PACS supporting image-based surrogates in clinical trials. Submitted to SIIM Annual Meeting 2015. 2015.
9. Haak D, Samsel C, Gehlen J, et al. Simplifying electronic data capture in clinical trials: Workflow embedded image and biosignal file integration and analysis via web services. J Digit Imaging. 2014;27(5):571–80.

Semi-automatische Segmentierung von Schädigungszonen in post-interventionellen CT-Daten

Jan Egger[1,2], Harald Busse[3], Michael Moche[3], Philipp Brandmaier[3],
Daniel Seider[3], Matthias Gawlitza[3], Steffen Strocka[3], Nikita Garnov[3],
Jochen Fuchs[3], Peter Voigt[3], Florian Dazinger[3], Philip Voglreiter[1],
Mark Dokter[1], Michael Hofmann[1], Alexander Hann[4], Bernd Freisleben[2],
Thomas Kahn[3], Dieter Schmalstieg[1]

[1]Institut für Maschinelles Sehen und Darstellen, TU Graz
[2]Verteilte Systeme, Philipps-Universität Marburg
[3]Klinik und Poliklinik für Diagnostische und Interventionelle Radiologie,
Universitätsklinikum Leipzig
[4]Klinik für Allgemeine Innere Medizin, Gastroenterologie, Hepatologie und
Infektiologie, Katharinenhospital, Stuttgart
egger@tugraz.at

Kurzfassung. Die perkutane Radiofrequenzablation (RFA) ist ein minimalinvasives Verfahren zur thermischen Koagulation von Tumorgewebe und stellt somit eine Alternative zur chirurgischen Entfernung dar. Die Erhitzung wird durch ein elektromagnetisches Wechselfeld erreicht, welches über eine spezielle Nadelanordnung im Gewebe erzeugt wird. Nach der Intervention wird mit Hilfe von CT-Aufnahmen überprüft, inwieweit die Ablation vollständig war, um so das Risiko eines Rezidivs zu minimieren. In diesem Beitrag wurden zwölf RF-Ablationszonen aus post-interventionellen CT-Aufnahmen semiautomatisch segmentiert, um die sehr zeitaufwändige manuelle Inspektion zu unterstützen. Dazu wurde ein interaktiver, graphbasierter Ansatz verwendet, der kugelförmige Objekte bevorzugt. Zur quantitativen und qualitativen Bewertung des Algorithmus wurden manuell segmentierte Schichten von klinischen Experten als Goldstandard verwendet. Zur statistischen Validierung wurde der Dice-Koeffizient herangezogen. Es konnte gezeigt werden, dass der vorgeschlagene Ansatz die Läsionen schneller mit ausreichender Genauigkeit segmentiert und somit für einen Einsatz in der klinischen Routine geeignet zu sein scheint.

1 Einleitung

Über die letzten Jahrzehnte tritt das Leberzellkarzinom weltweit verstärkt auf, was vor allem mit der hohen Rate an Hepatitis-C-Erkrankungen in Verbindung gebracht wird. Insbesondere Patienten mit primärem Leberkrebs (Hepatozelluläres Karzinom, HCC) haben aufgrund der späten Symptomatik eine schlechte Prognose, die unbehandelt eine mittlere Überlebenszeit von lediglich 4 bis 6

Monaten nach Diagnose zeigt. Gemäß der aktuellen Behandlungsrichtlinie [1] fungiert die Radiofrequenzablation (RFA) als First-Line-Therapie für HCCs im frühen Stadium mit Leberzirrhose. Nach Vorstellung der RFA in den 1990er Jahren zählt diese Technik mittlerweile zu den etablierten thermischen Therapieverfahren. Das Prinzip basiert auf der Reibung von Ionen im Gewebe, die sich periodisch entlang des elektrischen Wechselfelds bewegen. Dieses Feld wird durch im Gewebe bzw. im Tumor platzierte Elektroden erzeugt [2] (Abb. 1). Die resultierende Hitze führt zur Tumorkoagulation und zur Ausbildung einer Nekrose. Eine manuelle Schicht-für-Schicht-Konturierung der Ablationszone ist generell zeitaufwändig und in der klinischen Routine selten praktikabel. Daher sind bereits Algorithmen aus der medizinischen Bildverarbeitung vorgeschlagen worden, derartige Segmentierungen zu erleichtern bzw. zu beschleunigen [3, 4]. Passera et al. [3] z. B. haben einen Live-Wire-Algorithmus in 2D entwickelt, der allerdings bei einzelnen Schichten bis zu 10 Minuten benötigen kann. Das Verfahren von Weihusen et al. [4] basiert auf einem morphologischen Regionenwachstum in 3D, dessen Ergebnis jedoch anschließend noch manuell korrigiert werden muss. Bisher ist uns noch keine Arbeit bekannt, bei der die Ablationszonen auf post-interventionellen Aufnahmen segmentiert wurden, auf denen die Ablationsnadel noch enthalten ist. Solche interventionellen Kontrollaufnahmen werden vorgenommen, um zu überprüfen, ob der Tumor komplett abladiert wurde oder weitere Ablationsschritte notwendig sind.

2   Material und Methoden

Datenakquisition: Für diese retrospektive Studie wurden 12 post-interventionelle CT-Datensätze von 10 Patienten ausgewertet, die sich einer RFA in der Leber unterzogen hatten. Die Datensätze hatten eine Auflösung von 512x512 Voxeln (Pixelgrößen 0,68 bis 0,78 mm) und bestanden aus 52 bis 232 Schichten (Schichtdicke: 1 oder 2 mm, Schichtabstand: 1 bis 3 mm). Alle Datensätze wurden mit einem Multislice CT-Scanner (Brilliance oder Mx8000, Philips Healthcare, Best, Niederlande) aufgenommen. Manuelle Segmentierung: Zur Generierung der Ground Truth der Ablationszonen wurde ein Segmentierungsnetzwerk unter MeVisLab erstellt. Die RFA-Läsionen wurden ohne algorithmische Unterstützung Schicht für Schicht segmentiert, voxelisiert und zu einer 3D-Maske zusammengefasst (Abb. 2). Evaluationsmetrik: Zur Evaluation wurde der Dice Similarity Coefficient (DSC) [5] zwischen manuell (M) und interaktiv (I) bestimmter, bi-

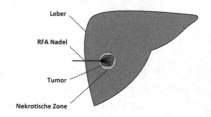

Abb. 1. Schematische Darstellung einer Radiofrequenzablation in der Leber mit im Tumor platzierter Nadel sowie umgebender Koagulationsnekrose.

närer 3D-Ablationsmaske berechnet:

$$DSC = \frac{2 \cdot V(M \cap I)}{V(M) + V(I)} \tag{1}$$

Hierbei ist $V(\cdot)$ das Volumen in cm^3 und $\cap$ gibt die Überschneidungen/Schnittmenge der Masken an. Das Gesamtvolumen ergab sich durch Summation der Voxelvolumina. Zusätzlich wurde noch die Zeit gemessen, die ein erfahrener Radiologe für die Konturierung bzw. interaktive Segmentierung benötigte. Interaktive Segmentierung: Bei der semiautomatischen Segmentierung wird ein Graph $G(V,E)$ aus Knoten $n \in V$ und Kanten $e \in N$ konstruiert. Im Unterschied zum Originalansatz von Li et al. [6] wird der Graph mit einer Kugel (und nicht mit einem Zylinder) aufgebaut, was zu einer Bevorzugung von rundlichen Objekten wie Ablationszonen (und nicht länglichen Gefäßstrukturen) führt. Im Anschluss an die Konstruktion separiert ein Min-Cut/Max-Flow-Algorithmus [7] den Graphen in zwei disjunkte Knotenmengen, der Ablationszone und den Hintergrund. Während Li et al. von einer Mittellinie (diskrete Anzahl von Punkten) ausgeht, benötigt unser Ansatz lediglich den Mittelpunkt einer Kugel [8, 9]. Dieser kann vom Benutzer innerhalb der Ablationszone verschoben werden. Bei jeder Änderung wird der Graph automatisch neu aufgebaut, der Min-Cut berechnet und die aktualisierte Segmentierung angezeigt. Diese Echtzeitsegmentierung erlaubt eine schnelle, benutzerkontrollierte Definition bzw. Volumetrie der Ablationszone.

3   Ergebnisse

Tab. 1 und 2 zeigen die Evaluationsergebnisse beim direkten Vergleich zwischen manueller Segmentierung durch zwei Radiologen und einer semiautomatischen, interaktiven Segmentierung. Dabei wurden für zwölf RF-Ablationszonen Minimum, Maximum, Mittelwert μ und Standardabweichung σ für Volumen, Voxelanzahl und DSC berechnet. Tab. 3 vergleicht die beiden manuellen Segmentierungen untereinander. Der Vergleich der manuellen Segmentierungen ergab einen DSC von 88,8%, während die interaktive Segmentierung DSCs zwischen 77,0 und 77,1% zeigten. Die jeweiligen Unterschiede waren statistisch nicht signifikant (Wilcoxon p=0,42 bzw. 0,30 für Radiologe 1 bzw. 2). Der interaktive

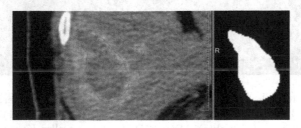

Abb. 2. Manuelle Volumetrie einer RFA-Läsion in der Leber. Links: Axiale CT-Schicht mit manueller Segmentierung (rot) der hypodensen Ablationszone. Rechts: Dazugehörige voxelisierte 2D-Maske (weiß).

Tabelle 1. Evaluation durch Radiologe 1: Minimum, Maximum, Mittelwert μ und Standardabweichung σ der Volumina von zwölf Ablationszonen.

	Volumen in cm^3		Anzahl der Voxel		DSC
	manuell 1	interaktiv	manuell 1	interaktiv	(%)
Bereich	10,0-122,6	6,3-104,0	5866-70806	3689-70208	71,8-83,5
$\mu \pm \sigma$	35,9±30,0	33,0±25,1	31294,8	30756,3	77,0±4,7

Segmentierungsalgorithmus wurde als eigenes C++ Modul unter Visual Studio 2008 für MeVisLab (Version 2.3) entwickelt. Auf einem Laptop (mit Intel Core i5-750 CPU, 4 x 2,66 GHz, 8 GB RAM, Win 7 Prof. x64) arbeitete die interaktive Segmentierung in Echtzeit und führte so in wenigen Sekunden zu einem zufriedenstellenden Ergebnis. Eine manuelle Konturierung dauerte zwischen 0:48 und 8:16 (Mittelwert 3:13) Minuten:Sekunden. Erste Ergebnisse wurden auf der RSNA 2014 präsentiert [10].

4 Diskussion

In diesem Beitrag wurde eine semi-automatische Segmentierung von RFA-Läsionen für die klinische Routine vorgestellt und evaluiert. Die Koagulationszone nach RFA der Leber zeigt sich als hypodenses Areal auf post-interventionellen CT-

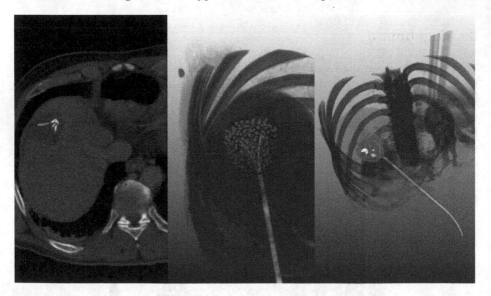

Abb. 3. Semiautomatische Volumetrie einer RFA-Läsion in der Leber. Links: Axiale CT-Schicht mit benutzerdefiniertem Saatpunkt (blau) für die interaktive Segmentierung samt Ergebnis (rote Punkte). Mitte: 3D-Darstellung aller Knoten (rot), welche die Oberfläche der segmentierten Ablationszone bilden. Rechts: Geschlossene Oberfläche der automatischen Segmentierung (grün). Der DSC ergibt sich aus dem Vergleich der Masken von automatischer und manueller Segmentierung.

Tabelle 2. Evaluation durch Radiologe 2: Minimum, Maximum, Mittelwert μ und Standardabweichung σ der Volumina von zwölf Ablationszonen.

	Volumen in cm^3		Anzahl der Voxel		DSC
	manuell 2	interaktiv	manuell 2	interaktiv	(%)
Bereich	11,1-117,7	6,3-104,0	6543-67963	3689-70208	68,1-85,3
$\mu \pm \sigma$	36,2±28,7	33,0±25,1	31240,1	30756,3	77,1±5,8

Tabelle 3. Vergleich der beiden manuellen Segmentierungen (Radiologe 1 und 2): Minimum, Maximum, Mittelwert μ und Standardabweichung σ der zwölf Ablationszonen.

	Volumen in cm^3		Anzahl der Voxel		DSC
	manuell 1	manuell 2	manuell 1	manuell 2	(%)
Bereich	10,0-122,6	11,1-117,7	5866-70806	6543-67963	82,4-92,6
$\mu \pm \sigma$	35,9±30,0	36,2±28,7	31294,8	31240,1	88,8±3,3

Aufnahmen. Die Segmentierungsgenauigkeit war in den meisten Fällen zufriedenstellend, wenngleich die manuelle Segmentierung weiterhin am genauesten bleibt. Der Vorteil einer algorithmischen Segmentierung liegt in dem deutlich geringeren Zeitaufwand, welcher die Methode zu einer attraktiven Alternative für zukünftige Routineanwendungen macht. In einem nächsten Schritt ist geplant, die interaktive Segmentierung in zwei Frameworks zur Unterstützung therapeutischer Ablationsverfahren zu integrieren, welche zurzeit im Rahmen zweier

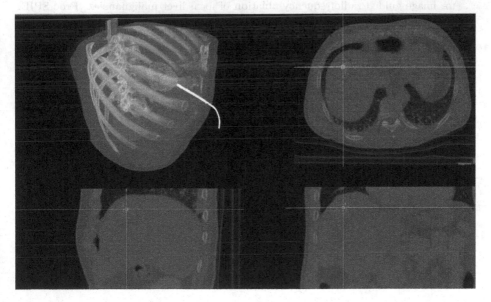

Abb. 4. Direkter Vergleich einer automatischen (rot) mit einer manuellen (grün) Segmentierung: 3D-Modell (oben links), axiale (oben rechts), sagittale (unten links) und koronare Schnittebene (unten rechts). Das gelbe Kreuz markiert den benutzerdefinierten Saatpunkt, von dem aus der Segmentierungsgraph generiert wurde.

EU-Projekte (www.gosmart-project.eu & www.clinicimppact.eu) entwickelt werden. Dabei soll die vorgestellte interaktive Segmentierung in den Fällen zum Einsatz kommen, bei denen eine vollautomatische Segmentierung keine zufriedenstellenden Ergebnisse liefert. Des Weiteren könnte der Ansatz für ein sogenanntes „Tumor Tracking"nach wiederholten Interventionen genutzt und mit anderen Segmentierungsverfahren [11] verglichen werden.

Danksagung. Diese Arbeit erhielt Förderung von der EU (FP7): ClinicIMPPACT (Grant Nr. 610886) und GoSmart (Grant Nr. 600641). Dank gilt auch Frau Edith Egger-Mertin für das Korrekturlesen des Beitrags. Videos der interaktiven Segmentierung finden sich in YouTube:
http://www.youtube.com/c/JanEgger/videos

Literaturverzeichnis

1. Graf D, Vallboehmer D, Knoefel WT, et al. Multimodal treatment of hepatocellular carcinoma. Eur J Intern Med. 2014;25(5):430–7.
2. Buscarini E, Savoia A, Brambilla G, et al. Radiofrequency thermal ablation of liver tumors. Eur Radiol. 2005;15(5):884–94.
3. Passera K, Selvaggi S, Scaramuzza D, et al. Radiofrequency ablation of liver tumors: quantitative assessment of tumor coverage through CT image processing. Biomed Chromatogr. 2013;13(3):1–10.
4. Weihusen A, Ritter F, Kroeger T, et al. Workflow oriented software support for image guided radiofrequency ablation of focal liver malignancies. Proc SPIE. 2007;6509(19):1–9.
5. Zou KH, Warfield SK, Bharatha A, et al. Statistical validation of image segmentation quality based on a spatial overlap index. Acad Radiol. 2004;2:178–89.
6. Li K, Wu X, Chen DZ, et al. Optimal surface segmentation in volumetric images: a graphtheoretic approach. IEEE PAMI. 2006;28(1):119–34.
7. Boykov Y, Kolmogorov V. An experimental comparison of min-cut/max-flow algorithms for energy minimization in vision. IEEE PAMI. 2004;26(9):1124–37.
8. Egger J, Bauer MHA, Kuhnt D, et al. A flexible semi-automatic approach for glioblastoma multiforme segmentation. Proc Biosignal. 2010;60:1–4.
9. Egger J, Bauer MHA, Kuhnt D, et al. Pituitary adenoma segmentation. Proc Biosignal. 2010;61:1–4.
10. Busse, et al. Novel Semiautomatic Real-time CT Segmentation Tool and Preliminary Clinical Evaluation on Thermally Induced Lesions in the Liver. Proc Rad Soc North Am. 2014; p. http://rsna2014.rsna.org/program/details/?emID=14017499.
11. Egger J, Kapur T, Fedorov A, et al. GBM volumetry using the 3D slicer medical image computing platform. Sci Rep. 2013;3(1364):1–7.

Automatic Segmentation of the Cerebral Falx and Adjacent Gyri in 2D Ultrasound Images

Jennifer Nitsch[1,2], Jan Klein[1], Dorothea Miller[2], Ulrich Sure[2], Horst K. Hahn[1]

[1]Fraunhofer MEVIS, Institute for Medical Image Computing, Bremen, Germany
[2]Department of Neurosurgery, University Clinic Essen, Germany
jennifer.nitsch@mevis.fraunhofer.de

Abstract. We present an automatic segmentation of the cerebral falx and adjacent gyri (perifalcine region) for B-mode 2D ultrasound (US) images. The movement of brain tissue during neurosurgery reduces the accuracy of navigation systems which provide image guidance based on preoperative MRI (preMRI). Thus, the segmentation of the falx and its adjoining gyri in navigated, intraoperative US (iUS) may be used to improve navigation within preMRI scans by providing additional, spatially updated image information of the patient's brain. The segmentation was tested on 50 2D US images and achieved on average a Dice coefficient of 0.79, a Hausdorff distance of 1.56 mm, and a Jaccard index of 0.64.

1 Introduction

The survival of brain tumor (glioma) patients correlates with the extent of the tumor resection, whereas the patient's quality of life depends on the functional outcome after the surgical intervention. Knowing the location of a tumor and its relation to eloquent structures is crucial for an optimal outcome after surgery. Neuronavigation systems offer image guidance through intraoperative navigation within the patient's brain, based on preMRI scans, and assist in identifying the position of a tumor and its borders to healthy tissue and other important anatomical/functional structures. However, the movement of brain tissue during surgery, i.e. caused by brainshift and tumor tissue removal, severely reduces the navigation accuracy. Therefore, additional intraoperative imaging modalities are used in order to improve the orientation within the operation field. For instance, iUS is widely available at low cost, easy to use intraoperatively, offers real-time information and does not cause any radiation which are important advantages when compared to intraoperative MRI or CT. A navigated US device can be tracked by the navigation system and its position in relation to the patient's head can be visualized within the preMRI scan. Currently scanned US images are typically shown on a secondary screen next to the preoperative scan. The surgeon has to track the changes between preMRI and the current intraoperative situation within the US images and has to correct the brainshift in the mind. But this is a challenging task especially due to the fact that the brainshift is not likely to be uniform in nature and, thus, implies a deformation of the image data that is difficult to (mentally) predict and model. The long-term goal of this project is to develop a system which automatically detects characteristic, anatomical structures within the iUS scans that can be equally good detected within the preMR scan in order to improve the image registration of both modalities and may even allow a partial fusion of MR and US data by using a scanned US volume. Hence the proposed automatic segmentation of the falx is one component within the project and represents an initial step towards a collection of US image features that can be used to achieve the project's objective. For the first instance, the segmentation of the falx was chosen on the basis of being a central, anatomical structure of the brain as a meningeal fold that separates the cerebral hemispheres. Due to this fact, the falx can usually be clearly depicted in 2D iUS images during neurosurgical procedures. Additionally the adjacent gyri to the falx are segmented to extract a more detailed collection of local image features that may allow a more precise registration of MRI and US images in future works, by providing more unique local image information. Using US images in order to enable or refine an initial image registration of two modalities, can i.e. be seen in [1] where vessels of the liver are segmented in US images to improve the registration of 3D CT and 2D US slices or in [2] where a registration of US and MR imaging is presented based on contextual conditioned mutual information that conditions mutual information on similar structures. A complete different approach for MR and US image fusion is proposed in [3] where the MRI image is modified in order to fit the image characteristics and features of US images and a pseudo US image is created. After the MRI image is made comparable to the 3D US image a registration of two images is performed.

2   Material and methods

2D US images were acquired using an US system (Alpha 10, Hitachi Aloka Medical, Japan) connected to a navigation system (Curve, Brainlab AG, Munich, Germany) via a video cable. A micro-convex multifrequency probe (mean frequency: 7.5 MHz, penetration depths: 8 cm) was used for image acquisition. An adapter for optical tracking was mounted onto the probe and calibrated. Before opening the dura an US scan was performed by manually moving the probe over the VOI. One scan included up to 200 2D B-mode US images which were stored on the navigation system with their positional information and reconstructed into a 3D volume before being sent to a standard laptop for postoperative image analysis.

We decided to process the acquired US volume in its original 2D US slices within the segmentation method, instead of a reconstructed volume, to avoid additional artifacts. Our segmentation method is outlined in Fig. 1.

The first step within the segmentation method is the application of a diffusion stick filter as proposed in [4, 5]. Two diffusion stick filters are applied sequentially (kernel size 15×15). The advantage of the diffusion stick filter is that it offers edge enhancement of voxel values along lines and edges, while smoothing homogeneous regions. Therefore, the line-type structures of the falx and gyri with strong edges are enhanced while speckles within the 2D US image are reduced (Fig. 1). The kernel size was determined by an automatic test and was varied from 5 to 31 in 25 US images. The kernel size of 15×15 offers a good compromise between smoothing and edge enhancement. The kernel achieved one of the highest average Dice coefficients and one of the lowest average Hausdorff distances within the test (Fig. 2). Followed by a histogram equalization to increase the global contrast between the falx and gyri (image content with strong edges; gray values with high intensities) and other structures (gray values with low intensities) within the image.

At this point the proposed method splits into two different parts. One part leads the resulting image, after speckle reduction and edge enhancement, into a Hessian filter. Whereas the other part is focused on defining the ROI, containing the image region of the falx and its adjacent gyri, and later used to mask the result image of the Hessian filter.

The Hessian filter is applied because it can detect the local strength and the direction of edges and lines. This has already been proven to be advantageous to segment anatomical structures such as vessels, bronchi, and pulmonary fissures [6, 7] which are line-type or tube-like structures that have a similar image representation and characteristics as the perifalcine region. The Hessian filter is

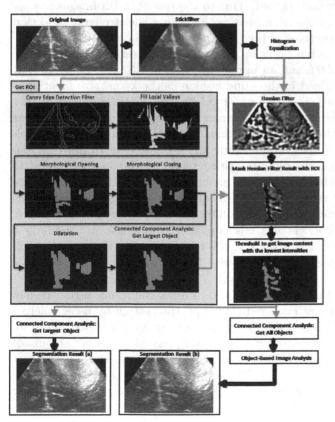

Fig. 1. Image processing pipeline of the proposed segmentation method. The two segmentation results at the bottom represent the result from the connected component analysis (a) compared to the result of the OBIA approach (b).

Fig. 2. Finding the optimal kernel size for two diffusion stick filters.

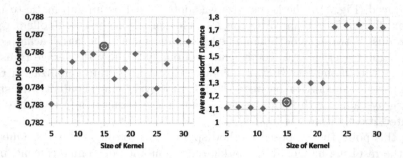

based on the eigendecomposition of the Hessian matrix that contains the second-order partial derivatives of the image intensities. The relation of the eigenvalues are used to describe the local image structure and enable an analysis of the strength and direction of lines and edges. The Hessian filter is applied on the whole preprocessed 2D US image and contains solely a pre-selection of possible candidates of lines and edges that may be structures of the falx and gyri. Thus, a ROI is determined, representing the image section that contains (ideally) solely the structures of the falx and its gyri. Due to the fact that US images are acquired to scan the perifalcine region, it is assumed that the strongest collection of edges represent the structures of the falx and gyri within the US image.

In order to identify this image region, a canny edge detection filter is applied with a lower threshold of 0.8 and an upper threshold of 2.8 (Fig. 1). Note that the thresholds are determined in the same fashion as the kernel size mentioned above and performed well on the 50 US images but might need further adaption and testing when applied to a larger amount of data sets. After that local valleys, present within the resulting binary image, are filled (Fig. 1). Followed by a morphological opening, a closing and a dilation to cut-off thin and small connections between the filled image contents, to fill small gaps, and to slightly dilate the filtered image content to enable that the resulting binary image covers the image content as well as the boundaries of the objects that should be segmented (Fig. 1). Kernel sizes for these filters where evaluated on 20 images. Finally, a connected component analysis is applied in order to get the largest image content from the binary image which is the region with the strongest collection of edges. This represents the ROI within the 2D US image that contains the structures of the falx and adjoining gyri.

The binary image of the ROI is then used to mask the result of the Hessian filter (Fig. 1). At first it was expected that a postprocessing by using solely a connected component analysis, in order to get the largest connected line from the image content, is sufficient. Nevertheless, after processing a larger amount of US images it turned out, that the falx and the gyri do not necessarily represent one connected region within the 2D US slices. Thus a further analysis of the image content of the masked result of the Hessian filter is necessary to correctly extract the structures of interest.

Table 1. Comparison of the overall achieved segmentation results: Minimum, maximum and results on average with standard deviation (SD) for the 50 US images with and without using the OBIA approach in a postprocessing step.

Postprocessing	Dice coefficient	Hausdorff distance (mm)	Jaccard index
With OBP			
Minimum	0.48	0.64	0.03
Maximum	0.89	7.33	0.81
Average ± SD	0.79 ± 0.07	1.56 ± 1.40	0.64 ± 0.14
Without OBP			
Minimum	0.48	0.64	0.31
Maximum	0.84	15.42	0.73
Average ± SD	0.68 ± 0.07	3.90 ± 3.41	0.60 ± 0.08

To assure this an OBIA approach is applied to the masked result image in order to correctly extract the perifalcine region by the following image features: positional features (x and y position of presegmented structures), shape features (circularity, elongation and size) and intensity statistics (mean intensity). A comparison of the segmentation results with and without using the OBIA can be seen in Fig. 1. The result image of the Hessian filter proved to be especially suitable as basic image from which characteristic features could be derived. The used OBIA approach has already shown to be a powerful method to extract and classify image features of US images [8].

3   Results

The quality of the segmentation was tested on 50 2D US images. The segmentation results are compared to reference segmentations of an expert. In 48 cases the falx and gyri could be correctly detected. On average a Dice coefficient of 0.79, a Hausdorff distance of 1.56 mm, and a Jaccard index of 0.64 could be achieved. It could be shown that the postprocessing with an OBIA approach could considerably improve the segmentation results, concerning the fact that the falx and adjacent gyri do not necessarily represent a single connected structure as mentioned above. A comparison of the results with and without the object-based postprocessing (OBP) can be seen in Tab. 2. Additional segmentation results for the perifalcine region are visualized in Fig. 3.

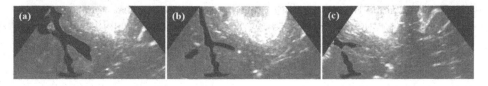

Fig. 3. Visualization of additional segmentation results (a)-(c). The images show the reference segmentation (red) with an overlay of the segmentation results of the proposed method with OBIA (green).

4 Discussion

The most challenging part in segmenting the cerebral falx and the adjacent gyri is that these structures do not provide a homogeneous representation within the US images. The falx itself is predominantly easily detected with its strong edges, whereas the adjacent gyri usually provide less contrast to the background and, therefore, less prominent edges. This momentarily minimizes the detection rate of the gyri and is the reason why the proposed method tends to undersegmentation when compared to the reference. In two cases the contrast of falx and gyri to the background of the US image was too weak and a segmentation of these structures could not be performed when based on prominent edges. OBIA has proven to be a powerful approach to allow a feature-based image segmentation. For future works it is planned to test the proposed method on more US images and to extend the falx/gyri specific image features in order to increase the general robustness of the approach.

Acknowledgement. This work is part of a research project sponsored by the Wilhelm Sander-Stiftung (grant no. 2013.109.1).

References

1. Heldmann S, Beuthien B, Olesch J, et al. Improved minimal-invasive laparoscopic liver surgery by registration of 3D CT and 2D ultrasound slices. Biomed Tech. 2010;55(1):84–6.
2. Rivaz H, Karimaghaloo Z, Fonov VS, et al. Nonrigid registration of ultrasound and MRI using contextual conditioned mutual information. IEEE Trans Med Imaging. 2014;33(3):708–25.
3. Kuklisova-Murgasova M, Cifor A, Napolitano R, et al. Registration of 3D fetal neurosonography and MRI. Med Image Anal. 2013;17:1137–50.
4. Xiao CY, Zhang S, Chen Y. A diffusion stick method for speckle suppression in ultrasonic images. Pattern Recognit Lett. 2004;25(16):1867–77.
5. Zoehrer F, Drexel J, Hahn HK. Speckle reduction for automated breast ultrasound. Proc BVM. 2010; p. 390–4.
6. Lassen B, Kuhnigk JM, Friman O, et al. Automatic segmentation of lung lobes in CT images based on fissures, vessels, and bronchi. Proc IEEE Int Symp Biomed Imaging. 2010;10:560–63.
7. Shikata H, McLennan G, Hoffman EA, et al. Segmentation of pulmonary vascular trees from thoracic 3D CT images. Int J Biomed Imaging. 2009; p. 1–11.
8. Schwier M, Hahn HK. Segmentation hierarchies and border features for automatic pregnancy detection in porcine ultrasound. Proc IEEE Int Symp Biomed Imaging. 2014;11:931–34.

Measurement of the Aortic Diameter in Plain Axial Cardiac Cine MRI

Marko Rak, Alena-Kathrin Schnurr, Julian Alpers, Klaus-Dietz Tönnies

Department of Simulation and Graphics, University of Magdeburg
rak@isg.cs.ovgu.de

Abstract. We address the task of aortic diameter measurement in (non-contrast-enhanced) plain axial cardiac cine MRI. To this end, we set up a likelihood maximization problem which allows us to recover globally optimal aorta locations and diameters of the cine sequence efficiently. Our approach provides intuitive means of manual post-correction and requires little user interaction, making large-scale image analysis feasible. Experiments on a data set of 20 cine sequences with 30 time frames showed (at least) pixel-accurate diameter measurements which are also highly stable against re-parameterization.

1 Introduction

Diameters of the ascending and descending aorta are potential medical markers for aortic dilatation and possibly a later dissection, cf. [1]. Currently, ongoing epidemiological studies such as the "Study of Health in Pomerania" (SHIP) [2] investigate such markers on a large scale, trying to discover populations at risk and relations to other parameters of general health. The aorta cannot be assessed manually here due to the sheer number of subjects. Therefore, computerized strategies with little to no manual interaction are needed.

For each time frame the task can be viewed as a circle detection problem with the additional constraint that circle parameters (center and diameter) change little over time. Exploiting the latter, we cast the task into a longest path problem on a directed acyclic graph (DAG), maximizing an aorta likelihood along time frames. To set up the likelihood we exploit the circularity by applying a filter bank of differently sized and sub-pixel-shifted ring templates to the gradient magnitude image of each time frame. Since other image structures show strong likelihood as well, we constrain the problem by manual interaction, letting the user select the correct solution in one (or two) time frame(s).

Related work is summarized in Tab. 1. We also included work that is intended to handle three-dimensional images slice-wise because this task is inherently similar to ours. Approaches range from clustering on intensity thresholdings [3] over dynamic programming on mixed cost functions [4, 5, 6] to fitting of active contour models [7]. It seems that research interest shifted from X-ray to MRI in recent years. However, since MRI usually lacks in resolution (and speed) it is unclear how accurate and stable approaches developed for CT perform on MRI data. Therefore, additional work is required on the MRI side in general.

Table 1. Summary of related work. Abbreviations: contrast-enhanced (CE), X-ray computed tomography (CT), phase-contrast (PC), magnetic resonance imaging (MRI).

Task		Modality	Anomal.	Interact.	Correct.	Optimal.	Resol. [mm]
Slices	Saur'08 [3]	CE-CT	Yes	None	No	Local	0.2–0.5
	Kurkure'08 [4]	CT	Yes	None	No	Local	0.5–0.5
	Avila'10 [5]	CT	Yes	None	No	Local	0.5–0.5
	Avila'13 [6]	CT	Yes	None	No	Local	0.68
Frames	Herment'10 [7]	PC-MRI	Yes	< 5 s	No	Local	1.1–1.8
	Our work	MRI	No	< 5 s	Yes	Global	1.41

The ability to cover anomalies (strong deviation from circularity) such as aneurysms or aortic dilatation is important for all other approaches, but is of minor interest for our particular task. Such cases would already be clinically relevant and are excluded for marker analysis. This enables us to use rather basic but certainly more reliable means of processing. It even allows us to find globally optimal solutions, while the related work is prone to local optimality. Another aspect is the possibility to introduce additional information to re-run the computation in case of wrong results. Our approach supports such means of guided post-correction quite naturally, while the other approaches do not.

2   Method

2.1   Aorta likelihood in parameter space

We seek to evaluate an aortic likelihood over the three-dimensional parameter space of all circles that measures how well any particular circle parameterization (center and diameter) resembles the ascending/descending aorta in a single time frame. Fig. 1 outlines how this is done. We first calculate a gradient magnitude image for the time frame which is then filtered with a bank of ring templates to form the parameter likelihood. Furthermore, we considered likelihoods based on cross-correlation with circle templates and circular Hough transformation, but experiments showed that the former is more computationally demanding and the latter is less accurate. We next go into more detail on the individual aspects.

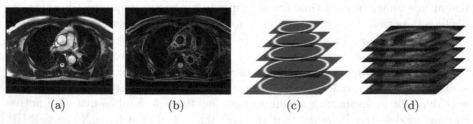

(a)   (b)   (c)   (d)

Fig. 1. Estimation of the aorta likelihood over the three-dimensional parameter space (center and diameter). For a time frame (a) we calculate its gradient magnitude image (b), filter it with a bank of ring templates (c) and thus obtain the aorta likelihood (d).

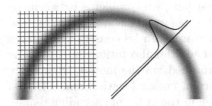

Fig. 2. Templates are defined by Gaussian profiles in polar coordinates with the rings' centers as origins. Function values are integrated over each template pixel to reflect the narrow ridge adequately.

We found that a ridge with a Gaussian profile is a suitable representation for the ring template, since its width neatly mimics the extent of the aorta boundary that is present due to partial volume effects. We choose a standard deviation σ of half the size of a pixel, i.e., $\sigma = \frac{1}{2}$ px, which can be motivated by the sampling theorem. As illustrated in Fig. 2, the ring is constructed by fixing the Gaussian profile at the desired radius in polar coordinates with the ring's center being the origin. To adequately reflect the rather narrow Gaussian ridge by a template we numerically integrate it over each template pixel using adaptive quadrature. We then normalize the overall template integral to unity, which makes results comparable across different diameters. By shifting the position of the ring's center inside the central template pixel (sub-pixel shift) we are able to pinpoint aorta centers beyond pixel accuracy. Thus, the center location as well as the diameter can be sampled up to a fraction (center: $\frac{1}{s_c}$ and diameter: $\frac{1}{s_d}$) of the pixel size. The derivation of the gradient magnitude image $\|\nabla I\|_2$ is another important aspect. As smoothing is already an integral part of the template, we do not consider gradient operators with intrinsic smoothing here. Therefore, central finite differences are the intuitive choice to estimate the gradient field ∇I.

2.2   Graph formulation and longest path

For each time frame we extract the local likelihood maxima from parameter space. Thus, we reduce the problem to a small number of parameter candidates per time frame, from which the actual ascending/descending aorta is to be identified next. To this end, we form a DAG on the candidates, which allows us to recover the likelihood-optimal parameter combination (along time frames) efficiently by longest path search. The DAG is constructed as illustrated in Fig. 3. Each parameter candidate is a node of the DAG, carrying it's likelihood as node weight. Directed edges link candidates of adjacent time frames if their difference in parameters is admissible according to thresholds t_c and t_d for variation in center location and diameter, respectively. Searching for the longest path (w.r.t. node weights) between the additional source and sink recovers the solution with maximum cumulative candidate likelihood. The problem can be solved in linear time via standard techniques based on topological ordering.

To distinguish the correct result from other strongly peaking image structures such as fat tissue boundaries, the user is required to select the correct solution among the parameter candidates in one (or two) time frame(s). All remaining candidate nodes of the same time frame(s) are simply removed from the DAG. Now, the problem splits into longest path sub-problems between the user-supplied constraints which can be solved as before. This also provides intuitive means of post-correction since the path search can be constrained further in case of wrong results by manual selection of additional solutions in other time frames. Interaction with a time frame is performed via the mouse, where only candidates are accessible that enclose the current cursor location and selection among them takes place by scrolling over them in the order of ascending diameter. For visual feedback we overlay the boundary of the current candidate to the time frame, which in combination with the intuitive mouse interaction allows to select the solution in less than five seconds per time frame for a trained user.

3   Experiments

3.1   Dataset and setup

For experiments we use a data set of 20 subjects from the SHIP, each covering a sequence of 30 time frames with a pixel size of 1.41 mm each (see [8] for further details). For every time frame, we were given annotations of the center and diameter for the ascending and descending aorta from a single reader. Using this ground truth we performed two experiments: (1) benchmarking accuracy under realistic circumstances; (2) assessing parameter influence on result quality.

In the first experiment, an expert interactively selected the correct solution for the ascending and descending aorta in the first and last time frame in each image sequence. Being familiar with the data set, this expert was also prompted to specify the admissible inter-frame variation, resulting in thresholds $t_c^r = 5.64$ mm and $t_d^r = 8.64$ mm. Sub-pixel sampling factors were fixed at $s_c^r = 2$ and $s_d^r = 2$, which means sampling the parameter space up to half the size of a pixel. Using this reference setup (superscript r) we applied our approach and compared the obtained centers and diameters to the ground truth in terms of L^2 error.

In the second experiment, we altered all parameters (one at a time) to more challenging values, applied our approach with each of the altered setups and compared results to ground truth using L^2 error as before. Altered parameter setups include sparser likelihood samplings according to sub-pixel sampling factors $s_c^- = 1$ and $s_d^- = 1$ as well as larger thresholds $t_c^+ = 11.28$ mm and $t_d^+ = 14.10$ mm for inter-frame variation. It should be noted that the latter were

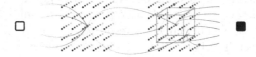

Fig. 3. Construction of the directed acyclic graph from the solution candidates (red dots) in parameter space. Candidates are linked forward in time between adjacent frames (left and right parameter grid) if their difference in parameters is admissible (blue box). Candidates of the first and last time frame are connected to source (empty square) and sink (filled square), respectively.

Fig. 4. Tukey box plots for the center (left plot) and diameter L^2 error (right plot) of the ascending (red) and descending aorta (blue) using reference (upper row) and more challenging parameterization (lower row).

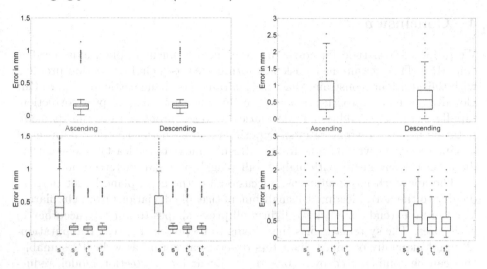

already quite spacious in the reference setup of the first experiment, since the maximal inter-frame variation in the ground truth was 2.21 mm and 3.66 mm for the center location and the diameter, respectively.

3.2 Results and discussion

The Tukey box plots range from the lower (Q_1) to the upper quartile (Q_3), while the median (Q_2) is marked green (Fig. 4). Whiskers extend to at most 1.5 times the inter-quartile range. Centers for ascending/descending aorta were estimated well beyond pixel accuracy $(Q_1$: 0.10/0.11 mm, Q_2: 0.15/0.16 mm and Q_3: 0.18/0.19 mm). Errors for diameters were significantly higher but still in the range of a pixel size $(Q_1$: 0.28/0.28 mm, Q_2: 0.56/0.56 mm and Q_3: 1.13/0.85 mm). Reviewing results more closely, we found that our approach systematically overestimated diameters of the manually annotated ground truth. A quick comparison showed a discrepancy to ground truth diameters of 0.29 mm on average.

Fig. 4 (lower row) depicts the results of our second experiment. Increasing the variation thresholds t_c^r and t_d^r to t_c^+ and t_d^+ did neither change center nor diameter errors noticeably. We reason that these can be set rather roughly without effecting the result quality. As expected, decreasing the center sub-pixel sampling factor s_c^r to s_c^- increases center errors, but results still remain pixel-accurate or better $(Q_1$: 0.30/0.39 mm, Q_2: 0.41/0.47 mm and Q_3: 0.59/0.59 mm). Interestingly, the equivalent does not hold true for decreasing the diameter sub-pixel sampling factor s_d^r to s_d^-, which left diameter errors almost unchanged $(Q_1$: 0.20/0.40 mm, Q_2: 0.60/0.60 mm and Q_3: 0.80/1.00 mm). This supports our hypothesis of a systematic bias that makes up a large portion of the observed diameter error.

4 Conclusion

We proposed a method for aortic diameter measurement in plain axial cardiac cine MRI. The measurement task was formulated as a circle detection problem with the additional constraint that circle parameters change little over time. Our globally optimal approach provides intuitive means of manual post-correction, rapidly introducing additional information into the problem to re-run the computation in case of wrong results. Experiments were performed on a data set of 20 cine sequences with 30 time frames. Results indicate (at least) pixel-accurate diameter measurements with high stability against re-parameterization.

The approach has limitations. Occasionally, the axial plane is not perpendicular to the aorta, leading to small but noticeable deviations from circularity. We plan to extend our work to slightly elliptical shapes to improve accuracy in such cases. The systematic bias that seems to be present between computationally and manually obtained diameters deserves attention as well. Presumably, this can be compensated by a constant or linear bias correction model, reducing errors in measurement even further. Here, more research is required since intra/inter-observer variations also play an important role in this context.

References

1. Mensel B, Hegenscheid K, Heßelbarth L, et al. Thoracic and abdominal aortic diameter measurement by MRI using plain axial volumetric interpolated breath-hold examination in epidemiologic research: a validation study. Acad Radiol. 2012;19:1011–7.
2. Völzke H, Alte D, Schmidt CO, et al. Cohort profile: the study of health in pomerania. Int J Epidemiol. 2011;40:294–307.
3. Saur SC, Kühnel C, Boskamp T, et al. Automatic ascending aorta detection in CTA datasets. Proc BVM. 2008; p. 323–7.
4. Kurkure U, Avila-Montes OC, Kakadiaris IA. Automated segmentation of thoracic aorta in non-contrast CT images. Proc IEEE Int Symp Biomed Imaging. 2008; p. 29–32.
5. Avila-Montes OC, Kukure U, Kakadiaris IA. Aorta segmentation in non-contrast cardiac CT images using an entropy-based cost function. Proc SPIE. 2010; p. 76233J.
6. Avila-Montes O, Kurkure U, Nakazato R, et al. Segmentation of the thoracic aorta in non-contrast cardiac CT images. IEEE J Biomed Health Inf. 2013; p. 936–49.
7. Herment A, Kachenoura N, Lefort M, et al. Automated segmentation of the aorta from phase contrast MR images: validation against expert tracing in healthy volunteers and in patients with a dilated aorta. J Mag Res Imaging. 2010;31:881–8.
8. Hegenscheid K, Kühn JP, Völzke H, et al. Whole-body magnetic resonance imaging of healthy volunteers: pilot study results from the population-based SHIP study. Fortschr Geb Rontgenstr Nuklearmed. 2009;181:748–759.

Detection of Facial Landmarks in 3D Face Scans Using the Discriminative Generalized Hough Transform (DGHT)

Gordon Böer[1], Ferdinand Hahmann[1], Ines Buhr[2], Harald Essig[3],
Hauke Schramm[14]

[1]Institute of Applied Computer Science, University of Applied Sciences Kiel
[2]Hannover Medical School
[3]University Hospital Zurich
[4]Faculty of Engineering, University of Kiel
gordon.boeer@fh-kiel.de

Abstract. This paper presents the Discriminative Generalized Hough Transform (DGHT) as a technique to localize landmarks in 3D face scans. While the DGHT has been successfully used for the detection of landmarks in 2D and 3D images this work extends the framework to be used with triangle meshes for the first time. Instead of edge features and their respective gradient direction, the relative positions and orientations of the mesh faces are utilized to describe the geometric structures which are relevant for the detection of a specific landmark. Implementing a coarse-to-fine strategy at first a decimated version of the mesh is used to locate the global region of the point of interest, followed by more detailed localizations on higher resolution meshes. The utilized shape models are created in an automated, discriminative training process which assigns individual weights to the single model points, aiming at an increased localization rate. The technique has been applied to detect 38 anthropometric facial landmarks on 99 3D face scans. With an average error of 1.9mm, the most accurate detection was performed for the right alare, the average error when considering all landmarks amounts to 5.1 mm.

1 Introduction

Stereo photogrammetry has drawn a lot of attention as a method for clinical surface imaging, given its possibility to generate 3D images rapidly and in a non-invasive manner. Medical applications for the recorded 3D surfaces include among many others the assessment of facial morphology [1] or the planning of surgical interventions [2].

It has been shown [3], that measurements using stereo photogrammetric images are reliable when compared to direct anthropometric measurements. The anthropometric landmarks defined by Farkas [4] play an important role to perform quantitative measurements. Those landmarks have to be identified on the 3D surface which is often done manually using an annotation tool. Since the manual annotation of landmarks is a tedious work, systems which could perform this task automatically and reliable are highly desirable.

Some of the technologies available in computer vision have been applied to detect anthropometric facial landmarks in 3D surfaces. In [5] a statistical facial feature model (SFAM) is employed for the localization of up to 19 anthropometric landmarks. The used model incorporates local properties (range and texture maps) as well as the global configurational relationships between the facial landmarks, achieving mean localization accuracies ranging from 2.7 mm to 12 mm. A recently published system [6] utilizes active appearance models combined with random forests to detect 14 landmarks in intensity and depth images, resulting in a mean error of 4.6 mm. Another approach [7] exploits the so called shape index and spin images to perform a detection of 8 landmarks. The system was evaluated thoroughly and achieved an mean localization error of 4.5 mm to 6.3 mm.

2 Materials and methods

The described system employs the DGHT, a general object localization technique, to detect landmarks in triangle meshes. Following a coarse-to-fine approach the detection is performed in three different detail levels, whereby each level provides the starting point for the subsequent, more precise localization step.

2.1 Discriminative generalized hough transform (DGHT)

The DGHT is a technique for the localization of arbitrary shapes using models that describe the appearance of an object in relation to a reference point. It extends the well-known Generalized Hough Transform (GHT) [8] by an iterative discriminative training procedure to generate shape models achieving a low error rate on the given training data. Besides learning the object appearance, the technique employs a weighted voting scheme with individually adjusted model point weights. This further expands the standard GHT approach where every model point has the same impact on the detection result.

The GHT tries to find the best match of a model in a given image by voting into a quantized parameter space, the so called Hough space H. Every cell c_i of the Hough space represents possible transformation parameters which map the model to a position in the image.

Note, that in the DGHT implementation at hand no other transformations than translation are used, resulting in a Hough space which is of equal dimension as the image. This restriction of the considered transformation parameters is possible since moderate variability may be well captured by the learned shape model. Consequently, after finishing the voting procedure, the searched for translation parameters are given by the cell $\hat{c}$ with the highest vote: $\hat{c} = \operatorname*{argmax}_{c_i} H(c_i)$

The models used by the DGHT are generated automatically from given training data in an iterative and supervised manner. Using a small training subset a first shape model is generated by overlaying the feature points, extracted from a specified region around the target point. The performance of this initial model is evaluated on the remaining training images. Considering the individual model point contributions to the N best localization hypothesis the weights are optimized using a Minimum Classification Error (MCE) approach. Subsequently the now weighted model is evaluated on the complete training set. It is assumed, that the images, on which the weighted model performs badly, contain an object variability which is not yet contained in the model. Hence the shapes extracted from those images will be incorporated into the model during the next iteration. In this way the model evolves iteratively until it performs with a predefined accuracy or all images have been used for the model generation. An extensive description of the DGHT training procedure is given in [9].

Usually the DGHT utilizes edge features to describe the shape of a target object, but since the voting procedure is a very general approach it is possible to use other one- to multi-dimensional features as well, which may also be combined to improve the localization result. For the detection of the anthropometric landmarks local features, based on the mesh faces, are employed. The centroid of each face is considered as the feature position while the orientation is given by the face normal. Fig. 1 illustrates the used models.

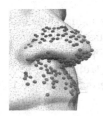

Fig. 1. Illustration of a 3D DGHT model for the localization of the columella point . The dots correspond to the several model points while their color refers to the individual weights assigned during the model training (with red color referring to a high weight). The direction of the face normal is depicted by the line.

2.2 Coarse-to-fine strategy

In previous work, an improved accuracy is achieved in the DGHT framework with a coarse-to-fine strategy, e.g. for the detection of epiphyseal regions in hand radiographs [10]. Generally spoken, the localization is carried out at several consecutive steps, aiming at a more precise detection by increasing the grade of detail and simultaneously narrowing down the considered image region within each step. At first, a subsampled version of the whole image is used which allows focusing on global and reliable structures to run a first rough localization. Using this first estimate for the landmark position as starting point, a more accurate detection is performed which is limited to a smaller region but uses a higher resolution image, hence focusing on more detailed structures. This process is repeated until the original image resolution is reached. It should be noted, that a separate localization model is generated for each of the localization steps, thus every model is tailored to level specific shapes, ranging from global but strong to local and fine details. When working with 2D images the level of detail can be reduced by a simple subsampling or low-pass-filtering, e.g. using a Gaussian kernel. In case of triangle meshes it is possible to achieve a similar effect by using a decimation algorithm, which tries to approximate the shape of a mesh using a reduced number of polygons. Within the current system an algorithm is employed which performs the polygon simplification using iterative pair contractions and quadric error metrics [11]. The effect of a mesh simplification is depicted in Fig. 2.

2.3   Experimental setup

To evaluate the performance of the described system a dataset provided by the Clinic for Cranio-Maxillo-Facial Surgery of the Hannover Medical School (MHH) has been used. It is constituted of 99 3D face scans of both female (32) and male (67) persons, ranging in age from 14 to 87 years. They were recorded in 2011 and 2012 utilizing a face scanner by the company 3D-Shape GmbH and subsequently converted to triangle meshes in the STL file format, consequently losing the color and texture information of the scanner. The data set excludes duplicate recordings for one and the same person as well as clinically relevant asymmetries and deformities. All provided 46 anthropometric facial landmarks per image where annotated manually by a member of the MHH, adding up to 4554 annotations in total.

The experiments were carried out for 38 landmarks always using the same experimental setup and parameter settings. All models were trained on 60 images and evaluated on the remaining 39 images. Since each image depicts an unique person, no individuals used in the final test were part of the training corpus. Regarding the coarse-to-fine strategy described above three different detail levels were employed, starting with a mesh-decimation by 66%.

3   Results

Using the DGHT to localize all considered landmarks an average localization error of 5.1 mm was achieved. With an error of 1.9 mm the right alare (alR) was localized most accurate while the system performed worst for the trachion with 10.7 mm. Detailed results for all landmarks are given in Tab. 1.

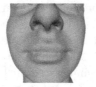   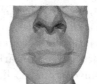

(a) Original mesh   (b) Decimated mesh

Fig. 2. Effect of mesh simplification. The original mesh (a) was decimated (b) by 90%, effectively reducing the number of faces from 44980 to 4497. In (b) the global face structure is well visible, while finer details are lost.

Table 1. Results of the localization experiments for all considered facial landmarks. Listed are the mean and standard deviation of the localization error in mm.

Landmark	$\bar{x} \pm \sigma_x$ (mm)	Landmark	$\bar{x} \pm \sigma_x$ (mm)
Alare left (alL)	3.2 ± 4.1	Alare right (alR)	1.9 ± 1.5
Alar curvature left (acL)	2.9 ± 2.0	Alar curvature right (acR)	3.5 ± 6.4
Subalare left (subalL)	7.5 ± 4.5	Subalare right (subalR)	7.3 ± 3.9
Nostril medial left (nmL)	3.4 ± 2.1	Nostril medial right (nmR)	5.5 ± 7.1
Nostril anterior left (naL)	2.9 ± 2.1	Nostril anterior right (naR)	4.2 ± 6.4
Nostril posterior left (npL)	2.8 ± 1.6	Subnasale (su)	7.5 ± 24.5
Chelion left (chL)	7.0 ± 7.4	Chelion right (chR)	5.4 ± 4.9
Stomion (sto)	3.8 ± 5.2	Crista philtre left (cpR)	5.8 ± 7.2
Labrale superius (ls)	4.3 ± 7.5	Sublabiale (sl)	3.9 ± 4.0
Endocanthium left (enL)	5.7 ± 6.5	Endocanthium right (enR)	4.0 ± 2.6
Zygoma right (zyR)	2.9 ± 3.1	Superciliar right (scR)	5.1 ± 5.0
Trachion (tr)	10.7 ± 8.7	Glabella (g)	4.2 ± 2.1
Nasion (n)	4.6 ± 12.4	Pronasale (pra)	6.8 ± 5.5
Columella point (cp)	3.0 ± 5.3	Gnathion (gn)	5.3 ± 3.4
Preaurale left (praL)	6.8 ± 7.4	Preaurale right (praR)	7.3 ± 8.8
Superaurale left (saL)	6.6 ± 9.6	Superaurale right (saR)	6.0 ± 7.5
Postaurale left (paL)	6.7 ± 5.5	Postaurale right (paR)	6.5 ± 4.5
Subaurale left (sbaL)	4.3 ± 2.5	Subaurale right (sbaR)	4.1 ± 3.0
Tragus left (traL)	6.8 ± 4.4	Tragus right (traR)	4.8 ± 4.2

4 Discussion and conclusion

In this paper, the DGHT was presented as a method to detect facial landmarks in 3D polygonal meshes of face scans. Therefor the previously existing system was extended to be used with this kind of data for the first time, by implementing a feature descriptor, based on the position and orientation of mesh faces, as well as the coarse-to-fine strategy by utilizing a mesh decimation algorithm. It has been shown that the DGHT system can be adopted to new application areas with relatively little effort.

Experiments were carried out for a substantial amount of clinical relevant anthropomorphic landmarks, achieving state-of-the art accuracy, however on a small set of data. It becomes obvious, that the localization success of the DGHT differs remarkably for several landmarks (ranging from a mean error of 1.9mm to 10.7mm). An explanation of this behavior is given by the usage of the same experimental setup for all landmarks. The automatic model generation can be adjusted by a lot of parameters to handle the landmark specific difficulties individually, rather than using a global setup that may be suitable only for several targets. E.g. the usage of more or less than three detail levels may improve the accuracy for some landmarks. It should as well be noted that the employed simple shape descriptor is not distinct enough for some landmarks, e.g. the trachion.

Further improvements of the system will include the usage of more complex feature descriptors, e.g. local curvature properties or spin images. It is imaginable that a specific feature descriptor is suitable to detect a landmark while it fails for another one or that a combination of several descriptors into one model is even more helpful. The localization results may be further improved by applying a confidence measure to reject candidate landmarks which receive a low confidence score. An implementation of a heuristic based confidence measure was already exploited successfully in [10].

Future evaluations should be carried out on more challenging datasets with an increased number of images, also incorporating rotations, occlusions or deformities.

References

1. Krimmel M. Three-dimensional assessment of facial development in children with unilateral cleft lip with and without alveolar cleft. J Craniofac Surg. 2013;24(1):313–6.
2. Ayoub AF, Siebert P, Moos KF, et al. A vision-based three-dimensional capture system for maxillofacial assessment and surgical planning. Br J Oral Maxillofac Surg. 1998;36(5):353–7.
3. Wong J, Oh A, Ohta E, et al. Validity and reliability of craniofacial anthropometric measurement of 3D digital photogrammetric images. Cleft Palate Craniofac J. 2008;45(3):232–9.
4. Farkas LG, Kolar JC. Anthropometric guidelines in cranio orbital surgery. Clin Plast Surg. 1987;14(1):1–16.
5. Zhao X, Dellandréa E, Chen L, et al. Accurate landmarking of three-dimensional facial data in the presence of facial expressions and occlusions using a three-dimensional statistical facial feature model. IEEE Trans Syst Man Cybern B Cybern. 2011;41(5):1417–28.
6. Fanelli G, Dantone M, van Gool L. Real time 3D face alignment with random forests-based active appearance models. IEEE Int Conf Automat Face Gesture Recognit. 2013; p. 1417–28.
7. Perakis P, Passalis G, Theoharis T, et al. 3D facial landmark detection under large yaw and expression variations. IEEE Trans Pattern Anal Mach Intell. 2013;35(7):1552–64.
8. Ballard DH. Generalizing the hough transform to detect arbitrary shapes. Pattern Recogn. 1981;13(2):111–22.
9. Ruppertshofen H. Automatic modeling of anatomical variability for object localization in medical images. Ph.D. Thesis: University Magdeburg; 2013.
10. Hahmann F, Böer G, Deserno TM, et al. Epiphyses localization for bone age assessment using the discriminative generalized hough transform. Proc BVM. 2014; p. 66–71.
11. Garland M, Heckbert PS. Surface simplification using quadric error metrics. Proc SIGGRAPH. 1997; p. 209–216.

Extraction of the Aortic Dissection Membrane via Spectral Phase Information

Cosmin Adrian Morariu[1], Daniel Sebastian Dohle[2], Konstantinos Tsagakis[2], Josef Pauli[1]

[1]Intelligent Systems Group, Faculty of Engineering, University of Duisburg-Essen
[2]Department of Thoracic and Cardiovascular Surgery, Universitätsklinikum Essen
adrian.morariu@uni-due.de

Abstract. Streak/ring/motion artifacts, unequal distribution of the intravenously injected contrast agent and the partial volume effect lead to significant differences in brightness and contrast between CTA datasets or even between slices of the same dataset. These issues affecting the segmentation of fine structures such as the aortic dissection membrane can be efficiently addressed only by applying a measure invariant to luminance and contrast. Towards this end, the analysis of local phase information in the frequency domain using Log-Gabor wavelets achieves sub-mm accuracy when segmenting the dissection membrane by 3 new approaches. In order to avoid under-segmentation, as well as the inclusion of artifacts, this contribution extends phase congruency by proposing a novel scale space strategy, which consists of combining low-frequent, "secure" structures only with adjoining filtering results of high-frequent nature. Our concept harmonizes with the principles of perceptual organization pertaining to the human visual cortex.

1 Introduction

A fissure in the intimal layer of the aortic wall can lead to intramural blood flow with consecutive formation of a so called false lumen, separated from the true lumen by the dissection membrane. Dynamic or static branch vessel occlusion with organ malperfusion arise when the blood flow is compromised by either the true lumen exerting pressure on the false lumen or the dissection membrane occluding the orifice of a branch vessel. A classification system based on the localization of the primary lesion and the longitudinal extent of the dissection membrane within the aorta has been contrived in order to guide the treatment strategy [1]. Segmentation of the dissection membrane has only recently emerged as an important image processing application field, due to the aforementioned insights gained by the medical community. A sheetness measure, derived from eigenvalue analysis of the Hessian matrix, serves in [2] for segmenting the dissection wall. The authors report an overall average error of 1.71 ± 1.89 mm. The approach highlighted in [3] utilizes the zero-crossing of the scalar product between the intensity gradient vector field and the field of eigenvectors with highest associated eigenvalues of the local structure tensors. This method yields an average absolute error of half a voxel after validation on 5 MDCT datasets.

2   Materials and methods

Segmentation of the dissection membrane within the aortic volume may be carried out following the automatic segmentation of the aorta, in case that no manually delineated ground truth for the aortic outer contours is available. Algorithms such as [4] have been proposed for segmenting the complete aortic volume affected by dissection. Varying contrast and brightness between CTA datasets or even between slices belonging to the same dataset conjures usage of a robust and dimensionless measure of feature significance. Kovesi [5] improved a model, which relies on the concept of salient features being perceived at those locations where local phase values from the Fourier spectrum are maximally congruent. Acquisition of undistorted local frequency information requires usage of linear-phase filters. Quadrature filter pairs enable computation of signal amplitude and phase for a certain frequency at a determined pixel. Log-Gabor wavelets fulfill these prerequisites and, in contrast to Gabor wavelets (1D Gabor filter in Fig. 1(a)), they allow for arbitrarily large bandwiths with no overlap in the low-frequent domain.

Three proposed approaches, namely uniform phase congruency (UPC), multiscale phase congruency (MSPC), respectively selective phase congruency (SPC) are being applied to each CTA axial slice (axial w.r.t. the volume). With respect to our UPC approach in the following we will outline the implemented $N \times M$ polar-separable frequency-domain filter bank

$$J_{\omega_n, \theta_m}(\omega, \theta) = G_{\omega_n} \cdot LP_{\omega_c} \cdot R_{\theta_m} = e^{\frac{-\log(\omega/\omega_n)^2}{2\log(\sigma/\omega_n)^2}} \cdot \left(1 + (\omega/\omega_c)^{2k}\right)^{-1} \cdot e^{-\frac{(\theta - \theta_m)^2}{2\sigma_\theta^2}} \quad (1)$$

for computing phase congruency using N Log-Gabor quadrature filter pairs $G_{\omega_n}(\omega)$ of center frequency ω_n, M directional filters $R_{\theta_m}(\theta)$ of orientation θ_m, as well as a Butterworth filter LP_{ω_c} with cutoff-frequency ω_c. The first exponential term in (1), denoting $G_{\omega_n}(\omega)$, represents the starting element in Fig. 2. Appropriate values of the ratio σ/ω_n, influencing the bandwith of the wavelet, for detecting the dissection membrane range from 0.3 to 0.8. Center frequencies ω_n for the n-th Log-Gaborfilter are obtained by scaling of a minimal wavelength $\lambda_{\min}$. Since the membrane in axial slices usually represents only a few pixels wide structure, the value of $\lambda_{\min}$ should be chosen accordingly. The exponential term representing $R_{\theta_m}(\theta)$ in (1) defines the orientation angle θ_m of the filter $J_{\omega_n, \theta_m}(\omega, \theta)$ within the polar frequency plane. Choosing $R_{\theta_m}(\theta)$ as a Gaussian in

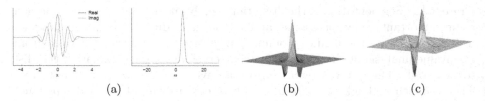

(a)   (b)   (c)

Fig. 1. 1D Gabor filter in spatial and frequency domain (a), via FFT^{-1} computed 2D quadrature filter pair $J_{n,m}^e$ and $J_{n,m}^o$ for even and odd in (b) and (c), respectively.

angular direction within the frequency plane has its justification in the fact that, transformed to the spatial domain, it will remain a Gaussian function, which will be subsequently convolved with the image. Thus, only the amplitudes of the original signal will undergo modulation, leaving the phase information undistorted. Please note that the standard deviation σ_θ influences the orientation spacing between the filters. Therefore, it should be tailored to the number M of directions in order to ensure an even spectral coverage of the spectrum. In conjunction with 6 main orientations of 30 degrees each, we choose $\sigma_\theta = 0.43$. Finally, the non-exponential term representing LP_{ω_c} in (1) describes the transfer function of the Butterworth lowpass filter, which removes excessively high frequencies aiming to avoid artifacts. The larger the order k of the filter, the steeper its slope at cutoff frequency ω_c. Fig. 2 illustrates the process of generating $J_{\omega_n,\theta_m}(\omega,\theta)$ within the spectral domain.

Subsequently, the Inverse Fourier Transform FFT^{-1} applied to $J_{\omega_n,\theta_m}(\omega,\theta)$ leads to the desired quadrature filter pair $[J^e_{n,m}, J^o_{n,m}] = FFT^{-1}(J_{\omega_n,\theta_m})$, with $J^e_{n,m}$ (Fig. 1(b)) the even filter component (real part) and $J^o_{n,m}$ (Fig. 1(c)) the odd filter term (imaginary part in spatial domain). We obtain the even and odd filter responses $[e_{n,m}(\boldsymbol{x}), o_{n,m}(\boldsymbol{x})] = [I(\boldsymbol{x}) * J^e_{n,m}, I(\boldsymbol{x}) * J^o_{n,m}]$ by convolving the image function $I(\boldsymbol{x})$ with the aforementioned spatial domain filter components. Estimating $F(\boldsymbol{x})$, which denotes the image function $I(\boldsymbol{x})$ without DC component, respectively $H(\boldsymbol{x})$, its Hilbert transformation (90 degree phase shift) and also the amplitudes of the filter responses by $F(\boldsymbol{x}) \approx \sum_{n,m} e_{n,m}(\boldsymbol{x})$, $H(\boldsymbol{x}) \approx \sum_{n,m} o_{n,m}(\boldsymbol{x})$ and $A_{n,m}(\boldsymbol{x}) \approx \sqrt{e_{n,m}(\boldsymbol{x})^2 + o_{n,m}(\boldsymbol{x})^2}$ allows for calculating the measure of phase congruency $PC(\boldsymbol{x}) = \frac{\sqrt{F^2(\boldsymbol{x}) + H^2(\boldsymbol{x})}}{\sum_{n,m} A_{n,m}(\boldsymbol{x})}$ at each image pixel $\boldsymbol{x}$ [5]. Fig. 3 depicts PC results of UPC for different orientations θ_m overlayed onto original ROI-images. The color code bar on the right side illustrates that very strong PC responses are marked in red, very weak responses in blue.

The MSPC approach for extracting the aortic dissection membrane is designed to mimic human perception. In particular, it resembles the concept of perceptual organization and uniform connectedness pertaining to the visual cortex. This concept states that our brain is able to perceive and organize two or more basic-level local elements with common attributes into global patterns as superordinate units [6]. A fine structure such as the dissection membrane

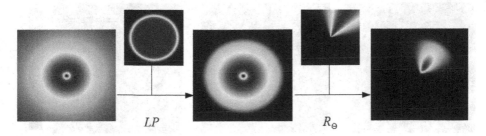

Fig. 2. Generating the polar-separable UPC filter $J_{\omega_n,\theta_m}(\omega,\theta)$ in frequency domain.

Table 1. Average distances (AD) in mm between manually delineated and automatically segmented dissection membrane within 7 CTA datasets reveal subvoxel accuracy.

Method	AD (manual → auto)	AD (auto → manual)	Mean AD
UPC	0.8887 ± 0.2162	0.9765 ± 0.2328	0.9326
MSPC	1.0000 ± 0.2533	0.8764 ± 0.1931	0.9382
SPC	1.0157 ± 0.2067	0.9626 ± 0.2451	0.9892

undergoes changes in width and intensity, nevertheless our visual cortex will perceive it as a global unit due to spatial continuity. Hence, different scale space representations of the membrane, which we can extract by different parameter values of $\lambda_{\min}$, can be connected subsequently, on a higher, additional level due to their spatial connectivity. Let R be the final extracted membrane region such as in Fig. 4(c), R_{λ_2} a high-frequent, "uncertain" spatial component extracted by the proposed UPC filter by a low value of $\lambda_{\min}$ (Fig. 4(b)) and finally, R_{λ_1} a low-frequent, coarse structure associated to a higher $\lambda_{\min}$ value (Fig. 4(a)). By defining

$$R_{\lambda_2} \in R \Leftrightarrow \exists R_{\lambda_1} | R_{\lambda_1} \cap R_{\lambda_2} \neq \varnothing, \text{ with } \lambda_2 < \lambda_1 \qquad (2)$$

only those fine structures R_{λ_2} will be maintained in R, for which an adjoining coarse structure R_{λ_1} exists.

3   Results

The third proposed approach, SPC, is aimed to avoid under-segmentation in axial slices where the minimal wavelength of the filterbank proves too high for detecting the membrane. Hence, a second calculation of phase conguency using a lower $\lambda_{\min}$ is prompted only for those slices j, which fulfill the criterion

$$\frac{MP_j}{\sqrt{AP_j}} < \frac{1}{q} \cdot \sum_{i=1}^{q} \frac{MP_i}{\sqrt{AP_i}} \qquad (3)$$

with q the total number of aorta slices in a dataset, MP the number of membrane pixels per slice and AP the number of aorta pixels within the same slice. Thus,

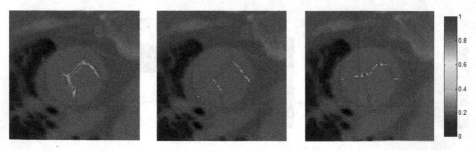

Fig. 3. UPC filter respones after combining all directional filters $R_{\theta_m}(\theta)$ of orientation angle θ_m (left), respectively only for $\theta_m = 45°$ (middle) and only for $\theta_m = 90°$ (right).

Table 2. Enlarged representation of the aorta within the dataset of 0.46 mm slice spacing automatically leads to parameters set to extract coarser structures.

Method	Parameters 6 CTAs 0.77 spacing	Parameters 1 CTA 0.46 spacing
UPC	$\lambda_{min} = 6$; $th_{fixed} = 0.1$	$\lambda_{min} = 15$; $th_{fixed} = 0.4$
MSPC	$\lambda_{m1} = 6.5$; $\lambda_{m2} = 5$; $th_{fixed} = 0.1$	$\lambda_{m1} = 14$; $\lambda_{m2} = 6$; $th_{fixed} = 0.5$
SPC	$\lambda_{m1} = 6.5$; $\lambda_{m2} = 4$; $th_{fixed} = 0.2$	$\lambda_{m1} = 14$; $\lambda_{m2} = 5$; $th_{fixed} = 0.6$

slices, in which the ratio between membrane and aorta pixels is lower than the average ratio per dataset following first iteration, undergo a subsequent filtering.

As a final processing step common to all proposed approaches (UPC, MSPC, SPC), we introduce an adaptive thresholding with

$$th_{adapt} = |PC_{max} - PC_{min}| \cdot th_{fixed} + PC_{min}, \text{ with } 0 \leq th_{fixed} \leq 1 \quad (4)$$

which permits selection of a certain percentage of filter responses between minimal value PC_{min} and maximal value PC_{max} of each individual slice.

Manual delineation of the dissection membrane, as well as of the aortic outer walls, effected by a vascular surgeon on 7 CTA datasets of aortic dissection, enables performance quantification of the 3 proposed approaches. Due to the lacerated nature of the dissection membrane within the ascending aorta, ground truth and evaluation are confined to the descending part. The average distance $AD(A \rightarrow B) = (\sum_{a \in A} \min_{b \in B} \{d(a,b)\})/|A|$ between two voxel sets A and B, denoting manual respectively automatic membrane segmentations, is employed as accuracy measure. $|A|$ represents the number of elements in the set A and $d(a,b)$ is the 3D euclidean distance between a and b. Considering the asymmetrical relation $AD(A \rightarrow B) \neq AD(B \rightarrow A)$ both distances have to be computed. Tab. 1 summarizes these distances for all 3 proposed approaches. UPC and MSPC perform equally well, yielding a mean AD of 0.93 mm. Due to the better $AD(\text{manual} \rightarrow \text{auto})$ of 0.89 mm, UPC proves advisable for applications where over-segmentation is rather desired, e.g. separate quantification of the true and

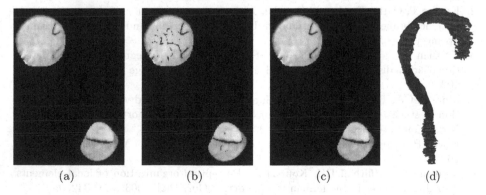

(a)   (b)   (c)   (d)

Fig. 4. MSPC approach: the final result (c) contains only those high-frequent structures from (b), which connect to a low-frequent spatial component from (a); and 3D reconstruction of the membrane volume (d).

false lumen by having an (even artificially) closed dissection membrane. On the other side, MSPC exposes greater AD(auto $\rightarrow$ manual) = 0.88 mm, recommending it in cases where over-segmentation is to be avoided, i.e. locating the entry and re-entry tears within the membrane. While 6 CTA datasets possess an axial within-slice resolution of 0.77 ± 0.03 mm, one dataset exhibits 0.46 mm, reflecting in an enlarged representation of all body tissues, including aorta and membrane. For this reason, the parameters for this dataset differ from those of the other 6 datasets (Tab. 2), as they get automatically set for the extraction of coarser structures. The scale parameter $N = 2$ regarding the number of quadrature filter pairs proves optimal for all approaches and datasets.

4   Discussion

In this study, we have addressed the issue of extracting fine structures in CTA data by analyzing spectral phase information. Application of a measure invariant to luminance and contrast allows for precise detection of the dissection membrane despite a high variability of image data and in the presence of artefacts. Since our datasets possess an average slice spacing of 2.1 mm (range: 0.7-6 mm), comparison with manual tracing reveals sub-mm accuracy for all 3 extraction techniques proposed by this contribution. Future research will be aimed at locating entry and re-entry tears within the membrane and define their morphology. This endeavor will be considerably sustained by the inherent benefits regarding over-segmentation brought by MSPC, an approach designed in compliance with the rules of uniform connectedness pertaining to the human visual cortex.

References

1. Erbel R, Alfonso F, Boileau C, et al. Diagnosis and management of aortic dissection, task force on aortic dissection. Eur Heart J. 2001;22(18):1642–81.
2. Kovács T, Cattin P, Alkadhi H, et al. Automatic segmentation of the aortic dissection membrane from 3D CTA images. In: Medical Imaging and Augmented Reality. Springer; 2006. p. 317–24.
3. Krissian K, Carreira JM, Esclarin J, et al. Semi-automatic segmentation and detection of aorta dissection wall in MDCT angiography. Med Image Anal. 2014;18(1):83–102.
4. Morariu CA, Terheiden T, Dohle DS, et al. Graph-based and variational minimization of statistical cost functionals for 3D segmentation of aortic dissections. Lect Notes Computer Sci. 2014;8753:511–22.
5. Kovesi P. Image features from phase congruency. J Computer Vis Res. 1999;1(3):1–26.
6. Altmann CF, Bülthoff HH, Kourtzi Z. Perceptual organization of local elements into global shapes in the human visual cortex. Curr Biol. 2003;13(4):342–9.

Fast Adaptive Regularization for Perfusion Parameter Computation
Tuning the Tikhonov Regularization Parameter to the SNR by Regression

Michael Manhart[1,2], Andreas Maier[2,3], Joachim Hornegger[2,3], Arnd Doerfler[1]

[1]Department of Neuroradiology, Universitätsklinikum Erlangen
[2]Pattern Recognition Lab, Friedrich-Alexander-Universität Erlangen-Nürnberg
[3]Erlangen Graduate School in Advanced Optical Technologies (SAOT), Erlangen
michael.manhart@cs.fau.de

Abstract. Computation of perfusion parameters by deconvolution from contrast-enhanced time-resolved CT or MR perfusion data sets is an ill-conditioned problem. Thus, adequate regularization and determination of corresponding regularization parameters is required. We present a novel method for Tikhonov regularization for perfusion imaging to locally adapt parameters to the SNR level by using a regression function. In an numerical evaluation our simple approach provided similar or even superior results compared to methods applying computationally more demanding L-curve analysis.

1 Introduction

Perfusion imaging techniques are widely used for diagnosis of cerebrovascular disease such as acute stroke as well as in the diagnostic work-up and therapy monitoring of brain tumors. Perfusion imaging is usually performed by contrast-enhanced time-resolved CT or MR imaging [1]. Recently, first results on inter-ventional perfusion imaging using flat detector CT have been presented [2, 3]. Perfusion parameters, such as the cerebral blood flow (CBF), can be computed by deconvolution techniques. In practice, the deconvolution process is performed by inversion of an ill-conditioned linear equation system (LES). To obtain a meaningful solution from the ill-conditioned inversion, Tikhonov regularization is commonly applied [1]. A crucial problem in regularization is how to choose the right parameter to control the trade-off between the regularization penalty and the data fit. In perfusion imaging, a fixed parameter independent of the contrast signal strength is usually used [1]. Salehi Ravesh et al. [4] showed that using an adaptive regularization parameter, which is tuned to the local signal-to-noise ratio (SNR), can improve MR lung perfusion measurements. The parameters are tuned locally by a modified version of the L-curve criterion (LCC) [5]. The LCC is a popular tool to find an appropriate parameter for Tikhonov regularization.

However, using L-curve analysis for determining adaptive regularization parameters causes a considerable amount of computational overhead. In this work, we present a novel technique to adapt the regularization parameter locally to the SNR in a computationally efficient way by regression and show its potential benefits in a numerical brain perfusion phantom study.

2 Materials and methods

2.1 Perfusion parameter computation using Tikhonov regularization

The indicator-dilution theory describes how CBF and other related perfusion parameters can be recovered from the acquired time series of contrast agent enhanced volumes. For a comprehensive introduction, please refer to the review paper by Fieselmann et al. [1]. In this work, we restrict the description to the deconvolution problem, which needs to be solved by algebraic methods. We assume that the contrast agent attenuation is sampled at t_i, $i = 1 \ldots N$ time points with a sampling distance Δt. Let matrix $\mathbf{A} \in \mathbb{R}_{[0,\infty)}^{N \times N}$ denote a convolution with the arterial input function (AIF), vector $\mathbf{c} \in \mathbb{R}_{[0,\infty)}^{N}$ a time-contrast-concentration curve (TCC) inside a tissue voxel, and vector $\mathbf{r} \in \mathbb{R}_{[0,\infty)}^{N}$ the corresponding residual function from which the essential perfusion parameters can be computed

$$
\mathbf{A} = \Delta t \begin{pmatrix} a\,(t_1) & 0 & \cdots & 0 \\ a\,(t_2) & a\,(t_1) & \cdots & 0 \\ \vdots & \vdots & \ddots & \vdots \\ a\,(t_N) & a\,(t_{N-1}) & \cdots & a\,(t_1) \end{pmatrix}, \; \mathbf{c} = \begin{pmatrix} c\,(t_1) \\ \vdots \\ \vdots \\ c\,(t_N) \end{pmatrix}, \; \mathbf{r} = \begin{pmatrix} r\,(t_1) \\ \vdots \\ \vdots \\ r\,(t_N) \end{pmatrix} \tag{1}
$$

For example, CBF can be computed from $\mathbf{r}$ using the relationship CBF $=$ $\max \mathbf{r}\,(t)\,/\rho_{\mathrm{T}}$, where ρ_{T} denotes the tissue density. The residual function $\mathbf{r}$ can be recovered by solving the deconvolution problem

$$
\mathbf{A}\mathbf{r} = \mathbf{c} \tag{2}
$$

However, the convolution matrix $\mathbf{A}$ is generally ill-conditioned [1]. Thus, slight errors in $\mathbf{c}$ (e.g., due to noise) result in large errors in $\mathbf{r}$ and solving LES 2 directly will result in physiologically not meaningful residual functions with strong oscillations and high energy. To obtain an improved solution, Tikhonov regularization can be applied, which penalizes solutions with a larger semi-norm $\|\mathbf{L}\mathbf{r}\|_2^2$

$$
\mathbf{r}_\lambda = \arg\min_{\mathbf{r}} \; \|\mathbf{A}\mathbf{r} - \mathbf{c}\|_2^2 + \lambda^2 \, \|\mathbf{L}\mathbf{r}\|_2^2 \tag{3}
$$

The matrix $\mathbf{L} \in \mathbb{R}^{N \times N}$ typically describes a discrete approximation to some derivative operator. In standard Tikhonov regularization, as conducted in this work, $\mathbf{L}$ corresponds to the identity matrix $\mathbf{L} = \mathbf{I}$ (i.e., solutions with lower energy are preferred). The strength of regularization is controlled by the parameter $\lambda \in \mathbb{R}_{[0,\infty)}$. The quadratic optimization problem 3 can be solved using singular value decomposition (SVD) [5], which decomposes $\mathbf{A}$ into the orthonormal left singular vectors $\mathbf{u}_i$, the orthonormal right singular vectors $\mathbf{v}_i$, and the non-negative singular values σ_i

$$\mathbf{A} = \sum_{i=1}^{N} \mathbf{u}_i \sigma_i \mathbf{v}_i^T \quad \text{with} \quad \sigma_1 \geq \sigma_2 \geq \ldots \geq \sigma_N \geq 0 \tag{4}$$

The regularized solution $\mathbf{r}_\lambda$ can be recovered using the SVD of $\mathbf{A}$ [5]

$$\mathbf{r}_\lambda = \sum_{i=1}^{N} f_i(\lambda) \frac{\mathbf{u}_i^T \mathbf{c}}{\sigma_i} \mathbf{v}_i \quad \text{with} \quad f_i = \frac{\sigma_i^2}{\sigma_i^2 + \lambda^2} \tag{5}$$

2.2 Adaptive regularization with the L-curve criterion

The L-curve is a convenient way to display information about solutions computed via Tikhonov regularization [5]. It is a log-log plot of the norm of a regularized solution $\eta(\lambda)$ versus the norm of the corresponding residual norm $\rho(\lambda)$ (Fig. 1a). The quantities of $\eta(\lambda)$ and $\rho(\lambda)$ can be efficiently computed via the SVD of $\mathbf{A}$ [5]

$$\eta(\lambda) = \|\mathbf{r}_\lambda\|_2^2 = \sum_{i=1}^{N} \left(f_i(\lambda) \frac{\mathbf{u}_i^T \mathbf{c}}{\sigma_i} \right)^2 \tag{6}$$

$$\rho(\lambda) = \|\mathbf{A}\mathbf{r}_\lambda - \mathbf{c}\|_2^2 = \sum_{i-1}^{N} \left((1 - f_i(\lambda)) \mathbf{u}_i^T \mathbf{c} \right)^2 \tag{7}$$

The L-curve criterion (LCC) states that the best trade-off between η and ρ is reached by a λ lying on the characteristic corner of the L-curve. A corresponding

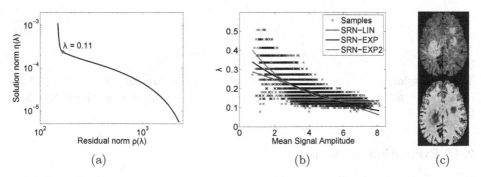

(a)　　　　　　　　　(b)　　　　　　　　　(c)

Fig. 1. (a) L-curve with λ selected at maximum curvature; (b) mean signal amplitude $\bar{c}$ and corresponding λ values determined using modified L-curve criterion (MLCC) (blue crosses) and corresponding regression functions using linear and exponential models; (c) top: plot of spatial distribution of λ determined with MLCC, bottom: corresponding mean signal amplitude.

λ can be found by identifying the maximum curvature $\kappa(\lambda)$ of the L-curve, where $\kappa(\lambda)$ is given as [5]

$$\kappa(\lambda) = 2\frac{\eta\rho}{\eta'}\frac{\lambda^2\eta'\rho + 2\lambda\eta\rho + \lambda^4\eta\eta'}{(\lambda^2\eta^2 + \rho^2)^{3/2}} \text{ with } \eta'(\lambda) = \sum_{i=1}^{N}(1 - f_i)^2 f_i \mathbf{u}_i^T \mathbf{c} \quad (8)$$

Salehi Ravesh et al. [4] discussed that the straightforward application of the LCC to MR lung perfusion data is not feasible. In many cases, $\kappa(\lambda)$ showed multiple maxima or no local maximum at all. In these cases, the λ chosen by the LCC were too small leading to noisy results. Therefore a modified LCC (MLCC) was introduced implying two additional criteria: if multiple maxima are present in $\kappa(\lambda)$, the maximum with the largest λ is chosen and if no local maximum is present, λ is set to a minimally allowed value $\lambda_{\min} = 0.1 \cdot \sigma_1$.

2.3 Adaptive regularization with SNR regression

The LCC based methods require to sample $\kappa(\lambda)$ in a sufficient density. In practice, typically 50 evaluations of Equations 6, 7 and 8 are required to determine the parameter for computing the residual function for one tissue voxel. This causes a considerable amount of computational overhead. Fig. 1c shows the average amplitude of the TCCs over time $\bar{c} = \frac{1}{N}\sum_{i=1}^{N} c(t_i)$, which is proportional to the average SNR, compared to the adaptive λ values determined using the MLCC. As expected, higher λ value were assigned to regions with low SNR and vice versa. This suggests to use simple regression functions to adapt the λ values to the SNR. In this work, we apply a linear regression model (SNR-LIN), as well as exponential models with one (SNR-EXP) and two (SNR-EXP2) basis functions

$$\lambda_{\text{SNR-LIN}} = a\bar{c} + b$$
$$\lambda_{\text{SNR-EXP}} = a\exp(b \cdot \bar{c}) \quad (9)$$
$$\lambda_{\text{SNR-EXP2}} = a\exp(b \cdot \bar{c}) + l\exp(m \cdot \bar{c})$$

The regression parameters were computed using the `fit` function of the MATLAB curve fitting toolbox. Fig. 1b shows examples for fitting the regression functions.

2.4 Evaluation methods

For evaluation of the discussed methods, a volumetric time series of TCCs was simulated with a realistic numerical brain perfusion phantom [6]. The time series consisted of 3 slices with 256×256 voxels and 44 temporal samples with sampling distance $\Delta t = 1\,\text{s}$. Accordingly, white Gaussian noise with standard deviation $\sigma_n = 20\,\text{HU}$ was added and finally the TIPS method [7] was applied for noise reduction before perfusion parameter computation. The convolution matrix $\mathbf{A}$ was computed from the simulated ground truth AIF to avoid any influence from

Table 1. Estimated regression parameters according to the models in Equation 9 using different subsets of data.

Method	(Parameters)	Slice 1	Slice 2	Slice 3	All slices
SNR-LIN	(a,b)	$(-0.30, 0.31)$	$(-0.31, 0.31)$	$(-0.31, 0.32)$	$(-0.31, 0.31)$
SNR-EXP	(a,b)	$(0.39, -0.19)$	$(0.40, -0.20)$	$(0.41, -0.20)$	$(0.40, -0.20)$
SNR-EXP2	(a,b,l,m)	$(0.50, -0.37,$	$(0.50, -0.37,$	$(0.51, -0.36,$	$(0.50, -0.37,$
		$0.04, 0.14)$	$0.03, 0.16)$	$0.03, 0.17)$	$0.03, 0.16)$

the AIF selection to the parameter computation. For quantitative evaluation, Lin's concordance correlation (CC) [8] between the computed values and the ground truth values in all tissue voxels was determined. In contrast to linear correlation the CC is sensitive to a shift and scaling in the estimates.

3   Results

Fig. 2 shows CBF maps calculated with different methods and corresponding CC results. Tab. 1 shows the variation of the regression parameters using different subsets of the data.

4   Discussion

The CBF map in Fig. 2 which was created using a high global regularization parameter $\lambda = 0.3$ results in a smooth map but severely underestimated CBF

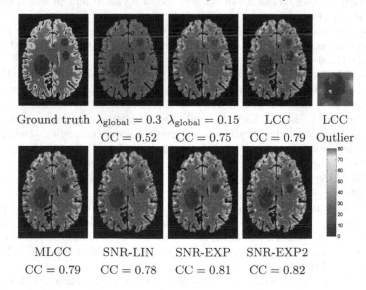

Ground truth $\lambda_{\text{global}} = 0.3$ $\lambda_{\text{global}} = 0.15$ LCC   LCC
                CC = 0.52   CC = 0.75   CC = 0.79   Outlier

MLCC   SNR-LIN   SNR-EXP   SNR-EXP2
CC = 0.79   CC = 0.78   CC = 0.81   CC = 0.82

Fig. 2. CBF maps computed using Tikhonov regularization with global and adaptive parameter settings and the corresponding CC to the ground truth. Units: ml/100 g/min.

values. If a smaller $\lambda = 0.15$ is used, the CBF values are less underestimated but the map gets noisy and the areas with reduced perfusion values are not as well separated. The adaptive methods can achieve maps with limited noise and limited underestimation at the same time. LCC produces some few outliers, which can be avoided using the MLCC. The regression based methods show similarly improved results as the LCC methods, with the SNR-EXP2 method showing the overall best CC value. A limitation of this work is that the regression functions were fitted with the same data as they were applied to in the evaluation. However, Tab. 1 shows that the parameters only vary slightly for different subsets of the data. This suggests that the parameters are stable over different data sets, but needs to be evaluated closely in future research.

In summary, the results suggest that using simple regression functions to locally adapt the λ parameter to the SNR can provide similar or even improved results compared to the computationally more expensive LCC based methods. From a clinical perspective, this approach could potentially provide quantitatively improved perfusion maps with less noise in a fast computation time.

Acknowledgement. The authors gratefully acknowledge funding of the Medical Valley, Erlangen, Germany, diagnostic imaging network, sub-project BD 16, grant nr. 13EX1212G.

References

1. Fieselmann A, Kowarschik M, Ganguly A, et al. Deconvolution-based CT and MR brain perfusion measurement: theoretical model revisited and practical implementation details. Int J Biomed Imaging. 2011.
2. Manhart M, Kowarschik M, Fieselmann A, et al. Dynamic iterative reconstruction for interventional 4-D c-arm CT perfusion imaging. IEEE Trans Med Imaging. 2013;32(7):1336–48.
3. Manhart M, Aichert A, Struffert T, et al. Denoising and artefact reduction in dynamic flat detector CT perfusion imaging using high speed acquisition: first experimental and clinical results. Phys Med Biol. 2014;59(16):4505–24.
4. Salehi Ravesh M, Brix G, Laun F, et al. Quantification of pulmonary microcirculation by dynamic contrast-enhanced magnetic resonance imaging: comparison of four regularization methods. Magn Reson Med. 2013;69(1):188–99.
5. Hansen PC. The L-Curve and its Use in the Numerical Treatment of Inverse Problems. IMM, Department of Mathematical Modelling, Technical University of Denmark; 1999.
6. Riordan AJ, Prokop M, Viergever MA, et al. Validation of CT brain perfusion methods using a realistic dynamic head phantom. Med Phys. 2011;38(6):3212–21.
7. Mendrik AM, Vonken E, van Ginneken B, et al. TIPS bilateral noise reduction in 4D CT perfusion scans produces high-quality cerebral blood flow maps. Phys Med Biol. 2011;56(13):3857–72.
8. Lin LIK. A concordance correlation coefficient to evaluate reproducibility. Biometrics. 1989;45(1):255–68.

Modellbasierte Simulation der Atembewegung für das Virtual-Reality-Training von Punktionseingriffen

Matthias Wilms[1], Dirk Fortmeier[1,2], André Mastmeyer[1], Heinz Handels[1]

[1] Institut für Medizinische Informatik, Universität zu Lübeck
[2] Graduate School for Computing in Medicine and Life Sciences, Universität zu Lübeck

wilms@imi.uni-luebeck.de

Kurzfassung. Virtual-Reality-Simulatoren bieten Medizinern eine virtuelle Trainingsumgebung, in der Eingriffe kostengünstig trainiert und geplant werden können, ohne hierbei reale Patienten zu gefährden. Eine Einschränkung der meisten VR-Trainingssimulatoren ist, dass sie von einem statischen Patienten ausgehen, dessen Anatomie im Bereich des simulierten Eingriffs während der Simulation keiner durch die Atmung verursachten Bewegung unterliegt. In diesem Beitrag wird gezeigt, wie Methoden zur Modellierung und Schätzung der Atembewegung aus dem Bereich der Strahlentherapie bewegter Tumoren genutzt werden können, um eine realistische Simulation komplexer, variabler Atembewegungen in VR-Trainingssimulatoren zu erreichen. Die entwickelte Methodik erlaubt eine Visualisierung der Atembewegung in Echtzeit und ermöglicht eine haptische Interaktion mit dem atmenden virtuellen Körper. Dies wird exemplarisch für das Szenario der Leberpunktion gezeigt.

1 Einleitung

Virtual-Reality-Simulatoren bieten Medizinern eine virtuelle Trainingsumgebung, in der Eingriffe kostengünstig trainiert und geplant werden können, ohne hierbei reale Patienten zu gefährden. Ein Schwerpunkt der Entwicklung von VR-Simulatoren lag in den letzten Jahren u.a. auf der Simulation von Nadelpunktionen. Es wurden beispielsweise Systeme und Verfahren zur Simulation der Punktion der Leber(-gefäße) [1, 2], der Prostata [3] und des Spinalkanals [4] entwickelt. Um ein realistisches Training zu ermöglichen, werden neben dem visuellen Rendering der Anatomie des virtuellen Patienten auch Techniken zur haptischen Interaktion mit dem Patienten eingesetzt. Spezielle haptische Eingabegeräte bieten hierfür neben der eigentlichen Steuerung von Werkzeugen auch die Möglichkeit am Werkzeug auftretende simulierte Kräfte an den Nutzer zurückzugeben.

Eine Einschränkung der meisten VR-Trainingssimulatoren ist, dass sie von einem statischen Patienten ausgehen, dessen Anatomie im Bereich der Punktion während der Simulation keiner Bewegung unterliegt. Dies ist beispielsweise für die Simulation von Lumbalpunktionen eine ausreichende Annahme, führt aber bei Punktionen von Organen im Abdomen oder Thorax zu einer zu starken Vereinfachung, da diese Strukturen in großem Maße durch die Atembewegung beeinflusst sind und deshalb starken Deformationen unterliegen, die für eine realistische Punktionssimulation berücksichtigt werden müssen. Bisher publizierte Ansätze (u.a. [2]) versuchen deshalb die Atmung mittels einfacher parametrischer Modelle, beispielsweise als sinusförmige Bewegung, zu simulieren, die nur eine grobe Annäherung an die wirkliche Atembewegung darstellen und keine Variabilität der Atmung berücksichtigen. Die realistische Modellierung und Simulation/Schätzung der Atembewegung ist ebenfalls Gegenstand aktueller Forschung im Bereich der Strahlentherapie von abdominalen und thorakalen Tumoren. In diesem Beitrag wird gezeigt, wie ein im Kontext der Strahlentherapie bewegter Tumoren entwickelter Ansatz zur Atmungsmodellierung [5] in Kombination mit einem innovativen Renderingverfahren für die realistische Simulation der Atembewegung in VR-Trainingssimulatoren genutzt werden kann.

2   Material und Methoden

2.1   VR-Simulator für das Training von Punktionseingriffen

Ausgangspunkt dieser Arbeit ist ein von uns für das Training verschiedener Punktionseingriffe (z.B. Leberpunktionen) entwickelter VR-Simulator [1]. Hardwareseitig nutzt das System ein Geomagic Phantom Premium 1.5 6DOF als haptisches Eingabegerät und eine Kombination aus Shutterbrille und Monitor, um eine stereoskopische 3D-Darstellung der Szene zu ermöglichen. Die Simulation des virtuellen Patienten basiert auf einem statischen 3D-CT-Datensatz, wobei für die Visualisierung ein direktes Volumenrenderingverfahren auf der Basis von Ray-Casting zum Einsatz kommt. Die durch die Interaktion der Nadel mit dem Körper hervorgerufenen Gewebedeformationen werden berechnet und visualisiert und die an der Nadel auftretenden Kräfte über das haptische Eingabegerät an den Nutzer zurückgegeben.

2.2   Modellbasierte Schätzung der Atembewegung

In den letzten Jahren haben im Bereich der Strahlentherapie von Lungen- und Lebertumoren vermehrt räumlich-zeitliche 4D-Bildgebungstechniken (4D-CT und 4D-MRT) Einzug gehalten, um die Therapie durch Analyse der patientenindividuellen Atembewegung zu verbessern [6]. Die klinisch häufig genutzten 4D-CT-Datensätze bestehen beispielsweise aus einer Sequenz von n 3D-CT-Bildern $I_{j\in\{1,...,n\}} : \Omega \to \mathbb{R}$ ($\Omega \subset \mathbb{R}^3$), welche die Anatomie des Patienten zu verschiedenen Phasen eines einzelnen Atemzyklus (u.a. max. Ein- und Ausatmung) abbilden. Für die Schätzung der komplexen Atembewegung auf Basis dieser Bilddaten kommen in der Regel spezialisierte Registrierungsverfahren zum Einsatz. Mit Hilfe dieser Verfahren können nicht-lineare Transformationen $\varphi_j : \Omega \to \Omega$ zwischen einer beliebigen Referenzphase I_{ref} und allen anderen Phasen I_j bestimmt werden, die die komplexe atmungsbedingte Bewegung der internen Strukturen zwischen den Bildern/Phasen beschreiben. Die auf diese Weise ermittelten Bewegungsinformationen können dann u.a. zur Optimierung der Bestrahlungsplanung und der Generierung von sog. Korrespondenzmodellen genutzt werden. Letztere kommen während der Bestrahlung in technischen Lösungen zur Kompensation der Atembewegung zum Einsatz.

Die Kompensation der Bewegung des Tumors während der Bestrahlung beispielsweise durch Nachführen der Strahlenquelle erfordert eine genaue Lokalisation des Zielgebiets und umgebender Risikostrukturen in Echtzeit über den kompletten Verlauf einer Behandlungssitzung, welche aufgrund des Strahlenschutzes und anderer Limitationen aktueller Bildgebungstechniken nicht bildbasiert erfolgen kann. Die Steuerung von Bewegungskompensationlösungen erfolgt deshalb zumeist durch externe Atemsignale in Verbindung mit patientenspezifischen Korrespondenzmodellen, die eine Schätzung der internen Bewegung auf Basis des externen Atemsignals (Surrogat) ermöglichen [5]. Als Atemsignale werden in der klinischen Praxis u.a. Bauchgurtsignale oder Spirometermessungen genutzt. In diesem Beitrag wird diese Technik eingesetzt, um auf der Basis eines gegebenen Atemsignals, welches patientenspezifische Variationen der Atmung repräsentiert, und eines gelernten Korrespondenzmodells die Atembewegung modellbasiert realistisch zu schätzen/simulieren.

Im Folgenden wird kurz unser Framework zur Korrespondenzmodellierung [5] vorgestellt. Als Atemsignal wird ein zweidimensionales Signal $\hat{\mathbf{z}}(t) = (s(t), s'(t))^T$ bestehend aus einem Spirometersignal $s(t)$ und dessen zeitlicher Ableitung $s'(t)$ eingesetzt. Hierdurch können sowohl verschiedene Tiefen der Atmung (Inter-Zyklen-Variabilität) berücksichtigt als auch generell Ein- und Ausatmung unterschieden werden, was die Modellierung der Intra-Zyklen-Variabilität der Atmung (Hysterese) erlaubt. Ausgehend von der verbreiteten Annahme, dass ein linearer Zusammenhang zwischen dem Atemsignal und der internen Bewegung besteht, werden die auf Basis eines 4D-CT-Datensatzes mittels nicht-linearer Registrierung bestimmten n Transformationen φ_j und die zugehörigen für die Rekonstruktion der 4D-Daten eingesetzten Atemsignalmessungen $\mathbf{z}_j$ genutzt, um mittels multivariater linearer Regression die Koeffizienten des patientenindividuellen linearen Modells

$$\hat{\varphi}(\mathbf{x}, t) = a_1(\mathbf{x})s(t) + a_2(\mathbf{x})s'(t) + a_3(\mathbf{x}), \quad \mathbf{x} \in \Omega \tag{1}$$

zu schätzen. Die gelernte Funktion $\hat{\varphi}(\mathbf{x}, t)$ liefert zeitabhäng für jede Messung des Atemsignals die zugehörige Verschiebung jedes Punktes $\mathbf{x} \in \Omega$ des Referenzbildes I_{ref}. Es können somit bei Vorliegen eines entsprechenden Atemsignals auch Zustände der Atmung simuliert werden, die nicht durch die 4D-CT-Daten abgebildet werden (z.B. tiefere und flachere Ein-/Ausatmung). Weiterhin ist zu beachten, dass die nicht-lineare Registrierung großer Bereiche des Thorax und des Abdomens, wie für eine VR-Simulation notwendig, spezielle Anforderungen an das eingesetzte Registrierungsverfahren stellt, da an Übergängen zwischen Strukturen Gleitbewegungen auftreten können, die die Annahme vieler Registerungsansätze, dass die Atembewegung glatt ist, verletzen. Deshalb verwenden wir das Verfahren von Schmidt-Richberg et al. [7], welches die durch die Gleitbewegung auftretenden Diskontinuitäten detektiert und explizit berücksichtigt.

2.3   Echtzeitfähige Visualisierung atembewegter virtueller Patienten

Ziel ist es nun den modellbasierten Ansatz zur Schätzung der Atembewegung anhand eines Atemsignals (Abschnitt 2.2) in den in Abschnitt 2.1 beschriebenen VR-Simulator zu integrieren, um die Atembewegung des virtuellen Patienten während einer Punktion realistisch zu simulieren. Im Folgenden gehen wir deshalb davon aus, dass für den zu visualisierenden Patienten anstatt eines statischen 3D-CT-Datensatzes ein 4D-CT-Datensatz vorliegt, um ein entsprechendes patientenindividuelles Korrespondenzmodell trainieren zu können. Basierend auf einem ebenfalls gegebenen Atemsignal kann dann das gelernte Modell genutzt werden, um für alle Zeitpunkte t der Simulation Transformationen $\hat{\varphi}_t$ zu erzeugen, mit Hilfe derer die visualisierte Referenzphase I_{ref} des 4D-CT-Datensatzes deformiert werden kann. Da die Anwendung der Transformation $\hat{\varphi}_t$ auf das komplette Bild I_{ref} zeitaufwendig ist und zusätzlichen Speicher benötigt, deformieren wir in unserer GPU-basierten Implementierung nicht das Bildvolumen, sondern die für das Ray-Casting ausgesendeten Strahlen entsprechend der Funktion $\hat{\varphi}_t$, um eine Visualisierung der Atembewegung in Echtzeit zu erreichen. Zusätzlich wird die Funktion auch auf die virtuellen Werkzeuge in der Szene angewendet, um eine Integration der Atembewegung in die Berechnung des haptischen Feedbacks zu erreichen.

2.4   Experimente

Die Fähigkeiten des beschriebenen Verfahrens zur Integration realistischer variabler Atembewegungen in einen VR-Trainingssimulator werden exemplarisch anhand der Leberpunktion gezeigt. Hierfür wird ein 4D-CT-Datensatz des Thorax und Abdomens mit 14 Atemphasen ($512{\times}512{\times}270$ Voxel, Voxelgröße: $1{\times}1{\times}1.5$ mm) genutzt. Als Referenzatemphase für die Registrierung und das anschließende Training des Korrespondenzmodells wird die Phase maximaler Einatmung gewählt. Für das Training des Modells und die Simulation der Atembewegung liegt für diesen Datensatz zudem auch ein zur Rekonstruktion genutztes Spirometersignal vor. Aufgrund des begrenzten Arbeitsspeichers der Grafikkarte unseres Demo-Systems (CPU: Intel i7 970 mit 3.20 GHz und 24 GB RAM; GPU: Nvidia

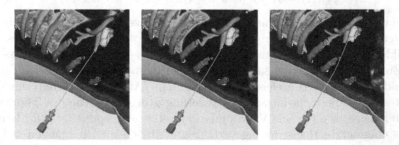

Abb. 1. Zeitliche Sequenz des Leberpunktionsszenarios bei simulierter Atmung mit zusätzlichem oberflächenbasierten Rendering zur verbesserten Darstellung der Rippen (grau), Gallengänge (grün) und einer simulierten Läsion (gelb).

GTX 680 mit 3 GB RAM), werden alle Daten auf eine Größe von 256^3 Voxeln gesampled.

3 Ergebnisse

Abb. 1 zeigt eine zeitliche Sequenz des Leberpunktionsszenarios bei simulierter Atmung. Es ist deutlich zu sehen, dass sich die Strukturen durch die Atmung bewegen und die Atembewegung zusätzlich zu einer Biegung der Punktionsnadel führt. Die Simulation variabler komplexer Atemmuster durch den modellbasierten Ansatz zur Schätzung der Atembewegung aller thorakalen und abdominalen Strukturen anhand eines variablen echten Atemsignals ist in Abb. 2 exemplarisch dargestellt. Es ist klar zu erkennen, dass durch das Atemsignal u.a. verschiedene Tiefen der Ein- bzw. Ausatmung realistisch simuliert werden können. Für das Ray-Casting mit simulierter Atembewegung wurden Renderingzeiten von

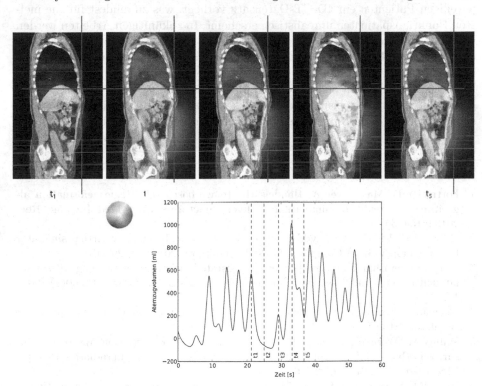

Abb. 2. Saggitale Ansicht der durch die simulierte Atmung deformierten CT-Daten des virtuellen Patienten (oben) zu den fünf markierten Zeitpunkten des für die Atmungssimulation genutzten Spirometersignals (unten). Die Richtung der Atembewegung ausgehend von der Referenzphase ist farbcodiert durch das HSV-Farbrad dargestellt, wobei die Amplitude der Bewegung durch die Deckkraft der Farbe angegeben ist (Transparenz: 0 mm; volle Deckkraft: $\geq$ 10 mm). Atemzugvolumen der Referenzphase des 4D-CT-Datensatzes: 600 ml. Die roten Linien dienen zur Orientierung für den Leser.

< 30 ms pro Einzelbild bei einer Viewportgröße von 1224×1014 Pixeln gemessen, was die Echtzeitfähigkeit zeigt.

4 Diskussion

Dieser Beitrag zeigt, wie Methoden zur Modellierung und Schätzung der Atembewegung aus dem Bereich der Strahlentherapie bewegter Tumoren genutzt werden können, um eine realistische Simulation komplexer variabler Atembewegungen in VR-Trainingssimulatoren zu erreichen. Die vorgestellte Methodik erlaubt eine Visualisierung der Atembewegung in Echtzeit und ermöglicht eine haptische Interaktion mit dem atmenden virtuellen Körper. Dies wurde exemplarisch für das Szenario der Leberpunktion gezeigt, wobei die in diesem Beitrag vorgestellte Methodik auch auf viele andere Trainings- und Planungsszenarien anwendbar ist. Eine Einschränkung des vorgestellten Vorgehens ist die Annahme, dass für den jeweiligen Patienten ein 4D-CT-Datensatz vorliegt, was zumindest für die meisten Punktionspatienten unrealistisch erscheint. In zukünftigen Arbeiten werden wir deshalb untersuchen, inwieweit gelernte Modelle auf Patienten für die nur ein statischer 3D-CT-Datensatz vorliegt übertragen werden können. Die Notwendigkeit der Aufnahme eines Atemsignals stellt unserer Meinung nach keine Einschränkung der Anwendbarkeit dar, da hierfür neben dem in diesem Beitrag genutzten Spirometer beispielsweise auch kostengünstige und berührungslose Lösungen auf Basis von Kamerasystemen existieren (z.B. Microsoft Kinect).

Literaturverzeichnis

1. Fortmeier D, Mastmeyer A, Handels H. Image-based soft tissue deformation algorithms for real-time simulation of liver puncture. Curr Med Imaging Rev. 2013;9:154–65.
2. Villard PF, Vidal FP, Cenydd L, et al. Interventional radiology virtual simulator for liver biopsy. Int J Computer Assist Radiol Surg. 2014;9(2):255–67.
3. Goksel O, Sapchuk K, Morris WJ, et al. Prostate brachytherapy training with simulated ultrasound and fluoroscopy images. IEEE Trans Biomed Eng. 2013;60(4):1002–12.
4. Gorman P, Krummel T, Webster R, et al. A prototype haptic lumbar puncture simulator. Stud Health Technol Inform. 2000;70:106–9.
5. Wilms M, Werner R, Ehrhardt J, et al. Multivariate regression approaches for surrogate-based diffeomorphic estimation of respiratory motion in radiation therapy. Phys Med Biol. 2014;59:1147–64.
6. Keall PJ, Mageras GS, Balter JM, et al. The management of respiratory motion in radiation oncology report of AAPM Task Group 76. Med Phys. 2006;33:3874–3900.
7. Schmidt-Richberg A, Werner R, Handels H, et al. Estimation of slipping organ motion by registration with direction-dependent regularization. Med Image Anal. 2012;16:150–9.

Rückenschmerz durch Übergewicht?
Biomechanische MKS-Modellierung der Belastungssituation der Lendenwirbelsäule bei unterschiedlichem Körpergewicht

Sabine Bauer, Eva Keller, Dietrich Paulus

MTI Mittelrhein, Universität Koblenz–Landau, Koblenz, Deutschland
bauer@uni-koblenz.de

Kurzfassung. In den letzten Jahrzehnten hat sich Übergewicht und Adipositas zu einem großen globalen gesundheitlichen Problem entwickelt. Während die Auswirkungen auf das kardiovaskuläre System im Fokus vieler Studien stehen, sind die Auswirkungen von Übergewicht und Adipositas auf die Strukturen der Wirbelsäule immer noch nahezu unbekannt. In dieser Studie wurden die Auswirkungen von Normalgewicht und Adipositas mit Hilfe der Mehrkörpersimulation (MKS) auf die Lendenwirbelsäule untersucht. Dazu wurden zwei MKS-Modelle, normalgewichtiger Mann und adipöser Mann, erstellt, die sowohl die biomechanischen Eigenschaften der Bandscheiben, der Facettengelenke und der Ligamente berücksichtigen, als auch die anthropometrischen Eigenschaften der zwei Körpergewichtsklassen. Zur Bestimmung der Auswirkungen dieser unterschiedlichen Gewichtsklassen auf die Strukturen der Wirbelsäule, wird die Lendenwirbelsäule jeweils mit der Gewichtskraft eines Normalgewichtigen und eines Adipösen belastet. Dabei werden insbesondere die Belastungsänderungen in den Bandscheiben und in den Facettengelenken untersucht.

1 Einleitung

Im Jahr 2012 betrug der prozentuale Anteil von Übergewicht und Adipositas unter den 18- bis 79-Jährigen 67,1% der männlichen und 53% der weiblichen Bevölkerung. Betrachtet man nun die Häufigkeit der gesundheitlichen Beschwerden bezüglich Rückenschmerzen, so stellt sich heraus, dass 70 bis 85% der Bevölkerung während ihres Lebens von Rückenschmerzen betroffen sind [1]. In [2] wird ein direkter Zusammenhang zwischen Rückenschmerz und Adipositas beschrieben. Wie genau aber die Belastungsänderungen innerhalb der verschiedenen Wirbelsäulenstrukturen sind, ist bis jetzt unzureichend erforscht. Daher wurden zwei MKS-Modelle, eines normalgewichtigen und eines adipösen Mannes erstellt, um die Auswirkungen von Normalgewicht und Adipositas während des natürlichsten Belastungsfalls des aufrechten Standes auf die Kinematik und die übertragenen Kräfte und Drehmomente der verschiedenen Wirbelsäulenstrukturen zu quantifizieren.

2   Material und Methoden

Die Modellierung wurde in drei Schritten durchgeführt (Abb. 1).

2.1   Erstellung eines MKS-Modells der Lendenwirbelsäule

Das MKS-Modell der Lendenwirbelsäule besteht aus os ilium, os sacrum und den Wirbelkörpern L1-L5. Die Wirbelkörper sind durch Bandscheiben mit entsprechenden Freiheitsgraden und 160 ligamentösen Strukturen, die an charakteristischen Punkten der knöchernen Wirbelkörperstrukturen befestigt sind, miteinander verbunden. Die Facettengelenke werden als 3D-Kontaktflächen so realisiert, dass die wirkenden Kontaktkräfte das Eindringen von zwei miteinander korrespondierenden Kontaktflächen vermeidet. Alle diese spinalen Strukturen sind mit ihren unterschiedlichen Materialeigenschaften und entsprechenden biomechanischen Eigenschaften modelliert, die im Detail aus [3] zu entnehmen sind. Dieses MKS-Modell der Lendenwirbelsäule wurde validiert, indem die berechneten kinematischen Größen mit Ergebnissen aus Finit-Elemente- und in vivo-Studien verglichen wurden [3, 4, 5, 6]. In Abb. 2 ist vergleichend der intervertebrale Druck der verschiedenen funktionalen Einheiten während des natürlichsten Belastungsfalls des aufrechten Standes dargestellt. Es ist zu sehen, dass der intervertebrale Druck der funktionalen Einheiten L5-Sac bis L2-L3 in gleicher Größenordnung sind. Offensichtlich ist hingegen der Druckunterschied in der funktionalen Einheit L1-L2 der MKS-Modellierung (Bauer_500N) im Vergleich zu der FE-Modellierung (Rohlmann). Der Grund hierfür kann eine kleinere Durchschnittsfläche der Bandscheiben im FE-Modell sein. Denn bei gleichgroßer einwirkender Kraft, ist der Druck umso höher, je kleiner die Durchschnittsfläche der Bandscheibe ist.

Wahrscheinlicher ist es jedoch, dass die verschiedenen intersegmentalen Rotationsrichtungen der Bandscheiben der Grund für die Diskrepanz der Druckwerte zwischen L1-L2 sind (Abb. 3). Während unter gleicher äußerer Kraft, in dem FE-Modell von Rohlmann alle funktionalen Einheiten Flexionsbewegungen durchführen, führt die oberste funktionale Einheit L1-L2 des MKS-Modells

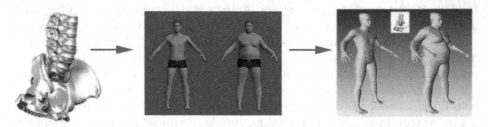

Abb. 1. Die drei Schritte der Modellierung beinhalten die Erstellung eines detaillierten MKS-Modells der Lendenwirbelsäule (links) und der Körpersilhouetten eines normalgewichtigen (mitte links) und eines adipösen Mannes (mitte rechts) und die Fusion der CAD-Körpersilhouette mit dem MKS-Lendenwirbelsäulenmodell (rechts).

Bauer_500N eine Extensionsbewegung durch. Dies führt zu einer Entlastung der Bandscheibe.

Zur weiteren Validierung des MKS-Lendenwirbelsäulen-Modells wurde eine ausführliche Sensibilitätsanalyse der Input-Parameter vorgenommen [7, 8, 9]. Die Intention dieser Analyse war die Identifizierung von Parametern, die bereits bei kleinen Wertänderungen einen signifikanten Einfluss auf die Simulationsergebnisse haben.

2.2 Erstellung von Oberflächenmodellen

Zur Erstellung der zwei Oberflächenmodelle inklusive deren anthropometrischen Eigenschaften wird zuerst das Körpergewicht eines 35-jährigen normalgewichtigen (75kg, BMI 22) und eines adipösen (Grad II, 127kg, BMI 37) Mannes über den Körpermassenindex (BMI) berechnet. Unter Berücksichtigung des berechneten Gewichts, des Geschlechts, des Alters, der Körpergröße (1,85m) und der Herkunft wurden zwei Oberflachenmodelle, ein normalgewichtiger Mann und ein adipöser Mann, mit Hilfe von Open-Source-Softwarelösungen zur Erstellung von menschlichen 3D-Oberflächen so kreiert, dass mittels eines Massenverteilungsmodells nach Zatsiorskj [10] die Massenverteilung der einzelnen Körpersegmente bestimmt werden kann.

2.3 Fusion des MKS-Lendenwirbelsäulenmodells mit den Oberflächenmodellen

Durch Fusion der Oberflächenmodelle mit dem detaillierten biomechanischen Modell der Lendenwirbelsäule entstehen zwei neue Simulationsmodelle, mit deren Hilfe nun die Auswirkungen eines normalgewichtigen und eines adipösen Mannes analysiert werden. Dabei sind die einzelnen Körpersegmente starr miteinander verbunden. Anzumerken ist, dass für die Simulation der gesamten Gewichtskraft ausschließlich die Körpersegmente berücksichtigt werden, die oberhalb des Sacrums liegen, da nur diese Strukturen auf die Lendenwirbelsäule

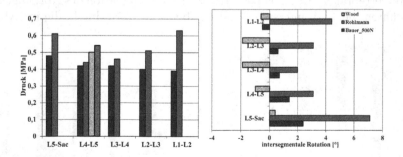

Abb. 2. Vergleich der Ergebnisse des intervertebralen Drucks und intersegmentalen Rotation aus MKS- und FE-Simluationen und in-vivo Experimenten, wobei positive Rotationswinkel einer Flexionsbewegung entsprechen.

einwirken. Als Kraftangriffspunkt der Gesamtgewichtskraft dieser einzelnen Körpersegmente ist der Mittelpunkt der Deckfläche des Lendenwirbels L1 definiert. Auf diesen Mittelpunkt der Deckfläche wirkt die Gewichtskraft aller Körpersegmente oberhalb des Sacrums mit ihren berechneten Massen. Diese auf die Deckfläche wirkende äußere Kraft löst die Kinematik des MKS-Modells aus und die Bewegungsgleichungen, die ein System gekoppelter Differentialgleichungen bilden, werden für jeden Zeitschritt integriert. Konkret bedeutet das, dass diese Gewichtskraft kleine Bewegungen in den spinalen Strukturen hervorruft und sie aus ihrem Gleichgewichtszustand herausgebracht werden. Die Reaktionskräfte der einzelnen spinalen Strukturen bauen sich auf, bis ein neuer Gleichgewichtszustand erreicht ist. Die folgenden Ergebnisse beziehen sich auf diesen neuen Gleichgewichtszustand und stellen nicht den zeitlichen Verlauf der kinematischen Werte dar.

3   Ergebnisse

Die in vertikaler Richtung auf die Deckfläche des Wirbelkörpers L1 gerichtet wirkende Gewichtskraft führt zu einer Deformation der Bandscheiben. Generell ist festzuhalten, dass die Deformationswerte bei den durch normalkörpergewichtbelasteten Bandscheiben relativ gering sind. In diesem Fall werden die Bandscheiben aller funktionalen Einheiten weniger als 0,02 cm deformiert, wobei die Bandscheibe der untersten funktionalen Einheit Sac-L5, sowohl bei Belastung mit Normalgewicht als auch bei Adipositas, die größte Deformation erfährt. Im direkten Vergleich der beiden Lastfälle ist zu sehen, dass die Bandscheiben einer adipösen Person mehr als 2,5-fach höher deformiert sind, als bei einer normalgewichtigen Person (Abb. 3 links).

Während des Deformationsprozesses entwickeln die Bandscheiben Kräfte, die entgegen der Deformationsrichtung wirken. Diese Belastungen der Bandscheiben eines adipösen Mannes, verglichen mit einem normalgewichtigen Mann, sind mehr als 3,5-mal höher (Abb. 3, rechts). Da die Gewichtskraft einen Hebelarm zu den einzelnen Drehzentren der Bandscheiben aufweist, entstehen Drehmomente, die intervertebrale Rotationen hervorrufen. In der Simulation des Normalgewichtigen führen die zwei untersten Bandscheiben Flexionen durch, die in (Abb. 4,

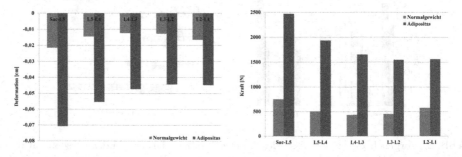

Abb. 3. Vergleich der Deformationen der Bandscheiben und Vergleich der Bandscheibenkräfte.

links) als positive Werte dargestellt werden. Die funktionale Einheit L4-L3 führt eine Extensionsbewegung durch und die darüber gelegenen funktionalen Einheiten wieder eine Flexionsbewegung. Bei den intervertebralen Rotationen eines adipösen Mannes handelt es sich ausschließlich um Flexionsbewegungen und diese sind in den untersten zwei funktionalen Einheiten fast dreimal, in der funktionalen Einheit L3-L2 nahezu achtmal und in der obersten funktionalen Einheit wieder dreimal so hoch, wie die eines normalgewichtigen Mannes.

Die verschiedenen Gewichtsklassen haben auch Einfluss auf die Belastungen der Facettengelenke. Es ist auffällig, dass nur in manchen funktionalen Einheiten die Facetten belastet werden (Abb. 4, rechts). Eine Kraft in den Facettengelenken entsteht nur, wenn zwei miteinander korrespondierende Gelenksflächen in Kontakt treten. Ob eine Kraftentwicklung stattfindet, hängt stark von der Bewegungsrichtung der einzelnen Wirbelkörper ab. Ein besonders hoher Belastungsanstieg verzeichnet die unterste funktionale Einheit Sac-L5. Eine mögliche Erklärung hierfür könnte die Orientierung die Facettenflächen dieser funktionalen Einheit sein. Während die darüber befindlichen Facettenflächen eher parallel zur Bewegungsrichtung der Wirbelkörper ausgerichtet sind und somit die Möglichkeit besteht, dass sie aneinander „vorbeigleiten", sind die untersten Facettenflächen Sac-L5 stärker orthogonal zu der Bewegungsrichtung ausgerichtet. Die mögliche Auswirkung dieser Ausrichtung kann eine erhöhte Belastung dieser untersten funktionalen Einheit Sac-L5 sein.

Bei beiden Gewichtsklassen werden die Facettengelenke der funktionalen Einheit L5-L4, L3-L2 und L2-L1 nur sehr gering bzw. gar nicht belastet. Dies kann eine Folge der zum Teil großen Flexionsbewegungen dieser funktionalen Einheiten sein. Durch die Vorwärtsrotation (Abb. 4) kommen die Kontaktflächen der entsprechenden Gelenkflächen nicht miteinander in Berührung, sodass keine Kontaktkraft in diesen Facettengelenken aufgebaut wird.

4 Diskussion

Es wurden zwei Computermodelle zur Berechnung der Belastungen auf die inneren Strukturen sowie zur Darstellung der Kinematik während der Belastungs-

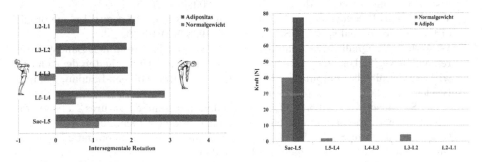

Abb. 4. Intervertebrale Rotationen der verschiedenen funktionalen Einheiten (links) und Kontaktkräfte der Facettengelenke (rechts)

situationen „Normalgewicht" und „Adipositas" erstellt. Es ist deutlich zu erkennen, dass die Gewichtszunahme starke Auswirkungen auf die Belastungen der Bandscheiben hat und diese erhöhten Belastungen zu langfristigen Schäden führen kann. Daher ist das Hauptziel unseres Forschungsprojekts, ein Werkzeug zur individualisierten Operationsplanung unter Berücksichtigung der sagittalen Balance bei natürlicher Körperbelastung von übergewichtigen und adipösen Patienten mit symptomatischen segmentalen Instabilitäten an der Wirbelsäule zu entwickeln. Da die Mehrkörpersimulation hocheffizient mit kurzen Rechenzeiten realisiert wird, ist eine spätere Nutzung in realen Systemen möglich. Eine besondere Bedeutung kommt der Validierung des Computermodells zu. Die berechneten Ergebnisse sind qualitativ so gut, wie es seine Modellierung zulässt. Es können anhand des Modells Aussagen getroffen werden, die jedoch schwierig anhand von aktuellen Publikationen zu belegen sind, da meist nicht alle Parameter veröffentlicht sind, die eine signifikante Auswirkung auf das Ergebnis haben. Die Kurvatur der Wirbelsäule hat beispielsweise eine starke Auswirkung auf die Verteilung der Belastung innerhalb der spinalen Strukturen [3]. Demzufolge ist es notwendig weitere Studien und somit weitere Parameter einzubeziehen, wozu auch die verbesserte Abbildung der Anteile von Muskulatur und Fettgewebe zählt. Dazu soll in unserem Forschungsprojekt eine Methode zur Fusionierung der Körpersilhouette und Massenverteilung mittels Aufrecht-Scan und MRT-Aufnahmen entwickelt werden.

Literaturverzeichnis

1. Andersson G.   Epidemiological features of chronic low-back pain.   Lancet. 1999;354(9178):581–5.
2. Djurasovic M, Bratcher KR, Glassman SD, et al. The effect of obesity on clinical outcomes after lumbar fusion. Spine. 2008;33(16):1789–92.
3. Wilke HJ, Neef P, Caimi M, et al. New InVivo measurement of pressure in the interverte-bral disc in daily life. Spine. 1999;24:755–62.
4. Sato K, Kiuchi S, Yonezawa T. In Vivo intradiscal pressure measurement in healthy individuals and in patients with ongoing back problems. Spine. 1999;24:2468–74.
5. Rohlmann A, Zander T, Bergmann G. Applying a follower load delivers realistic results for simulating standing. J Biomech. 2009;49:1520–6.
6. Wood K, Kos P, Schendel M, et al. Effects of position on the sagittal-plane profile of the thoracolumbal spine. J Spinal Disord. 1996;9(2):165–9.
7. Wasserhess C. Qualitative Analyse des Einflusses der Kräfte in den Bandstrukturen auf Beweglichkeit und Belastung einzelner funktionaler Einheiten der Lendenwirbelsäule mittels Computermodellierung. Universität Koblenz-Landau, Campus Koblenz; 2012.
8. Bauer S, Hausen U, Gruber K. Effects of individual spine curvatures - a comparative study with the help of computer modelling. Biomed Tech. 2012.
9. Gruber K, Juchem S. Realisation of physical properties in a computer model of the lumbar spine. J Biomechanics. 2008; p. 358.
10. Zatsiorskj VM. Massengeometrie des menschlichen Körpers. Theorie und Praxis Körperkultur. 1982;31:416–423.

Markov Random Field-Based Layer Separation for Simulated X-Ray Image Sequences

Peter Fischer[1], Thomas Pohl[2], Andreas Maier[1], Joachim Hornegger[1]

[1] Pattern Recognition Lab and Erlangen Graduate School in Advanced Optical
Technologies (SAOT), Friedrich-Alexander Universität Erlangen-Nürnberg
[2] Siemens Healthcare, Forchheim
peter.fischer@fau.de

Abstract. Motion estimation in X-ray images is a challenging task due
to transparently overlapping structures from different depths. We propose to separate an X-ray sequence into a static and a dynamic layer to
facilitate motion estimation. The method exploits the idea to use the
minimum intensity over time and a spatial smoothness prior for both
layers. For numerical optimization, we propose a conditional Markov
random field. In experiments on synthetic data, we achieve a root mean
squared intensity difference of 36.7 ± 8.4 to the ground truth static layer.
In addition, we show qualitative results that demonstrate an improved
layer separation compared to state-of-the-art algorithms.

1 Introduction

X-ray images are 2D projection images formed by accumulated attenuation along
a line through a 3D volume. This leads to a transparency effect that enables
physicians to examine the interior of the human body. However, it also means
that structures from different depths overlap transparently in the images. In
many cases, some of the projected structures are unnecessary or even hinder
interpretation and processing of the images. In particular, motion estimation is
substantially complicated [1]. Many image registration algorithms are based on
intensity similarities. Hence, the estimated motion is dominated by the high-
contrast structures. However, the motion of the soft tissue that is investigated
in the intervention is required. A separation of X-ray images into independent
layers is therefore desired.

In literature, multiple approaches to layer separation in X-ray images have
been proposed. Early methods were restricted to rigid motion of the layers and
separated the layers by averaging the stabilized X-ray sequences [2]. Preston
et al. alternate between non-rigid motion estimation and layer separation [3].
Layer separation is easier for dual-energy X-ray, where additional spectral information is available. In this domain, separation can be performed without motion
estimation based on minimizing the mutual information between the layers [4].
Transparent layer separation has also been treated in computer vision. Szeliski
et al. iteratively estimate parametric motion and layers, using the minimum over

time to extract the static layer from a stabilized sequence [5]. Weiss separates the reflectance from the temporally changing illumination using an independence assumption and the sparsity of natural images in the gradient domain [6].

The contribution of this work is a new method for layer separation. It builds on the idea to use the pixel-wise minimum over time of a X-ray sequence to extract layers. However, in some cases the minimum does not correspond to semantically meaningful images. Prior knowledge, e.g., spatial smoothness and non-negativity, is useful to restrict the layers. We introduce a combined formulation for spatial smoothness of both transparent layers. The model is formulated as a conditional Markov random field (CRF). In the experiments, we show that our method separates X-ray sequences into two motion layers on synthetic data.

2   Materials and methods

2.1   Layered X-ray model

X-ray images are generated by X-ray photons that are attenuated on their path through an imaged volume. We assume monochromatic X-ray. Attenuation is an exponential process, which can be transformed to a linear relationship between image intensities and attenuation using logarithmic processing [7]. We are interested in separating X-ray images into differently moving layers. Therefore, all tissues that undergo a similar motion are summarized into a single layer I_l. The image $I^t \in [0, 255]^{W \times H}$ at time $t \in \{1, \ldots, T\}$ is then computed from the layers as

$$I^t(x) = \sum_{l=0}^{L-1} I_l^t(x) \tag{1}$$

with the image pixel $x \in \mathbb{R}^2$ and the number of layers L. In this work, we limit ourselves to $L = 2$ transparent layers, a static $I_0 = S$ and a dynamic $I_1 = D$ layer. The whole sequence of X-ray images is denoted as I.

2.2   Layer separation using a conditional markov random field

The basic assumption of our layer separation model is that the layer S is static. A straightforward method to remove a static layer from an X-ray sequence is to compute the pixel-wise minimum over time

$$S^{\min}(x) = \min_t I^t(x) \tag{2}$$

because the dynamic layer can only increase attenuation. This min-composite yields an upper bound on the static layer [5]. Its major problem is that artificial edges are introduced. If an object is larger than the motion it performs in the sequence, a part of the object is assigned to the static layer (Fig. 1). In particular in medical images, moving structures are physically a better explanation than appearing and disappearing structures. To this end, we penalize the creation of artificial edges by introducing a spatial smoothness prior on both layers.

We formulate the layer separation problem in a CRF model. Due to the assumption of a static layer, it is sufficient to represent each static layer pixel with a random variable. The intensity of the dynamic layer can be calculated directly from the static layer and the image

$$D^t(\boldsymbol{x}) = I^t(\boldsymbol{x}) - S(\boldsymbol{x}) \tag{3}$$

The random variables have discrete labels $z \in \mathcal{Z}$ representing the intensity $z_i = S(\boldsymbol{x}_i)$. The labels of all random variables are denoted as $\boldsymbol{z}$. $\mathcal{Z}$ contains equally distributed intensities in $[0, 255]$ without loss of generality.

In the CRF, we incorporate unary potentials Φ_v for nodes $v \in \mathcal{V}$ and pair-wise potentials Ψ_{ij} for edges $(i,j) \in \mathcal{E}$

$$E(\boldsymbol{z}, \boldsymbol{I}) = \sum_{v \in \mathcal{V}} \Phi_v(z_v, \boldsymbol{I}(\boldsymbol{x}_v)) + \sum_{(i,j) \in \mathcal{E}} \Psi_{ij}(z_i, z_j, \boldsymbol{I}(\boldsymbol{x}_i), \boldsymbol{I}(\boldsymbol{x}_j)) \tag{4}$$

The unary potential function

$$\Phi_v(z_v, \boldsymbol{I}(\boldsymbol{x}_v)) = \begin{cases} \alpha \min\left\{\beta, \sum_{t=1}^{T} \|z_v - I^t(\boldsymbol{x}_v)\|_1\right\} & \text{if } z_v \le I^t(\boldsymbol{x}_v)\,\forall t \\ \infty & \text{otherwise} \end{cases} \tag{5}$$

with parameters $\alpha, \beta \in \mathbb{R}$ penalizes deviations from the min-composite using a truncated L_1-norm. The unary potential ensures the non-negativity constraint of the X-ray generation model in the dynamic layer. The static layer is non-negative by definition of the label set $\mathcal{Z}$. Φ_v prevents the static layer from being larger than any of the images $I^t(\boldsymbol{x}_v)$ by assigning infinite weight, thus avoiding a negative dynamic layer. Note that the minimum of the unary potential is achieved by the min-composite.

The potential Ψ_{ij} consists of pair-wise terms $(i,j) \in \mathcal{E}$ in a 4-neighborhood

$$\Psi_{ij}(z_i, z_j, \boldsymbol{I}(\boldsymbol{x}_i), \boldsymbol{I}(\boldsymbol{x}_j)) = \|z_i - z_j\|_1 + \sum_{t=1}^{T} \left\|(z_i - z_j) - (I^t(\boldsymbol{x}_i) - I^t(\boldsymbol{x}_j))\right\|_1 \tag{6}$$

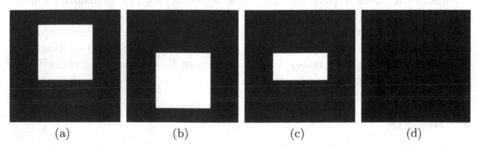

| (a) | (b) | (c) | (d) |

Fig. 1. Visualization of the artificial edge creation problem of the min-composite. The inputs are a white rectangle moving on a black background (a,b). Areas that are covered in all images by the rectangle are assigned to static layer for the min-composite (c). The desired result is a reached by our method (d).

A common image prior is to penalize gradients, e.g., using the L_1-norm to promote sparsity. (6) jointly encodes smoothness of both layers. This is straightforward for the static layer using $\|z_i - z_j\|_1$. It needs to be added only once, because the pixel values of the static layer are perfectly statistically dependent $p\left(\boldsymbol{S}(\boldsymbol{x})\right) = p\left(S(\boldsymbol{x})\right)$ over time. For the dynamic layer, we reformulate $\|D^t\left(\boldsymbol{x}_i\right) - D^t\left(\boldsymbol{x}_j\right)\|_1$ using (3), thus removing the need to directly model D^t. Assuming statistical independence of the gradients over time $p\left(\boldsymbol{D}(\boldsymbol{x})\right) = \prod_{t=1}^{T} p\left(D^t(\boldsymbol{x})\right)$, different time steps can be combined by summation in the energy. With the assumption of independence of the static and the dynamic layer $p\left(\boldsymbol{S}(\boldsymbol{x}), \boldsymbol{D}(\boldsymbol{x})\right) = p\left(\boldsymbol{S}(\boldsymbol{x})\right) \cdot p\left(\boldsymbol{D}(\boldsymbol{x})\right)$, the individual layer contributions can be added (6). Note that the minimum of the pair-wise potential is achieved by the median gradient over time [6].

To perform the layer separation in a new X-ray sequence, the maximum a posteriori (MAP) estimate of the CRF model is obtained by

$$z^* = \operatorname*{argmin}_{z} E\left(\boldsymbol{z}, \boldsymbol{I}\right) \tag{7}$$

This yields the statistically optimal layer under this model given the input sequence. For inference, sequential tree-reweighted message passing (TRWS) [8] in the OpenGM framework is used [9].

2.3   Experiments

In the experiments, we compare the proposed algorithm to the min-composite [5] and Weiss method [6]. Min-composite and Weiss method do not have any parameters. The parameters of our method were set empirically to $\alpha = 0.1, \beta = 10$. TRWS optimization is run for 40 iterations, using $\|\mathcal{Z}\| = 256$ labels.

As experimental data, we use four simulated X-ray sequences. Simulated images resemble real X-ray images, but ground truth is still available. They are created by adding two independent layers, where one is static and the other one dynamic. Layers are created by segmenting 3D volumes and projecting the parts independently to 2D. The 3D volumes are created by clinical CT scanners or simulations using CONRAD [10]. The dynamic layer is transformed with artificial motions, which are interpolated from manually specified control point motions using thin-plate splines. The error is computed as the root mean squared difference (RMSD) of the image intensities. Before the RMSD, we subtract the mean from the compared layers, because it cannot be uniquely determined and is not relevant for motion estimation.

3   Results

The RMSD error for the min-composite is 42.1 ± 8.4, for the Weiss method 42.2 ± 6.9, and for our method 36.7 ± 8.4 (mean $\pm$ standard deviation). These results indicate a better performance of our method compared to the others.

Two X-ray sequences from different views including the spine, diaphragm, ribs, heart, and lungs are depicted in Fig. 2. The images are already preprocessed to fit the additive model. The sequence in the first row is created using CONRAD. Note that the static structures are removed from the dynamic layer in all cases. The main difference is how well the soft tissue is preserved. There, the problem of artificial edges is clearly visible in the min-composite. In the second sequence created from a 3D CT, more structure is present in the soft tissue. Nevertheless, the same problems occur in the min-composite. Our approach and Weiss method perform similarly well. Both have problems with inconsistent gradient estimates, e.g., visible in the liver in the first sequence. The main differences is that Weiss method does not ensure non-negativity of the dynamic layer, which corresponds to physically impossible negative attenuations. Non-negativity of the static layer can be achieved by simple postprocessing. Another difference is an offset of the mean intensity, which cannot be uniquely determined from gradient information alone, but is irrelevant for subsequent motion estimation.

The runtime of the method depends linearly on the number of pixels. For images of size $W = H = 256$ and a sequence of length $T = 50$, the runtime is about 200 s.

4   Discussion

We propose a novel approach to separate an X-ray image sequence into static and dynamic layers. This intermediate representation can facilitate further processing. In particular, soft tissue motion estimation would not be possible without it due to overlapping structures from different depths. The separation is based on the min-composite, which is only an upper bound on the static layer. Our method adds a smoothness term to suppress artificial edges in either layer.

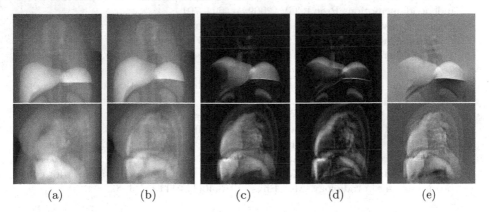

(a)   (b)   (c)   (d)   (e)

Fig. 2. Qualitative results on simulated X-ray sequences are shown, one per row: two images of the input sequence (a,b), a dynamic layer extracted using our (c), min-composite (d), and Weiss (e) method. Contrast is enhanced for better display.

The current runtime of the method is not yet sufficient for clinical use. However, real-time performance is not feasible by design, as a whole image sequence is postprocessed. The goal can only be to reduce the latency to a minimum.

In future work, the method needs to be transferred to and tested on clinical X-ray data. The validity of a static layer is questionable for clinical X-ray images. Some structures, e.g., ribs, move slightly, although from an application point of view they should be in the static layer. Additionally, patient body motion is possible. Consequently, the robustness of the method to these challenges needs to be evaluated. In the future, the use of the dynamic layer for motion estimation should be investigated. Furthermore, substantial speed ups of the method are possible for example using an inference method that is amenable to parallelization and a GPU implementation.

Acknowledgement. The authors gratefully acknowledge funding by Siemens Healthcare and of the Erlangen Graduate School in Advanced Optical Technologies (SAOT) by the German Research Foundation (DFG) in the framework of the German excellence initiative. The concepts and information presented in this paper are based on research and are not commercially available.

References

1. Klüppel M, Wang J, Bernecker D, et al. On feature tracking in X-ray images. Proc BVM. 2014; p. 132–7.
2. Close RA, Abbey CK, Morioka CA, et al. Accuracy assessment of layer decomposition using simulated angiographic image sequences. IEEE Trans Med Imaging. 2001;20(10):990–8.
3. Preston JS, Rottman C, Cheryauka A, et al. Multi-layer deformation estimation for fluoroscopic imaging. Lect Notes Computer Sci. 2013;7917:123–34.
4. Chen Y, Chang TC, Zhou C, et al.; IEEE. Gradient domain layer separation under independent motion. Proc ICCV. 2009; p. 694–701.
5. Szeliski R, Avidan S, Anandan P. Layer extraction from multiple images containing reflections and transparency. Proc ICCVPR. 2000;1:246–53.
6. Weiss Y. Deriving intrinsic images from image sequences. Proc ICCV. 2001;2:68–75.
7. Buzug TM. Computed Tomography: From Photon Statistics to Modern Cone-Beam CT. Springer; 2008.
8. Kolmogorov V. Convergent tree-reweighted message passing for energy minimization. IEEE Trans Pattern Anal Mach Intell. 2006;28(10):1568–83.
9. Andres B, Beier T, Kappes JH. OpenGM: a C++ library for discrete graphical models. arXiv. 2012;1206.0111:1–5.
10. Maier A, Hofmann H, Berger M, et al. CONRAD: a software framework for cone-beam imaging in radiology. Med Phys. 2013;40(11):111914–1–8.

Image Registration with Sliding Motion Constraints for 4D CT Motion Correction

Alexander Derksen[1], Stefan Heldmann[1], Thomas Polzin[2], Benjamin Berkels[3]

[1]Fraunhofer MEVIS Project Group Image Registration, Lübeck
[2]Institute of Mathematics and Image Computing, University of Lübeck
[3]Aachen Institute for Advanced Study in Computational Engineering Science, RWTH Aachen University

alexander.derksen@mevis.fraunhofer.de

Abstract. A common assumption in medical image registration is that the estimation of a globally continuous deformation field is plausible in reality. However, a sliding behavior of adjacent organ boundaries (e.g. lung and ribcage) cannot be described in a plausible way by a continuous deformation field. In this paper, we address this issue with a novel registration framework that explicitly models sliding of interfaces and can preserve discontinuities in the deformation field along predefined organ boundaries. Incorporated methods involve constrained nonlinear registration and a finite element discretization on unstructured tetrahedral meshes. Evaluation is based on the freely available DIR-Lab datasets.

1 Introduction

Image registration aims at establishing correspondences between two given images. One of many possible applications is follow-up evaluation, of e.g. pre- and postoperative scans to determine surgery success [1]. Here, we focus on registration of thoracic CT scans from different respiration phases. The established correspondences allow e.g. to detect local lung volume changes during respiration for COPD screening [2, 3] and improved treatment planning for radiotherapy [4].

Numerous sliding organ interfaces are located inside the human body. Certainly, the respiratory motion induced sliding of lung and ribcage is one of the well-known cases of sliding motion. An accurate estimation of lung motion is critical e.g. for an effective radiotherapeutic treatment of tumors. Particularly for targets near the ribcage sliding motion should be modeled adequately. A characteristic property of sliding motion is that deformations along the sliding interface cannot be described in a continuous way. However, common registration techniques assume global continuity of the deformation and thus are unsuitable for sliding motion. Closing this gap is an active research topic and several registration techniques have been proposed recently in this context.

Schmidt-Richberg et al. [5] used diffusive regularization and a distance measure similar to Thirions demons forces to register in regions without a sliding interface. Near the interface, the deformation is split into tangential and normal motion and regularized direction-dependently to recover a smooth motion in the normal component while allowing for discontinuities in the tangential part. Pace et al. augment these ideas by the possibility to control the direction of regularization with the usage of diffusion tensors [6]. They also used diffusion regularization which is now locally adaptive based on the construction of the tensors but the penalized energy is globally defined. This is beneficial for instance if several sliding organs are considered. Recently, the usage of individual biomechanical models allowing for sliding motion followed by a deformable registration was proposed by Han et al. [7]. The main volume change and motion is captured by physical modeling of pressures and applying them to a finite element mesh of tetrahedra. Free-form deformation with the Mutual Information distance measure and B-spline transformations is subsequently performed to handle inaccuracies.

In this paper, we propose a novel registration framework, incorporating a constraint designed for registration of organs with sliding interfaces.

2   Materials and methods

In this work we extend a general variational image registration approach with an explicit model for sliding organs via additional constraints and evaluate it on publicly available 4D CT data.

2.1   Modeling

Variational approach Given a reference image $R\colon \mathbb{R}^d \to \mathbb{R}$, a template image $T\colon \mathbb{R}^d \to \mathbb{R}$, and a domain $\Omega \subset \mathbb{R}^d$ ($d = 2,3$) the goal is to find a reasonable deformation field $y\colon \Omega \to \mathbb{R}^d$ such that $R(x) \approx T(y(x))$ for $x \in \Omega$. To this end, we minimize a joint functional $\mathcal{J}(y) := \mathcal{D}(y) + \alpha \mathcal{S}(y)$, where $\mathcal{D}$ is a distance measure quantifying the similarity of images and $\mathcal{S}$ is a regularizer ensuring smoothness of the deformation, see e.g. [8] for details. Without loss of generality here we consider the sum-of-squared-differences [8] distance measure and hyperelastic regularization given by

$$\mathcal{D}(y) := \frac{1}{|\Omega|} \int_{\Omega} (T(y(x)) - R(x))^2 \; \mathrm{d}x \tag{1}$$

$$\mathcal{S}(y) := \int_{\Omega} \frac{\lambda}{2} \operatorname{tr}(E)^2 + \mu \operatorname{tr}(E^2) \; + \beta \log(\det(\nabla y))^2 \mathrm{d}x \tag{2}$$

with Green-St-Vernant tensor $E := \frac{1}{2}(\nabla y^\top \nabla y - I)$ and $\log(a) := \infty$ for $a \le 0$.

Sliding motion For sake of simplicity in the following we model sliding motion at the boundary of a single organ. The extension to multiple organs is straightforward. However, let $\Omega_{\mathrm{in}} \subset \Omega$ be the subdomain that is occupied by the organ and let $\Omega_{\mathrm{out}} := \Omega \setminus \overline{\Omega_{\mathrm{in}}}$. We further assume that Ω_{in} is strictly inside the image domain Ω such that $\partial\Omega_{\mathrm{in}} \cap \partial\Omega = \emptyset$. Then sliding shall be possible along the joint interface $\Sigma := \partial\Omega_{\mathrm{in}}$ of Ω_{in} and Ω_{out}. Clearly, the desired deformation y

cannot be smooth. To still be able to work with smooth deformations, we split the deformation and the registration problem, respectively. Instead of one deformation, we now are looking for two smooth deformations $y_{in} : \Omega_{in} \cup \Sigma \to \mathbb{R}^d$ and $y_{out} : \Omega_{out} \cup \Sigma \to \mathbb{R}^d$ such that

$$y_{in}(\Sigma) = y_{out}(\Sigma) \tag{3}$$

and $y(x) := y_{in}(x)$ for $x \in \Omega_{in} \cup \Sigma$ and $y(x) := y_{out}(x)$ for $x \in \Omega_{out}$. Thus both deformations are independent from each other but linked on the interface Σ. Note that the sliding constraint $y_{in}(\Sigma) = y_{out}(\Sigma)$ is not a point-wise but set-valued constraint, since $y_{in}(\Sigma) = \{y_{in}(x) \colon x \in \Sigma\}$ and $y_{out}(\Sigma) = \{y_{out}(x) \colon x \in \Sigma\}$. Hence, we consider two separate registration problems linked via the constraint (3)

$$\left. \begin{array}{ll} \text{Minimize} & \mathcal{D}(y_{in}) + \mathcal{D}(y_{out}) + \alpha\big(\mathcal{S}(y_{in}) + \mathcal{S}(y_{out})\big) \\ \text{subject to} & y_{in}(\Sigma) = y_{out}(\Sigma) \end{array} \right\} \tag{4}$$

with the implicit understanding that the integrals (1) and (2) in $\mathcal{D}$ and $\mathcal{S}$ are defined on Ω_{in} and Ω_{out}, respectively, rather than on the whole domain Ω.

Discretization The deformations y_{in} and y_{out} are discretized independently. We use finite elements to resolve the geometries of Ω_{in} and Ω_{out} reasonably and discretize deformations as piecewise linear functions on tetrahedral meshes (Delaunay triangulation). Then, $\mathcal{S}$ can be computed exactly and $\mathcal{D}$ is discretized by common mid-point rule quadrature on a rectangular regular grid.

For the discretization of the constraint we exploit the tetrahedral mesh structure. The sliding interface Σ is already discretized by the boundary of the tetrahedral meshes for Ω_{in} and Ω_{out} (Fig. 1, middle and right). Thus we have two sets of faces Σ_{in} and Σ_{out} that represent Σ. In general, the polyhedral structure of the discretization prevents continuous sliding of the faces if $y_{in}(\Sigma_{in}) = y_{out}(\Sigma_{out})$ is enforced. Therefore we introduce the penalty function

$$\mathcal{P}(y_{in}, y_{out}) := \sum_{x \in N_{in}} d(y_{in}(x), y_{out}(\Sigma_{out}))^2 + \sum_{x \in N_{out}} d(y_{out}(x), y_{in}(\Sigma_{in}))^2 \tag{5}$$

with $d(z, A) := \inf_{a \in A} \|z - a\|_2$ and the node sets $N_{in} := \text{Nodes}(\Sigma_{in})$ and $N_{out} := \text{Nodes}(\Sigma_{out})$. Summarizing, we solve the optimization problem

$$\text{Minimize} \quad \mathcal{D}(y_{in}) + \mathcal{D}(y_{out}) + \alpha\big(\mathcal{S}(y_{in}) + \mathcal{S}(y_{out})\big) + \gamma\mathcal{P}(y_{in}, y_{out}) \tag{6}$$

with regularization parameter $\alpha > 0$ and penalty parameter $\gamma > 0$.

2.2 Data and evaluation

For evaluation, the well-known DIR-Lab 4D CT data sets were used [9]. Additionally to each of the five 4D scans, 300 landmarks were annotated by medical

338   Alexander Derksen[1], Stefan Heldmann[1], Thomas Polzin[2], Benjamin Berkels[3]

Fig. 1. Example of a 2D Delaunay triangulation discretizing Ω and Σ, in the decompositions Ω_{in} and Ω_{out}. The interface Σ is drawn as red ellipse.

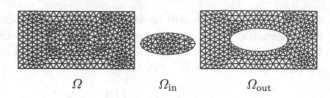

Ω Ω_{in} Ω_{out}

experts [9] in the end-inhale (EI) and end-exhale (EE) phase. For all conducted experiments, we used EE as template image and EI as reference image.

The proposed method was compared with the same registration without the soft penalty $\mathcal{P}$ and partition of Ω, i.e. $\Omega_{out} = \Omega$, $\Omega_{in} = \Sigma = \emptyset$ and $\gamma = 0$. For comparison, one-sided Wilcoxon rank sum tests were performed with level of significance $\alpha_W = 0.05$ to investigate if the difference in median expert landmark error is significant for sliding versus non-sliding motion registration. Furthermore, results were compared quantitatively on the landmarks to the sliding motion registration approaches [5] and [6], which use a similar distance measure.

Our implementation uses a mesh for each lung leading to two separate sliding interfaces (Fig. 2). To generate an appropriate mesh the lungs were segmented according to [10]. Surface mesh generation was performed using MeVisLab and volume mesh generation has been done via the Matlab package *iso2mesh*[1]. On average the left lung meshes consisted of 2146 tetrahedra and the right lung meshes consisted of 2435 tetrahedra. The complementary mesh on Ω_{out} consisted of 18062 elements. For the scenario without sliding motion, a single connected mesh with 21161 elements was used. All registrations were performed in Matlab.

Fig. 2. Example of lung surface meshes representing two separate sliding interfaces, i.e. the lungs were treated as two separate sliding organs. Meshes were generated from DIR-Lab data set 5.

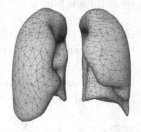

Parameters were equal for all tests and have been determined empirically as $\lambda = 0$, $\mu = 1$, $\alpha = 10^{-2}$ and $\beta = 10^{-8}$. Problem (6) was solved iteratively with increasing $\gamma = 10^{-2}, 10^{-1}, \ldots, 10^2$ to allow for a good alignment with less cohesive meshes for lower values of γ but generating tightly connected meshes in the final result.

3   Results

Accuracy of the registration was measured as landmark target registration error (TRE) on the DIR-Lab data sets, cf. [5]. The resulting means and standard

---

[1] http://iso2mesh.sourceforge.net

Table 1. Comparison of DIR-Lab landmark distances before and after registration. All values are given in mm as mean ± standard deviation. Significant lower median TRE for sliding motion compared to no sliding registration is indicated by an asterisk.

Case	Initial [9]	Pace et al. [6]	DDR detect [5]	No Sliding	Sliding
1	3.89 ± 2.78	1.06 ± 0.57	1.22 ± 0.64	1.72 ± 1.30	1.02 ± 0.50*
2	4.34 ± 3.90	1.45 ± 1.00	1.14 ± 0.65	2.46 ± 2.28	1.12 ± 0.59*
3	6.94 ± 4.05	1.88 ± 1.35	1.36 ± 0.81	4.15 ± 3.08	1.49 ± 0.96*
4	9.83 ± 4.86	2.04 ± 1.40	2.68 ± 2.79	5.78 ± 3.82	1.99 ± 1.53*
5	7.48 ± 5.51	2.73 ± 2.13	1.57 ± 1.23	4.47 ± 3.50	2.08 ± 1.81*
average	6.50 ± 4.22	1.83 ± 1.29	1.59 ± 1.22	3.72 ± 2.80	1.54 ± 1.08*

deviations are given in Tab. 1. Deformed template images $T(y)$ and deformation fields y of all data sets were visually inspected to ensure that the sliding motion of the lungs could be successfully recovered. Fig. 3 shows a central coronal slice of the registration result of the fourth DIR-Lab data set together with the corresponding deformation field.

R with sliding contour Σ T $|T - R|$

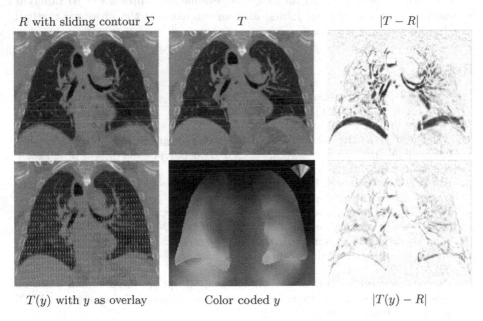

$T(y)$ with y as overlay   Color coded y $|T(y) - R|$

Fig. 3. Registration result of DIR-Lab data set 4. Note the respiratory motion induced discontinuity in y at the lung boundary Σ. Absolute difference image plots are inverted such that white areas are well aligned. Deformation y was in the direction of the depicted quarter cycle. Hue describes magnitude of motion (bright means large motion).

4 Discussion

We have presented a constrained registration framework designed to recover discontinuities in the deformation field caused by sliding organ interfaces. The proposed method was evaluated on 4D inhale/exhale thoracic CT scans. In all cases, the respiratory motion induced discontinuities in the deformation field at the lung boundary could be recovered, leading to more plausible registration results. The TRE could be improved significantly ($p < 10^{-9}$) in all cases compared to the proposed registration approach without sliding constraint. Furthermore, for each case the TRE is in the range of results computed by Schmidt-Richberg et al. and Pace et al. This is reflected in an average of 1.54 ± 1.08 mm over all test cases whereas the reported values are 1.59 ± 1.22 mm [5] and 1.83 ± 1.29 mm [6], respectively.

The proposed sliding registration framework is by design highly modular, i.e. standard choices of regularization can be integrated without modification. The same holds for the distance measure which might be beneficial for data sets with more breathing motion induced or disease related intensity changes.

For future work, we plan an extended evaluation, application to different anatomical sites (e.g. liver or joints) and an extension of the proposed method to a hard constraint approach.

References

1. Murphy K, van Ginneken B, Reinhardt JM, et al. Evaluation of registration methods on thoracic CT: the EMPIRE10 challenge. IEEE Trans Med Imaging. 2011;30:1901–20.
2. Galbán CJ, Han MK, Boes JL, et al. Computed tomography-based biomarker provides unique signature for diagnosis of COPD phenotypes and disease progression. Nat Med. 2012;18:1711–5.
3. Rühaak J, Heldmann S, Kipshagen T, et al. Highly accurate fast lung CT registration. Proc SPIE. 2013;8669:86690Y–1–9.
4. Werner R, Ehrhardt J, Schmidt R, et al. Patient-specific finite element modeling of respiratory lung motion using 4D CT image data. Med Phys. 2009;36:1500–11.
5. Schmidt-Richberg A, Werner R, Handels H, et al. Estimation of slipping organ motion by registration with direction-dependent regularization. Med Image Anal. 2012;16:150–9.
6. Pace D, Aylward S, Niethammer M. A locally adaptive regularization based on anisotropic diffusion for deformable image registration of sliding organs. IEEE Trans Med Imaging. 2013;32:2114–26.
7. Han L, Hawkes D, Barratt D. A hybrid biomechanical model-based image registration method for sliding objects. Proc SPIE. 2014;9034:90340G–1–6.
8. Modersitzki J. FAIR: Flexible Algorithms for Image Registration. SIAM; 2009.
9. Castillo R, Castillo E, Guerra R, et al. A framework for evaluation of deformable image registration spatial accuracy using large landmark point sets. Phys Med Biol. 2009;54:1849–70.
10. Lassen B, Kuhnigk JM, Schmidt M, et al. Lung and lung lobe segmentation methods at fraunhofer MEVIS. Proc Int Workshop Pulmon Image Anal. 2011; p. 185–99.

The Cell-Shape-Wizard
User Guidance for Active Contour-Based Cell Segmentation

Daniela Franz[1,2], H. Huettmayer[1], Marc Stamminger[2], Veit Wiesmann[1], Thomas Wittenberg[1]

[1]Fraunhofer Institute for Integrated Circuits (IIS), Erlangen
[2]Computer Graphics Group, University of Erlangen-Nuremberg
daniela.franz@iis.fraunhofer.de

Abstract. Cell segmentation on fluorescent micrographs requires preprocessing, cell-background separation and cell-cell separation. The presence of touching or overlapping cells requires more sophisticated segmentation methods – such as Active Contours (AC) – for cell-cell separation, but the usage and parametrization of these methods is often infeasible for users with no image processing expertise. We present the Cell-Shape-Wizard which introduces an abstraction layer between a complex AC approach and the users. It couples tight user guidance with the benefits of interactive cell segmentation of fluorescence micrographs. We have evaluated the wizard in a small user study with four subjects. Results show, that the wizard concept is well applicable to cell segmentation. Segmentation results are compared to manual reference annotations and result in a mean Jaccard index of 0.72. With the Cell-Shape-Wizard life scientist are able to segment their fluorescence micrographs semi-automatically on their own, without being forced to acquire additional knowledge in image processing.

1 Introduction

Within virology or microbiology research, fluorescent cell micrographs are often evaluated manually. This approach is error-prone, not reproducible and only a small subset of the recorded images can be assessed within limited time. Automated cell segmentation methods increase the number of evaluated images and cells and increase validity and reproducibility of fluorescence micrograph evaluation. These methods typically consist of three steps: preprocessing, cell-background and cell-cell separation. When cells touch or overlap in the micrographs, cell-cell separation requires to use model knowledge about the cell shape [1]. To integrate such model knowledge in the segmentation process we use an active contours (AC) approach, enhanced by an active shape model (ASM). Sophisticated segmentation methods, like our method, are most often quite difficult to use and the parameter adaptations do not always lead to predictable changes in the segmentation. Especially, a naive user regarding image processing methods will not be able to fine-tune the parameters [2], because there exists a "semantic gap" between image processing methods and their life scientist users. We bridge this "semantic gap" with the Cell-Shape-Wizard based on the concepts presented in [3]. The wizard is an abstraction layer between the image processing algorithms and the user and deals with parameter adaptation through interactive corrections. It separates a complicated task into a series of steps, each easy to solve [4]. The advantages of wizard-based segmentation are a reduced orientation phase within a new software tool and increased reproducibility of segmentation results. The disadvantage is a reduced flexibility, as the task's structure and parameters are hidden. For our application scenario – cell segmentation tasks performed by life scientist – this is no disadvantage, because users are mainly interested in a correct, easy and quick solution. The Cell-Shape wizard uses cell nuclei as seed points for an initial cell segmentation on the cytoplasm and refines it with an ASM-supported AC approach.

In literature only a few cell segmentation tools provide explicit user guidance. The users of CellProfiler [5] design their own image processing pipelines from modules. A "help button" for each parameter describes the parameter and related guidelines for the adjustment of the parameter. MiToBo is a plugin for ImageJ and guides the user by grouping functionalities due to cell segmentation applications [6]. Both tools provide a high amount of functionality and wizards for parameter tuning or a problem oriented menu structure. In contrast to that, the presented Cell-Shape-Wizard is deliberately restricted in functionality and flexibility and tightly guides the user through a cell segmentation task.

2 Methods and materials

In the next section we give a brief overview of the used segmentation methods and their integration into the Cell-Shape-Wizard. Afterwards, we describe the used fluorescence micrographs and introduce our initial user study.

2.1 Segmentation approach

We enhance an AC approach with model knowledge from an ASM. The standard AC minimizes the energy function

$$E_{AC} = k_{int}E_{int} + k_{ext}E_{ext} \tag{1}$$

where the internal energy E_{int} is influenced by features of the contour, like contour and curvature energy, and the external energy E_{ext} is influenced by image features, such as edges [7]. We extend the standard AC cell segmentation pipeline with an energy term from an ASM.

$$E_{AC} = k_{int1}E_{Contour} + k_{int2}E_{Curvature} + k_{ext1}E_{Edge} + k_{ext2}E_{ASM} \tag{2}$$

$E_{Contour}$ and $E_{Curvature}$ are internal energies. The contour energy $E_{Contour}$ directs the AC to a smaller shape, the curvature energy $E_{Curvature}$ directs the AC to a more round shape. E_{Edge} and E_{ASM} are external energies. E_{Edge} directs the AC towards image edges and E_{ASM} directs the AC towards the ASM mean shape weighted with ASM model variances.

2.2   Wizard structure

The wizard is divided into four standard wizard pages (Fig. 1), which correspond
to cells segmentation steps. Micrographs are loaded on the first page. On the
second page ("Nuclei Segmentation" Fig. 1) the nuclei are segmented on the
nuclei image with a combination of Gaussian smoothing, k-means clustering and
a watershed approach, they serve as seed points for the cell segmentation. On the
third page ("Cell Segmentation" Fig. 1) the initial and refined cell segmentation
are performed on the cytoplasm image. The segmentation is similar to the nuclei
segmentation, but with a seeded watershed instead of the watershed approach.
Initial cell segmentation is input to the refined cell segmentation with our ASM-
enhanced AC approach. In the wizard three aspects of the AC segmentation can
be adjusted (Fig. 2): "Adjust Size" changes parameter k_{int1}, "Adjust Circularity"
changes parameter k_{int2} and manual "Annotations" updates the ASM model and
with that the E_{ASM} energy. The other parameters are kept constant.

With the corrections and manual annotations, the wizard provides a control
loop to iteratively adapt the energy function of the AC.

2.3   Fluorescence micrographs

To test the applicability of the Cell-Shape-Wizard to different cell types, we used
two sets of fluorescence micrographs (Fig. 3, left). The first dataset contains
three micrographs with a total of 52 macrophages, the second dataset contains
three micrographs with a total of 60 HeLa cells. Both datasets were captured
with a Zeiss Axio Scan.Z1 and each image had a size of 1388×1040 pixels with a
pixel size of $0.16 \times 0.16 \mu m$ in the macrophages images and $0.32 \times 0.32 \mu m$ for the
HeLa cells images. Nuclei of both sets were stained with DAPI. The cytoplasm of
the HeLa cells was stained with DiD and the cytoplasm of the macrophages was
stained with API. For both sets, hand-labelled expert annotations of multiple
observes were available.

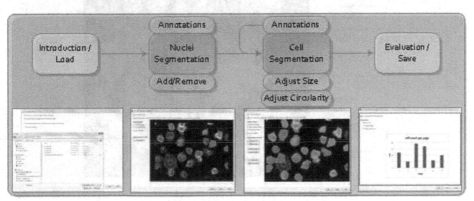

Fig. 1. Page structure of the Cell-Segmentation-Wizard.

2.4   User study

To evaluate the performance of the Cell-Shape-Wizard, we carried out an initial user study with two biologists and two computer scientists with no cell segmentation experience. The task was to perform a complete cell segmentation of a HeLa and Macrophages set of fluorescence micrographs (Sec. 2.3). After they completed the segmentation task the test users filled in a questionnaire about the appropriate time requirement, the complexity of the segmentation tasks and with five additional groups of questions (Tab. 1). The "Usability" group included questions about user guidance, intuitiveness and orientation within the software. The "Tutorial" group asked, if the tutorial page was meaning- and helpful. The "Segmentation" groups asked about the users content with the segmentation results and how easy it was to achieve the results. The "Wizard concept" group tested, whether the program was too rigid and facilitates cell segmentation. The users' answers range between 1 and 4, from "disagree" over "weak disagree" and "weak agree" to "agree"À short interview offered the possibility to give precise feedback and suggest changes to the wizard. To analyse the duration of the procedure, we captured the time the subjects needed to use the program. To assess segmentation quality, we matched each cells from the users' segmentations C_U to a cell from the manual annotations C_A, compared them pixel-wise with the Jaccard index $J(C_U, C_A) = |C_U \cap C_A| / |C_U \cup C_A|$ and averaged the results.

3   Results

Two groups of users were assessed: Users with a background in biology had no experience with image processing, cell segmentation and cell segmentation tools

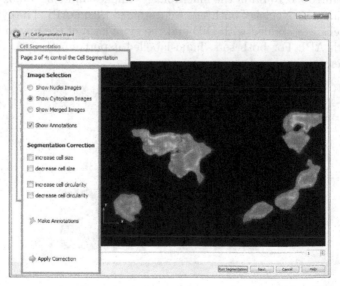

Fig. 2. Cell segmentation page (right) with enlarged corrections section and instructions (orange boxes).

Table 1. Rating results for the question groups with mean and standard deviation. Values range is [1,4]. One subject did not use the tutorial, hence $n = 3$ for the tutorial group.

Category	Mean	Std. dev. ($\sigma =$)	Rating
Usability	3.4	0.5	"weak agree"
Tutorial ($n = 3$)	4.0	0.0	"agree"
Segmentation macrophages	3.6	0.5	"agree"
Segmentation HeLa	3.3	0.8	"weak agree"
Wizard Concept	3.4	0.5	"weak agree"

and users with a background in computer science had experience with image processing but no experience with cell segmentation and cell segmentation tools. The time needed for a Cell-Shape-Wizard run for one dataset was 20 minutes on average and was perceived as appropriate with a mean agreement value of 3.8 (σ =0.4, "agree"). The complexity of the segmentation tasks was perceived as high 3.5 (σ =0.5, "agree"). Tab. 1 depicts the results of the questionnaire evaluation.

Feedback from the users showed, that they liked the rigid concept of wizard-based segmentation in general. They appreciated the reduced flexibility but would have liked a more precise feedback how they could improve segmentation results. The idea of an iterative segmentation improvement with corrections ("Adjust Size/Circularity") was not used as often as manual corrections ("Annotations"). Fig. 3 (right) exemplarily depicts a result segmentation for both cell

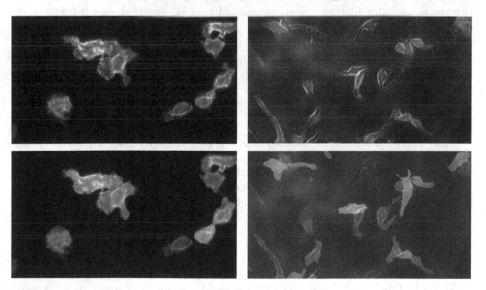

Fig. 3. Images examples for Macrophages (left) and HeLa cells (right) in a combined view of nuclei and cytoplasm dye (top) and with exemplary segmentation results in green (bottom).

sets. The mean Jaccard index for all subject on the macrophages dataset was 0.72 (σ =0.05).

4 Discussion

Compared to an inter-observer variance of 0.78 and intra-observer variance of 0.74, a Jaccard index of 0.72 is sufficiently high. The results of the questionnaire showed an appropriate "Usability" of the Cell-Shape-Wizard. When subjects used the "Tutorial" page, they perceived it as help- and meaningful. The "Segmentation" results for the different image sets show, that the HeLa segmentation was more difficult than the Macrophages segmentation. This is because AC tends to produce compact cell segmentations and Macrophages are more compact than HeLa cells. That fact was only perceived by the biologists, that have a better idea about the necessary quality of a cell segmentation. The difference between both subject groups is reflected by a larger standard deviation (Tab. 1). The "Wizard Concept" is applicable for the given application scenario: User rating and feedback showed, that the segmentation tool was not perceived as too rigid and the users felt well guided in the wizard. This tendency was also noticeable in the users' feedback.

Also the feedback revealed, that segmentation correction by manually drawing cells was much more intuitive to the user (especially the biologists), than using the corrections. This might partially be due to the large run-time of the corrections. Drawing new cells seems easy, intuitive and leads to perfect results whereas the iterative enhancement cannot be precisely defined by the user. Future work includes further improvements of the AC method and a larger user study on the Cell-Shape-Wizard.

Acknowledgement. This work has been supported by the DFG CRC 796 "Reprogramming of host cells by microbial effectors", subproject A4.

References

1. Zhao T, Murphy RF. Automated learning of generative models for subcellular location: building blocks for systems biology. Cytometry A. 2007;71:978–90.
2. Wiesmann V, Franz D, Held C, et al. Review of free software tools for image analysis of fluorescence cell micrographs. J Microsc. 2014; p. online.
3. Franz D, Wiesmann V, Stamminger M, et al. Cell-shape wizard: a concept for user-guidance for active shape segmentation in fluorescence cell micrographs. Biomed Tech. 2014;59(s1):77–80.
4. Tidwell J. Designing Interfaces. O'Reilly; 2007.
5. Carpenter AE, Jones TR, Lamprecht MR, et al. CellProfiler: image analysis software for identifying and quantifying cell phenotypes. Genome Biol. 2007; p. 7:R100.
6. Möller B, Posch S. A framework unifying the development of image analysis algorithms and associated user interfaces. Proc MVA. 2013; p. 447–50.
7. Kass M, Witkin A, Terzopoulus D. Snakes: active contour models. Int J of Comput Vis. 1988; p. 321–31.

Tumorsegmentierung in CD3/CD8-gefärbten Histopathologien

Anqi Wang[1,2], Matthias Noll[1,2], Stefan Wesarg[1]

[1]Visual Healthcare Technologies, Fraunhofer IGD, Darmstadt, Germany
[2]GRIS, Technische Universität Darmstadt, Germany
anqi.wang@igd.fraunhofer.de

Kurzfassung. Segmentierung von bestimmten Gewebetypen in Histopathologien ist eine oft untersuchte Fragestellung. Üblicherweise werden dafür Gewebeproben mit Hämatoxylin-Eosin(HE)-Färbung verwendet. CD3/CD8-Färbungen hingegen sind nötig zur Sichtbarmachung von Immunzellen, differenzieren aber nur wenig zwischen unterschiedlichen Gewebearten. Vorteilhaft wäre es, wenn aus nur einem Gewebeschnitt mit einer bestimmten Färbung beide Informationen extrahiert werden könnten. In dieser Arbeit stellen wir ein Segmentierungsverfahren auf CD3/CD8-gefärbten Gewebeproben vor, das effizient zu berechnende und gleichzeitig aussagekräftige Features als Eingabe für einen Clustering-Algorithmus verwendet. In der Evaluation wird ein durchschnittlicher Accuracy-Wert von 94,44% erzielt. Dieser Wert ist vergleichbar mit den Ergebnissen verwandter State of the Art Methoden, die HE-gefärbte Proben einsetzen.

1 Einleitung

Es existieren zwar bereits Ansätze zur Segmentierung von Tumorbereichen in Aufnahmen von HE-gefärbtem Gewebe (siehe etwa [1, 2]), jedoch sind uns keine Arbeiten bekannt, die hierbei CD3/CD8-gefärbte Proben verwenden. Die unterschiedlichen Ergebnisse dieser beiden Färbeverfahren sind in Abb. 1 zu sehen. In der CD3-gefärbten Gewebeprobe werden Immunzellen als bräunliche, gut segmentierbare Punkte abgebildet, während das Gewebe selbst in Struktur und Textur wesentlich weniger differenziert dargestellt wird. In der HE-gefärbten Probe hingegen sind überhaupt keine Zellen erkennbar. Für ein System, das in CD3/CD8-gefärbten Proben automatisch die in und um einen Tumorbereich enthaltenen Immunzellen zählen soll, wurde das hier vorgestellte Tumor-Segmentierungsverfahren entwickelt.

Zwar sind oft zu den vorliegenden Proben auch HE-gefärbte Nachbarschnitte verfügbar, eine Übertragung von erfolgter Segmentierung ist jedoch kein triviales Problem. Hierzu ist eine exakte Registrierung der Schnitte nötig, wobei die Gewebestruktur sehr unterschiedlich sein kann. Um das Registrierungsproblem zu vermeiden, wird daher in dieser Arbeit der Tumorbereich direkt in CD3/CD8-gefärbten Gewebeschnitten segmentiert. In verwandten Arbeiten, die mit HE-gefärbten Proben arbeiten, werden mehrheitlich Supervised Machine Learning-basierte Verfahren verwendet [1, 3]. Diese setzen komplexe, oft zellstruktur-basierte Features ein und benötigen große Mengen an annotierten Trainingsdaten. Da uns hierfür nicht genügend Trainingsdaten vorliegen, wird ein Clustering-Ansatz aus dem Bereich Unsupervised Machine Learning gewählt.

2   Material und Methoden

2.1   Verwendete Daten

Insgesamt 8 histopathologische Aufnahmen von Gewebeproben von Darmkrebspatienten, die gleichmäßig in Entwicklungs- und Testset aufgeteilt werden, sind bei der Verfahrensentwicklung verfügbar. Zu jedem Bild existiert eine gelabelte Ground Truth-Segmentierung. Die Gewebeproben wurden mit einem Hamatsu NanoZoomer Scanner digitalisiert und liegen in 3 Auflösungen vor: x1,25-, x5- und x20-fache Vergrößerung. In der höchsten Auflösung (x20) sind die Bilder ca. 60.000 × 40.000 Pixel groß und benötigen rund 5 bis 6 GB Speicher. Bereits ab der x5-Auflösung ist es aufgrund beschränkter Arbeitsspeichergröße praktisch nicht mehr möglich, ganze Bilder zu verarbeiten. Nicht nur wegen der Performanz, sondern auch weil das Clustering Verfahren Bildinformationen des ganzen Bildes benötigt, wird mit der kleinsten Auflösung gearbeitet. Die Bearbeitung des vorliegenden Segmentierungsproblems erfolgt in drei Schritten, bestehend aus Vordergrunddetektion, anschließender Tumorsegmentierung und Entfernung der gesunden Darmwand.

2.2   Vordergrunddetektion

Im ersten Schritt muss auf der Aufnahme die größte zusammenhängende Gewebekomponente im Vordergrund detektiert werden, damit im nächsten Schritt dort der Tumor segmentiert werden kann. In verwandten Arbeiten [1, 3] wird diese Aufgabe mit Schwellwertverfahren gelöst. Bei den hier verwendeten CD3/CD8-

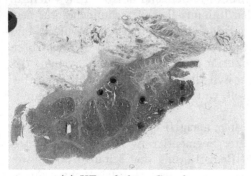
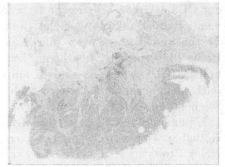

(a) HE-gefärbtes Gewebe   (b) CD3-gefärbtes Gewebe

Abb. 1. HE- und CD3-gefärbte Nachbarschnitte.

gefärbten Proben können damit jedoch keine zufriedenstellenden Ergebnisse erzielt werden, da der Farbunterschied zwischen Vorder- und Hintergrund wesentlich kleiner ist als bei HE-gefärbten Proben. Stattdessen wird das K-Means Clustering Verfahren gewählt, da es gemäß [4] im Vergleich mit 4 anderen bewährten Clustering Algorithmen große Datenmengen am effizientesten und mit gutem Ergebnis verarbeiten kann. Das Clustering wird pixelweise ausgeführt, wobei die Pixelwerte der Farbkanäle L, U und V des CIELUV-Farbraums als Features verwendet werden. Der die Anzahl der entstehenden Cluster festlegende Parameter K wird mit 7 gewählt nach experimenteller Evaluation für K $\in$ [2, 40]. Da Clustering-Verfahren keine Zuordnung der sich ergebenden Cluster-Label vornehmen, geschieht dies in einem nachträglichen Schritt. Hierfür wird angenommen, dass die meisten Pixel aus den Bildecken Hintergrundpixel sind. Daher wird das am häufigsten vorkommende Cluster-Label der Bildecken als Hintergrundlabel angenommen. Pixel mit diesem Label werden im Ergebnisbild auf 0, die übrigen auf 1 gesetzt. Anschließend wird ein Closing ausgeführt und verbleibende Löcher morphologisch geschlossen. In Abb. 2 sind die jeweiligen Zwischenergebnisse und das Endergebnis der Vordergrunddetektion dargestellt.

2.3 Tumorsegmentierung

Da die Datengrundlage zu wenig Bildmaterial enthält, um ein verlässliches Ergebnis mit einem Supervised Learning Verfahren zu erzielen, wird ein Clustering Verfahren für die Lösung des Problems ausgewählt. Wegen der überlegeneren Ergebnisse bei sehr großen Featuresets wird in diesem Schritt ebenfalls der K-Means Algorithmus verwendet. Das Clustering erfolgt jedoch nicht pixelweise, denn für die Tumorsegmentierung müssen neben Farbwerten auch Struktur und Textur betrachtet werden. Das Bild wird in Kacheln der Größe 16x16 Pixel unterteilt, der Parameter K wird mit 3 gewählt. Bei den sich ergebenden Clustern wird dasjenige als Tumorcluster bestimmt, welches zwei Kriterien erfüllt. Zunächst muss es mehr als 30% der gesamten Gewebefläche einnehmen. Außerdem muss die Summe von seinem Kantendichte-Mittelwert und Farbmittelwert des V-Kanals aus dem CIELUV-Farbraum von allen drei Clustern am höchsten sein.

Features, die in verwandten Arbeiten gute Ergebnisse erzielen und nicht gewebespezifisch sind, sind vor allem statistisch oder texturbasiert. Statistische Features können sowohl mit Grau- als auch mit Farbwerten berechnet werden und bestehen aus Mittelwert, Median, Modus, Maximum, Minimum und Standardabweichung der Pixelwerte innerhalb einer Bildregion. Bei den texturbasier-

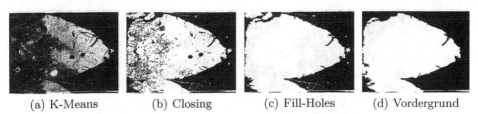

(a) K-Means   (b) Closing   (c) Fill-Holes   (d) Vordergrund

Abb. 2. Schritte der Vordergrunddetektion.

ten Features sind vor allem Local Binary Pattern und der Gaborfilter von Bedeutung. Für die Featureextraktion werden verschiedene Featuremengen in Form von multidimensionalen Histogrammen kombiniert. Hierdurch wird die wertvolle Zusatzinformation über gemeinsames Vorkommen bestimmter Werte gewonnen. In [5] wurde bereits festgestellt, dass eine solche Kombination von Werten zu großer Verbesserung der Genauigkeit bei der Messung von Bildähnlichkeit führt. Da bei der vorliegenden Arbeit durch den Einsatz von Clustering Bildregionen nach ihrer Ähnlichkeit gruppiert werden, sind multidimensionale Histogramme eine effektive Art der Featurekombination. Nach erfolgtem Clustering und der Bestimmung des Tumorclusters werden hier die gleichen morphologischen Nachverarbeitungsschritte durchgeführt wie bei der Vordergrunddetektion. Sofern neben dem Haupttumor noch kleinere Tumorherde im Bild enthalten sind, werden diese ebenfalls entsprechend des Vorgehens in den Ground Truth Daten nicht berücksichtigt. Die jeweiligen Zwischenergebnisse und das Endergebnis einer Tumorsegmentierung sind in Abb. 3 zu sehen.

2.4 Entfernung von gesunder Darmwand

Das oben vorgestellte Verfahren unterscheidet zwar mit hohem Accuracy-Wert die Tumorregion von normalem Darmgewebe, aber (bei K = 3) nicht zwischen gesunder Darmwand und der Tumorregion, da diese sich optisch stark ähneln. Zur Entfernung der gesunden Darmwand kann die spezifische Gewebetextur, bestehend aus runden und elliptischen Zellen, genutzt werden. Im ersten Schritt wird eine Kantendetektion ausgeführt. In dem resultierenden Kantenbild sind die Zellen als Kreise und Ellipsen sichtbar. Das Kantenbild wird anschließend invertiert, sodass die Kreise und Ellipsen zu ausgefüllten, voneinander abgetrennten Flächen werden. Von den nun sichtbaren Strukturen werden nur diejenigen beibehalten, die einerseits einen Schwellwert für Rundheit oder Ellipsenartigkeit erfüllen, und andererseits einen überdurchschnittlichen Abstand zum Gewebemittelpunkt aufweisen. Auf den verbleibenden Strukturen wird wiederum ein Closing ausgeführt und verbleibende Löcher morphologisch geschlossen, um dichte Ansammlungen zu zusammenhängenden Regionen zusammenzufassen. Anschließend wird eine Filterung nach Größe ausgeführt. Nur Regionen mit überdurchschnittlich vielen Pixeln werden behalten. Diese sind mit hoher Wahrscheinlichkeit Teile der gesunden Darmwand und werden aus der segmentierten Tumorregion entfernt. Die Zwischenergebnisse dieses Verarbeitungsschritts sind in Abb. 4 zu sehen.

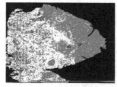 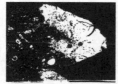 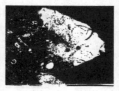 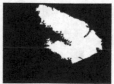

  (a) K-Means   (b) Tumorcluster   (c) Closing   (d) Endergebnis

Abb. 3. Schritte der Tumorsegmentierung.

Abb. 4. Detektion der gesunden Darmwand.

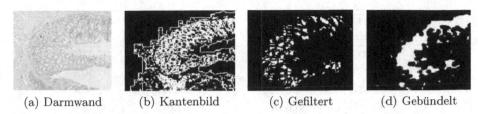

(a) Darmwand   (b) Kantenbild   (c) Gefiltert   (d) Gebündelt

3 Ergebnisse

Bei der Evaluation des entwickelten Systems wird die Tumorsegmentierung auf dem Testset ausgeführt. Zur Bewertung der dabei erzielten Ergebnisse wird der Accuracy-Wert als Metrik verwendet. In Abb. 5 sind die erzielten Segmentierungen des Systems (obere Reihe), jeweils mit dem zugehörigen Ground Truth Bild im Vergleich (untere Reihe), zu sehen. Das Verfahren erreicht einen durchschnittlichen Accuracy-Wert von 94,44% als direktes Ergebnis der Tumorsegmentierung, und 95,99% mit zusätzlicher Entfernung der Darmwand (Tab. 1). Das direkte Ergebnis ist vergleichbar mit den Ergebnissen von verwandten Arbeiten, die mit HE-gefärbten Proben arbeiten und dabei Supervised Learning Verfahren einsetzen [1, 6]. Das Ergebnis nach Entfernung der Darmwand ist hingegen leicht überlegen.

4 Diskussion

In dieser Arbeit wurde ein Algorithmus zur Segmentierung von Tumorgewebe in CD3/CD8-gefärbten Histopathologien vorgestellt. Im Gegensatz zu existierenden Lösungen zur Gewebeanalyse können damit in ein und demselben Schnittbild das Gewebe klassifiziert und enthaltene Immunzellen gezählt werden. Das hat Vorteile bezüglich des Workflows der Gewebeanalyse und vermeidet Ungenauigkeiten, die bei der sonst notwendigen Registrierung benachbar-

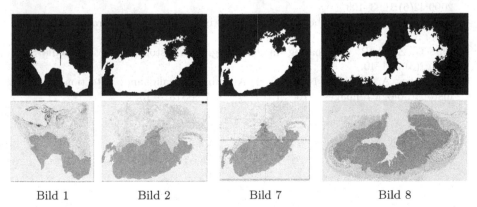

Bild 1   Bild 2   Bild 7   Bild 8

Abb. 5. Segmentierungen des Systems und Ground Truth Bilder im Vergleich.

Tabelle 1. Ergebnisse der Tumorsegmentierung.

Bild-Nr.	Vor Darmwandentfernung		Nach Darmwandentfernung	
	Accuracy	F_1	Accuracy	F_1
Bild 1	99,09%	97,71%	98,98%	97,41%
Bild 2	94,05%	90,48%	95,46%	92,56%
Bild 7	94,42%	91,03%	95,52%	92,66%
Bild 8	90,21%	85,68%	94,01%	90,55%
Durchschn.	94,44%	91,22%	95,99%	93,29%

ter HE- und CD3/CD8-Schnitte auftreten können. Je nach verwendeten Daten kann der zusätzliche Zuordnungsschritt, der für ein Klassifizierungsergebnis benötigt wird, problematisch sein, da dessen Korrektheit nicht für alle ungesehenen Fälle garantiert werden kann. Trotz weniger zur Verfügung stehender Daten konnte ein Unsupervised Learning-basiertes Segmentierungsverfahren mit überdurchschnittlich guter Genauigkeit entwickelt werden. Das implementierte System stützt sich ausschließlich auf allgemeine Textur-Unterschiede zwischen Tumorregionen und gesundem Gewebe, zudem verwendet es keine gewebespezifischen Features. Durch diese Datenunabhängigkeit ist zu erwarten, dass es auch bei neuen Aufnahmen mit bislang ungesehenen Gewebearten gute Ergebnisse erzielt.

Literaturverzeichnis

1. Homeyer A, Schenk A, Arlt J, et al. Practical quantification of necrosis in histological whole-slide images. Comp Med Imag Graph. 2013;37(4):313–22.
2. Khan AM, El-Daly H, Rajpoot N. Ranpec: andom projections with ensemble clustering for segmentation of tumor areas in breast histology images. Med Image Understand Anal. 2012; p. 17–23.
3. Sertel O, Kong J, Shimada H, et al. Computer-aided prognosis of neuroblastoma on whole-slide images: classification of stromal development. Pattern Recognit. 2009;42(6):1093–103.
4. Abbas OA. Comparisons between data clustering algorithms. Int Arab J Inf Technol. 2008; p. 320–5.
5. Pass G, Zabih R. Comparing images using joint histograms. Multimedia Syst. 1999;7(3):234–40.
6. Chekkoury A, Khurd P, Ni J, et al. Automated malignancy detection in breast histopathological images. Proc SPIE. 2012;8315:831515–13.

Segmentierung von zervikalen Lymphknoten in T1-gewichteten MRT-Aufnahmen

Florian Jung, Julia Hilpert, Stefan Wesarg

Fraunhofer IGD, Fraunhoferstr. 5, 64283 Darmstadt
`florian.jung@igd.fraunhofer.de`

Kurzfassung. Die Untersuchung von Größe und Aussehen eines Lymphknotens kann ein entscheidender Indikator für die Existenz eines Tumors sein und ist außerdem ein probates Mittel, um Verlaufsanalysen bei einem Patienten durchzuführen, welche wiederum maßgeblichen Einfluss auf die Behandlung haben können. Um die Größe und andere Parameter des Lymphknotens bestimmen zu können, ist zuerst eine Segmentierung vonnöten. Wir präsentieren ein neues Verfahren für die halbautomatische Segmentierung von Lymphknoten auf MR-Datensätzen. Unser Ansatz verwendet eine Wasserscheidentransformation als Grundlage und kombiniert diese mit einem Radialstrahlbasierten Verfahren, um eine möglichst akurate Segmentierung des Lymphknotens zu erhalten. Für die Evaluation wurden 95 Lymphknoten-Segmentierungen aus 17 verschiedenen, kontrastverstärkten T1-gewichteten Patientendatensätzen verwendet. Das durchschnittliche Dice Ähnlichkeitsmaß lag bei 0.69 ± 0.15 und die mittlere Oberflächendistanz bei 0.65 ± 0.54mm.

1 Einleitung

Der menschliche Körper besitzt mehr als 600 einzelne Lymphknoten, (davon mehr als 300 zervikale Lymphknoten, die sich im Kopf-Hals-Bereich befinden) die das Lymphsystem bilden, welches Bestandteil des menschlichen Immunsystems ist. Standardmäßig haben Lymphknoten eine Größe von 5-10mm und im Kopf-Hals Bereich von bis zu 20mm. Lymphgefäße verbinden die einzelnen Lymphknoten zu diesem Lymphsystem. Kommt es zu einem Tumorbefall, besteht die Gefahr, dass einzelne Tumorzellen in das Lymphsystem gelangen und von dort aus Lymphknoten infiltrieren können. Ein wichtiger diagnostischer Faktor in der Krebstherapie ist daher häufig die Analyse und Volumenabschätzung von Lymphknoten. Werden verdächtige Lymphknoten ausgemacht, werden diese einer Biopsie unterzogen, um festzustellen, ob eine bösartige Veränderung vorliegt.

Im Bereich der automatischen Segmentierung von Lymphknoten im Kopf-Hals-Bereich gibt es für CT-Aufnahmen bereits einige Verfahren. Steger et al. [1] verwenden ein radialstrahlbasiertes Verfahren für die halbautomatische Segmentierung der Lymphknoten. Maleike et al. [2] verwenden ein elliptisches Formmodell für Segmentierung von Lymphknoten und Dornheim et al. [3] verwenden ein 3D Masse-Feder-System. Im Bereich der Lymphknoten-Segmentierung auf MR-Datensätzen gibt es bisher deutlich weniger Arbeiten. So haben Unal et al. [4] ein Verfahren zur semi-automatischen Segmentierung von Lymphknoten im Bereich der Prostata, in MR-Datensätzen vorgestellt, verwenden dafür jedoch das Lymphotropic Nanoparticle-enhanced Magnetic Resonance Imaging (LN-MRI). Debats et al. [5] haben ein Verfahren zur halbautomatischen Segmentierung von Beckenlymphknoten vorgestellt, bei dem sie jedoch 4 verschiedene MR-Sequenzen verwenden. Unseres Wissens nach gibt es bisher kein Verfahren, was sich konkret mit der Segmentierung der Lymphknoten im Kopf-Hals-Bereich auf T1-gewichteten MR-Datensätzen beschäftigt.

2   Methodik

Die Segmentierung von Lymphknoten in MR-Datensätzen stellt eine besondere Herausforderung dar. Einerseits sind Lympknoten in MR-Datensätzen besser sichtbar, andererseits variiert die Intensität der Lymphknoten signifikant zwischen unterschiedlichen Datensätzen und selbst innerhalb eines MR-Datensatzes kommt es häufig zu deutlichen Abweichungen bei der Intensität des Lymphknotengewebes. Deshalb lassen sich die Ansätze aus dem Bereich der CT-Aufnahmen, die mehrheitlich auf feste Schwellwerte zurückgreifen können, nicht ohne weiteres auf MR-Aufnahmen übertragen. Analog zu [6] diente für unser Verfahren eine Wasserscheidentransformation als Grundlage. Zusätzlich waren jedoch noch einige Vorverarbeitungsschritte notwendig, um brauchbare Ergebnisse zu erzielen. Für die Segmentierung eines Lymphknotens wird ein einzelner Klick in die Mitte des Lymphknoten benötigt, welcher dann als Initialisierungspunkt für die automatische Segmentierung verwendet wird.

2.1   Schwellwertverfahren von Otsu

Die erste Hürde bei der Segmentierung von Lymphknoten in MR-Datensätzen, ist die fehlende Normierung der Intensitätswerte, wie sie bei CT Datensätzen üblicherweise vorliegt. Diese ließen sich ansonsten dazu verwenden, eine Abschätzung bzgl. der Grenzen der Lymphknoten, als Vorwissen in den Ansatz einfließen zu lassen. Um die Intensitätswerte des aktuell vorliegenden Lymphknoten und

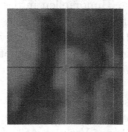

Abb. 1. Binarisierung des Ausschnitts, das den Lymphknoten enthält. Es ist deutlich zu erkennen, dass große Bereiche des Auschnitts ähnliche Intensitätswerte besitzen wie der Lymphknoten.

dessen Grenze abschätzen zu können, verwenden wir das Schwellwertverfahren von Otsu [7]. Dadurch wird das Bild in Vorder- und Hintergrund unterteilt und wir erhalten ein Binärbild, welches den Lymphknoten und andere Strukturen mit ähnlicher Intensität enthält (Abb. 1).

2.2 Radialstrahlbasiertes Verfahren zur Oberflächenbestimmung

Für eine initiale Abschätzung der Form des Lymphknotens verwenden wir ein radialstrahlbasiertes Verfahren. Hierfür werden von dem Saatpunkt ausgehend Radialstrahlen in alle 3 Raumrichtungen ausgesandt. Dazu werden 8 Azimuthwinkel θ und 10 Inklinationswinkel φ verwendet. Die Strahlen werden 40 mal in Abständen von 0.5mm abgetastet, solange bis ein Übergang von Vordergrund zu Hintergrund innerhalb des Binärbildes erkannt wird. Dies hat sich für uns als geeignete Annahme über die Größe der Lymphknoten erwiesen. Weicht die Länge eines Strahls signifikant von der der anderen Strahlen ab, wird dieser nach folgender Formel (Eq. 1) als Ausreißer deklariert und korrigiert. Abb. 2 zeigt solch eine Korrektur.

$$m(\theta_j, \varphi_k) = \begin{cases} \bar{m}_k & \text{if } 2 * \bar{m}_k < m(\theta_j, \varphi_k) \\ m(\theta_j, \varphi_k) & \text{sonst} \end{cases} \tag{1}$$

Wobei $m \in [1, ..., 40]$ die Position auf einem Radialstrahl angibt und $\bar{m}_k = \frac{1}{8} \sum_{j=1}^{8} m(\theta_j, \varphi_k)$ mit $k \in [1, ..., 10]$ gilt.

2.3 Bestimmung der Minima im Binärbild

Im Laufe der Arbeit kristallisierte sich heraus, dass die alleinige Verwendung des Radialstrahlbasierten Verfahrens als Input für die Wasserscheidentransformation häufiger Übersegmentierungen produziert oder die Segmentierung in andere Strukturen ausläuft. Um dem vorzubeugen, bestimmen wir in einem weiteren Schritt, mithilfe einer Distanzkarte, Minima in unserem Binärbild. Die Distanzkarte enthält den minimalen Abstand eines jeden Voxels im Binärbild zum Hintergrund. Die Voxel, die in der Mitte einer Struktur liegen, sollten nun den größten Wert aufweisen. Die Idee, die dahinter steckt, ist, dass die Minima des

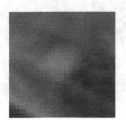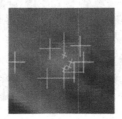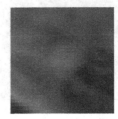

Abb. 2. Radialstrahlbasiertes Verfahren zur Ermittlung einer lymphknotenähnlichen ellipsoiden Oberfläche.

Lymphknotens als Include Marker und die Minima, die zu anderen Strukturen gehören als Exlude Marker für die Wasserscheidentransformation verwendet werden sollen. Diese Information kann nun verwendet werden, um sicher zu stellen, dass der Lymphknoten Teil der finalen Segmentierung ist und andere Strukturen mit identischen Grauwerten ausgeschlossen werden.

2.4 Generieren der Include- und Exclude-Masken

Die Resultate der beiden vorherigen Methoden können nun für die Erstellung von Include- und Exclude Masken für die Wasserscheidentransformation verwendet werden. Dazu werden die beiden Masken mit einem logischen UND überlagert, woraus die Include Maske resultiert. Alle weiteren Voxel aus dem Minima Bild, die keine Überlappung mit der Maske aus dem Radialstrahlbild besitzen, werden einer Exclude Maske hinzugefügt (Abb. 3). Diese beiden Masken dienen nun als Input für die Wasserscheidentransformation.

2.5 Wasserscheidentransformation

Bei der Wasserscheidentransformation wird ein Datensatz als topographische Oberfläche betrachtet. In unserem Fall dient die Distanzkarte unseres original Bildes als Eingabe. Aus diesem wird ein Gradientenbild berechnet. Das Labeln des Bildes läuft wie folgt ab. Es wird ein Fallen von Regentropfen auf das Relief simuliert. Diese bewegen sich in Richtung des steilsten Abstiegs und sammeln sich in unterschiedlichen Basins. Deren Wasserspiegel steigt kontinuierlich bis sie irgendwann in Berührung mit einem weiteren Basin kommen. Infolgedessen wird dann ein Damm zwischen diesen beiden Becken konstruiert, der die beiden Becken voneinander trennt und später dafür sorgt, dass diese unterschiedliche Label erhalten. Dieser Prozess wird solange durchgeführt, bis alle Becken geflutet wurden und man ein Bild mit n verschiedenen Labeln erhält (Abb. 4).

3 Evaluation

Für die Evaluation standen uns 17 T1-gewichtete Patientendatensätze mit insgesamt 95 Goldstandard-Lymphknotensegmentierungen zur Verfügung. Das Spacing der Datensätze lag zwischen [0.47mm x 3.3mm x 0.47mm] und [0.62mm x

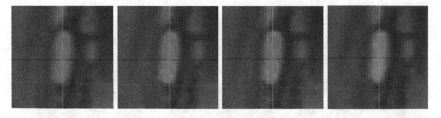

Abb. 3. Aus der Vereinigung der Oberfläche des radialstrahlbasierten Verfahrens (links) und den Minima der Distanzkarte (2.v.l.), ergibt sich die Include Maske (2.v.r) und die exclude Maske (rechts) für die Wasserscheidentransformation.

Abb. 4. Wasserscheidentransformation eines Bildausschnitts.

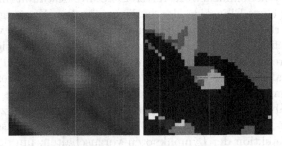

4.4mm x 0.62mm]. Die komplette Segmentierung benötigt weniger als 1 Sekunde und wurde infolgedessen keinen weiteren Benchmarks unterzogen. Abb. 5. zeigt das DICE Ähnlichkeitsmaß der 95 Segmentierungen. Insgesamt ergab sich ein durchschnittlicher DICE, mit einer Standardabweichung von 0.69 ± 0.15. Der durchschnittliche Oberflächenabstand (ASD) betrug 0.65 ± 0.55mm. Im Falle einer Fehlsegmentierung kristallisierte sich heraus, dass die berechnete Oberfläche, die als Include-Maske verwendet wurde, nicht genau genug war.

4   Fazit

Die Evaluation hat gezeigt, dass eine Großzahl der Segmentierungen bereits sehr gut ist. Optimierungsbedarf gäbe es noch bei der Wahl der Kontur, die basierend auf den Ergebnissen des Radialstrahlverfahrens, konstruiert wird. Diese

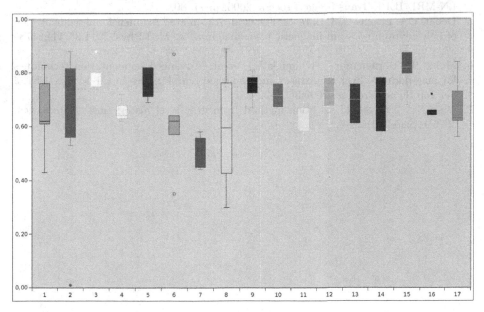

Abb. 5. Dice-Ähnlichkeitsmaß für die 95 Segmentierungen auf den 17 T1-gewichteten Patientendatensätzen.

wird aktuell mit einer einfachen Ausreißererkennung bestimmt und könnte durch die Verwendung eines Ellipsoids, der an die ermittelten Konturgrenzpunkte angepasst wird, verbessert werden. Die Berechnungdauer beträgt weniger als eine Sekunde für die finale Segmentierung und ist somit vernachlässigbar. Ein nächster Schritt wäre die Überprüfung, in wie weit das Verfahren invariant bzgl. der Saatpunktwahl ist. Hier wäre zu erwarten, dass das Verfahren bei schlechter Wahl des Saatpunkts unzureichende Ergebnisse liefert. Das ließe sich verbessern, indem das Verfahren mehrere Iterationen durchläuft, in denen zuerst ein geeigneter Saatpunkt ermittelt wird. Schließlich wäre es noch wünschenswert, eine automatische Detektion der Lymphknoten vorzuschalten, um das Verfahren zu einem vollautomatischen Ansatz zu erweitern.

Literaturverzeichnis

1. Steger S, Bozoglu N, Kuijper A, et al. Application of radial ray based segmentation to cervical lymph nodes in CT images. IEEE Trans Med Imaging. 2013;32(5):888–900.
2. Maleike D, Fabel M, Tetzlaff R, et al.; International Society for Optics; Photonics. Lymph node segmentation on CT images by a shape model guided deformable surface methodh. Med Imaging. 2008; p. 69141S.
3. Dornheim J, Seim H, Preim B, et al. Segmentation of neck lymph nodes in CT datasets with stable 3D mass-spring models: segmentation of neck lymph nodes. Acad Radiol. 2007;14(11):1389 – 99.
4. Unal G, Slabaugh G, Ess A, et al. Semi-automatic lymph node segmentation in LN-MRI. IEEE Trans Image Process. 2006; p. 77–80.
5. Debats OA, Litjens GJS, Barentsz JO, et al. Automated 3-dimensional segmentation of pelvic lymph nodes in magnetic resonance images. Med Phys. 2011;38(11):6178–87.
6. Moltz JH, Bornemann L, Kuhnigk JM, et al. Advanced segmentation techniques for lung nodules, liver metastases, and enlarged lymph nodes in CT scans. IEEE J Sel Top Signal Process. 2009;3(1):122–34.
7. Otsu N. A threshold selection method from gray-level histograms. Automatica. 1975;11(285-296):23–7.

Dynamic Programming for the Segmentation of Bone Marrow Cells

Sebastian Krappe[1], Christian Münzenmayer[1], Amrei Evert[1],
Can Fahrettin Koyuncu[2], Enis Cetin[2], Torsten Haferlach[3],
Thomas Wittenberg[1], Christian Held[1]

[1]Fraunhofer Institute for Integrated Circuits IIS, Erlangen
[2]Bilkent University, Ankara
[3]MLL Munich Leukemia Laboratory, Munich
sebastian.krappe@iis.fraunhofer.de

Abstract. For the diagnosis of leukemia the morphological analysis of bone marrow is essential. This procedure is time consuming, partially subjective, error-prone and cumbersome. Moreover, repeated examinations may lead to intra- and inter-observer variances. Therefore, an automation of the bone marrow analysis is pursued. The automatic classification of bone marrow cells is highly dependent on the preceding segmentation of the nucleus and plasma parts of the cell. In this contribution we propose a dynamic programming approach for the segmentation of already localized bone marrow cells and evaluate the method with 1000 manually segmented cells. With this approach the segmentation quality for whole cells is 0.93 and 0.85 for the corresponding nucleus parts.

1 Introduction

For the diagnosis of leukemia the morphological analysis of bone marrow is essential. Such a cytological examination is used as clarification of variations in a blood smear. It is the starting-point for a patient's diagnosis and decision support for a subsequent treatment. For a cytological analysis the bone marrow aspirate smear is stained and evaluated with the help of a light microscope. In the beginning the cell density, the bone marrow fat content and qualitative differences of the cells are detected in a mid-level magnification. Subsequently, cells of different types are recognized and counted. This phase is time consuming, partially subjective, error-prone and cumbersome. Moreover, repeated examinations may lead to intra- and inter-observer variances. Therefore, an automation of the bone marrow analysis is pursued. The staining variance, the variety of the smear quality of the samples, the accumulation of cells in cell clusters and the differentiation of immature cells are difficulties and challenges of automated image based analysis of bone marrow samples. The applied analysis pipeline contains the following steps: image acquisition, smear detection, cell localization and segmentation, feature extraction and cell classification. As the classification of bone marrow cells is highly dependent on the preceding segmentation of the nucleus and plasma parts of the cell, this contribution focuses on a fast and accurate segmentation approach using dynamic programming.

In literature there exist several algorithms dealing with the segmentation of bone marrow cells. The approach of Zerfaß et al. [1] can be divided into four phases. In the first phase images are preprocessed to remove low-frequency inhomogeneities in the background. Then regions containing leukocyte cells are estimated. In the third phase leukocyte cells are detected and segmented. In the last phase leukocyte cells are separated by using Fast Marching methods. Nilsson et al. [2, 3] describe a method for the segmentation of complex cell clusters. At first a background/foreground separation is done by thresholding. In order to separate the nuclei from each other a distance transform followed by a watershed algorithm is applied. The cytoplasm surrounding the nuclei is located by thresholding and fast marching method. Over-segmentation is reduced by merging regions belonging to the same cell. Reta et al. [4] use a two stage approach for the morphological classification of acute leukemia. In this method the CIE L*a*b color space and a texture model are used. The color and texture information is modeled by a random markov field. For the extraction of nucleus and cytoplasm parts color and shape information are used. Overlapping cells are separated by using a polar transformation. In [5] the image is normalized in order to avoid variations in different images at first. After that an adaptive thresholding method in the HSI color space is used to separate foreground and background. Then a distance transform is applied on the foreground. Thresholding that image produces seeds for a subsequent region growing algorithm. The segmentation of the cells is then represented by the grown regions. Leukocytes and erythrocytes in blood smear images are segmented in a simultaneous way in [6]. Pixel-wise classification is combined with template matching to locate erythrocytes. In order to get the exact cell contours of leukocyte nucleus and plasma regions a level-set approach is used. Nandy et al. [7] apply a dynamic programming approach for the segmentation of DAPI-stained nuclei. Gradient magnitude and direction information is used for the delineation of the detected nuclei.

In this work we propose a dynamic programming approach for the segmentation of bone marrow cells and evaluate the method with 1000 manually segmented cells. Our approach incorporates expert knowledge (e.g. cell size and color information) and assumptions about the appearance of the cells (especially the roundness of the cells) as well as SLIC Superpixels [8] which is not extensively used in the described literature.

2   Materials and methods

2.1   Image data

For the development and evaluation of the segmentation approach 1100 automatically localized cells [9] are used. These micrographs were acquired with a CCD-camera mounted on a microscope (Zeiss Axio Imager Z2). The size of the images is 400×400 pixels and the pixel size of the camera is $3.45~\mu m \times 3.45~\mu m$. For image acquisition a $40\times$ oil objective with a numerical aperture of 1.4 (Zeiss Plan-Apochromat) is applied. 100 cell images are used for training and 1000 cell images are used for the evaluation of the proposed approach. For each cell the nucleus and the boundary of the whole cell were annotated manually. The images contain images from 16 different cell bone marrow cell classes and the class distribution of the considered images is almost equal. These images were taken from regions on the slide which are suitable for a morphological analysis and had been confirmed by experienced experts (Fig. 1).

2.2   Segmentation of the contour

An automatically localized cell (Fig. 2(a)) is unrolled with respect to the detected cell center with the help of a polar transform [10] (Fig. 2(b)). For the image the corresponding cost image is calculated (Fig. 2(c)). This cost function is a weighted sum of six different components: For the gradient component the color image is smoothed with a Gaussian kernel and the gradient is calculated on the multi-channel image [11]. The radius component is modeling the size of a cell by assuming a specific minimum and maximum radius. The third component uses color information for the determination and weighting of foreground pixels. Hence the arctangent of the blue and green color component of the RGB color information of the pixel is used. The background penalty component is a distance transform on the background pixels of the thresholded gray image. The fifth part is the foreground penalty component. It is a distance transform on the foreground pixels of the thresholded gray image. The sixth component uses SLIC Superpixels [8] and a subsequent distance transform as a weighting component.

Based on the cost image the segmentation of the bone marrow cell is done. The path with the lowest cost from left to right is found by means of dynamic programming [12] (Fig. 2(d)). The segmentation result is obtained by applying an inverse polar transformation (Fig. 2(e)). Discontinuous transitions in the segmentation are avoided by a threefold unrolling.

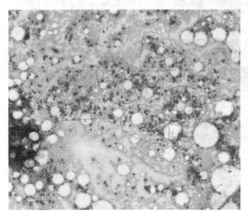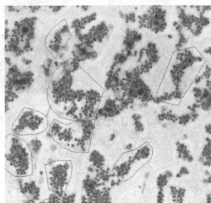

Fig. 1. Example regions on the slide which are suitable for a morphological analysis and had been confirmed by experienced experts.

362   Krappe et al.

2.3   Separation of nucleus and plasma parts

The separation of nucleus and plasma parts is based on the segmentation result
of the contour segmentation. The original color image is transformed into a gray
level image by using the arctangent of the blue and green color component of
the RGB color information of the pixel within the found contour. For these
pixels a gray value histogram is calculated. Based on the histogram a threshold
separating the pixels into two classes (nucleus and plasma) is computed by using
Otsu's method. Using this threshold the gray level image is then reduced to a
binary image.

2.4   Parameter optimization through genetic algorithms

The segmentation algorithm has several configurable parameters which were optimized by a steady state genetic algorithm [13]. Six parameters represent the

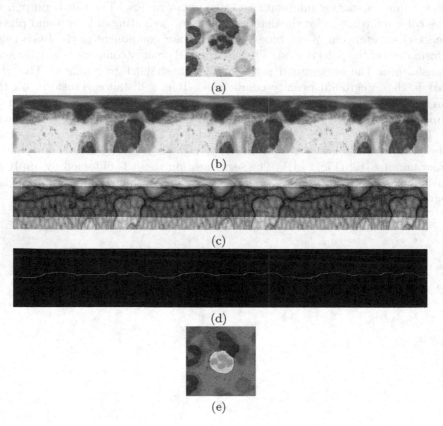

Fig. 2. Processing steps for segmentation of bone marrow cells using the dynamic programming approach: (a) cell to segment is in the center of the image (b) unrolled cell
image using polar transform (c) cost image (d) path with minimum cost (e) superimposed segmentation result for the whole cell after inverse polar transformation.

weights of the components of the cost function. Furthermore, parameters for the diagonal penalty and the minimum and maximum radius for the dynamic programming approach are used. For the optimization 100 manually segmented cells are used to minimize the differences between the output of the automatically segmented cell contours and the manually segmented cell contours. The similarity of these two regions of interest (ROIs) is computed with a combination of three measures which contribute equally: the Jaccard coefficient [14], a measure for oversegmentation and a measure for undersegmentation.

2.5 Segmentation quality evaluation

The quality of this segmentation approach is evaluated for the contours of the whole cell (nucleus and plasma part together) and for the nucleus part of 1000 cells where the ground truth data is generated by a manual segmentation.

3 Results

With the proposed approach the mean segmentation quality is 0.93 for the whole cell and 0.85 for the corresponding nucleus part. In Fig. 3 some visual results are presented. The relevant cells are in red boxes. Automatically segmented cell contours are painted in black, the corresponding nucleus parts are painted in red.

4 Discussion

Within the scope of the development of an automated analysis system for bone marrow aspirates the automatic segmentation of bone marrow cells including the separation of nucleus and plasma is essential for subsequent feature extraction and cell classification. For the segmentation of bone marrow cells it is possible to incorporate expert knowledge (e.g. cell size and color information) and different

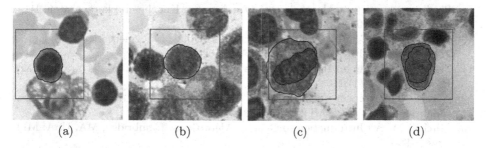

| (a) | (b) | (c) | (d) |

Fig. 3. Visual results for the automatic nucleus and plasma segmentation using the dynamic programming approach: In Figs. 3(a)–3(b), example segmentation results for the segmentation of the whole cell are shown, in Figs. 3(c)–3(d), both nucleus and plasma parts are automatically segmented.

assumptions about the appearance of the cells (e.g. shape) with the proposed dynamic programming approach. The results show that this approach is promising with regard to the segmentation quality. The segmentation is of prime importance and is further developed (for example by incorporating texture features) in order to increase the performance of the automatic morphological bone marrow analysis. Furthermore, automatically segmented bone marrow cells could be used for training and quality assurance purposes [15].

Acknowledgement. This work was funded through the MAVO-project Multi-NaBel from the Fraunhofer-Gesellschaft. A.E. Cetin and C.F. Koyuncu's work was funded by TUBITAK with project number 113E069.

References

1. Zerfass T, Haßlmeyer E, Schlarb T, et al. Segmentation of leukocyte cells in bone marrow smears. Comput Base Med Syst. 2010; p. 267–72.
2. Nilsson B, Heyden A. Model-based segmentation of leukocytes clusters. Proc ICPR. 2002;1:727–30.
3. Nilsson B, Heyden A. Segmentation of complex cell clusters in microscopic images: application to bone marrow samples. Cytometry A. 2005;66(1):24–31.
4. Reta C, Altamirano L, Gonzalez J, et al. Segmentation of bone marrow cell images for morphological classification of acute leukemia. Fla Artiff Intell Res Soc Conf. 2010.
5. Hengen H, Spoor SL, Pandit MC. Analysis of blood and bone marrow smears using digital image processing techniques. Proc SPIE. 2002;4684:624–35.
6. Bergen T, Steckhan D, Wittenberg T, et al. Segmentation of leukocytes and erythrocytes in blood smear images. Proc EMBS. 2008; p. 3075–8.
7. Nandy K, Gudla PR, Lockett SJ. Automatic segmentation of cell nuclei in 2D using dynamic programming. Proc Second Workshop Microsc Image Anal Appl Bio. 2007.
8. Achanta R, Shaji A, Smith K, et al. SLIC superpixels compared to state-of-the-art superpixel methods. IEEE Trans Pattern Anal Mach Intell. 2012;34(11):2274–82.
9. Krappe S, Macijewski K, Eismann E, et al. Lokalisierung von Knochenmarkzellen für die automatisierte Morphologische Analyse von Knochenmarkpräparaten. Proc BVM. 2014; p. 403–8.
10. Elter M, Held C, Wittenberg T. Contour tracing for segmentation of mammographic masses. Phys Med Bio. 2010;55(18):5299.
11. Zenzo SD. A note on the gradient of a multi-image. Computer Vis Graph Image Process. 1986;33(1):116 – 25.
12. Cormen T, Leiserson C, Rivest R, et al. Introduction to Algorithms. 2nd ed. Cambridge, MA, USA: MIT Press; 2001.
13. Mitchell M. An Introduction to Genetic Algorithms. Cambridge, MA, USA: MIT Press; 1998.
14. Tanimoto T. An Elementary Mathematical Theory of Classification and Prediction. International Business Machines Corporation; 1958.
15. Krappe S, Efstathiou E, Haferlach T, et al. Training und Qualitätssicherung für die morphologische Analyse von Knochenmarkpräparaten. Proc GMDS. 2013.

Colonic Polyp Classification in High-Definition Video Using Complex Wavelet-Packets

M. Häfner[1], M. Liedlgruber[2], A. Uhl[2]

[1]Department for Internal Medicine, St. Elisabeth Hospital, Vienna
[2] Department of Computer Sciences, University of Salzburg, Austria
mliedl@cosy.sbg.ac.at

Abstract. In this work, we extend different wavelet-packet based feature extraction methods to use the dual-tree complex wavelet transform. This way we aim at alleviating shortcomings of the different algorithms which stem from the use of the underlying discrete wavelet transform. The derived features are used to classify still-images extracted from HD colonoscopy videos to conduct poly staging. While some techniques cannot benefit from the extension to the dual-tree complex wavelet transform, other benefit in terms of classification accuracy.

1 Introduction

In the past, various different wavelet-based feature extraction methods have already been successfully applied to the problem of classifying endoscopic images. However, since most of the approaches are based on the discrete wavelet transform (DWT) or the discrete wavelet packets transform (DWPT), they also inherit two major shortcomings inherent to the DWT when used for image processing and classification. First, the DWT is not able to capture directional information. As a consequence it is not possible to distinguish between image details oriented at $+45°$ and $-45°$. Second, the DWT lacks shift-invariance. Thus, small shifts within an image may have a significant influence on the resulting wavelet coefficients around a singularity (i.e. an edge) due to the downsampling.

An extension to the pyramidal DWT, which aims at coping with these problems, is the dual-tree complex wavelet transform (DT-CWT) [1]. The original DT-CWT uses 2^D pyramidal DWTs for a D-dimensional transform (i.e. for a 2-D DT-CWT four DWTs are needed). The outcomes of these transforms are then combined to obtain six complex-valued subbands in the 2-D case. These subbands capture image details at $\pm15°, \pm45°$, and $\pm75°$. In addition, the DT-CWT is approximately shift-invariant. In the past it has already been shown that features based on the DT-CWT are able to deliver superior classification results as compared to the pyramidal DWT and other feature extraction methods [2, 3, 4].

However, for some methods we need a full wavelet-packet transform but analyticity gets lost for deeper decomposition levels if the DT-CWT is just extended to decompose the high-frequency subbands too [5]. But it has already been shown that a solution to this problem can be obtained fairly easily [5, 6]. We decided to use the method proposed in [5] due to its simplicity when it comes to integrate it into an existing DT-CWT implementation.

To exploit the benefits of the DT-CWT we extend a set of approaches to use the dual-tree complex wavelet packet transform (DT-CWPT). We then use the methods to extract features from a colonic polyp image database and investigate the classification performances as compared to the original (i.e. non-complex) version of the algorithms.

2   Material and methods

The high-definition (HD) color images used in this work are taken from 56 videos acquired during colonoscopy sessions between the years 2011 and 2013 at the anonymous Department (anonymous hospital) using an HD colonoscope (Pentax HiLINE HD+ 90i Colonoscope) with a resolution of 1280×1024 pixels. In order to acquire the videos 54 patients underwent endoscopy.

We extracted patches with a size of 256×256 pixels from the original images in order to get the final image set containing 85 images. For our experiments these are converted to grayscale prior to the actual feature extraction.

Lesions found during colonoscopy have been examined after application of dye-spraying with indigocarmine, as routinely performed in colonoscopy. Biopsies or mucosal resection have been performed in order to get a histopathological diagnosis. The Pentax i-SCAN image enhancement has been enabled in addition to the topical staining (i.e. i-SCAN mode 3, which enhances the visibility of pit pattern and vascular features).

Details on the image databases used are provided in Tab. 1. The columns N_O, N_E, and N_P denote the number of original images, the number of extracted patches, and the number of patients, respectively. We notice that the total number of patients given is slightly higher as compared to the number of patients who underwent endoscopy. The reason for this is that in case of some patients different types of pathologies showed up across the patient images. As a consequence a patient may be contained in more than one class.

In addition, we distinguish between a 2-classes case and a 3-classes case. In the former we distinguish between normal mucosa (non-neoplastic) and mucosal changes which need a medical intervention (neoplastic). A more fine-grained classification was proposed in [7]. In this classification scheme the images are divided into three classes: normal lesions, non-invasive lesions, and invasive lesions. This classification scheme is of particular importance since normal mucosa needs not to be removed, non-invasive lesions must be removed endoscopically, and invasive lesions must not be removed endoscopically.

We chose a set of four feature extraction methods, which have already been successfully used for the classification of endoscopic images in the past [8]:

- *WPC:* Each image is decomposed using the DWT. The features to be classified are then extracted based on coefficients in the resulting high-frequency subbands.

Table 1. The detailed ground truth information for the image database used.

Image Class	3 Classes			2 Classes		
	N_O	N_E	N_P	N_O	N_E	N_P
Normal	23	31	19	23	31	19
Non-Invasive	44	49	42	49	54	47
Invasive	5	5	5			
Total	72	85	66	72	85	66

- *WT-BB:* Using the DWPT and the Best-basis algorithm [9], each image is de-composed into an optimal basis with respect to a cost function. The features are then extracted from all resulting subbands, ignoring the approximation subband. Since the optimal bases among different images most likely will differ, the feature vectors from different images are adjusted to make them directly comparable (i.e. by using zero-filling, such that each position in a feature vector corresponds to a certain subband).
- *WT-BBCB:* This method also relies on the DWPT and the Best-basis algo-rithm. Hence, each image is decomposed into an optimal basis. Considering the decomposition trees for the resulting bases, the decomposition tree which on average is most similar to all other decomposition trees is searched for (we call this tree the centroid). To compute the similarity between two decomposition trees we employ the quadtree distance metric used in [8].
  Once the centroid has been found, all images are decomposed into the re-spective basis. The features are then extracted from the resulting subbands, ignoring the approximation subband.
- *WT-LDB:* Using the Local discriminant bases algorithm [10], which is based on the DWPT, an optimal basis with respect to the discriminant power of subbands among different image classes is computed. The discriminant power is similar to the cost function used in the Best-basis algorithm.
  Once the optimal basis has been found, all images are decomposed into the respective basis and the features are extracted from the resulting subbands, except for the approximation subband.

These methods are then extended to employ a complex transform. In case of WPC, the originally proposed DT-CWT already corresponds to a pyramidal transform and we use the magnitudes of the complex coefficients for feature extraction. For methods, which rely on the DWPT, we can use the complex variant DT-CWPT. Similar to the complex WPC, we again extract the features based on the magnitudes of the complex coefficients. For all complex methods features are extracted for negative and positive feature angles separately and stored in an interleaved fashion.

To extend the WT-LDB method to a complex one, the so-called time fre-quency energy map (TFEM) used in the Local discriminant bases algorithm must also be extended. We do this by simply computing two different TFEMs for each class, one for each direction. The discriminant power for a quadtree node is then computed by taking the sum over the TFEMs for the different directions.

Regarding the wavelet transform setup, we use Kingsbury's Q-Shift (14,14)-tap filters (for decomposition stages ≥ 2) in combination with (13,19)-tap near-orthogonal filters (for the first decomposition stage) in case of the complex methods. For the DT-CWPT we use the Q-Shift filters for the decomposition nodes needing special treatment (using the methodology proposed in [5]). To make the real and complex methods more comparable, we use the Q-Shift filters also for the real methods (i.e. just one of the filter banks). We chose a maximum decomposition level of 5 to have enough coefficients at the last decomposition stage (subband size 8×8).

For methods which are based on the Best-basis algorithm we use the entropy as cost function. For the Local discriminant bases algorithm we use the l^2-norm as discriminant measure. The feature we use for all methods is the entropy which is computed from the coefficients in the high-frequency subbands. We also evaluated other features, but on average the entropy yielded the highest classification accuracies. In case of complex methods the entropy is computed based on the magnitudes of the complex coefficients.

Since the adaptive methods usually yield far more leaf nodes than the pyramidal transform, the feature vectors are rather high-dimensional when features are extracted from all resulting leaf nodes This especially applies to the complex variants of the methods. Hence, we perform a principal component analysis (PCA) to reduce the dimensionality of the feature vectors. Prior to applying the PCA to the features, we center the training feature vectors by subtracting the feature-wise mean from each feature. After computing the eigenvalues and eigenvectors from the training features, these are sorted descending with respect to the eigenvalues. This is followed by computing the number of components p to retain from the cumulative sum of the eigenvectors, such that the cumulative sum for the first p largest eigenvalues is above 0.99.

Once the validation features have been extracted and centered (using the means from the original training features), the feature projection computed from the training features is also applied to the validation features. This preprocessing is applied to all real and complex methods (adaptive as well as pyramidal).

For the classification we use the k-Nearest neighbors (k-NN) classifier. This rather weak classifier has been chosen to emphasize more on the effect of extending the methods to complex methods. During our experiments the k-value for the classifier has not been fixed to some certain value. Instead, we carried out experiments with different values for k (i.e. $k = 1, \ldots, 25$).

To estimate the classification accuracies we use the leave-one-patient-out cross-validation (LOPO-CV). In this setup one image out of the database is considered to be an unknown image. The remaining images are used to train the classifier (omitting those images which originate from the same patient as the image left out). The class of the unknown image is then predicted by the system (i.e. the images from a single patient are considered as the validation images while the images from all other patients are considered as training images).

Table 2. The detailed classification results for our experiments.

Method	Mode	2 Classes	3 Classes
WT-BB	R	65.3 ± 3.6	59.0 ± 3.4
	C	69.6 ± 2.5	66.7 ± 3.2
WT-BBCB	R	64.2 ± 3.3	58.4 ± 3.7
	C	64.0 ± 1.4	58.0 ± 1.5
WT-LDB	R	67.6 ± 2.5	60.1 ± 2.8
	C	64.4 ± 2.3	60.6 ± 1.9
WPC	R	67.0 ± 1.9	60.9 ± 2.5
	C	63.1 ± 2.4	57.2 ± 3.0

These steps (training and prediction) are repeated for each image, yielding an estimate of the overall classification accuracy.

For the computation of the distances between feature vectors we use the l^1-norm. We also evaluated other distances metrics as well, but on average this metric delivered the highest classification results.

3   Results

A summary of the experimental results can be found in Tab. 2. In this table the mean overall classification rates are shown, along with the standard deviations over all choices for k. The column labeled "Mode" shows whether the respective row shows the results for a real method (R) or a complex method (C).

We notice that switching to the complex domain in most cases leads to a drop in terms of the mean overall classification rates. Only in case of WT-BB a consistent improvement can be observed (about 4% and 7% in the 2-classes case and the 3-classes case, respectively). Another method, which at least slightly benefits from switching to the complex domain in the 3-classes case is WT-LDB. But the improvement is negligible. In all other cases the complex variant of the methods leads to a result drop. While the result drops are only marginal in case of WT-BBCB, they are noticeably higher in case of WPC and WT-LDB (in the 2-classes case) with up to about 4%.

In addition, the complex version of WT-BB delivers the highest mean overall classification rates as compared to all other methods.

4   Discussion

In this work we investigated whether it is meaningful to extend a chosen set of wavelet-based feature extraction methods to use a complex wavelet transform instead of a real one. For this purpose we evaluated the extended methods on a colonic polyp image databases.

The results we obtained showed that at least one method (WT-BB) is able to consistently improve the classification rates when using the complex version of it. For all other methods the complex versions mostly lead to result drops. The complex WT-BB method also delivers the highest mean classification rates.

In future work we will investigate the use of all color information available as this work was restricted to grayscale images only. In addition a larger image database and a broader set of methods should be evaluated in order to be able to make robust statements about the benefit of the complex transform.

Acknowledgement. This work has been supported by the Austrian Science Fund (FWF), under Project No. TRP-206.

References

1. Selesnick IW, Baraniuk RG, Kingsbury NG. The dual-tree complex wavelet transform: a coherent framework for multiscale signal and image processing. IEEE Signal Process Mag. 2005;22(6):123–51.
2. Kwitt R, Uhl A. Modeling the marginal distributions of complex wavelet coefficient magnitudes for the classification of zoom-endoscopy images. Proc MMBIA. 2007.
3. Kwitt R, Uhl A. Image similarity measurement by Kullback-Leibler divergences between complex wavelet subband statistics for texture retrieval. Proc ICIP. 2008; p. 933–6.
4. Häfner M, Kwitt R, Uhl A, et al. Feature-extraction from multi-directional multi-resolution image transformations for the classification of zoom-endoscopy images. Pattern Anal Appl. 2009;12(4):407–13.
5. Bayram I, Selesnick IW. On the dual-tree complex wavelet packet and m-band transforms. IEEE Trans Signal Process. 2008;56(6).
6. Weickert T, Kiencke U. Analytic wavelet packets: combining the dual-tree approach with wavelet packets for signal analysis and filtering. IEEE Trans Signal Process. 2009;57(2).
7. Kato S, Fu KI, Sano Y, et al. Magnifying colonoscopy as a non-biopsy technique for differential diagnosis of non-neoplastic and neoplastic lesions. World J Gastroenterol. 2006;12(9):1416–20.
8. Liedlgruber M, Uhl A. Statistical and structural wavelet packet features for pit pattern classification in zoom-endoscopic colon images. Proc WSEAS, WAMUS). 2007; p. 147–152.
9. Coifman RR, Wickerhauser MV. Entropy based methods for best basis selection. IEEE Trans Inf Theory. 1992;38(2):719–46.
10. Saito N, Coifman RR. Local discriminant bases. Proc SPIE. 1994; p. 2–14.

Selection of Seeds for Resting-State fMRI-Based Prediction of Individual Brain Maturity

Norman Scheel[1,2], Andrea Essenwanger[1], Thomas F. Münte[2],
Marcus Heldmann[2], Ulrike M. Krämer[2], Amir Madany Mamlouk[1]

[1]Institute for Neuro- and Bioinformatics, Universty of Lübeck
[2]Department of Neurology, University of Lübeck
norman.scheel@neuro.uni-luebeck.de

Abstract. The analysis of resting-state brain connectivity allows unraveling the fundamentals of functional brain organization. Especially changes of network connectivity related to age or diseases promise to serve as early biomarkers. After control of subject movement, we found that, when reaching a critical number of subjects, age prediction is reproducible for all seed selection strategies tested here (functional, anatomical and random based seeds). On the Enhanced Rockland Community Sample, we use support vector regression (SVR) and intense permutation testing for statistical validation.

1 Introduction

Since its introduction, resting state functional MRI (rs-fMRI) has become an increasingly used tool to study functional brain connectivity. Functional rs-fMRI connectivity matrices are typically based on seeds using diverse brain atlases or points of interest (POIs). They describe the functional interactions of brain regions and can be used to document their changes. For example, Dosenbach et al. introduced a set of 160 POIs [1]. These points likely represent nodes of functional networks as they have been created on a meta study of task experiments. Using these special POIs, they were able to show, that age specific differences in functional brain organization allow the prediction of individual brain maturity.

This study set out to answer two questions: First we want to examine the predictive power of Dosenbach's points after careful removal of head-motion artifacts, as these can contribute substantially to the rs-fMRI signal and produce systematic but spurious patterns in functional connectomes [2]. Secondly, we evaluated the importance of seed point selection for the given age prediction scenario by testing the following established seeds against random POIs: The Automated-Anatomical-Labeling (AAL) atlas by Tzourio-Mazoyer [3], Dosenbach's POIs [1] and the resting state network (RSN) maps of Shirer et al. [4].

2   Materials and methods

2.1   The enhanced rockland community sample

Our dataset was kindly provided by the Nathan Kline Institute, Orangeburg, NY [5]: The Enhanced Rockland Community Sample. It provides diverse scanning protocols, simultaneous recording of cardiac and respiratory signals, as well as a multitude of healthy subjects. In four releases, 202 complete error-free resting-state recordings of subjects with an age-distribution of 43 ± 20 years, 131 women and 71 men are provided. Using a Siemens Magnetom TrioTim 3T scanner, a standard resting-state session of 5 minutes with a repetition time of 2.5s was acquired. Each volume has 38 slices (interleaved acquisition) of 3mm thickness and an in plane voxel resolution of 3×3 mm.

2.2   Preprocessing

Our preprocessing routine is carried out using physiological noise regression, SPM8 and DPARSFA[6]. It starts with RETROICOR RVHR[7], removing cardiac and respiratory noise using the provided physiological recordings. Reorientation of all images in setting the origin to the anterior comissure is then followed by realignment and New Segment + DARTEL[6]. The nuisance regression step removes linear trends, 6 rigid body as well as scrubbing head motion regressors and the signal of white matter and cerebro-spinal fluids. Normalization was carried out using DARTEL and the results where smoothed with a $fwhm = 4mm$ isotropic kernel. Bandpass filtering was carried out at $0.01 \sim 0.08$Hz. See SPM 8 Manual and [6] for details on single preprocessing methods used here.

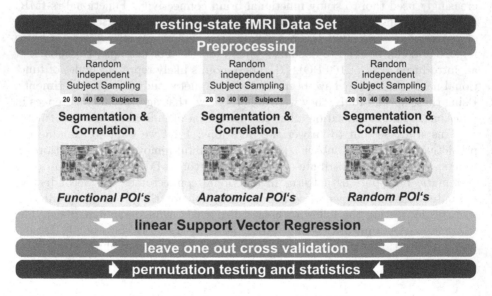

Fig. 1. Overview of our processing pipeline

2.3   Random independent subject sampling

When comparing the phenotopic data with movement parameters from the preprocessing step, we found a slight anti-correlation of subject movement with age progression, indicating that younger subjects tend to move more during scanning than older ones. To account for this problem we applied an additional step to motion and scrubbing parameter regression. We only use subsets of subjects, generated iteratively by randomly choosing 20, 30, 40 or 60 out of the 202 base subjects. Each set of subjects is then tested whether the sets movement parameters are correlated with the sets age distribution. If a correlation was found, the algorithm draws a new random set of subjects and tests again until an independent set ist found. The resulting sets have the following age distributions: 20 Subj.: 51±21; 30 Subj.: 43±20; 40 Subj.: 44±18; 60 Subj.: 45±18.

2.4   Seed selection

We used three main seed selection approaches. Firstly anatomical: Using the AAL-atlas we calculated either the mean activation time course of each region or the time course of centroids of each region with a sphere of 10 mm. Secondly functional: Using either the Dosenbach POIs with a 10 mm sphere or the RSN maps of Shirer et al., which provide 14 maps comprised of 90 local regions of which we again took the mean time course. Finally, we used 50, 70, 90, 120 and 160 random POIs, again with a 10 mm sphere. For each number of random POIs we drew 100 sets to create a cumulative distribution.

2.5   Age prediction and significance testing

After connectome generation we used linear support vector regression (SVR – from libSVM library) to find differences in brain connectivity due to aging. The regression accuracy is derived by using a leave-one-out cross validation (CV) and calculating the root mean squared error (RMSE). For significance testing, we estimated the empirical cumulative distribution, by calculating the RMSE 10.000 times for random label permutations. p-values are defined through the empirical probability. $p < 0.05$ implies that regression results differ significantly from chance. Our complete processing pipeline is depicted in Fig. 1.

3   Results

3.1   Age prediction

Randomly scattered POIs yield significant RMSEs (Fig. 2). Using more than 20 subjects and a minimum of 70 points consistently produced significant results. The result of 40 subjects using 50 points could be interpreted as an outlier. In general, the prediction error declines with the increase of nodes as well as subjects. Also the 95% interval of the empirical cumulative distribution narrows

Fig. 2. Overview of Random Points: 30 or more subjects allow significant age prediction. Shown here are mean cross validation (CV) results with standard deviation (SD), expected value (E) and the 95% interval.

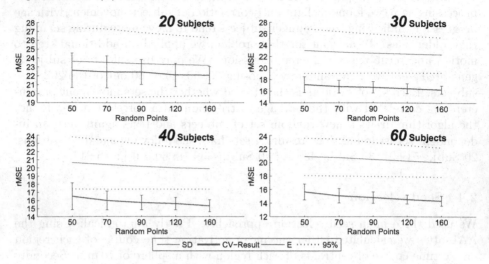

with more points. Age prediction for standard seeds (Fig. 3) also yields significant RMSEs. For 30 subjects AAL-Centroids seem to be most stable (RMSE = 13.7 / p = 0.0001) closely followed by Dosenbach POIs (RMSE = 14.4 / p = 0.0002) and AAL means (RMSE = 14 / p = 0.0003). Shirer/Greicius RSN 90 regions reach RMSE = 16.1 / p = 0.0079.

3.2 Connections

We used the normal vector of the support vector regression to analyze connections most discriminant for aging. Here, we report the results of the 60 subjects

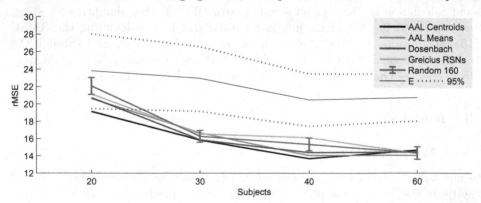

Fig. 3. Overview of all parcellation approaches: Shown here are the cross validation results of all seeds in different color, the mean expected value (E) and the mean 95% interval.

Table 1. Top 5 connections of the SVR normal vector, *strengthening* with age.

Region A	⇔ Region B	Region A	⇔ Region B
Feature: *AAL Means*		Feature: *AAL Centroids*	
Precentral R	⇔ Postcentral R	Postcentral R	⇔ Paracentral Lobule L
Frontal Sup. L	⇔ Supp. Motor Area L	Postcentral R	⇔ Paracentral Lobule R
Postcentral L	⇔ Postcentral R	Postcentral L	⇔ Postcentral R
Precentral L	⇔ Postcentral R	Cingulum Mid. R	⇔ Postcentral R
Precentral R	⇔ Postcentral L	Postcentral L	⇔ Paracentral Lobule L
Feature: *Dosenbach POIs*		Feature: *Random POIs*	
Postcentral L	⇔ Precentral R	Frontal Sup. L	⇔ Frontal Sup R
Precentral R	⇔ Precentral L	Postcentral L	⇔ Postcentral R
Precentral L	⇔ Precentral R	Precentral R	⇔ Postcentral L
Postcentral L	⇔ Precentral L	Frontal Sup. R	⇔ Frontal Mid. L
Frontal Sup. R	⇔ Postcentral R	Precentral L	⇔ Postcentral R

run. For random sets we used 160 POIs and mapped the connections of each connectome to the AAL standard map and calculated the mean normal connectome. Most prominent connections, that grow stronger with age can be found in Tab. 1 and resp. grow weaker with age in Tab. 2. Fig. 4 shows these connections for each feature set depicting strengthening connections in red and weakening connections in blue.

4 Discussion

We have shown that the results of Dosenbach et. al. can be reproduced when using stringent subject movement control. Surprisingly, age prediction is even possible for randomly selected seeds, just as it is for all other approaches tested here.

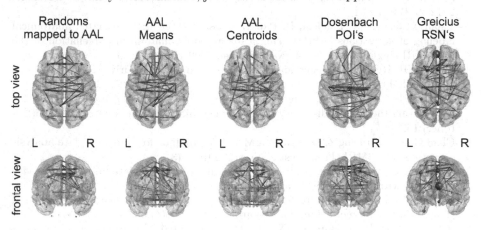

Fig. 4. Strongest connections of the SVR normal vector. Red connections decrease and blue connections increase with aging.

Table 2. Top 5 connections of the SVR normal vector, *weakening* with age.

Region A	⇔ Region B	Region A	⇔ Region B
Feature: *AAL Means*		Feature: *AAL Centroids*	
Insula R	⇔ Cingulum Mid. R	Putamen R	⇔ Pallidum R
Pallidum L	⇔ Pallidum R	Fusiform L	⇔ Fusiform R
Rolandic Oper. L	⇔ Insula R	Frontal Sup. L	⇔ Angular L
Frontal Sup. Orb. R	⇔ Frontal Inf. Orb. R	Occipital Mid. L	⇔ Occipital Inf. L
Cingulum Post. L	⇔ Cingulum Post. R	Frontal Sup. Orb. L	⇔ Amygdala R
Feature: *Dosenbach POIs*		Feature: *Random POIs*	
Occipital Mid. L	⇔ Occipital Mid. L	Supp. Motor Area L	⇔ Insula R
Rolandic Oper. R	⇔ Temporal Sup. L	Insula R	⇔ Cing. Mid. R
Temporal Sup. R	⇔ Temporal Mid. L	Supp. Motor Area R	⇔ Insula R
Putamen R	⇔ Putamen L	Insula R	⇔ Cing. Mid. L
Frontal Mid. L	⇔ Occipital Mid. R	Putamen L	⇔ Putamen R

Interestingly, primary motor and somatosensory cortex connections strengthen while connections with Pallidum and Putamen weaken with age. Quantitatively, these connections are consistent regardless of the underlying seeds and appear to be biologically plausible [8], [9]. Interpretation and comparison of single connections should be subject to further investigation and also should be compared over multiple subject groups.

References

1. Dosenbach NUF, Nardos B, Cohen AL, et al. Prediction of individual brain maturity using fMRI. Science. 2010;329(5997):1358–61.
2. Power JD, Barnes Ka, Snyder AZ, et al. Spurious but systematic correlations in functional connectivity MRI networks arise from subject motion. NeuroImage. 2012;59(3):2142–54.
3. Tzourio-Mazoyer N, Landeau B, Papathanassiou D, et al. Automated anatomical labeling of activations in SPM using a macroscopic anatomical parcellation of the MNI MRI single-subject brain. NeuroImage. 2002;15(1):273–89.
4. Shirer WR, Ryali S, Rykhlevskaia E, et al. Decoding subject-driven cognitive states with whole-brain connectivity patterns. Cereb Cortex. 2012;22(1):158–65.
5. Nooner KB, Colcombe SJ, Tobe RH, et al. The NKI-rockland sample: a model for accelerating the pace of discovery science in psychiatry. Front Neurosci. 2012;6(October):152.
6. Chao-Gan Y, Yu-Feng Z. DPARSF: a MATLAB toolbox for "pipeline" data analysis of resting-state fMRI. Front Syst Neurosci. 2010;4:13.
7. Chang C, Glover GH. Time-frequency dynamics of resting-state brain connectivity measured with fMRI. NeuroImage. 2010;50(1):81–98.
8. Mattay VS, Fera F, Tessitore A, et al. Neurophysiological correlates of age-related changes in human motor function. Neurology. 2002;58(4):630–5.
9. Salat DH, Tuch DS, Greve DN, et al. Age-related alterations in white matter microstructure measured by diffusion tensor imaging. Neurobiol Aging. 2005;26(8):1215–27.

Local Surface Estimation from Arbitrary 3D Contour Sets for Aortic Quantification

Cosmin Adrian Morariu[1], Daniel Sebastian Dohle[2], Tobias Terheiden[1],
Konstantinos Tsagakis[2], Josef Pauli[1]

[1]Intelligent Systems Group, Faculty of Engineering, University of Duisburg-Essen
[2]Department of Thoracic and Cardiovascular Surgery, Universitätsklinikum Essen
adrian.morariu@uni-due.de

Abstract. Possible future endovascular repair of aortic Type A dissections, which always also involve the ascending aorta (AA), implies custom-designed stent-grafts for each patient. Extraction of morphological parameters such as aortic diameters from an accurately reconstructed aortic volume proves essential for accomplishing this goal. Our contribution introduces a novel approach to local surface and normal estimation via implicit models. Given a sparse set of randomly positioned and oriented contours in 3D, we adapt a multi-level partition of unity (MPU) method, rescinding the existing MPU-related restriction of having contours in parallel planes. Radii and diameter measurements are evaluated based on a ground truth aortic volume for 11 patient CTA datasets.

1 Introduction

Intramural blood flow leads to the development of a false lumen in aortas affected by acute dissections [1]. Separate quantification of the true and false lumen addresses the task of reconstructing surfaces from non-convex contour sets, as the false lumen often discloses concave cross-sectional shapes. Hence, adequate alternatives to linear interpolation methods such as the quickhull algorithm [2], able to accurately reconstruct surfaces from sparse, yet only convex contour sets, are of special interest.

The local surface estimation proposed by this contribution relies on the multi-level partition of unity (MPU) method described in [3]. This approach assumes a dense point set, regularly distributed in 3D space. Moreover, it demands the existence of surface normals in each point, which might be obtained from range acquisition devices or by least-squares fitting. However, this is not feasible in cases of non-dense point sets such as isolated contour sets. Reference [4] adapts computation of normals to the requirements of a point set consisting of contours within parallel 2D planes, stemming from e.g. histological imaging. We expand the method in [4] by allowing surface reconstruction based on randomly positioned and oriented contours in 3D. In particular, we introduce a novel scheme for determining surface normals. Subsequently, we account for the average, minimal and maximal radii and diameters per aortic cross-section. These key morphological parameters are required for manufacturing patient-specific stent-grafts.

2   Materials and methods

Regarding the MPU approach [3], local piecewise quadratic functions serve for approximating a surface from a point cloud consisting of S points $\mathcal{P} = p_1, \ldots, p_S$. As mentioned before, a set of S surface normals $\mathcal{N}$ is additionally required. The result of the MPU corresponds to an implicit function $f(x)$, with its zero-level-set implicitly representing the surface. As suggested by its terminology, the partition-of-unity approach, achieves a partition of the definition domain Ω in m subdomains. The global approximation of $f(x)$ corresponds to the weighted sum of local approximations $Q_i(x)$

$$f(x) \approx \sum_{i=1}^{m} \varphi_i(x) Q_i(x) \qquad \forall x \in \Omega \tag{1}$$

Partition-of-unity-weights $\varphi_i(x)$ get assigned to each i-th subdomain, whereby their sum equals to one: $\sum_{i=1}^{m} \varphi_i(x) = 1$, $\forall x \in \Omega$. MPU-implicits utilize an adaptive, octree-based decomposition technique to refine areas with a higher density of detail. The first octree cell consists of a bounding box around all data points. A local approximation $Q(x)$ for the data points contained in each cell is determined. In case of a high deviation ϵ of the local approximation from the data points of the cell, the approximation $Q(x)$ is considered too vague and the octree cell is further divided into eight cells.

Computation of the required set of surface normals $\mathcal{N}$ is restricted in [4] to a point cloud consisting of contours within parallel axial slices. Normals are obtained by firstly creating a binary volume, which represents a trivial undertaking in case of contours in axial slices. Subsequently, a 3D Gaussian function serves for volume filtering (blurring) in order to retrieve the gradient information leading to normals in each input contour point.

With respect to our field of application, *arbitrary* contour sets originate from automatic aortic segmentations carried out within multiplanar reformatted (MPR) planes [5]. Therefore, we contrive another scheme, which allows us calculating the normals. In order to fulfill the condition, that all normal vectors associated with each MPR's contour points are oriented outwards, we compute two orientation vectors for each MPR-contour $\mathcal{M}$ in such manner, that the plane normals $\overrightarrow{N}_{\mathcal{M}}$ exhibit similar orientation w.r.t. the MPR-contours. Let an MPR-contour consist of k points with 3D coordinates. The first orientation vector will be defined by the contour points at location 1 and $\frac{k}{4}$ and the second vector by the points at $\frac{k}{2}$ and k. Consequently, the plane's normals, obtained via cross product, will always reveal the same orientation w.r.t. the contours. Finally, surface normal

$$\overrightarrow{N}_j = \overrightarrow{N}_{\mathcal{M}} \times (\overrightarrow{P_{j+1} - P_{j-1}}) \quad \text{with} \quad j \in \{1, ..., k\} \text{ and } P_0 = P_k, P_{k+1} = P_1 \tag{2}$$

associated with an MPR contour point P_j results as the cross product between plane normal $\overrightarrow{N}_{\mathcal{M}}$ and vector $\overrightarrow{P_{j+1} - P_{j-1}}$. The ends of the vascular segment to be reconstructed can be closed by the insertion of additional points in the point

Table 1. Mean, minimal and maximal measurement errors for the average radii and diameters in cross-sectional MPRs belonging to the evaluated 11 CTA datasets.

Error type (in mm)	Average radii	Average diameters
$\bar{e}_{mean}$	0.5740 ± 0.1784	1.2383 ± 0.3398
$\overline{std}_{mean}$	0.5336 ± 0.1978	1.0784 ± 0.3502
$\bar{e}_{min}$	0.0047 ± 0.0048	0.0155 ± 0.0178
$\bar{e}_{max}$	2.5860 ± 1.0348	5.3800 ± 1.9278

cloud. For this purpose, all points constituting the interior of both contours in the first, respectively last MPR, will be added to the point cloud. Normals associated with points *inside* the first MPR contour $\mathcal{M}_1$ point in opposite direction to the normal $\overrightarrow{N}_{\mathcal{M}_1}$ of the corresponding MPR plane. Point normals *inside* the last MPR contour $\mathcal{M}_n$ are identical with the plane normal $\overrightarrow{N}_{\mathcal{M}_n}$.

The mean, minimal and maximal radii and diameters per aortic cross-section represent clinically valuable entities with regard to enabling minimally invasive techniques within the AA. We obtain these values in planes orthogonal to the aortic centerline, which is provided by the prior segmentation step (not subject of this contribution, please refer to [5]). The spline is sampled equidistantly (2 mm spacing) and the orthogonal MPRs are extracted from the binary 3D matrix containing the aortic volume (not from the 3D image data, as for aortic segmentation). The aortic volume stems directly from the estimated surface, which has been obtained from contours in 5 mm spacing. Due to the mostly noncircular nature of aortic cross-sections bearing severe pathologies such as dissections, assuming a constant cross-sectional radius would not prove feasible. Therefore we compute all the distances from each region center to the outer

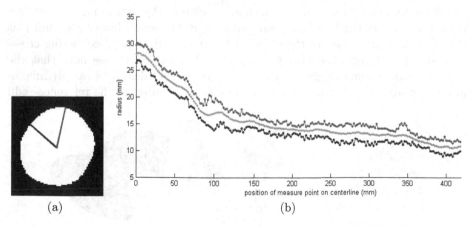

(a)   (b)

Fig. 1. a) MPR with minimal (blue) und maximal (red) radius. b) Radius measurement within cross-sectional MPRs of a CTA dataset: mean radius (green), minimum (blue), maximum (red). The position of each MPR along the aortic centerline (sampled in 2 mm steps) is represented on the abscissa axis, starting in the AA just above the heart.

Table 2. Computation times for surface reconstruction via convex hull, respectively using the proposed approach with different grid parameter values g.

Approach	t_{min}	t_{max}	$\varnothing$ (s)
Convex hull	2.77	19.12	5.68
MPU-implicits ($g = 5$)	3.51	11.0	5.80
MPU-implicits ($g = 2$)	6.87	20.46	10.38
MPU-implicits ($g = 1$)	17.90	42.10	24.63

boundaries in order to determine the radii. Fig. 1(a) illustrates an MPR with the minimal radius marked in blue and the maximal radius depicted in red. Fig. 1(b) shows a plot of the measured distances for all MPRs within a patient's dataset, wherein the abscissa axis evolves from above the heart in the AA towards the iliac bifurcation in the descending aorta. The average of all measured distances per MPR is depicted in green, in addition to the minimum (blue) and maximum (red) radius. The diameters (min, mean and max) are calculated by pairwise matching the slopes associated to each radial segment.

The measurements have been evaluated on 11 CTA datasets from patients with aortic Type A dissection. The datasets contain 87 to 1034 axial slices with a slice spacing ranging from 0.7 to 5 mm and a within-plane resolution between 0.445 and 0.863 mm.

3 Results

Tab. 1 summarizes the errors when measuring the average aortic radii and diameters along the aortic centerline. The gold standard regarding the radii and the diameters is obtained in an automated manner, by extracting a centerline from the ground truth volume, sampling it at the same interval (2 mm) as the centerline associated to the estimated surface and, finally, extracting cross-sectional MPRs from the binary ground truth volume. Please note that the ground truth volume originates from contours in parallel slices (axial), manually annotated by a vascular surgeon. The quantification of the reference-radii

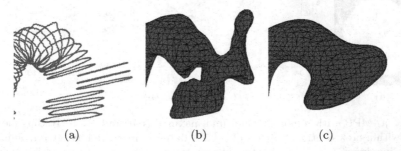

| (a) | (b) | (c) |

Fig. 2. Faulty point cloud (a) with 3 deliberately shifted contours (by 25 mm in each MPR plane). MPU-implicits with $\max_{level} = 15$ leads to erroneous results (b). Diminishing $\max_{level} = 3$ increases octree cell size but reveals surface artifacts (c).

and reference-diameters within these MPRs ensues in a similar manner to the approach described in previous section for the automatically segmented volume. Previous to evaluating radii and diameter quantification, the ground truth aortic volume and the automatically segmented volume have been cropped to a common segment with regard to starting and ending positions within the datasets. The mean radial error $\bar{e}_{mean,r} = 0.57$ mm, averaged within and also over all 11 CTA datasets, reveals subvoxel resolution. Fig. 4 c) illustrates the mean radii within all MPRs of a dataset along the centerline, extracted from the segmented volume (red), as well as from the ground truth volume (blue).

The depth of the octree decomposition is mainly steered by the parameters ϵ and $\max_{level}$. While the latter defines the maximum recursion depth of the tree (Fig. 2), the first parameter, ϵ, limits the permissible errors of local approximations. Despite a short distance to the input data points, small ϵ-values lead to overfitting and, consequently, the surface will deviate from a smooth, organic shape (Fig. 3(a)). High error tolerance results in a less deep octree subdivision. However, inclusion of more data points in a cell provides a strong shape distortion (Fig. 3 c)). Based on a further parameter g, we adjust the resolution of the polygonized triangle mesh pertaining to the implicit function $f(x)$. Fig. 3(d–f) depicts the aortic surface for 3 different g values. Tab. 2 reveals that the computation time, averaged over all 11 datasets, for surface reconstruction (including computation of normals) via our proposed implicit approach (with $g = 5$) is similar to that of linear interpolation by the convex hull method (2.66 GHz Intel Core i5, 8 GB RAM and Matlab). The quickhull algorithm, depicted in Fig. 4 a) and b) reconstructs convex 3D surfaces regardless of the initial contours shapes. In contrast to the convex hull-based surface reconstruction [2], our approach is also suitable for tubular structures having non-convex cross-sections. As an example within our application field, the false lumen pertaining to aortic dissections often implies non-convex cross-sections. We achieve a good compromise between accuracy of estimation and computation time by setting $\epsilon = 0.05$, $\max_{level} = 15$ and $g = 5$ mm.

4   Discussion

Concerning theoretical foundations, based on the implicit MPU approach, we present a novel local surface estimation relying on a sparse set of 3D contours

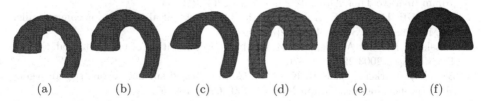

| (a) | (b) | (c) | (d) | (e) | (f) |

Fig. 3. Influence of the error parameter ϵ on the accuracy of the reconstruction: (a) $\epsilon = 0,005$, (b) $\epsilon = 0,05$ and (c) $\epsilon = 0,2$. MPU-implicits with different grid sizes: (d) $g = 10$mm, (e) $g = 5$ mm und (f) $g = 2$ mm.

Fig. 4. 3D point set of the segmentation results for two consecutive MPRs (a). Triangle mesh of the convex hull belonging to the vessel segment between both MPRs (b). Comparison of the mean radius in cross-sectional MPRs (c) extracted from the reconstructed surface (red) with ground truth (blue). The position of each MPR along the aortic centerline (sampled in 2 mm steps) is represented on the abscissa axis.

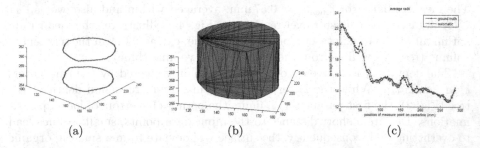

|(a)|(b)|(c)|

of arbitrary position and orientation. The proposed computation of normals to each contour point, needed by the MPU method, widely applies to tubular structures with convex and, mostly important, also non-convex cross-sections. By approximation instead of interpolation, noise in the input point set can be efficiently suppressed and a smooth surface will be reconstructed. Control over smoothness, accuracy and resolution of the reconstruction allow generation of natural-looking vascular models. However, a limitation of our algorithm resides in yielding inaccurate surface estimations in cases where two consecutive contours significantly deviate from each other. Increasing the robustness of the proposed approach with respect to cases such as in Fig. 2, where we deliberately shifted 3 contours, defines the direction of our future research on this topic. On application level, the accurately estimated surface serves for enabling minimally invasive therapy in case of Type A dissections by accounting for the average, minimal and maximal radii and diameters per cross-section. These cannot be assumed constant due to the non-circular cross-sectional shape of aortas affected by severe pathology.

References

1. Wendt D, Thielmann M, Melzer A, et al. The past, present and future of minimally invasive therapy in endovascular interventions: a review and speculative outlook. Minim Invasive Ther Allied Technol. 2013;22(4):242–53.
2. Barber CB, Dobkin DP, Huhdanpaa H. The quickhull algorithm for convex hulls. ACM Trans Math Softw. 1996;22(4):469–83.
3. Ohtake Y, Belyaev A, Alexa M, et al. Multi-level partition of unity implicits. ACM Trans Graph. 2003;22(3):463–70.
4. Braude I, Marker J, Museth K, et al. Contour-based surface reconstruction using MPU implicit models. Graph Models. 2007;69(2):139–57.
5. Morariu CA, Terheiden T, Dohle DS, et al. Graph-based and variational minimization of statistical cost functionals for 3D segmentation of aortic dissections. Lect Notes Computer Sci. 2014;8753:511–22.

Multithreading-Support für die Programmiersprache Julia

Tobias Knopp[1,2]

[1]Abteilung für Biomedizinische Bildgebung, Universitätsklinikum
Hamburg-Eppendorf
[2]Technische Universität Hamburg-Harburg
t.knopp@uke.de

Kurzfassung. Julia ist eine junge, für das wissenschaftliche Rechnen
entworfene Programmiersprache. Mit ihrer Matlab verwandten Syntax
ist Julia insbesondere für die Forschung im Bereich der medizinischen
Bildverarbeitung von Interesse. Trotz einer einfachen Syntax und eines
dynamischen Typsystems erreicht Julia Programmlaufzeiten wie äquivalenten C-Programme. Eine Limitierung von Julia ist die fehlende Unterstützung für das Schreiben von Multithreading-Programmen. In dieser
Arbeit stellen wir unser unseren experimentellen Patch vor, der das Ausführen von Julia Code in mehreren Threads ermöglicht.

1 Einleitung

Julia ist eine vielversprechende Programmiersprache, die seit 2009 von Jeff Bezanson, Stefan Karpinski und Viral Shah [1, 2] entwickelt wurde. Julias Fokus
liegt im Bereich des wissenschaftlichen Rechnens wobei Julia sehr flexibel eingesetzt werden kann, wie z.B. für Webanwendungen [3] und graphische Benutzungsschnittstellen [4]. Besonders interessant ist Julia für die Forschung im Bereich der medizinischen Bildverarbeitung. In dem Julia Paket *Images.jl* wurden
bereits zahlreiche Bildverarbeitungmethoden implementiert [5].

Das besondere an Julia ist, dass die Benutzung ähnlich einfach wie bei den
meisten dynamisch typisierten Programmiersprachen (Matlab, Python, R) ist,
jedoch Ausführungsgeschwindigkeiten wie bei kompilierten C Programmen er-
reichbar sind. In vielen Bereichen wird die langsame Ausführungsgeschwindigkeit
dadurch umgangen, dass zeitkritische Bereiche in C-Code ausgelagert werden.
Bekannte Beispiele sind Matlab mit dem *MEX-Interface* und Python mit *ctypes*
oder *Cython* [6]. Die Verwendung und Integration mehrere Programmiersprachen benötigt jedoch viel Erfahrung und die Wartbarkeit der Programme wird
anspruchsvoller. Mit Julia ist es nicht nötig zeitkritische Programmteile in C zu
programmieren. Somit wird die Entwicklungszeit verkürzt, was insbesondere in
der Forschung von großer Wichtigkeit ist.

Die hohe Ausführungsgeschwindigkeit von Julia-Programmen liegt an dem
speziell entworfenen Typsystem, welches die Erzeugung von hocheffizienten Maschinencode ermöglicht. Hierzu nutzt die Referenzimplementierung von Julia

LLVM [7]. Das Hauptfeature von Julia ist die Nutzung von Multiple-Dispatch, welches es ermöglicht verschiedene Funktionen basierend auf den Typen der Funktionsargumente auszuführen. Durch ein parametrisches Typsystem können zusätzlich generische Funktionen geschrieben werden, ohne hierbei Performance-Einbußen hinnehmen zu müssen.

Asynchrone Programmierung kann in Julia mittels sogenannter *tasks* erreicht werden (siehe *co-routine* oder *green thread* [8]). Für das Ausnutzen mehrerer CPU-Kerne bietet Julia jedoch nur einen Mechanismus für verteilte Anwendungen, die mehrere Prozesse nutzen. In der Praxis ist es jedoch häufig deutlich einfacher Programme zu schreiben, welche native Threads nutzen. Insbesondere im Bereich des wissenschaftlichen Rechnens ist die Verwendung mehrerer Threads Standard.

In dieser Arbeit werden wir unseren Patch vorstellen, der Multithreading-Support für Julia implementiert. Betrachtet man andere dynamische Programmiersprachen, wie z.B. Matlab, Python und R sieht man, dass die Implementierung von Multithreading sehr anspruchsvoll sein kann, da eine enge Kopplung zwischen dem Nutzer-Code und der Laufzeitumgebung besteht. Z.B. verhindert der Global Interpreter Lock (GIL) in Python, dass Programme bei der Verwendung von Threads auch tatsächlich schneller ausgeführt werden.

2   Material and Methoden

2.1   Architektur von Julia

In Abb. 1 ist ein Überblick über die interne Struktur von Julia gegeben. Ganz grundlegend besteht Julia aus drei Teilen:

- Julia REPL (d.h. das ausführbare *julia* Programm)
- Julia Core
- Julia Base

julia (*julia.exe* unter Windows) ist das ausführbare Hauptprogramm, welches eine *Read Eval Print Loop* kurz REPL implementiert. Die Julia REPL ist dynamisch gegen die C Bibliothek *libjulia* gelinkt, welche die Kernfunktionalität von Julia bereitstellt. *libjulia* nutzt für die Codegenerierung LLVM [7], ein C++ Compiler Framework, welches hocheffizienten Maschinencode generierten kann und einen Just-In-Time (JIT) Compiler bereitstellt.

Mit nur ca. 15000 Zeilen an C/C++ Code [1] ist Julias Kern relativ klein. Der Großteil an Basisfunktionalität ist in Julia selbst geschrieben und Teil des *Base* Moduls, welches in das sogenannte *System Image* (sysimg.{so,dll,dylib}) vorkompiliert wird.

2.2   Threadsicherheit der Laufzeitumgebung

Threadsicherheit wurde bislang bei der Entwicklung von Julia nicht berücksichtigt, sodass *libjulia* derzeit nicht threadsicher ist. Um dies zu ändern mussten die folgenden Module gegen Race-Conditions geschützt werden:

– Codegenerierung
– Speicherallokierung
– Garbage-Collection

In unserem Multithreading-Patch [9] verwenden wir die Threading- und Mutex-Implementierung der Bibliothek *libuv*, welche statisch in *libjulia* gelinkt ist, sodass keine zusätzliche Binärabhängigkeit eingeführt wurde.

Im Gegensatz zu anderen dynamischen Programmiersprachen wird Julia Code nicht interpretiert sondern zur Laufzeit in Maschinencode kompiliert. Dies führt dazu, dass die Interaktion zwischen dem kompilierten Code und der Laufzeitumgebung auf ein Minimum reduziert werden kann. Im Bereich der Codegenerierung musste lediglich der globale Methoden-Cache mit einem Mutex geschützt werden, sodass immer nur ein Thread zur Zeit Code generieren und in den Methoden-Cache hinzufügen kann.

Julia verwendet einen einfachen *Mark-And-Sweep* Garbage-Collector, der an bestimmten Stellen aufgerufen wird, z.B. bei Speicherallokationen. Hier mussten in unserem Multithreading-Patch mehrere globale Variablen geschützt werden. Hierzu wurden atomare Operationen verwendet (z.B. unter GCC / LLVM `__sync_fetch_and_add` bzw. unter Windows `_InterlockedExchangeAdd`). Größere Speicherallokierungen werden mit einem Mutex geschützt. Für die Allokierung kleiner Speicherblöcke verwendet Julia einen Speicherpool, der durch einen Mutex geschützt werden kann. In unseren Experimenten führte dies jedoch zu deutlichen Performanceverlusten. Aus diesem Grund haben wir in unserem Multithreading-Patch einen parallelen Speicherpool implementiert, bei dem mehrere Speicherbereiche für jeden Thread separat bereitgestellt werden. Hierdurch können mehrere Threads gleichzeitig kleine Speicherblöcke allokieren.

Den Garbage-Collector threadsicher zu machen ist eine anspruchsvolle Aufgabe. In unserem Multithreading-Patch haben wir eine einfache Lösung implemen-

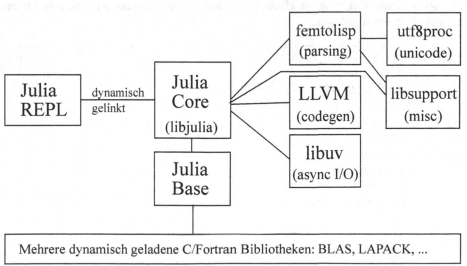

Abb. 1. Überblick über die interne Struktur von Julia.

tiert, welche in vielen Situationen effektiv funktioniert, jedoch nicht bei jedem Problem praktikabel ist. Die Idee ist, den Garbage-Collector auszuschalten, wenn mehrere Threads ausgeführt werden. Daher sollten Speicherallokierung innerhalb des nebenläufigen Codes vermieden werden.

2.3   Multithreading-Implementierung

Die eigentlichen Threadingroutinen wurden in C implementiert und nutzen die Bibliothek *libuv*. Von Julia aus werden die Funktionen durch Julias Foreign-Function-Interface (FFI) `ccall` aufgerufen.

Auf der Julia Seite wurde ein einfaches Interface implementiert, das aus der Funktion `parapply` besteht. Als Argument wird `parapply` ein Callback übergeben, sowie ein Bereich über dem die übergebene Funktion nebenläufig ausgeführt werden soll. Hierbei wird der Bereich in mehrere Subbereiche aufgeteilt. Das Aus- und Anstellen des Garbage-Collectors wird automatisch von `parapply` übernommen. Standardmäßig nutzt `parapply` soviele Threads wie CPU-Kerne verfügbar sind.

2.4   Testprogramm

Um die Performance unserer Multithreading-Implementierung zu testen betrachten wir eine parallele Implementierung der vektorisierten `tanh` Funktion. Sie akzeptiert als Argument einen Vektor und berechnet elementweise den Tangens Hyperbolicus berechnet. Die parallele Implementierung nutzt die `parapply` Funktion und ist im Folgende angegeben.

Hierbei ist `tanh_core` die Kernfunktion, welche einen Bereich als Eingabe bekommt und den Tangens Hyperbolicus über den angegebenen Bereich berechnet. Das `@inbounds` Makro ist ein Hinweis für den Compiler, dass keine Indexgrenzen überprüft werden müssen.

```
function tanh_core(r,x,y)
    for i in r
        @inbounds y[i] = tanh(x[i])
    end
end

function ptanh(x)
    y = similar(x)
    N = length(x)
    parapply(tanh_core, 1:N, x, y)
    return y
end
```

3   Ergebnisse

In Abb. 2 sind die Ergebnisse nach Anwendung der `ptanh` Funktion und der
nicht-parallelen `tanh` Funktion auf Vektoren unterschiedlicher Länge gezeigt.
Das Testprogramm wurde auf einem Apple Macbook (Intel Core 2 Duo P7350)
mit zwei Kernen ausgeführt. Die Funktionsaufrufe wurden 20 mal wiederholt
und die schnellste Ausführung wurde gewertet.

Wie man in Abb. 2 sieht ist die nicht-parallele `tanh` Funktion bis zu einer Vek-
torlänge von ca. 4000 schneller. Dies ist typisch für ein Multithreading-Programm
da sich durch die Threaderzeugung ein Overhead nicht vermeiden lässt. Für Vektoren mit mehr als 4000 Elementen ist die `ptanh` Funktion schneller als die `tanh`
Funktion. Ab einer Länge von ca. 5×10^4 wird der volle Speedup erreicht.

4   Diskussion

In dieser Arbeit wurde eine Multithreading-Implementierung für die Programmiersprache Julia vorgestellt. Die Implementierung ist noch als Proof-of-Principle
zu sehen, da für eine Integration in Julia noch einige Hürden zu nehmen sind.
Derzeit muss der Garbage-Collector noch ausgeschaltet werden, wenn mehrere
Threads laufen. Dies ist bei vielen Anwendungen kein Hindernis. Bei der Programmierung von interaktiven graphischen Oberflächen ist es aber üblich Hinte-
grundthreads laufen zu lassen, was mit unserer Implementierung problematisch
werden kann, falls Speicher allokiert wird.

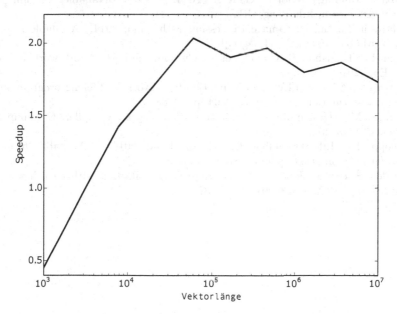

Abb. 2. Speedup der Funktion `ptanh` im Vergleich zur `tanh` Funktion bei der Verwendung von zwei Threads.

Um den Garbage-Collector auch laufen zu lassen, wenn mehrere Threads ausgeführt werden, ist es nötig die Garbage-Collector-Heaps für jeden Thread getrennt zu erstellen (thread local), siehe [10].

In unserer Implementierung der `parapply` Funktion wurden standardmäßig so viele Threads wie CPU-Kerne genutzt. In der Praxis wäre es besser eine zentrale Stelle innerhalb der Julia-Laufzeitumgebung zu haben, welche die Anzahl laufender Threads berücksichtigt, so dass nicht zu viele Threads für eine Aufgabe verwendet werden.

Während unsere `parapply` Funktion Callbacks nutzt, wäre in der Praxis eine Implementierung wünschenswert, die auf beliebigen Code-Blöcken operieren kann, ähnlich wie es in C/C++ mit OpenMP möglich ist. In Julia könnte dies sogar ohne Erweiterung der Sprache implementiert werden, da Julia über ein sehr mächtiges Makrosystem verfügt. Beispielsweise gibt es in Julia bereits das `@simd` Makro, welches for-Schleifen so modifiziert, dass effiziente SIMD-Instruktionen von dem LLVM-Vektorisierer generiert werden können.

Literaturverzeichnis

1. Bezanson J, Karpinski S, Shah V, et al. Julia: a fast dynamic language for technical computing. Comput Res Reposit. 2012;abs/1209.5145.
2. Bezanson J, Chen J, Karpinski S, et al. Array operators using multiple dispatch. Proc ARRAY. 2014; p. 6.
3. Julia Webstack; 2014. Available from: http://juliawebstack.org.
4. Julia Bindings for GTK; 2014. Available from: https://github.com/JuliaLang/Gtk.jl.
5. Images.jl: Package for Image Processing with Julia; 2014. Available from: https://github.com/timholy/Images.jl.
6. Behnel S, Bradshaw R, Citro C, et al. Cython: the best of both worlds. Comput Sci Eng. 2010.
7. Lattner C, Adve V. LLVM: a compilation framework for lifelong program analysis and transformation. Proc CGO. 2004; p. 75–88.
8. Conway ME. Design of a separable transition-diagram compiler. Commun ACM. 1963;6(7):396–408.
9. Knopp T. Multi-Threading Branch of Julia; 2014. Available from: https://github.com/tknopp/julia/tree/jlthreading.
10. Marlow S, Peyton Jones S. Multicore garbage collection with local heaps. Proc Int Symp Mem Manage. 2011; p. 21–32.

Data-Parallel MRI Brain Segmentation in Clinical Use

Porting FSL-FASTv4 to GPGPUs

Joachim Weber[1], Christian Doenitz[2], Alexander Brawanski[2],
Christoph Palm[1,3]

[1]Regensburg – Medical Image Computing (ReMIC)
Ostbayerische Technische Hochschule Regensburg (OTH Regensburg), Regensburg
[2]Department of Neurosurgery, University Medical Center Regensburg, Regensburg
[3]Regensburg Center of Biomedical Engineering (RCBE),
OTH Regensburg and Regensburg University, Regensburg
christoph.palm@oth-regensburg.de

Abstract. Structural MRI brain analysis and segmentation is a crucial part in the daily routine in neurosurgery for intervention planning. Exemplarily, the free software FSL-FAST (FMRIB's Segmentation Library – FMRIB's Automated Segmentation Tool) in version 4 is used for segmentation of brain tissue types. To speed up the segmentation procedure by parallel execution, we transferred FSL-FAST to a General Purpose Graphics Processing Unit (GPGPU) using Open Computing Language (OpenCL) [1]. The necessary steps for parallelization resulted in substantially different and less useful results. Therefore, the underlying methods were revised and adapted yielding computational overhead. Nevertheless, we achieved a speed-up factor of 3.59 from CPU to GPGPU execution, as well providing similar useful or even better results.

1 Introduction

For the segmentation of 3D Magnetic Resonance Imaging (MRI) brain data the software FMRIB's Automatic Segmentation Tool (FAST) of FMRIB's Segmentation Library (FSL) [2] is frequently used in the field of neurosurgery. For interventional planning, the results of FSL-FASTv4 have shown to be advantageous compared to other releases. FSL-FASTv4 classifies the voxels into five tissue types: white matter, two gray matter compartments, CSF and vessels. In order to support the neurosurgeon's workflow, the aim was to speed up the overall segmentation process by providing a GPGPU implementation, to benefit from the parallel processing power of modern GPGPU architectures. The re-implementation makes use of the Insight Toolkit (http://www.itk.org), which delivers a parallel execution model harnessing OpenCL. FSL-FAST shows a mixture of data-parallel (DP) and data-dependent (DD) algorithms. DP algorithms are well suited for execution on GPGPUs, whereas DD algorithms are not. In this work, we propose methods to port FSL-FASTv4 to GPGPUs, explore implications on the volume segmentation results and introduce methods to convert DD to DP methods.

2   Material and methods

In this section, a basic overview of FSL-FASTv4 is given. Furthermore, the parts suitable for parallelization are identified and necessary changes of the code base are introduced.

2.1   Software structure

FSL-FAST consists of two main parts. First, an tree k-means clustering delivers initial tissue class parameters for tissue segmentation. Secondly an Expectation-Maximization loop (EMLoop)(Fig. 1) performs a lowpass filtering and Bias field correction (Init). This contains a further loop (HMRFIter) to re-segment the dataset with an iterated-conditional-modes (ICM) algorithm to update the tissue classes (Update). We added an error adaption routine for our special purposes, which is not present in the original implementation. Details of the segmentation algorithm can be found in [2]. Here, we only discuss those parts relevant for the parallelization task.

2.2   Data parallelization

The original software's execution model in the HMRFIter is inherently sequential, prohibiting general parallel execution. Transforming the HMRFIter to use DP execution is the factor of exploiting speed-up by using a GPGPU. Therefore two parts of the original software have to be changed (ICM and summation).

ICM   The original ICM algorithm re-labels a voxel x according to a weighted sum of probabilities regarding the spatial neighborhood information N and voxel intensity i_x with weighting factor β. Thus, it calculates a label $l_x^{(t)}$ according to Eq. 1, where L indicates the number of classes. $N_{1,2}$ are different neighborhoods according to Fig. 2

$$l_x^{(t)} = \arg\max_{l \in \{1...L\}} \left\{ \beta \log \left(P(l \mid N_1^{(t-1)}, N_2^{(t)}) \right) + \log \left(P(l \mid i_x) \right) \right\} \qquad (1)$$

Fig. 1.   Overview of EM-Loop. HMRFIter is the part of the code, where the most execution time is spent, which is parallelized completely on a GPGPU.

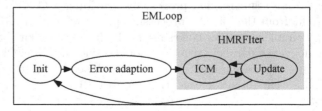

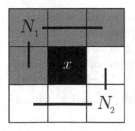

Fig. 2. The original ICM treats the neighboring label information differently (N_1 and N_2) depending on their relativ position to the current voxel x. Note, that this is only a schematic view in 2D whereas the algorithm is performed in 3D. In a raster scan fashion, the relabeled voxels are instantly written back and re-used to label the next voxel.

Note, that the data in the voxel raster are examined row-wise. After re-labeling, the new information is written instantly and used in the optimization procedure (1) of the subsequent voxel. Therefore, a mixture of neighboring labels generated at time t and at time $t-1$ is taken into account (Fig. 2). For DP execution (1) is transformed to

$$l_x^{(t)} = \arg\max_{l \in \{1...L\}} \left\{ \beta \log \left(P(l \mid N_1^{(t-1)}, N_2^{(t-1)}) \right) + \log \left(P(l \mid i_x) \right) \right\} \qquad (2)$$

Since the DP ICM method (Eq. 2) makes different use of neighboring labels, the weighting β has to be adapted as well.

Summations For the computation of(3) and (4), linear sums of floating-point numbers of IEEE754-2008 format in single precision [3] are used. After re-labeling, the model parameters $\mu_l^{(t)}$ and $\sigma_l^{(t)}$ are updated, which define mean and variance of a Gaussian distribution related to l at time t, respectively

$$\mu_l^{(t)} = \frac{\Sigma_{x \in X} P^{(t-1)}(l \mid i_x) i_x}{\sigma_{x \in X} P^{(t-1)}(l \mid i_x)} \qquad (3)$$

$$\sigma_l^{(t)} = \frac{\Sigma_{x \in X} P^{(t-1)}(l \mid i_x)(i_x - \mu_l)^2}{\sigma_{x \in X} P^{(t-1)}(l \mid i_x)} \qquad (4)$$

However, this kind of computation is not only DD (Fig. 3, (a)) but also prone to rounding errors [4]. Transforming the DD floating point summation to a DP variant, a tree-wise summation is applied (Fig. 3, (b)). Thus, not only the time complexity is reduced from linear to logarithmic, also the rounding error is reduced from $O(n)$ to $O(\log n)$ [4]. Remarkably, the change of summation pro-

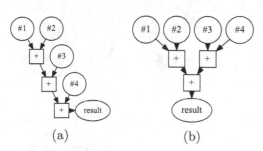

(a)   (b)

Fig. 3. Schematic comparison of different summation methods: (a) linear summation, (b) tree-wise summation.

cedure has a strong impact on segmentation results. Unfortunately, the results based on lower rounding errors by tree-wise summation are worse compared to the original method (Sec. 3). Therefore, we propose a compensation of the error reduction and, hence, raise the rounding error artificially. Error adaption is done once before each HMRFIter by subtraction of Kahan's summation [4] and linear summation yields $c_{\mu,l}$ and $c_{\sigma,l}$ for μ and σ, respectively, given label l. Therefore, the error corrected mean $\mu_{l,\mathrm{corr}}^{(t)}$ and variance $\sigma_{l,\mathrm{corr}}^{(t)}$ substitute $\mu_l^{(t)}$ and $\sigma_l^{(t)}$ in (3) and (4), respectively

$$\mu_{l,\mathrm{corr}}^{(t)} = \mu_l^{(t)} - c_{\mu,l}, \quad \sigma_{l,\mathrm{corr}}^{(t)} = \sigma_l^{(t)} - c_{\sigma,l} \tag{5}$$

3   Results

In this section, segmentation results are presented according to the parallelization steps (Sec. 2.2). Furthermore, execution time (ET) between the different configurations and speed-up using a GPGPU are examined. The results base on nine contrast enhanced T1-weighted MRI brain data sets from clinical routine (eight data sets with voxel spacing of $1.0 \times 0.97 \times 0.97$ and $8.1 \cdot 10^6$ voxels; one dataset with voxel spacing of $0.5 \times 0.5 \times 1.3$ and $2.7 \cdot 10^7$ voxels). Skull is removed using FSL-BET as a pre-processing step for all data.

3.1   Segmentation quality

The segmentation results were quantified by the Dice coefficient (DC) measuring the normalized overlap between labels. Since the goal of this work was a speed-up of segmentation preserving the labels of the sequential algorithm, the resulting labels of the original FSL-FASTv4 were taken as ground truth. Since the execution on a GPGPU is not only parallel but incorporates additional differences like compiler optimization etc., most of the segmentation results are computed on the CPU to enable direct comparison to FSL-FASTv4. Switching from DD (Fig. 4(b)) to DP (Fig. 4(c)) causes substantially different segmentation results. The main reason for differing labels are the differing mean and variance values

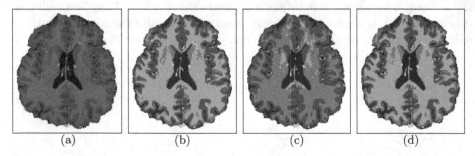

| (a) | (b) | (c) | (d) |

Fig. 4. Comparison of a transversal section of data set 1. (a) original (unsegmented T1-MRI), (b) segmentation result of original FSL-FASTv4, (c) segmentation result with DP execution, (d) segmentation result with DP execution and additional change of weighting factor ($\beta = 0.08$ instead of 0.1) and error adaption.

		DC	ET
(a)	Original	1.0	125.11 s
(b)	DP	0.85	168.22 s
(c)	+ Error Adaption	0.90	169.77 s
(d)	+ $\beta = 0.08$	0.93	171.78 s
(e)	+ GPGPU	0.93	34.78 s

Table 1. Average DC of all data and all labels according to the algorithmic modifications. (a) original FSL-FASTv4, (b) with activated DP execution, (c) additional error adaption, (d) (Fig. 4 (d)) additional change of β, (e) execution on GPGPU.

of the Gaussian distributions characterizing the class probabilities. Fig. 5 (a), (b) shows the evolution of both parameters depending on the iteration depth of EMLoop exemplarily for data set 1 and label 1. Especially the mean value keeps constant approximately and declines applying DP and DD, respectively. Including the error adaption (Sec. 2.2) the DP curve becomes similar to the DD curve. The overall DCs give also evidence to the positive effect of error adaption on the segmentation results. While DC is reduced to 0.85 using DP, it raises again to 0.90 including error adaption (Tab. 1 (b,c)). The impact of the weighting factor β (originally: 0.1 in (2)) is shown by the further increase of DC to 0.93 using the optimum β (Tab. 1 (d)), which was determined by the median of leaving one out experiments (median: 0.08; mean: 0.086; variance: 0.0003).

3.2   Speed-up

ET varies heavily due to changes in the code basis, because these changes causes different convergence times of the underlying EM algorithm. The measured ETs in Tab. 1 are based on a Intel Xeon X5675 and Nvidia Tesla C2075. Changing to DP the average ET increases from 125.11 s to 168.22 s. Obviously, the convergence is worse due to the parallelization steps introduced here. This is in line with the statements of Besag [5]. However, the execution on the GPGPU reverses this effect completely resulting in a speed-up of 3.59 regarding the original algorithm and a speed-up of 4.93 regarding the modified CPU version (Tab. 1 (d)).

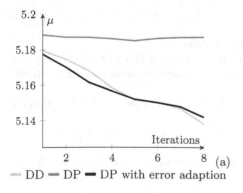
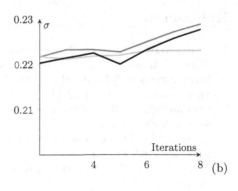

Fig. 5. Evolution of mean (a) and variance (b) of data set 1, according to the original DD execution, DP execution and DP with error estimation.

The speed-up seems to depend on the structure of the data and the convergence behavior of the algorithm than the number of voxels.

4 Discussion

Transforming FSL-FASTv4 to utilize the parallel computation power of a modern GPGPU enforces modifications to enable data parallel execution. However, data parallelism resulted in drastic changes of the segmentation results. We introduced two modifications to reduce this effect: error adaption taking the rounding error of summations into account and a change of weighting of the neighborhood probabilities. We showed that the modifications helped to get reasonable results to the original algorithm with DC values well above 0.9.

In general, the rounding error changing from linear to tree-wise summation decreases. However, the segmentation results get worse. This contradiction is explainable by some modifications (e.g. iteration numbers, constants, etc.) between the theory described in [2] and the actual implementation. Obviously, the original implementation is experimentally optimized for the very specific task of MRI brain segmentation. In this optimization the rounding error was existent and was taken into account. Reducing this error by tree-wise summation decrease the quality of result. Therefore, we adapted the error meaning to add an error artificially to meet the assumptions of the algorithm. Alternatively, all modifications and constants of the implementation have to be optimized for a smaller rounding error.

The change of weighting was necessary to underweight the probabilities of neighboring voxels. However, the convergence of the EMLoop is affected and might cause troubles. Nevertheless, in our experiments the EMLoop converged.

In this work, the dramatic effect of apparently small changes due to DP was shown and solutions were introduced allowing the use of FSL-FASTv4 on GPGPUs.

References

1. Group KOW. The OpenCL Specification 1.1; 2008.
2. Zhang Y, Brady M, Smith S. Segmentation of brain MR images through a hidden Markov random field model and the expectation-maximization algorithm. IEEE Trans Med Imaging. 2001;20(1):45–57.
3. Committee MS. IEEE Standard for Floating-Point Arithmetic. IEEE Computer Society; 2008.
4. Higham NJ. The accuracy of floating point summation. SIAM J Sci Comput. 1993;14(4):783–99.
5. Besag J. On the statistical analysis of dirty pictures. J R Stat Soc Ser B. 1986;48(3):259–302.

GraphMIC
Medizinische Bildverarbeitung in der Lehre

Alexander Eduard Szalo[1], Alexander Zehner[1,], Christoph Palm[1,2]

[1]Regensburg – Medical Image Computing (ReMIC) Ostbayerische Technische
Hochschule Regensburg (OTH Regensburg), Regensburg
[2]Regensburg Center of Biomedical Engineering (RCBE) OTH Regensburg und
Universität Regensburg, Regensburg

info@graphmic.org

Kurzfassung. Die Lehre der medizinischen Bildverarbeitung vermittelt
Kenntnisse mit einem breiten Methodenspektrum. Neben den Grundla-
gen der Verfahren soll ein Gefühl für eine geeignete Ausführungsreihenfolge und ihrer Wirkung auf medizinische Bilddaten entwickelt werden.
Die Komplexität der Methoden erfordert vertiefte Programmierkenntnisse, sodass bereits einfache Operationen mit großem Programmierauf-
wand verbunden sind. Die Software GraphMIC stellt Bildverarbeitungs-
operationen in Form interaktiver Knoten zur Verfügung und erlaubt das
Arrangieren, Parametrisieren und Ausführen komplexer Verarbeitungssequenzen in einem Graphen. Durch den Fokus auf das Design einer Pipeline, weg von sprach- und frameworkspezifischen Implementierungsdetails,
lassen sich grundlegende Prinzipien der Bildverarbeitung anschaulich er
lernen. In diesem Beitrag stellen wir die visuelle Programmierung mit
GraphMIC der nativen Implementierung aquivalenter Funktionen gegenüber. Die in C++ entwickelte Applikation basiert auf Qt, ITK, OpenCV,
VTK und MITK.

1 Einleitung

Die Medizinische Bildverarbeitung nutzt ein breites Methodenspektrum von der
Bildverbesserung, der Merkmalsextraktion und Klassifikation, über die Bild-
segmentierung und Bildregistrierung bis hin zur Visualisierung der Ergebnisse.
Die Besonderheiten medizinischer Bilder, insbesondere die unzureichende Abgrenzung von Gewebetypen, die Vielzahl an bildgebenden Modalitäten und die
Varianz der Bildinhalte bei verschiedenen Patienten, aber auch beim gleichen
Patienten zu verschiedenen Zeitpunkten macht die besondere Herausforderung
aus. Immer komplexere Verfahren versuchen, ärztliches Vorwissen für die automatisierte und damit objektive Verarbeitung nutzbar zu machen, verschiedene Modalitäten zu kombinieren oder Lösungsansätze verschiedener Problemfel-
der gemeinsam zu bearbeiten. Ein Schlüssel zur Medizinischen Bildverarbeitung
liegt damit in der detaillierten Kenntnis der gebräuchlichen Verfahren in ihrer
Wirkung, der geeigneten Kombination und vor allem der problemspezifischen
Parametrisierung. Dabei müssen viele Methoden nicht von Grund auf implementiert werden. Vielmehr haben sich mehrere Programmbibliotheken etabliert,

die den Entwicklungsprozess vereinfachen sollen. Allerdings sind diese Bibliotheken in hohem Maße komplex und auf Programmierebene nur mit großem Aufwand kombinierbar. Die Lehre der Medizinischen Bildverarbeitung ist damit konfrontiert, nichttriviale Methoden zu vermitteln und in praktischen Übungen zu vertiefen. Die Nutzung der professionellen Bildverarbeitungsbibliotheken zur praktischen Umsetzung der Konzepte erfordert aber mitunter tiefgehende Programmierkenntnisse, die sich erst im Lauf des Studiums und der beruflichen Praxis entwickeln. So sind schon einfache Vorverarbeitungsverfahren mit einem nicht unerheblichen Aufwand zur Umsetzung verbunden, was schnelle Erfolgserlebnisse erschwert. Die Software GraphMIC soll den Zugang zur Bildverarbeitung im Rahmen der Lehre erleichtern. Durch die Interaktion mit visuellen Komponenten ist es möglich, Operationen aus den Bibliotheken ITK [1] und OpenCV [2] in einem Graphen zu arrangieren, zu parametrisieren und auszuführen. Features wie Multithreading, die integrierte Visualisierung von zweidimensionalen (2D) und dreidimensionalen (3D) Bilddaten und die Verarbeitung von Bildsequenzen erlauben das Erlernen von Methoden der Bildverarbeitung mit besonderem Schwerpunkt auf den Einsatz in der Medizin.

2   Material und Methoden

2.1   Stand der Technik

Die Anwendungen MevisLab [3] und CASSANDRA (www.cassandra-vision.com) setzen ebenfalls auf die visuelle Darstellung von Bildoperationen. MevisLab bietet neben eigenen Modulen große Teile der Funktionen aus ITK und VTK [4]. Allerdings setzt ein effizientes Arbeiten umfangreiche Kenntnisse der Bibliothken voraus. CASSANDRA integriert OpenCV zur Bildverarbeitung. Relevante Eigenschaften für den Einsatz im medizinischen Bereich wie die Verarbeitung von 3D Bilddaten oder die Unterstützung bekannter Bildformate wie DICOM sind nicht vorhanden. Das vielfach in der Lehre verwendete Programm ImageJ [5] bietet zahlreiche Funktionen zur Interaktion mit Bilddaten, darunter die Erstellung von Java Plugins, um die Wirkung eigener Methoden zu vermitteln [6]. In ImageJ geht jedoch schnell aufgrund der gewachsenen Struktur die Übersicht und der Zusammenhang zwischen den Methoden verloren.

Die in GraphMIC verwendeten Bibliotheken ITK und OpenCV zeigen verschiedene Anwendungsschwerpunkte. ITK ist für die Verarbeitung medizinischer Bilddaten ausgelegt und konzentriert sich insbesondere auf die Registrierung und Segmentierung. Die Zahl der in ITK verfügbaren Bildoperationen beläuft sich aktuell auf über 700. OpenCV stellt ca. 2500 Algorithmen insbesondere für die Echtzeitbildverarbeitung bereit.

2.2   Konzept

Ziel von GraphMIC ist die Entkopplung vom Verständnis der Methoden der Medizinischen Bildverarbeitung und vertiefter Programmierkenntnisse. Das wird durch die Abbildung der Bildoperationen auf einen Graphen erreicht, in dem Operationen als Knoten und Kommunikationswege zum Datenaustausch von Bildern und Parametern als Kanten darstellt werden. Durch Interaktion mit visuellen Komponenten lassen sich Parameter und die Reihenfolge der Operationen anpassen und erlauben so das Erlernen der Wirkung von Funktionen aus ITK und OpenCV auf experimentellem Wege.

Vereinfachung durch Visuelle Programmierung Nachfolgend stellen wir die native Programmierung auf Basis des ITK Frameworks der visuellen Programmierung mit GraphMIC anhand eines einfachen Beispiels gegenüber.

ITK nutzt das Template-Konzept von C++ sehr intensiv. Der Vorteil besteht in der Wiederverwendbarkeit von Code für diverse Bilddatentypen und Bilddimensionen. Allerdings muss spätestens beim Einsatz der Bildverarbeitungsklassen in einer Applikation der Typ des tatsächlich zu verwendenden Bildtypen festgelegt werden (Abb. 1(1)). Mittels typedef wird dieser Typ auch für die verwendeten Operationen weitergegeben (Abb. 1(2)). Der Instantiierung der beteiligten Klassen (Abb. 1(3)) folgt die Spezifikation des zu verarbeitenden Bildes (Abb. 1(4)). Durch die Verknüpfung der Ausgänge (GetOutput) mit den Eingängen (SetInput) wird die Ausführungsreihenfolge festgelegt (Abb. 1(5-7)). In dem Sinne ist ein Pipelinekonzept in ITK bereits angelegt. Der Parametrisierung der Operationen (Abb. 1(5-7)) folgt die Ausführung der gesamten Pipeline (Update) (Abb. 1(7)). Umfangreiche Verarbeitungssequenzen sind im Code schwierig nachzuvollziehen und zu warten. Änderungen der Pipeline erfordern ein Anstoßen des Buildprozesses: z.B. Anwendung auf einen anderen Bildtypen, einer anderen Verarbeitungsreihenfolge oder einer anderen Parametrisierung. Das

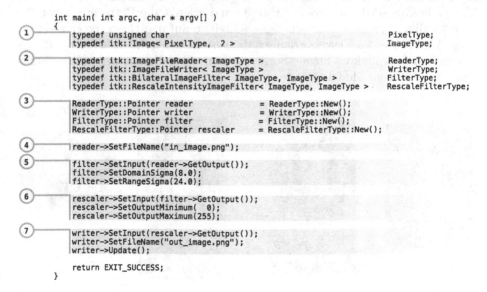

Abb. 1. Beispielprogramm zum ITK BilateralImageFilter (vgl. [1]).

Ergebnis der Pipeline ist nur durch Nutzung eines externen Viewers nachvoll-
ziehbar, Zwischenergebnisse müssen separat persistiert werden.

Abb. 2 zeigt die Umsetzung des Beispiels aus Abb. 1 mit GraphMIC. Bildoperationen werden als Knoten und ihre Beziehungen als Kanten sofort erkennbar. Ändert sich die Konfiguration eines Knotens, werden entsprechende Verbindungen farbig markiert. Damit wird der Verarbeitungszustand der Pipeline
verdeutlicht. Parameter einer Operation werden je nach Datentyp als Textbox,
Dropdown bzw. Checkbox abgebildet. Ausgeführte Knoten geben die Berech-
nungszeit an und optionale Vorschaubilder liefern einen schnellen Überblick über
die Wirkung einer Methode. Im Gegensatz zum nativen Code bleibt der Bildtyp
in GraphMIC variabel, so dass der Graph z.B. durch Auswahl eines 3D Daten-
satzes eine unveränderte Nutzung erlaubt, sofern die Operationen kompatibel
sind.

Performance durch Native Operationen Die Datenstruktur eines Knotens
besitzt neben Logiken zur Thread- und Parameterverwaltung eine Referenz auf
die zugrundeliegende ITK bzw. OpenCV Operation. Alle Knoten können sowohl
mit Einzelbildern als auch Bildserien umgehen und wenden die Bildoperation für
jedes in der Bildsequenz vorliegende Bild an. Bei der Verarbeitung wird grundsätzlich mit dem Datentypen des Eingabebildes gearbeitet. Typkonversionen sind
möglich, müssen aber explizit vom Benutzer in den Graphen eingebunden werden.

Integrierte Visualisierung Um bei der Betrachtung gewonnener Bilddaten
nicht auf externe Anwendungen angewiesen zu sein, ist ein auf VTK basierter
Viewer in GraphMIC integriert (Abb. 3) und erlaubt die Betrachtung von 2D
und 3D Bilddaten ohne ein vorheriges Schreiben auf den Datenträger zu erfordern. Werkzeuge des Viewers erlauben die verschiedenen Interaktionen z.B. das
Setzen von Saatpunkten für die Segmentierung oder die manuelle Vorregistrie-
rung verschiedener Modalitäten.

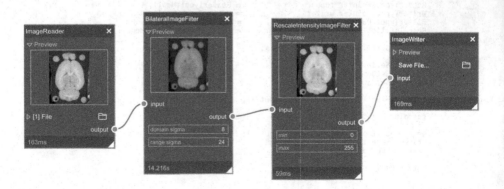

Abb. 2. Umsetzung des ITK Beispiels aus Abb. 1 in GraphMIC.

Moderne Frameworks Die Applikation basiert auf dem Qt5 Framework und erlaubt die plattformunabhängige Programmierung (www.qt.io). Die QtQuick Technologie ermöglicht die Umsetzung eines modernen User Interfaces durch Hardwarebeschleunigung. Der Anwendungskern profitiert von vielen High-Level Komponenten wie der Qt Meta Language und dem signal-slot Konzept. MITK [7] erlaubt es, die verschiedenen Kombinationen von Templateparametern in ITK für die dynamische Verwendung durch Makros zu umgehen.

3 Ergebnisse

Als Proof of Concept wurde die Software exemplarisch mit einer Reihe von Methoden aus den Bibliotheken ITK (110) und OpenCV (40) umgesetzt, die sich gemeinsam in einer Pipeline nutzen lassen. Abb. 3 zeigt das zugehörige User Interface von GraphMIC. Die linke Seite bietet eine Übersicht der angelegten Pipelines. Der mittlere Bereich integriert den Editor zum Arrangieren der Knoten. Die abgebildete Pipeline zeigt ein Beispiel für die kombinierte Verarbeitung von ITK und OpenCV Modulen. So wird die Kreisdetektion mit Hilfe eines Moduls aus OpenCV berechnet, während die Vorverarbeitung aus ITK Modulen besteht. Der rechte Fensterbereich enthält den Viewer, der die Analyse von Ergebnisbildern bzw. Bildserien durch verschiedene Interaktionsmöglichkeiten unterstützt.

4 Diskussion

GraphMIC hat derzeit den Entwicklungsstand eines Prototyps und soll in Zukunft ausgebaut werden. Neben der Integration von weiteren Modulen aus ITK

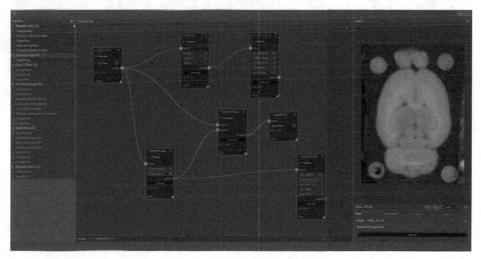

Abb. 3. Umsetzung einer Pipeline in GraphMIC zur Landmarkendetektion in Blockfaceaufnahmen eines Rattenhirnschnittblocks. Die Landmarken dienen zur Registierung der 2D Bilder zu einem 3D Modell.

und OpenCV sollen vor allem zwei Aspekte weiterentwickelt werden: der Viewer und benutzerdefinierte Knoten.

MITK stellt eine API für einen Viewer mit umfangreicher Funktionalität zur Verfügung. Sobald eine stabile Integration in Qt5 verfügbar ist, wird die MITK Viewer API für GraphMIC adaptiert und ersetzt den derzeitigen rudimentären VTK Viewer. Ein weiteres Ziel ist die Implementierung benutzerdefinierter Operationen mithilfe von Python. Diese sollen die Erstellung eigener Knoten erlauben und nahtlos in die Bildverarbeitungspipeline integriert werden können. In Zukunft soll GraphMIC die Lehre der medizinischen Bildverarbeitung unterstützen. Dazu ist es geplant die Software frei zur Verfügung zu stellen.

Danksagung. Erst- und Zweitautor lieferten den gleichen Beitrag zu dieser Arbeit

Literaturverzeichnis

1. Ibanez L, Schroeder W, Ng L, et al. The ITK Software Guide Second Edition. Kitware Inc; 2005.
2. Bradski G, Kaehler A. Learning OpenCV: computer vision with the OpenCV library. Cambridge, MA: O'Reilly; 2008.
3. Koenig M, Spindler W, Rexilius J, et al. Embedding VTK and ITK into a visual programming and rapid prototyping platform. Proc SPIE. 2006; p. 61412O.
4. Schroeder W, Martin K, Lorensen B. VTK Textbook 4th edition. Kitware, Inc; 2006.
5. Rasband W. ImageJ. U.S. National Institutes of Health, Bethesda, Maryland, USA; 1997-2014.
6. Burge M, Burger W. Digitale Bildverarbeitung: Eine Einführung mit Java und ImageJ. 2nd ed. Heidelberg: Springer Verlag; 2006.
7. Wolf I, Nolden M, Boettger T, et al. The MITK approach. Insight J. 2005.

A Modular Framework for Post-Processing and Analysis of Fluorescence Microscopy Image Sequences of Subcellular Calcium Dynamics

Daniel Schetelig[1], Insa M.A. Wolf[2], Björn-P. Diercks[2],
Ralf Fliegert[2], Andreas H. Guse[2], Alexander Schlaefer[3], Rene Werner[1]

[1]Department of Computational Neuroscience
[2]Department of Biochemistry and Molecular Cell Biology,
University Medical Center Hamburg-Eppendorf
[3]Institute of Medical Technology, Hamburg University of Technology
r.werner@uke.de

Abstract. Calcium (Ca^{2+}) signaling is essential for activation of T-lymphocytes and can be understood as fundamental on-switch for the adaptive immune system. The activation is supposed to start by initial spatially and temporally localized Ca^{2+} signals. Imaging and analysis of these signals require high spatio-temporal resolution fluorescence microscopy – which, in turn, results in the need for an efficient and reliable post-processing and analysis workflow of the acquired image data. Started with a well established but time-consuming post-processing process, we report on our efforts to automatize and optimize it. The efforts led to a modular post-processing and analysis framework, which is presented. In addition, the influence of instances of the main blocks of the framework (e.g. bleaching correction, deconvolution) on Ca^{2+} dynamics analysis measures is evaluated.

1 Introduction

Calcium (Ca^{2+}) is a versatile intracellular second messenger associated with the activation of a wide range of cellular functions. The increase of the free cytosolic Ca^{2+} concentration ($[Ca^{2+}]_i$) mediates the activation of T-lymphocytes and is therefore essential for the specific immune response. The mechanisms underlying the initial formation of Ca^{2+} signals and the signal dispersion within the cells that precede the global $[Ca^{2+}]_i$ increase are, however and especially in T cells, still not entirely understood [1]. A more profound understanding could eventually lead to the development of advanced therapeutic treatment options for immunological diseases [2].

Initial Ca^{2+} signal formation and dispersion can be examined by single cell fluorescence microscopy. As signal formation and dispersion take place within fractions of a second, high spatial and temporal resolution imaging is required – which, in turn, results in the need for an efficient and reliable workflow for post-processing and analysis of the generated large image data volume. The current workflow at our facility is well established [3] but depends on multiple third-party applications, with the data transfer between them and the corresponding user interaction leading to a time consuming process (1-2h/cell). Even more importantly, some of the third-party applications are proprietary and, consequently, the image processing results are in detail of limited comprehensibility.

To overcome the limitations of the current workflow, we developed a modular framework for flexible and fast post-processing of high spatio-temporal resolution fluorescence image data and basic analysis tasks, which is to be presented. The main contributions of our presentation will be: In line with the BVM workshop character, we report on our experiences during the process of automatizing and optimization of the existing workflow. The influence of the implemented variants of the main blocks of the post-processing chain (e.g. bleaching correction, deconvolution) is evaluated and their impact on the identification of short-lived subcellular Ca^{2+} signals and their spatio-temporal propagation investigated; the respective results are, to our knowledge, novel.

2   Materials and methods

2.1   Image acquisition and data description

The Ca^{2+} concentration image sequences are acquired by ratiometric fluorescence microscopy: The cells under investigation (human Jurkat T cells, diameter $\approx 15\mu m$) are loaded with two fluorescent dyes (Fluo-4, FuraRed). These bind to the Ca^{2+}, which allows to indirectly monitor changes in $[Ca^{2+}]_i$. Light with a wavelength of 472/30 nm is used for excitation, resulting in the emission of two distinct wavelengths by the dyes (measured: $\lambda_{Fluo} = 542/50$ nm, $\lambda_{FuraRed} = 647/57$ nm; split into two channels by an optical beam splitter). The two channels are simultaneously recorded by an EMCCD-camera (Hamamatsu C9100-02; framerate: 38.5 Hz; theoretically achievable spatial resolution: 153×153 nm/px). In our setup, the focal length is kept constant and temporal $[Ca^{2+}]_i$ changes in a single slice of the cell measured, with the period after stimulation of the cells ($\approx$ 300 frames; in total 2 min acquisition time; stimulation by addition of a bead coated with anti-CD3 mAb OKT3) being of primary interest. The two channel setup prevents misinterpretation of $[Ca^{2+}]_i$ caused by, e.g., intra- and inter-cellular variations in dye concentration; these effects cancel out by working on ratio images of the channels instead of using a single dye [4].

2.2   Post-processing blocks and implemented instances

The post-processing chain applied to the fluorescence microscopy data includes the implemented variants (MATLAB, MathWorks) of the main blocks (Fig. 1). Four blocks are subsequently detailed.

1. *Cell/ROI extraction & background correction:* As part of the original workflow, a rectangular region of interest (ROI) has been defined for subsequent

Fig. 1. Illustration of the post-processing pipeline applied to the acquired fluorescence microscopy data and overview of the implemented variants of the main pipeline blocks.

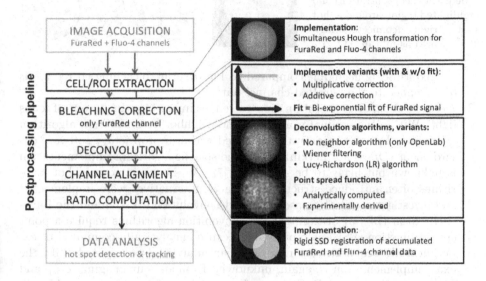

processing and a background correction performed by applying an user-defined threshold. Thresholding, however, led to erroneous zero intensity pixels within the cell regions. We therefore implemented an automatic cell detection approach by spherical Hough transformation (assumption of spherical cell shape; simultaneously performed in corresponding FuraRed and Fluo-4 frames), which allowed us to generate a binary cell (precisely: increased Ca^{2+} concentration) mask. Only intensity values outside the masks are labeled as background and set to zero.

2. *Bleaching correction:* Fluorescent dyes appear to bleach in case of continuous excitation. To compensate for the related decline in signal intensity, four approaches were implemented. The first two are based on a bi-exponential fit of the frame-by-frame arithmetic mean signal intensity in the specified ROI [5]. The original approach was to multiply the pixel intensities of a specific frame by the factor between the initial value of the curve progression and the fit value corresponding to the frame (multiplicative correction). As negative side-effect, signal noise is also amplified (critical for analysis of highly localized spatio-temporal signal patterns). We, therefore, replaced the multiplicative by a conservative additive correction strategy (frame-by-frame elevation of pixel intensities by the difference between the initial value of the curve progression and the fit value of the specific frame). Additionally, we implemented a multiplicative and an additive correction approach that is directly based on the frame-specific arithmetic mean intensity values instead of the corresponding fit values (Fig. 1). As bleaching of Fluo-4 can be con-

Fig. 2. Image data and Ca^{2+} dynamics. entire cell (left, color coded: Ca^{2+} concentration) and highlighted region around a 'hot spot' (right, connected high $[Ca^{2+}]_i$ area as in Tab. 1).

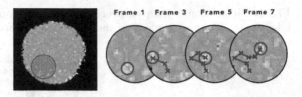

sidered as being negligible compared to FuraRed [6], bleaching correction is only applied to the FuraRed-channel data.

3. *Deconvolution:* Deconvolution aims to reduce image blur due to out-of-focus light. Within the original workflow, a no-neighbor deconvolution algorithm is applied. Deconvolution was performed within a proprietary software environment (OpenLab, PerkinElmer); the specific algorithm implementation is unknown but likely to be similar to [7]. As, however, no-neighbor algorithms often introduce structural artifacts, alternatives were implemented and investigated – in this case Wiener deconvolution (WNR) and the Lucy-Richardson (LR) algorithm. The deconvolution algorithms require a point spread function (PSF) as input, which can be analytically computed or experimentally acquired. OpenLab uses an analytically computed PSF; the exact implementation is, again, unknown. To model our imaging setup and to analytically derive a PSF for our framework, we followed [8]. In addition, we also acquired experimentally point spread functions for our system and applied them for comparison purposes.

4. *Channel data alignment:* The last step before ratio computation of the Fluo-4 and the FuraRed channel data is the alignment of the images of the two channels. Originally done manually and guided by visual inspection, this step is automatized by a rigid sum-of-squared-differences-based registration, simultaneously performed on the first ten frames of the image sequences.

2.3   Experiments and evaluation strategy

The experiments for evaluation and comparison of the implemented variants of the main pipeline blocks were divided into three parts: First, the deconvolution approaches (OpenLab, {Wiener, LR}×{exp. PSF, analyt. PSF}) were tested by imaging fluorescent beads, which act as point-like structures (diameter ≈ 200 nm). Evaluated parameters were signal-to-noise ratio (SNR) before and after deconvolution as well as in-slice spreading of the bead images, quantified by the Full Width at Half Maximum (FWHM) of the intensity profile of the imaged bead. Second, we evaluated the impact of the deconvolution approaches on measures frequently used for characterization of Ca^{2+} dynamics (see, e.g., [9]): number and diameter of local 'hot spots' (high $[Ca^{2+}]_i$ areas) and maximum observed path lengths when tracking the hot spots over time. The same parameters were evaluated in the third step: the analysis of the influence of the bleaching correction strategies. The results of the variants of the new were compared to the corresponding numbers for the original workflow.

Table 1. Influence of deconvolution and bleaching correction strategies on Ca^{2+} dynamics analysis quantities: number and diameter of 'hot spots'; length of observable hot spot paths (mean numbers over considered cells). Hot spot: approx. circular connected component of > 4 px. with a Ca^{2+} concentration of at least 63 nM ($= 3\times$noise amplitude) higher than the mean Ca^{2+} cell concentration. *: significant differences compared to the corresponding numbers of the original workflow (paired t-test, $p< 5\%$).

	Hot spots		Path length statistics	
Post-proc. pipeline	#	diam. [μm]	frames$_{max}$	length$_{max}$ [μm]
Original (= reference)	1169±1271	0.49±0.04	5.63±5.37	1.32±1.08
Experiments part 2: variation of deconvolution parts [Bleaching correction: bi-exp. fit + multipl. correction]				
LR + analyt. PSF	2118±883	0.51±0.01	10.13±3.72*	3.29±1.09*
LR + exp. PSF	1070±539	0.50±0.02	8.25±2.49	2.61±0.82*
WNR + analyt. PSF	3291±2205	0.50±0.02	11.25±3.62*	3.65±1.27*
WNR + exp. PSF	9182±5356*	0.49±0.03	7.00±2.00	2.39±0.72*
Experiments part 3: variation of bleaching correction strategy [Deconvolution: LR algorithm + analyt. PSF]				
Bleaching: fit + multipl.	2118±883	0.51±0.01	10.13±3.72*	3.29±1.09*
Bleaching: fit + add.	927±750	0.48±0.04	5.13±2.53	1.73±1.35
Bleaching: no fit, multipl.	1969±851	0.49±0.05	10.00±2.00*	3.20±0.97*
Bleaching: no fit, add.	908±739	0.48±0.04	5.75±3.28	1.67±1.31

3   Results

An example of a Ca^{2+} concentration image of a Jurkat T cell after stimulation and a subcellular propagation of a Ca^{2+} concentration 'hot spot' is shown in Fig. 2. The influence of the implemented deconvolution and bleaching correction strategies on the related measures are summarized in table 2.3; the numbers are based on the investigation of 8 cells. It can be seen that – applying the original fit-based multiplicative bleaching correction – the LR deconvolution with the experimentally acquired PSF resulted in a similar number of detected hot spots with an also similar mean hot spot diameter compared to the original workflow. Applying the analytically derived PSF, the LR algorithm led to a larger number of hot spots, accompanied by a superior SNR and bead spreading behavior compared to the other deconvolution approaches (FWHM reduced by $> 40\%$!).

As, in addition, WNR deconvolution failed to clearly separate signal and noise, the third part of the experiments was based on the combination 'LR + analyt. PSF'. The lower part of table 1 then illustrates the expected behavior of the conservative additive bleaching correction schemes and the potentially noise-amplifying multiplicative strategies: For the additive approaches, less hot spots were found and the observed hot spot paths were shorter. Differences between the fit- and non-fit-based approaches were rather small, although artificial hot spots were observed to be introduced by sub-optimal fitting of the FuraRed signal.

4 Discussion

We presented a modular framework for post-processing and analysis of fluorescence microscopy image sequences, with the framework being applied to the analysis of initial subcellular calcium signals in T cells. The focus of the work was to evaluate the influence of especially different deconvolution and bleaching correction approaches on respective analysis results – always with regard to the well-established workflow at our facility. The original results were approximately reproduced using LR deconvolution combined with a conservative additive bleaching correction – accompanied by a decrease of single cell processing times from 1-2 h to 5-10 min and control about algorithm implementations.

For the near future, we intend to extend our framework by integrating especially more sophisticated deconvolution algorithms [10] as well as additional methods for the analysis of the generated data.

Acknowledgement. The study was supported by the Forschungszentrum Medizintechnik Hamburg (to IMAW, AS and RW) and the Deutsche Forschungsgemeinschaft (grant no GU 360/15-1 to AHG).

References

1. Ernst IMA, Fliegert R, Guse AH. Adenine dinucleotide second messengers and T-lymphocyte calcium signaling. Front Immunol. 2013;4:259.
2. Cordiglieri C, Odoardi F, Zhang B, et al. Nicotinic acid adenine dinucleotide phosphate-mediated calcium signalling in effector T- cells regulates autoimmunity of the central nervous system. Brain. 2010;133:1930–43.
3. Kunerth S, Mayr GW, Koch-Nolte F, et al. Analysis of subcellular calcium signals in T-lymphocytes. Cell Signal. 2003;15:783–92.
4. Lipp P, Niggli E. Ratiometric confocal Ca2+-measurements with visible wavelength indicators in isolated cardiac myocytes. Cell Calcium. 1993;14:359–72.
5. Vicente NB, Zamboni JED, Adur JF, et al. Photobleaching correction in fluorescence microscopy images. J Phys Conf Ser. 2007;90.
6. Thomas D. A comparison of fluorescent Ca2+indicator properties and their use in measuring elementary and global Ca2+signals. Cell Calcium. 2000;28:213–23.
7. Monck JR, Oberhauser AF, Keating TJ, et al. Thin-section ratiometric Ca2+ images obtained by optical sectioning of fura-2 loaded mast cells. J Cell Biol. 1992;116(3):745–59.
8. Pankajakshan P, Blanc-Feraud L, Kam Z, et al. Point-spread function retrieval for fluorescence microscopy. Proc ISBI. 2009; p. 1095–8.
9. Lipp P, Niggli E. Fundamental calcium release events revealed by two-photon excitation photolysis of caged calcium in Guinea-pig cardiac myocytes. J Physiol. 1998;508:801–9.
10. Arigovindan M, Fung JC, Elnatan D, et al. High-resolution restoration of 3D structures from widefield images with extreme low signal-to-noise-ratio. Proc Natl Acad Sci USA. 2013;110(43):17344–9.

Automated Whole Slide Analysis of Differently Stained and Co-Registered Tissue Sections

Ralf Schönmeyer[1], Nicolas Brieu[1], Nadine Schaadt[2], Friedrich Feuerhake[2], Günter Schmidt[1], Gerd Binnig[1]

[1]Definiens AG, München
[2]Medizinische Hochschule Hannover, Institut für Pathologie
rschoenmeyer@definiens.com

Abstract. Digital pathology enables applications that are not possible using traditional microscopy and facilitates new ways of handling and presenting whole slide image data, along with quantitative evaluation. Differently stained tissue, highlighting specific biological functions, contains a vast amount of spatial information that must be interpreted by a pathologist. With automated image analysis, some of this information can be quantified and made available for computations such as stain expression analysis. In this contribution we present an automated workflow where quantitative image analysis results of consecutive, differently stained tissue sections are locally fused by co-registration. The results are spatially resolved feature vectors containing features like the densities of positively marked cell types for different stains, which are – in this sense – hyperspectral. Heat maps with many layers (hyperspectral) are generated from this data, revealing relationships between different stains that would not be evident from single stains alone. These hyperspectral data are also a starting point for further investigations; in supporting biomarker discovery in oncology, a systematic search for properties that correlate with clinical data for a patient cohort can be performed in an highly automated way.

1 Introduction

The advent and increasing availability of whole slide imaging (WSI) from stained tissue sections are key enablers for new developments and make digital pathology an exciting area of research. The digital revolution already dramatically changed other imaging and medical fields. For example radiology allows today for powerful applications not realizable with analogous data. One kind of new development [1, 2] addresses the handling and user presentation of digital pathology imagery to aim for more efficient and optimized workflows in a pathologist's lab by replacing traditional microscopes with digital equipment. On the other hand, completely new procedures – such as automated image analysis – can assist pathologists by providing relevant data to further improve diagnostics. A very fascinating approach, made feasible with WSIs of consecutive tissue sections, is their virtual realignment in a z-stack. Since single sections are typically only 3μm thick, which is small compared to most relevant objects, corresponding regions can be co-registered. When tissue sections are differently stained they contain information about specific biological functions. With co-registration the information of many such markers becomes available for each particular region of a WSI. In this contribution we go further than just providing a user interface for visual analysis of co-registered digital slides [3]; the prototype presented here is capable of producing quantitative results through computational work in form of image analysis. The established workflow lets us apply image analysis algorithms on high-resolution WSIs and join results of related regions in different stains, making them available for all types of calculations. To achieve this, extensions of Definiens' image analysis software Developer XD [4] were used and combined – automated landmark detection, image layer transformation with landmarks, generic nuclei detection for immunohistochemical (IHC) stains, and result containers to store (intermediate) image analysis results. An application was created to demonstrate protein co-expression analysis using IHC stains from consecutive tissue sections – heat maps are generated which, for example, display the difference in densities between proliferating cells positively marked by Ki67 staining and estrogen-expressed cells positively marked by PR staining. Since such heatmaps have the power to unveil spatial dependancies between biological properties derived from involved stainings, this is a tool for pathologists to gain new insights about healthy and/or diseased tissues.

2   Materials and methods

A cohort of ten cases, representing ten different patients, was taken from a repository of breast cancer biopsies provided by Hannover Medical School. For each case consecutive tissue sections with the following seven stains have been produced: Hematoxylin and eosin (H&E), progesterone (PR), estrogen (ER), Ki-67

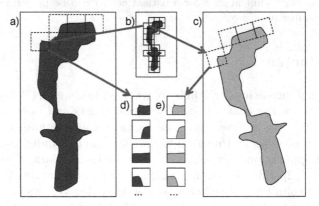

Fig. 1. A selected WSI of a case is assigned to be the master slide (a). A smaller version (b) is generated and tile objects are created. The corresponding regions of each tile in the master slide (a) and a slide to be co-registered (c) are copied to separate working maps (d) and (e) where image analysis at native resolution can be performed.

protein, cluster of differentiation 8 (CD8), cytokeratin 5 & 14 (CK5&14), and basal membrane protein p63. Each slide was scanned by an Aperio AT2 scanner at 40x resolution (0.253μm per pixel), resulting in WSIs of up to 10^5 x 10^5 pixels of 24-bit RGB data with file sizes of up to 4GB. In the latest version of Developer XD, new co-registration features are available, with automated landmark detection capable of identifying common landmarks in sets of consecutive tissue sections. We formulate the global rigid registration of the whole tissue sections as an optimization problem, in which the cost function is defined as the normalized-cross correlation of the brightness. A set of landmarks is automatically defined at the border of the tissue sections and the rigid transformation is locally refined on this set using block matching, therefore defining a set of pairs of corresponding landmarks [5]. These landmarks are used to align rectangular portions of whole slide images; for the portion's center, a virtual landmark is calculated by linear interpolation of all other landmarks and the co-ordinate system of one slide is taken as master co-ordinate system. Corresponding portions of the slides to be co-registered are then copied by a rigid transformation to the master slide image portion (Fig. 1). Another recent and ongoing development available to this contribution is a general nuclei detection module for WSIs of IHC-stained tissue based on machine learning algorithms. The procedures are taken here as is and the publication of the algorithm is in preparation. Finally, an extension has been integrated to flexibly store and retrieve image analysis results – for example layers of segmented and classified objects together with meta-information – to and from a result container file per slide. These are based on the HDF5 [6] data model and, from a user perspective, automatically organize from which portion or scale of an image the results are written or read. With these software modules

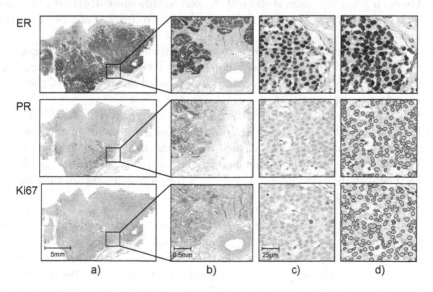

Fig. 2. WSIs of different stains (a) are co-registered tile-by-tile (b). Detailed view (c) of image analysis results (d) with automated nuclei detection in IHC stains.

in place, a workflow to analyze sets of consecutive tissue sections of a case has been implemented with the following main processing steps:

1. One slide is assigned as master (Fig. 1a) and determines the main co-ordinate system.
2. For heat map production a demagnified copy master_small of master is created (Fig. 1b).
3. A simple region of interest (ROI) identification on master_small is performed, mainly by thresholding tissue area against a white background.
4. In the ROI of the master_small tile objects are created. These later constitute the pixels of a heat map.
5. For each tile on the master_small the corresponding region in the master with full resolution is automatically defined (Fig. 1a).
6. The region's co-ordinates are then projected according the current transformation parameters into each WSI to be co-registered (Fig. 1c) and the contained image raster data portion is copied to a separate image working storage (tile_map) (Fig. 1e). They are now in the same co-ordinate system as the corresponding tile region of master (Fig. 1d) and therefore co-registered.
7. For each tile_map the image analysis procedure for nuclei detection (Fig. 2d) is applied and the resulting segmented objects are stored in a result container.
8. The nuclei objects on the tile_map are classified for IHC-positive cases according to a brown detection method. An approved measure for the brownness of objects is given by the RGB layer value statement:
   brownness $= (R > G) \ \& \ (G > B) * (R-(G+B)/2)$.
   If brownness > 0, then nuclei objects are classified as positively stained.
9. For each tile_map some statistical measurements are calculated and stored. This comprises number and total area of positive (brown) and negative (non-brown) nuclei.
10. The results are collected as feature vectors attached to the tile_map's corresponding tile object of master_small. They later constitute the pixels of a heat map visualization when computations based on the values of the feature vectors are displayed (Fig. 3).
11. Steps 6-10 are repeated for all WSIs to be co-registered. In this way, the feature vector for each tile object on master_small is complemented with the statistical results from the detailed image analysis procedure of each stain. We call the result after processing all tiles a hyperspectral image since for each heat map-pixel (corresponding to a tile) a feature vector with values of different co-registered stains is available.

The sizes of tiles used for image analysis and statistical evaluation (heat map pixels) are not necessarily the same, because they can be independently generated and gathered to or from the result containers available for each slide and stain. The analysis tiles in principle should be as big as possible without creating memory issues, whereas the statistic tiles should be as small as possible for a high resolution of the heat maps without being smaller than small groups of relevant objects. This decoupling of image analysis, statistical evaluation and heat map creation also allows us to save processing time when a new statistical evaluation is based on previously available image analysis results. Typically the image analysis is performed on tiles of 2,048 x 2,048 pixels and the heat map pixels represent the local statistics of a tile with 256 x 256 pixels.

3   Results

This workflow has been applied to the cohort with 10 cases à 7 stains. The majority of processing time is consumed by the detailed nuclei detection procedures which take an average of about ten hours per slide. As we utilize a Win64 cluster environment made up of more than ten engines (Intel Xeon E5-2690, 16 cores, 3.8 GHz, 256GB RAM), all cases can be processed in parallel. For preprocessing (landmark creation) and heat map production (data retrieval from result containers and statistics calculations) approximately one hour of processing time per case is required. Based on visual inspection, we can verify that the accuracy of co-registration and the quality of nuclei detection is sufficient to demonstrate this prototype workflow: Fig. 2 shows an example tile for co-registered images and results of nuclei segmentation. In Fig. 3 some sample heat maps are displayed. They show differences of positive nuclei densities for multiple stain combinations.

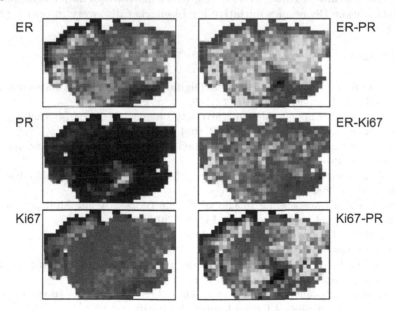

Fig. 3. Heat maps showing IHC-positive nuclei densities for ER, PR, and Ki67 staining (Fig. 2), which have been normalized to exhibit intensities of comparable magnitude. The differences between density maps are displayed in the right column and feature structures not evident in heat maps of single stains.

4   Discussion

This workflow is an example of an innovative application [7, 8] made possible by the availability of WSIs and automated image analysis. It provides features to display and uncover non-linear relationships across the specific structures highlighted in different IHC stains, which are not evident for a human observer analyzing single stains with a traditional microscope. Heat maps can be designed by combinatorial calculations with values of different stains to unveil spatially resolved properties – such as protein co-expression or more general cell-type co-occurrence – in tissue sections and thus guide pathologists to new insights. In the current development the image analysis procedures do not support artifact removal for inconsistent regions, such as blurred image regions or folded tissue. Anyway, for co-registration a high quality of consecutive tissue sections is required to allow for valid spatially resolved calculations. The accuracy of co-registration must be better than the size of a full-resolution tile represented by a pixel in a heat map, in order to obtain reasonable results. The availability of hyperspectral data is only a pre-requisite for further developments and applications. We are currently developing methods to further segment and classify the pixels of heat maps and systematically search for objects with properties that correlate to clinical outcome data of patient cohorts [9]. Together with data mining and machine-learning procedures, this constitutes a major component of Definiens' Tissue Phenomics initiative for biomarker discovery in oncology.

References

1. Al-Janabi S, Huisman A, Van Diest PJ. Digital pathology: current status and future perspectives. Histopathology. 2012;61:1–9.
2. Rohde G, et al. Carnegie Mellon University bioimaging day 2014: challenges and opportunities in digital pathology. J Pathol Inform. 2014;5:32.
3. Schönmeyer R, et al. Visualization and navigation platform for co-registered whole tissue slides. Proc BVM. 2014; p. 13–8.
4. Schäpe A, et al. Fraktal hierarchische, prozeß- und objektbasierte Bildanalyse. Proc BVM. 2003; p. 206–10.
5. Brieu N, et al. Coregistering Images of Needle Biopsies Using Multiple Weighted Landmarks. ; 2014. US Patent App. 13/764,539.
6. The HDF Group. Hierarchical Data Format, Version 5. ; 2014. Http://www.hdfgroup.org/HDF5/.
7. Schönmeyer R, et al. Generating artificial hyperspectral images using correlated analysis of co-registered images. ; 2014. EP Patent 2,546,802.
8. Cucoranu IC, Parwani AV, Vepa S, et al. Digital pathology: a systematic evaluation of the patent landscape. J Pathol Inform. 2014;5:16.
9. Schönmeyer R, Binnig G, Schmidt G. Generating Image-Based Diagnostic Tests By Optimizing Image Analysis and Data Mining Of Co-Registered Images. ; 2014. US Patent App. 14/197,197.

Band-Pass Filter Design by Segmentation in Frequency Domain for Detection of Epithelial Cells in Endomicroscope Images

Bastian Bier[1], Firas Mualla[1], Stefan Steidl[1], Christopher Bohr[2],
Helmut Neumann[3], Andreas Maier[1], Joachim Hornegger[1]

[1]Pattern Recognition Lab
[2]Department of Otorhinolaryngology
[3]Department of Medicine I
Friedrich-Alexander-Universität, Erlangen-Nürnberg, Germany
bastian.bier@fau.de

Abstract. Voice hoarseness can have various reasons, one of them is a change of the vocal fold mucus. This change can be examined with micro endoscopes. Cell detection in these images is a difficult task, due to bad image quality, caused by noise and illumination variations. In previous works, it was observed that the repetitive pattern of the cell walls cause an elliptical shape in the Fourier domain [1, 2]. A manual segmentation and back transformation of this shape results in filtered images, where the cell detection is much easier [3]. The goal of this work is to automatically segment the elliptical shape in Fourier domain. Two different approaches are developed to get a suitable band-pass filter: a thresholding and an active contour method. After the band-pass filter is applied, the achieved results are superior to the manual segmentation case.

1 Introduction

A hoarse voice can have various reasons, such as structural changes or changes in the mucus of the vocal folds, leading to an influence on the voice signal [4]. One method to examine the vocal fold mucus is to use micro endoscopes in vivo and investigate the resulting epithelial cell images. Compared to normal microscopes, micro endoscope images have a poor image quality with much noise and brightness changes across the image. This lack of image quality makes the detection of cells a difficult task.

In the literature, several cell detection approaches exist [5, 6, 7, 8]. The cell images we use have the property that no separation of background and foreground has to be done, because cells cover the whole scene. Furthermore, the cell walls form a repetitive pattern. This property is used in [1, 2], where they observed a circular shape in the Fourier domain of cell images, representing the pattern of the cell walls in the image. Furthermore, this approach is used in [3], where the ellipse is segmented manually in the Fourier domain. The filtered cell image has less noise and cell detection is then easier and more robust. The goal of this work is to find a method which automatically segments the elliptical shape in the Fourier domain. Two different methods are presented: one thresholding approach and an approach using geodesic active contour segmentation.

2   Material and methods

Nine images of epithelial cells of the vocal fold acquired with a micro endoscope of a Cellvisio probe-based confocal laser endomicroscope (pCLE) system are used in this work, same images as in [3] (Fig. 1(a)). In order to avoid artificial frequencies of the black circle around the cells, the original images are cropped (Fig. 1(b)). Image resolution after cropping is 405×397 pixels. In Fig. 1(c), the Fourier transform of the cropped image is shown. In the middle of the image, one can see clearly an elliptical shape corresponding to the repetitive pattern of the cell walls. The following presented methods segment this circle to get a band-pass filter mask. The methods are implemented in C++ with ITK [9]. Cell detection is performed by detecting intensity minima in the filtered image.

2.1   Labeling of the reference data and evaluation

To be able to evaluate the new methods, ground truth is needed. This is done by manually labeling the cropped cell images with the program ImageJ. In the labeling procedure, each cell center is clicked and the coordinate of these reference cells are stored. These coordinates are used for evaluation.

Due to the bad image quality caused for example by dirt on the lens and illumination changes, it is not easy to recognize all cells properly during the labeling process. Consequently, one has to have in mind that even the ground truth contains some mistakes. The average number of cells per image after cropping is 294.

In order to be able to evaluate the methods quantitatively, the detected cells have to be matched with the reference cells. This is done with a standard

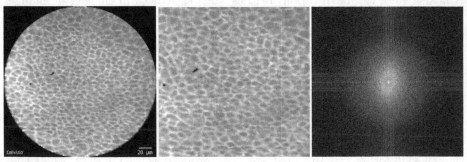

(a) Epithelial cell image   (b) Cropped input image   (c) Fourier transform of (b)

Fig. 1. Sample epithelial cell image and its Fourier transform. In the Fourier transform an elliptical shape in the center of the image can be seen.

algorithm for such problems, the Hungarian algorithm. This matching algorithm allows a maximum distance of 8 pixels between the reference and the detected cells. This is the same evaluation method used in [3].

2.2 Thresholding method

The thresholding method is based on finding a suitable threshold. Experimentally, a relative threshold of 0.988 is estimated, meaning that the highest 1.2% of the values in the Fourier image are set to one, and the other 98,8% to zero

$$M(\mathbf{x}) = \begin{cases} 1 & \text{if } |F(\mathbf{x})| > \text{threshold} \\ 0 & \text{otherwise} \end{cases} \tag{1}$$

$M(\mathbf{x})$ describes the mask at coordinate $\mathbf{x}$ and F is the input Fourier image. After applying this threshold, many pixels inside the elliptical shape are zero (Fig. 2(a)). In order to get a nice ellipse, a median filter with size 12 is used to smooth the pixel cloud. The brightness and illumination changes in the images can be reduced by cutting out the low frequencies. This is done by setting a circle with radius of three pixels in the center of the image mask to zero. The resulting band-pass filter mask is shown in Fig. 2(b).

2.3 Geodesic active contours segmentation

The geodesic active contour filter needs a feature image on which it can find a contour iteratively, according to the energy term [10]

$$\frac{d}{dt}\Psi = -\alpha \mathbf{A}(\mathbf{x}) \cdot \nabla\Psi - \beta B(\mathbf{x})|\nabla\Psi| + \gamma Z(\mathbf{x})\kappa|\nabla\Psi| \tag{2}$$

$\mathbf{A}(\mathbf{x})$ describes the advection term to the edge in the image, $B(\mathbf{x})$ describes the propagation term and $Z(\mathbf{x})$ is the spatial modifier term for the mean curvature κ. α, β and γ are weights defining the influence of each term. The algorithm then finds the optimal contour, where the level-set function Ψ equals 0.

To get a feature image, a filter is used which calculates the gradient of the image by convolving it with the first derivative of the Gaussian. The smoothing size of the Gaussian is determined experimentally and set to $\sigma = 0.9$ (Fig. 2(c)). Afterwards, the derivative image is multiplied by -1 and scaled between zero and one, required for the geodesic filter. For Eq. (2) this results that $B(\mathbf{x})$ and $Z(\mathbf{x})$ are equal to the the negative and scaled gradient magnitude image. $\mathbf{A}(\mathbf{x})$ is the negative gradient of the feature image. The geodesic active contour filter is then applied with the weights $\beta = 1.0$, $\gamma = 1.0$ and $\alpha = 4.0$. Furthermore, the filter needs an initial contour, set here to a circle around the center of the image with a radius of 24 pixels. Same as in the thresholding method, the low frequencies are cut out of the mask center with a circle of radius three pixels. The resulting band-pass filter mask is shown in Fig. 2(d).

Table 1. Recall, Precision and the F-measure results averaged over all images.

Method	Recall	Precision	F-measure
Original Images	98.2 ± 0.9	24.3 ± 4.0	38.8 ± 5.1
Manual Segmentation [3]	94.6 ± 3.7	70.0 ± 7.3	80.2 ± 4.7
Thresholding Method	83.6 ± 2.2	83.9 ± 3.3	83.7 ± 2.0
Geodesic Segmentation	83.5 ± 5.1	83.1 ± 4.1	83.3 ± 4.1

3   Results

In Tab. 3, the results achieved with the thresholding and the geodesic method are compared with minima detection on the original unprocessed image and with the results of the manual segmentation presented in [3]. The two presented methods achieved almost the same results. In addition, they were considerably superior to minima detection on the unprocessed image and approximately 3% better than [3] in F-measure.

Qualitative results are shown in Fig. 3. In Figs. 4(a) and 4(b), the cell image before and after the processing is shown with a zoomed region of the same ROI

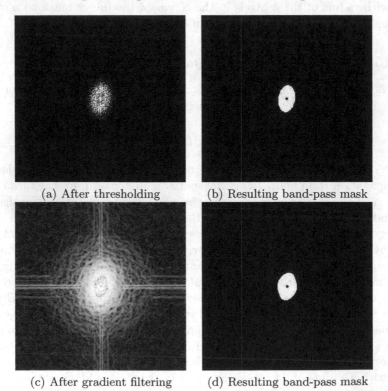

(a) After thresholding   (b) Resulting band-pass mask

(c) After gradient filtering   (d) Resulting band-pass mask

Fig. 2. Intermediate steps and final masks of the thresholding method (upper row) and the geodesic segmentation (lower row).

Fig. 3. Qualitative comparison between minima detection on an unprocessed image and on an image filtered with the band-pass filter designed by the thresholding method. In Figs. 4(c) and 4(d), reference cells are marked with a red plus sign and the automatically detected cells with a green plus sign. The yellow lines in Fig. 4(d) connect matched cells.

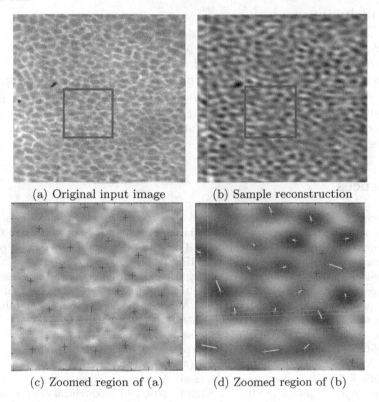

(a) Original input image	(b) Sample reconstruction
(c) Zoomed region of (a)	(d) Zoomed region of (b)

(Fig. 4(c) and 4(d)). Here, one can see that the band-pass filtered image contains less noise and the cell walls and centers are well visible.

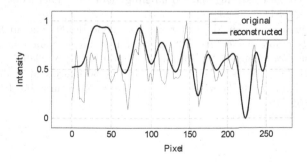

Fig. 4. Line profile comparison of the original and the reconstructed image.

The effect of the enhanced cell walls can be seen in Fig. 4, where two normalized line profiles of the original and the reconstructed image are shown. The noise is removed and only the cell walls remain.

4   Conclusion

In [3], it was shown that detection of epithelial cells in endomicroscope images of the vocal folds is possible with basic image processing techniques when an image is preprocessed with a band-pass filter which corresponds to the repetitive pattern of cells inside the image. In this paper, we showed that it is possible to automatically design this filter by segmenting an ellipse which shows up in Fourier domain, even though segmentation parameters were manually set or experimentally found.

References

1. Ruggeri A, Grisan E, Jaroszewski J. A new system for the automatic estimation of endothelial cell density in donor corneas. Br J Ophthalmol. 2005; p. 306–11.
2. Foraccia M, Ruggeri A. Estimating dell density in corneal endothelium by means of fourier analysis. Proc Second Jt EMBS/BMES. 2002; p. 1097–8.
3. Mualla F, Schöll S, Bohr C, et al. Epithelial cell detection in endomicroscopy images of the vocal folds. Proc Int Multidisciplin Microsc Congr. 2013; p. 1097–8.
4. Klemuk SA, Riede T, Walsh EJ, et al. Adapted to roar: functional morphology of tiger and lion vocal folds. PLoS One. 2011;6(11):e27029.
5. Long X, Cleveland W, Yao Y. Automatic detection of unstained viable cells in bright field images using a support vector machine with an improved training procedure. Comput Biol Med. 2006;36(4):339–62.
6. Mualla F, Schöll S, Sommerfeldt B, et al. Automatic cell detection in bright-field microscope images using SIFT, random forests, and hierarchical clustering. IEEE Trans Med Imaging. 2013;32(12):2274–86.
7. Mualla F, Schöll S, Sommerfeldt B, et al. Unsupervised unstained cell detection by SIFT keypoint clustering and self-labeling algorithm. Lect Notes Computer Sci. 2014;8675:377–84.
8. Pan J, Kanade T, Chen M. Heterogeneous conditional random field: realizing joint detection and segmentation of cell regions in microscopic images. Proc IEEE Comput Soc Conf Comput Vis Pattern Recognit. 2010; p. 2940–7.
9. Johnson HJ, McCormick M, Ibáñez L. The ITK Software Guide. 3rd ed.; 2013.
10. Caselles V, Kimmel R, Sapiro G. Geodesic active contours. Int J Computer Vis. 1997;22(1):61–79.

Foreground Extraction for Histopathological Whole Slide Imaging

Daniel Bug[1], Friedrich Feuerhake[2], Dorit Merhof[1]

[1]Institute of Imaging and Computer Vision, RWTH Aachen
[2]Institute of Pathology, Hannover Medical School
daniel.bug@lfb.rwth-aachen.de

Abstract. Segmentation of histopathological whole-slide images is a challenging task that requires dedicated approaches. In this paper, the fore- and background segmentation problem is addressed by a combination of basic filters, which is evaluated against the established methods GrabCut and Watershed. It is shown that our computationally efficient, dedicated approach performs better than the technically more advanced methods. The main lesson is that dedicated solutions built on prior knowledge can out-compete advanced algorithms.

1 Introduction

In medical image analysis, segmentation of input data often forms a crucial pre-processing step, e.g. to reduce the amount of input to the advanced and often computationally costly main processing. In recent research, Watershed (WS) segmentation is commonly applied in cell-segmentation or cell-nuclei identification [1], GrabCut / GraphCut (GC) for the segmentation of image regions [2, 3] and Markov-Random-Fields (MRF) for both segmentation and classification of regions [4]. For the purpose of foreground extraction, WS is not particularly suited as standalone solution due to its tendency to over-segment [5]. GC on the other hand, is particularly designed for foreground extraction and abstracts models for fore- and background, which can even be adapted iteratively [2]. MRFs form another model-based approach. The training of MRF models implicitly includes a-priori knowledge into the algorithm, but an MRF is computationally costly if large neighborhoods have to be analyzed.

In this work, a rather basic approach to split histopathological brightfield-microscopic images of tissue samples into fore- and background is introduced. Such preprocessing is a necessary step for detailed analysis in digital pathology and computer-aided diagnosis. The proposed method aims at providing a reliable and easy to implement, automatic foreground selection, tolerant to artifacts and noise, without creating a large computational overhead to any further processing. The method is compared to WS and GC for evaluation purposes.

2   Materials and methods

As input data, 43 images of tissue samples are available, which are stained with different methods, i.e. H&E staining and specific immunological markers. The files contain images at three scales, subsampled by the factors 1, 4 and 16 and have a size of approximately 2500, 150 and 5 mega-pixels, respectively. For the purpose of foreground extraction, the lowest scale (strongest subsampling) is used. It is characteristic for the images to have a bright background, slightly disturbed by noise, dust particles and occasional markings on the object slide. Visually, fore- and background can already be distinguished very well by looking at the color and the „structuredness" of a region. As a measure for structure, the standard-deviation in a region or the Laplacian operator can be used. The algorithm suggested here is a combination of basic methods, such as Median-Filtering, Thresholding, Erosion and Dilation, which are well explained in [6]. The pipeline proposed in the following is the result of extensive analysis, which has shown that the structure information provides a superior segmentation compared to a color-based approach.

2.1   Foreground extraction from structure information (FESI)

Based on the gray-scale image, the absolute value of the Laplacian is calculated and blurred by a strong Gaussian filter. This gives an average measure for the structure in an image, with a high response in textured regions and a low response in homogenous background regions. By applying the mean of the blurred image as a global threshold, we obtain an initial mask and the inverse threshold will be used later to find a reliable background point for flood-filling. On the initial mask, morphological operations and median-blurring are used to open the foreground mask and suppress noise. Still, there will be some remaining gaps inside the tissue area. In order to identify the outer contours, we apply flood-filling, starting at the maximum of the distance transform of the inverse initial mask, which reliably belongs to the background, even after morphological operations. The result already provides a good segmentation, but includes several artifacts.

At this point, further prior knowledge needs to be introduced: in the majority of applications using serial tissue sections or similar types of samples, the tissue areas on a slide are consistently about the same size and relatively large compared to the artifacts. This implies that we can use the size of each region to separate tissue from artifacts for this type of WSI scans. To measure the size of a region, the distance transform is used and we start iterating over the distance maxima, deleting visited ones with flood-filling and at the same time flood-filling the accepted maxima into the final mask. Sometimes small tissue regions will occur separated from the maximum, but close to it. Therefore, we still accept small regions if they are close to a large maximum. FESI in pseudo-code:

```
laplace = abs(laplace(grayim(image)))
blurred = GaussianBlur(laplace, midsizeKernel, largeSigma)
```

```
mask = threshold(blurred, blurred.mean(), val=150)
dseed = distanceTransform(...
        ...threshold(blurred, blurred.mean(), val=255, 'inverse'))
mask = medianBlur(mask, 'strong')+100
mask = morphOpen(mask)
floodFill(mask, seed=dseed.argmax(), newVal=0)
mask[mask > 1] = 255
distance = distanceTransform(mask)
final_mask = mask.copy()
dmax = distance.max()
globalMax = distance.max()
seeds = []
while (dmax > 0):
    start = distance.argmax()
    seeds.append((start, dmax))
    cv2.floodFill(mask, seed=start, newVal=0)
    distance[mask == 0] = 0
    dmax = distance.max()
    if (dmax > 0.6*globalMax) or isClose(seeds, start):
        floodFill(final_mask, start, newVal=200)
    final_mask[final_mask != 200] = 0
    final_mask[final_mask == 200] = 255
return final_mask
```

The algorithm was implemented in Python using the NumPy, and OpenCV (Python) libraries. Matplotlib was applied to display the results. The WS and GC implementations were taken from OpenCV. The initial mask for WS was the threshold of the mean-blurred gray-scale image. GC gets a mask based on the gray-scale image as input and is postprocessed with a median-blur for noise reduction.

3   Results

For evaluation, the intersection-to-union area ratio, i.e. Jaccard-index, is used to measure the overlap of the calculated mask C to the ground-truth G, i.e. $r = (C \cap G)/(C \cup G)$, where $r = 1$ (or 100%) represents a perfect overlap with the ground-truth. The ground-truth was labeled manually in advance as a reference mask. Fig. 1 shows the resulting histograms for WS, GC and our algorithm.

For 34 out of 43 images, our algorithm matches the areas without visually notable differences and an area overlap of more than 95%. In the remaining 9 images, the algorithm responds to noise or artifacts and includes additional material. In none of the investigated cases, our algorithm missed relevant parts of the tissue. With a deviation of 3.2% in the overlap, FESI shows a consistent foreground/background separation.

WS on the other hand is only able to segment the image without any major deviations from the ground truth segmentation in 7 out of 43 cases. The mean overlap of 82.3% is significantly lower than for our approach and the higher deviation suggests less reliability. In many cases the mistakes include examples of tissue regions that are discarded by WS as background.

GC matches the area slightly better, with an average overlap of 85.9% and a standard-deviation of 8.7%. In most cases, GC manages to reliably subtract the background, but tends to include many artifacts into the foreground. The overall number of erroneously segmented images is 24, out of which only 5 are missing small parts of the tissue (which would still be an acceptable range).

In terms of the processing time, FESI is the fastest algorithm with 0.59s on average to segment an images. WS runs quite fast, too, with an average duration of 0.95s and GC is by far the slowest algorithm with 14.3s. All performance tests were run on a machine with a 3.5GHz processor and 32GB RAM. Tab. 1 summarizes all results and an example for the segmentation output is given in Fig. 2.

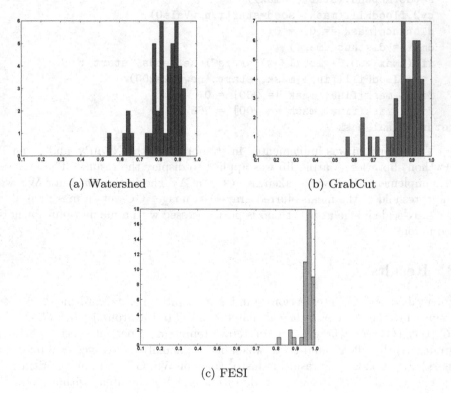

(a) Watershed   (b) GrabCut

(c) FESI

Fig. 1. Histogram of the area overlaps, measured as intersection-to-union ratio for Watershed, GrabCut and FESI.

Table 1. Results and comparison of the Algorithms. The mistakes are the cases in which relevant parts were incorrectly marked as fore- or background. In total, 43 tissue samples were tested.

Algorithm	Mean	Std	Time [s]	Mistakes
Watershed	82.3%	8.9%	0.95	36
GrabCut	85.9%	8.7%	14.29	24
FESI	95.9%	3.2%	0.59	9

4 Discussion

As initially assumed, WS proved not to be suitable to solve the fore- and background segmentation task. According to our experience, the algorithm performs well on identifying potential regions of interest, if this implies a strong change in appearance in the image. The challenge in our application, however, is to identify tissue even in regions that display weak staining intensity due to the less compact tissue composition, or due to technical characteristics of the staining method. Discarding these regions may result in loss of information for the main processing. Depending on the scientific or clinical question to digital histopathology evaluation, this is in most cases not acceptable. The risk of a mistakenly retained artifact is less severe, as it can easily be excluded further downstream in the analysis process.

In contrast, GC tends to include many artifacts, which then *have* to be processed in later steps. Although the high number of false-positives will likely affect the overall processing time in later processing stages, GC seems to be

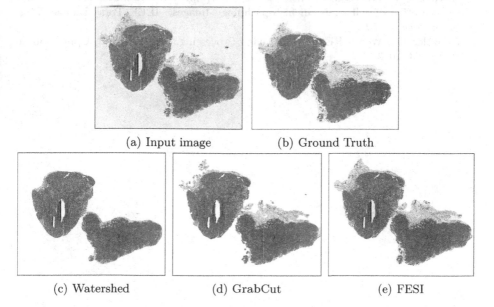

(a) Input image   (b) Ground Truth

(c) Watershed   (d) GrabCut   (e) FESI

Fig. 2. Comparison of the segmentation results in case of a H&E stained tissue sample.

more suited to solve the task than WS. Basically, the assumptions about the region size and spatial relations could be used to improve the result of the GC algorithm, as well. However, the relatively high processing time of GC plus the anticipated increased processing time in later analysis stages, constitute severe limitations of GC for clinical use.

FESI actually performs best on the whole-slide image data set and manages the foreground extraction accurately and reliably. It has the tendency of rather including (slightly) too much background as tissue than discarding relevant content, but at the same time provides a good selectivity. As fore- and background segmentation sets the stage for the subsequent more detailed WSI analysis, it can have important impact on quality and speed of image processing. FESI might represent a promising component of large-scale WSI processing, given the importance of performance and speed in the emerging field of digital pathology.

References

1. Veta M, Huisman A, Viergever MA, et al. Marker-controlled watershed segmentation of nuclei in H&E stained breast cancer biopsy images. Proc ISBI. 2011; p. 618–21.
2. Rother C, Kolmogorov V, Blake A. Grabcut: interactive foreground extraction using iterated graph cuts. ACM Trans Graph. 2004; p. 309–14.
3. Boykov YY, Jolly MP. Interactive graph cuts for optimal boundary & region segmentation of objects in ND images. Proc ICCV. 2001;1:105–12.
4. Xu J, Monaco JP, Madabhushi A. Markov random field driven region-based active contour model (MaRACel): application to medical image segmentation. Proc MICCAI. 2010; p. 197–204.
5. Al-Kofahi Y, Lassoued W, Lee W, et al. Improved automatic detection and segmentation of cell nuclei in histopathology Images. IEEE Trans Biomed Eng. 2010;57(4):841–52.
6. Gonzalez RC, Woods RE. Digital Image Processing. Prentice Hall, Upper Saddle River, NJ; 2002.

Sharp as a Tack

Measuring and Comparing Edge Sharpness in Motion-Compensated Medical Image Reconstruction

Oliver Taubmann[1,2], Jens Wetzl[1,2], Günter Lauritsch[3], Andreas Maier[1,2],
Joachim Hornegger[1,2]

[1]Pattern Recognition Lab, Friedrich-Alexander-University Erlangen-Nuremberg
[2]Graduate School in Advanced Optical Technologies (SAOT), Erlangen, Germany
[3]Siemens AG, Healthcare, Forchheim, Germany
oliver.taubmann@fau.de

Abstract. Organ motion occuring during acquisition of medical images can cause motion blur artifacts, thus posing a major problem for many commonly employed modalities. Therefore, compensating for that motion during image reconstruction has been a focus of research for several years. However, objectively comparing the quality of different motion compensated reconstructions is no easy task. Often, intensity profiles across image edges are utilized to compare their sharpness. Manually positioning such a profile line is highly subjective and prone to bias. Expanding on this notion, we propose a robust, semi-automatic scheme for comparing edge sharpness using an ensemble of profiles. We study the behavior of our approach, which was implemented as an open-source tool, for synthetic data in the presence of noise and artifacts and demonstrate its practical use in respiratory motion-compensated MRI as well as cardiac motion-compensated C-arm CT.

1 Introduction

Motion artifacts such as image blurring are caused by movements of the imaged objects during acquisition, leading to inconsistent raw data. To obtain high-quality images using all of the acquired data—as opposed to a retrospective gating—this inconsistency must be addressed during image reconstruction. A typical approach is to estimate the motion from an initial reconstruction and subsequently or jointly perform another motion-compensated reconstruction from all data [1, 2]. Comparing the quality of motion-compensated reconstructions in terms of common measures such as the signal-to-noise ratio of the reconstructed image is of limited value: A noise-free image may be obtained even if the motion was estimated incorrectly. In fact, many pixel-wise distance measures used in phantom studies are dominated by homogeneous regions as well. Therefore, it makes sense to attempt to directly measure the entity that is supposed to be improved, i. e. the sharpness of an edge. For this purpose, analyses of modulation transfer functions (MTF) of slanted edges [3] used to be common, but they are not applicable to non-linear reconstruction methods which are dependent on the imaged object. Here, the measurements need to be performed on the representative object itself. Typically, in order to perform such measurements, intensity profile lines across edges are considered [4]. Proper selection of these lines is crucial, but typically amounts to visual inspection based on personal experience.

We propose a more robust, objective approach, comparable to e. g. [5], that aims to measure edge sharpness reliably from a large number of semi-automatically placed profile lines and is explained in section 2. In section 3, its merits are demonstrated using a synthetic phantom and shown exemplarily for respiratory motion-compensated 3-D whole-heart coronary magnetic resonance imaging (MRI) [2] and cardiac motion-compensated C-arm computed tomography (CT) of the heart [1]. We discuss and conclude the paper in section 4.

2   Materials and methods

Let us first identify the main problems of manual placement of a profile line:

P1 *Susceptibility to noise.* Even noise that is incoherent with the signal and randomly distributed will influence the measurement if it cannot be separated reliably in the 1-D profile, which is often the case. As this influence is generally not consistent for different reconstructions, comparing a profile line across images may be problematic.

P2 *Susceptibility to artifacts.* For similar reasons, artifacts pose a problem to this approach. In contrast to (moderate) noise, however, they may completely render a profile invalid in one image but not the other. For instance, consider a streak artifact coinciding with the profile line in one image, which happens to appear at a different position along the same edge in the other.

P3 *Placement bias.* With no automated process for positioning the profiles, there is no way to avoid a subjective placement, potentially unconsciously biased toward a certain outcome.

P4 *Mismatch of desired and measured entity.* This is a more abstract, conceptual issue than (P1) through (P3). The entity we are interested in is the sharpness of an originally motion blurred edge. Reducing this problem to measuring the sharpness of a profile is a simplification which may or may not be valid

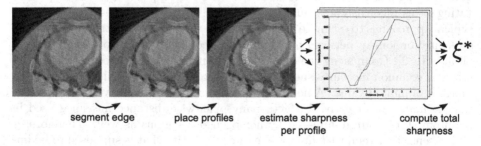

segment edge   place profiles   estimate sharpness   compute total
                                     per profile   sharpness

Fig. 1. A schematic overview of our approach to measuring edge sharpness from a large number of semi-automatically placed intensity profile lines.

in any given case. The closer we can get to measuring the relevant entity, i. e. the less we have to simplify, the more trustworthy our results.

We address each of these problems with our approach, which is summarized below and illustrated in Fig. 1. An obvious and common choice for alleviating the susceptibility to noise and artifacts is using multiple profile lines and some form of averaging of the measurements for increased robustness. Manually choosing a large number of lines, though, is time-consuming and may even increase the effect of placement bias. If they are to be averaged, it also requires the chosen profiles to be somewhat comparable. Therefore, starting from the core idea behind (P4), the first and only manual step in our method is to select the desired edge by roughly tracing it with a connected sequence of line segments. Along this segmentation, profile lines of equal length are generated at short equidistant steps, oriented orthogonally to the segmented line. They cover the edge densely and completely, eliminating placement bias. Naturally, there still remains a possibility for bias while choosing the edge, although we believe that it is considerably less dangerous than manually placing profiles. For each profile, an estimate of its sharpness is obtained. For this purpose, the image is sampled densely along the profile line, which is subsequently reoriented, if necessary, such that the intensities are rising. A region of interest is defined starting at the location of the minimum intensity in the first half of the profile and ending at that of the maximum in the second. In this region, the slope of the least squares regression line fit is computed as

$$\xi_\ell = \frac{\text{cov}[\boldsymbol{s}_\ell, \boldsymbol{I}_\ell]}{\text{var}[\boldsymbol{s}_\ell]} = \frac{\sum_i (s_{\ell,i} - \frac{1}{N_\ell} \sum_j s_{\ell,j})(I_{\ell,i} - \frac{1}{N_\ell} \sum_j I_{\ell,j})}{\sum_i (s_{\ell,i} - \frac{1}{N_\ell} \sum_j s_{\ell,j})^2} \tag{1}$$

where $\boldsymbol{s}_\ell$ contains the distances in physical units of the N_ℓ sample locations within the region of interest and $\boldsymbol{I}_\ell$ the corresponding intensities along profile line ℓ. The slope ξ_ℓ serves as a rough measure of the edge sharpness locally, but as explained above, we do not expect it to be very robust. Averaging all the ξ_ℓ would now reliably eliminate susceptibility to noise, yet artifacts can be the cause of outliers strongly affecting the mean value. Hence, we select the

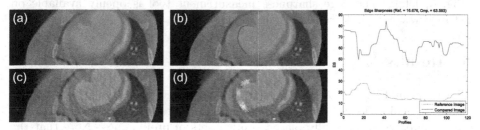

Fig. 2. The upper row shows a motion-blurred image (a) and the edge selected for comparison (b). Below, a motion-compensated reconstruction (c) and the edge sharpness increase (d) can be seen, with stronger hues of red indicating a larger relative change. The plot shows the corresponding sharpness estimates along the edge for both images.

total edge sharpness as $\xi^* = \mathrm{median}[\boldsymbol{\xi}]$, where $\boldsymbol{\xi} = [\xi_0, \xi_1, \ldots, \xi_{M-1}]^\top$ with M the number of profiles. For two comparable images showing the same edge, the sharpness can now be compared quantitatively using the ratio of their respective ξ^*. Our approach can also support a qualitative, visual comparison. Instead of computing a single sharpness value for the whole edge, we can alternatively restrict the median computation to a smaller window to retain the spatial information, i. e. apply a median filter to $\boldsymbol{\xi}$. Plotting the color-coded ratios of two vectors filtered in that manner on top of the corresponding edge shows in which regions the sharpness has increased the most (Fig. 2). It facilitates an intuitive understanding and "sanity check" of the performed measurements.

2.1 Experiments

For a first validation of our method, we use a Gaussian-blurred Shepp-Logan phantom as well as a slightly sharper version (Fig. 3, left). The latter is additionally corrupted with noise or artifacts to obtain test images for which we expect roughly the same relative increase in edge sharpness compared to the original blurred image. Next, we assess the performance in real-world scenarios by comparing measured edge sharpness values to scores assigned by people working in the field of medical image reconstruction (hereafter referred to as experts). The first data set we use for this purpose is a C-arm CT acquisition of a porcine model [6]. Over 14.5 s, 381 projection images are acquired in a single sweep. Right atrial pacing and systemic injection of contrast agent ensure a sufficient quality of the initial electrocardiography-gated reconstructions. Each phase is deformably registered to the reference phase using a uniform B-Spline motion model [1, 7]. Subsequently, a motion-compensated reconstruction is performed for the reference phase (Fig. 4, left). The second data set stems from an in-vivo volunteer experiment using a 1.5 T clinical MR scanner. The measurement was taken with electrocardiography triggering to avoid cardiac motion artifacts, but in free breathing. Respiratory motion is taken into account with a motion-compensated reconstruction [2] using displacement fields computed with Demons at half resolution and Bilateral Demons [8] (Fig. 5, left). The edge sharpness measurement tool is openly available on http://www5.cs.fau.de/research/software/.

3 Results

The table in Fig. 3 shows the results of our phantom study. The proposed approach achieved the most consistent measurements (smallest standard deviation) compared to manually placed smaller sets of profile lines. Note that the sets in (ii) and (iv) do not touch the simulated artifact; hence, they measure the same values in the corresponding case (d). Nevertheless, they show higher standard deviations due to the noise case (c) alone. In the tables of Figs. 4 and 5, the sharpness scores given to each image by experts are compared to the computed edge sharpness estimates. Expert annotation was performed without any prior knowledge of the employed reconstruction algorithms or the computed estimates. In both experiments, the sharpest (least sharp) image according to our measurements also received the highest (lowest) score. The difference between the uncompensated and the motion compensated images is larger than the difference between the two motion compensated versions consistently in both scores and measurements. For the C-arm CT images, even the relative distances are preserved well. As there still is a slight slope present in the uncompensated reconstructions despite the edge appearing strongly blurred visually, our approach yields comparatively larger values here.

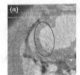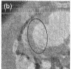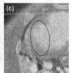
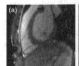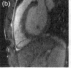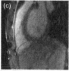

Image	Profiles			
	(i)	(ii)	(iii)	(iv)
(b) vs. (a)	1.477	1.504	1.412	1.345
(c) vs. (a)	1.459	1.936	1.334	1.487
(d) vs. (a)	1.463	1.504	0.133	1.345
Std. dev.	**0.0095**	0.25	0.72	0.082

Fig. 3. The top row shows a blurred phantom image (a) and a sharper version (b) corrupted with noise (c) and a large artifact (d). In the bottom row, profile lines covering the whole edge (i) or parts of it (ii, iii, iv) are plotted on top of the blurred image. The table on the right lists the edge sharpness increase as described in the text for different combinations of images and profile lines used to measure the sharpness.

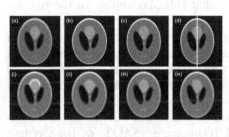

Image	Edge sharpness	Expert score
(a)	0.0402	3.43 ± 0.53
(b)	0.0296	2.14 ± 0.69
(c)	0.0114	0.00 ± 0.00

Fig. 4. Two different motion-compensated C-arm CT images (a,b) of a porcine model are shown together with an uncompensated FDK reconstruction (c) for comparison. B-Spline based deformable motion estimation [7] was performed with a control point spacing of 8 mm (a) and 16 mm (b). The table lists the computed sharpness as well as the average scores (4 = very sharp, 0 = blurred) of 7 experts for the highlighted edge.

Image	Edge sharpness	Expert score
(a)	0.0604	2.00 ± 0.58
(b)	0.0724	3.57 ± 0.53
(c)	0.0367	0.29 ± 0.49

Fig. 5. Two different motion-compensated MR images (a,b) of a volunteer are shown together with an uncompensated reconstruction (c) for comparison. Demons at half resolution (a) and Bilateral Demons [8] (b) motion estimation was performed. The table lists the computed sharpness as well as the average scores (4 = very sharp, 0 = blurred) of 7 experts for the highlighted edge.

4 Discussion

In summary, the edge sharpness values computed by our method are in agreement with the visual impression and exhibit increased robustness compared to the manual approach. Artifacts and noise still have an influence on the measurements as they locally affect the observed sharpness, but it is reduced considerably. A limitation of our method lies in reconstruction methods that enforce sharp edges. In this case, the sharpness of an edge is no longer a clear indication that the motion of this edge was indeed estimated correctly, eliminating the validity of our main criterion. However, note that this also applies to the manual placement of profile lines we compare our method with. Further improvements of our approach in the future could include an integrated intensity normalization scheme, the use of higher-order splines instead of line segments for representing the edge, a pre-segmentation step to automatically generate a set of edges to select from, as well as a variety of different per-profile estimators of sharpness.

Acknowledgement. The authors gratefully acknowledge funding of the Erlangen Graduate School in Advanced Optical Technologies (SAOT) by the German Research Foundation (DFG) in the framework of the German excellence initiative, and would like to thank S. De Buck, J.-Y. Wielandts and H. Heidbüchel from the University of Leuven for providing the C-arm image data. The concepts and information presented in this paper are based on research and are not commercially available.

References

1. Müller K, Maier A, Schwemmer C, et al. Image artefact propagation in motion estimation and reconstruction in interventional cardiac c-arm CT. Phys Med Biol. 2014;59(12):3121–38.
2. Forman C, Grimm R, Hutter J, et al. Free-breathing whole-heart coronary MRA: motion compensation integrated into 3D cartesian compressed sensing reconstruction. Proc MICCAI. 2013; p. 575–82.
3. Reichenbach SE, Park SK, Narayanswamy R. Characterizing digital image acquisition devices. Opt Eng. 1991;30(2):170–7.
4. Chung YC, Wang JM, Bailey RR, et al. A non-parametric blur measure based on edge analysis for image processing applications. IEEE Int Syst Cybern. 2004;1:356–60.
5. Schwemmer C, Forman C, Wetzl J, et al. CoroEval: a multi-platform, multi-modality tool for the evaluation of 3D coronary vessel reconstructions. Phys Med Biol. 2014;59(17):5163.
6. De Buck S, Dauwe D, Wielandts JY, et al. A new approach for prospectively gated cardiac rotational angiography. Proc SPIE. 2013;8668.
7. Klein S, Staring M, Murphy K, et al. Elastix: a toolbox for intensity based medical image registration. IEEE Trans Med Image. 2010;29(1):196–205.
8. Papież BW, Heinrich MP, Risser L, et al. Complex lung motion estimation via adaptive bilateral filtering of the deformation field. Lect Notes Computer Sci. 2013;8151:25–32.

Gestenbasierte Interaktionsmethoden für die virtuelle Mikroskopie
Anforderungen und Implementierung in der Pathologie am Beispiel des Leap Motion Sensors

Arend Müller[1,2], Thorsten Knape[2], Peter Hufnagl[2]

[1]Hochschule für Technik und Wirtschaft, Berlin
[2]Institut für Pathologie, Charité–Universitätsmedizin Berlin
arend.mueller@charite.de

Kurzfassung. Im Fokus dieses Beitrages liegt die Ermittlung von Anforderungen, die prototypische Implementierung sowie die Verifizierung einer neuartigen Benutzerschnittstelle für die virtuelle Mikroskopie. Zentrale Fragestellungen sind hierbei: Welche Anforderungen werden an die Gestaltung des Arbeitsplatzes eines Pathologen im Nutzungskontext der virtuellen Mikroskopie und insbesondere an die Benutzerschnittstelle des virtuellen Mikroskops gestellt? Inwieweit kann eine berührungslose Steuerung diese Vorgaben erfüllen? Zur Beantwortung der Fragen werden Alternativen zur klassischen Bedienung mittels Maus und Tastatur aufgezeigt. Als Methode kommt die nutzerorientierte Gestaltung zum Einsatz, wobei semi-strukturierte Interviews, Personas und Szenarien als Basis für die Ermittlung der Nutzungsanforderungen dienen. Das Ergebnis dieser Arbeit ist eine gestenbasierte Steuerung des virtuellen Mikroskops mittels des Leap Motion Sensors unter Verwendung hierfür entwickelter Gestensets.

1 Einleitung

Ziel dieser Arbeit sind Entwurf und Implementierung einer berührungslosen, gestenbasierten Interaktion im Kontext der virtuellen Mikroskopie. Als virtuelles Mikroskop wird eine Software bezeichnet, die speziell für die Betrachtung der hochauflösenden, digitalen Schnittbilder (Whole Slide Images – WSIs) entwickelt ist. Die bisherigen Interaktionsmöglichkeiten per Maus und Tastatur sind nicht zufriedenstellend [1, 2]. Ursache hierfür sind unter anderem Ermüdungserscheinungen des Anwenders, resultierend aus langen Navigationswegen in den hochauflösenden, virtuellen Schnitten.

Es wird untersucht, ob die Leap Motion (www.leapmotion.com) als optischer, gestenerkennender Sensor ein geeignetes Eingabegerät für die virtuelle Mikroskopie in der Routinediagnostik der Pathologie darstellt. Weiterführend wird analysiert, ob eine gestenbasierte Interaktion die Nutzungsfreundlichkeit im Vergleich zur Bedienung mit der Maus verbessert. Anhand von drei Szenarien aus der Routinediagnostik in der Pathologie sowie drei Personas werden Anwendergruppen identifiziert und deren Bedürfnisse analysiert. Die Anforderungen an die technische Implementierung werden aus den Szenarien und Personas abgeleitet. Eine vergleichbare Anwendung der Mensch Computer Interaktion (Human Computer Interaction, HCI) stellt die berührungslose Gesteninteraktion, speziell in einer sterilen Umgebung wie einem Operationsaal, dar. Hierzu gibt es bereits wissenschaftliche Untersuchungen zu unterschiedlichen Sensoren wie Time-of-Flight Kameras, der Microsoft Kinect oder der Nintendo Wii Mote [3, 4, 5]. Die Leap Motion ist ein optischer Infrarot Sensor, welcher ausschließlich für die Erkennung von Händen und Fingern, sowie fingerähnlichen Werkzeugen (wie bspw. Stiften) konzipiert ist. Der Sensor verfügt über eine geringere Reichweite, jedoch über eine höhere Genauigkeit ($< 1,0\,\text{mm}$) als die oben genannten Geräte [6].

2   Material und Methoden

Die Entwicklung der gestenbasierten Interaktionsmethoden für die prototypische Software erfolgt iterativ und orientiert sich an dem Prozess der nutzerorientierten Gestaltung (User Centered Design – UCD), vgl. ISO 9241-210 [7]. Zu Beginn der Arbeit werden Interviews mit den Nutzern geführt, Szenarien und Personas erstellt [8]. Aus diesen Untersuchungen leiten sich folgende Nutzungsanforderungen an die zu entwickelnde Gestensteuerung ab: einfache Nutzung, ermüdungsarme, schnelle, präzise Navigation, Zuverlässigkeit, Robustheit und schnelle Erlernbarkeit. Die Platzierungsmöglichkeiten des Leap Motion Sensors wurden mehrfach untersucht, um eine, den Anforderungen entsprechende, Interaktion zu ermöglichen. Vom Hersteller primär intendiert ist eine Platzierung des Sensors auf dem Tisch liegend (Abb. 1).

Die Implementierung erfolgt prototypisch in drei Iterationen in der Programmiersprache C# als Plugin für das virtuelle Mikroskop (Slide Explorer 4.0, VMscope GmbH, www.vmscope.de). In allen Iterationen werden Gesten für die Funk-

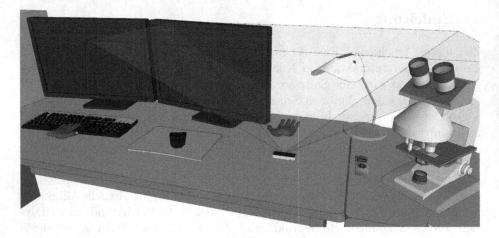

Abb. 1. Platzierung des Leap Motion Sensors liegend auf dem Tisch.

tionen der Translation, des Vergrößerns und Verkleinerns des Bildauschnitts sowie dem Wechsel zwischen verschiedenen virtuellen Schnitten entworfen. Zur Abgrenzung zu den jeweils anderen Funktionalitäten werden zusätzlich Gesten für die Aktivierung und Deaktivierung entworfen. Der Entwurf der Gesten der ersten Iteration erfolgt für eine Platzierung des Sensors auf dem Tisch. In der zweiten Iteration wird die Nutzung des Sensors bei einer Platzierung hängend über dem Tisch evaluiert. Für die dritte Iteration werden die Gesten für das Zoomen speziell für die hängende Platzierung entworfen.

In den folgenden Abbildungen werden in der dritten Iteration entworfene Gesten gezeigt. Die Gestenabfolge für die initiale Aktivierung aller anderen Funktionen besteht aus dem Platzieren der Hand im Sichtfeld des Sensors, dem Bilden einer Faust für 0,5 s (Abb. 2a) und dem anschließenden Ausstrecken von einem bzw. mehreren Fingern (Abb. 2b).

Dies ist nötig, um beabsichtigte Eingaben von zufällig ausgeführten Bewegungen abzugrenzen. Welche Finger gestreckt werden bestimmt, welche Funktion im Anschluss aktiv ist. Diese zeitbasierte Aktivierung muss nur wiederholt werden, wenn die Hand des Nutzers den Sichtbereich des Sensors verlässt.

Die Auswertung der Szenarien und der Interviews mit den Nutzern zeigt, dass der Nutzungsbedarf für die Translation am höchsten von allen berücksichtigten Funktionalitäten ist. Es folgt der Bedarf für das Vergrößern und Verkleinern, für den Schnittwechsel ist der am Bedarf geringsten. Entsprechend dieses ermittelten Bedarfs sowie der oben aufgeführten Anforderungen der Nutzer werden die Gesten entworfen. Für die Translation, als die am häufigsten genutzte Funktion, wird das Ausstrecken des Zeigefingers als Aktivierung genutzt. Diese Bewegung ist leicht mit der im alltäglichen Gebrauch üblichen Zeigegeste assoziierbar und lässt sich intuitiv ausführen. Die Translation selbst erfolgt durch das Bewegen der Hand horizontal auf dem Tisch (Abb. 3a), die Deaktivierung der Translation erfolgt durch Bewegen des Zeigefingers in Richtung Handfläche (Abb. 3b).

Die Zoom Funktionalität wird durch das Ausstrecken des Daumens und des Zeigefingers aktiviert. Eine Bewegung der Hand nach oben, während die Finger gestreckt sind, vergrößert das Bild (Abb. 4a). Eine Bewegung der Hand nach unten verkleinert das Bild entsprechend. Um für das Verkleinern die Hand nicht erst anheben zu müssen, dann die Finger zu strecken und die Hand anschließend

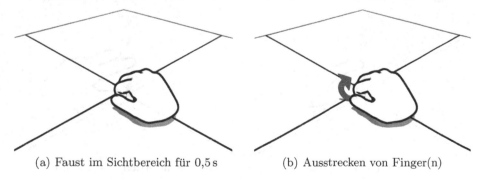

(a) Faust im Sichtbereich für 0,5 s   (b) Ausstrecken von Finger(n)

Abb. 2. Gesten für die Aktivierung der Steuerung.

Abb. 3. Gesten für die Translation.

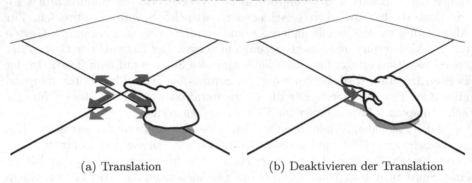

(a) Translation   (b) Deaktivieren der Translation

abzusenken, besteht die Möglichkeit, die Richtung des Zooms umzukehren, indem Daumen, Zeige- und Mittelfinger ausgestreckt werden (Abb. 4b). Wird die Hand mit diesen drei gestreckten Fingern nach oben bewegt, wird das Bild verkleinert. Die Deaktivierung des Zooms geschieht analog zur Translation durch das Bewegen der Finger in Richtung Handfläche.

Der Schnittwechsel wird durch ein Drehen der Handfläche nach innen aktiviert (Abb. 5a) und durch das Bewegen der Hand nach links bzw. rechts ausgeführt (Abb. 5b). Die Deaktivierung des Schnittwechsels erfolgt durch das Drehen der Handfläche in die Ausgangsposition, Richtung Tischplatte.

Das Deaktivieren des Trackings erfolgt durch das Bilden einer Faust. Anschließend kann der Sichtbereich des Sensors verlassen werden, ohne dass sich der dargestellte Bildausschnitt ändert. Um die Steuerung erneut zu aktivieren, wird die oben beschriebene Aktivierungsgeste für alle Funktionen ausgeführt. Mit den beschriebenen Gesten wird eine Steuerung des virtuellen Mikroskops ermöglicht, welche einen flüssigen Wechsel zwischen den einzelnen Funktionen erlaubt.

3   Ergebnisse

Ergebnis der Arbeit ist eine iterativ entwickelte, prototypische Implementierung einer gestenbasierten Steuerung eines virtuellen Mikroskops. Die Nutzungseva-

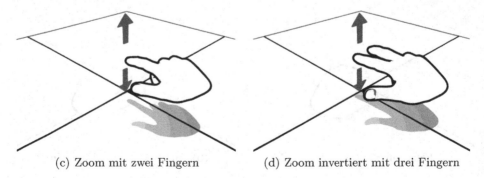

(c) Zoom mit zwei Fingern   (d) Zoom invertiert mit drei Fingern

Abb. 4. Gesten für den Zoom.

Abb. 5. Gesten für den Schnittwechsel.

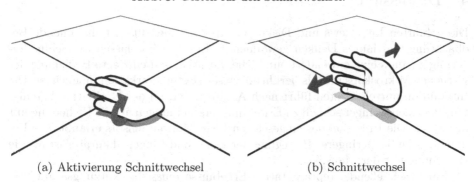

(a) Aktivierung Schnittwechsel   (b) Schnittwechsel

luation der einzelnen Iterationen erfolgt mit drei Anwendern durch Interviews, lautes Denken und teilnehmende Beobachtung. Die Evaluierung des Sensors unter Beachtung bestimmter Umgebungsbedingungen zeigt, dass eine andere Platzierung als die liegende Platzierung auf dem Tisch möglich ist. Für eine hängende Platzierung oberhalb des Schreibtisches in etwa 300 mm Höhe muss die Tischplatte mit einem matten Infrarotlicht absorbierenden Material von etwa $600 \times 600 \, \text{mm}^2$ versehen werden, beispielsweise schwarzem Plakatkarton. Diese Platzierung ermöglicht eine ermüdungsarme Bedienung des virtuellen Mikroskops mit dem Sensor, da die Hand auf dem Tisch abgelegt werden kann (Abb. 6).

Durch die entworfenen Gesten lässt sich die Navigation in einem virtuellen Schnitt nutzerfreundlicher als mit der Maus gestalten, da das Gedrückthalten der Maustaste und das Drehen des Mausrades entfallen.

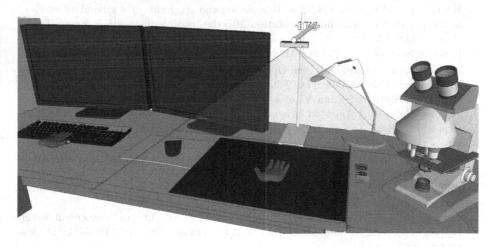

Abb. 6. Platzierung des Leap Motion Sensors hängend über dem Tisch.

4   Diskussion

Die geführten Interviews und Diskussionen sowie die, durch teilnehmende Beobachtung und lautes Denken gewonnenen, Erkenntnisse lassen die Schlussfolgerung zu, dass eine anwenderfreundliche, intuitive und effiziente Bedienung des virtuellen Mikroskops mittels berührungsloser Gesteninterkation möglich ist. Die Interaktion mittels Gesten führt nach Angaben der, an der Evaluation beteiligten, Personen weniger schnell zu Ermüdungserscheinungen als die Bedienung mit der Maus. Die Präzision des eingesetzten Leap Motion Sensors erlaubt eine Bedienung, die bei geringerer Bewegung der Hand und Finger akkurater ist als die Bedienung mit der Maus.

Für abschließende, repräsentative Ergebnisse muss die Nutzungsevaluation mit einer größeren Personengruppe durchgeführt werden. Hierfür ist die Entwicklung einer frei konfigurierbaren Gestensteuerung zweckmäßig. Die Möglichkeiten der Annotation und der Vermessung mittels Gesten oder durch trackbare Werkzeuge gilt es zu untersuchen. Die Verwendung des Leap Motion Sensors in sterilen Umgebungen, wie beispielsweise im Operationssaal, stellt ein interessantes Anwendungsgebiet für die Gestensteuerung dar, welches Gegenstand zukünftiger Untersuchungen sein kann.

Literaturverzeichnis

1. Hufnagl P, Schlüns K. Virtuelle Mikroskopie und Routinediagnostik. Pathologe. 2008;29(2):250–4.
2. Wienert S, Beil M, Saeger K, et al. Integration and acceleration of virtual microscopy as the key to successful implementation into the routine diagnostic process. Diagn Pathol. 2009;4(3):1–8.
3. Penne J, Soutschek S, Stürmer M, et al. Touchscreen ohne Touch BerÃ¼hrungslose 3D Gesten-Interaktion fÃ¼r den Operationssaal. i-com Zeitschrift fÃ¼r interaktive kooperative Medien. 2009;8(1):19–23.
4. Wachs JP, Stern HI, Edan Y, et al. A gesture-based tool for sterile browsing of radiology images. J Am Med Inform Assoc. 2008;15(3):321–3.
5. Graetzel C, Fong T, Grange S, et al. A non-contact mouse for surgeon-computer interaction. Technol Health Care. 2004;12(3):245–57.
6. Weichert F, Bachmann D, Rudak B, et al. Analysis of the accuracy and robustness of the leap motion controller. Sensors. 2013;13(5):6380–93.
7. ISO. 9241-210:2010 Ergonomics of Human-System Interaction. Part 210: Human-Centred Design for Interactive Systems. ISO; 2010.
8. Zimmermann D, Grötzbach L, Freymann M. Ansatz zur nutzerzentrierten Requirement-Analyse und Evaluation: Ein Framework-Entwurf. Usability Professionals. 2007.

Spherical Ridgelets for Multi-Diffusion Tensor Refinement
Concept and Evaluation

Simon Koppers[1], Thomas Schultz[2], Dorit Merhof[1]

[1]Institute of Imaging and Computer Vision, RWTH Aachen University, Germany
[2]Department of Computer Science, University of Bonn, Germany
`simon.koppers@lfb.rwth-aachen.de`

Abstract. High angular resolution diffusion imaging (HARDI) improved many neurosurgical areas due to its ability to represent complex intra-voxel structures, but is limited for clinical use mainly due to long acquisition times, but also due to noise.
To transcend these limits, our work addresses these problems by combining a state-of-the-art multi diffusion tensor model enhanced with spherical ridgelets. Spherical ridgelets are able to reconstruct a signal based on a limited number of measured directions by utilizing compressed sensing. This concept shows that combining spherical ridgelets with a multi diffusion tensor model can improve the accuracy in case of low signal-to-noise ratios and makes it possible to use less than 15 directional measurements per voxel.

1 Introduction

High angular resolution diffusion imaging (HARDI) is able to characterize complex intra-voxel structures such as crossing fibers. Various multi diffusion models (MDM) for HARDI reconstruction have been proposed [1, 2, 3]. Additionally, Schultz et al. [2] presented a novel approach that fits the commonly used Ball-and-Stick (BS) MDM via spherical deconvolution [2] to the signal. This allows to combine the highly accurate BS model with the computationally efficient spherical deconvolution.

As a downside, all current MDM methods require the measurement of a multitude of diffusion directions per voxel for maximum accuracy. This results in an increased scan duration and thereby reduces the applicability of these approaches in clinical scenarios.

To address this issue, we evaluate a combination of methods that fit the BS model to previously refined directions using spherical ridgelets (SR) [4]. SR are able to recover the original signal with fewer measured directions and a lower SNR by applying methods of compressed sensing [5].

2   Material and methods

2.1   Data

The presented methods have been developed and tested on synthetic diffusion weighted MRI data.

Data generation was performed using a multi diffusion tensor model which combines two diffusion tensors, with non-zero real diffusion estimated eigenvalues. Random eigenvectors and volume fractions were generated uniformly. This generation progress was repeated with random fiber sets for 10 to 50 equidistantly sampled directions [6] and a b-value of $b = 3000 \frac{s}{mm^2}$. Additional Rician noise with $SNR_0 = [3, 30]$ was added in a subsequent step. For each combination of parameters we simulated 500 random two-fiber voxels with an fix inter-fiber angle of 90 degrees.

2.2   Multi-tensor fitting with spherical ridgelets

Our new approach combines two state-of-the-art algorithms and can be divided into five different processing steps (Fig. 1). In the first part (Block A), the SR, which incorporate a-priori knowledge of occurring signal shapes, are used to reconstruct the signal. This allows to reduce noise and to reconstruct a good signal quality even in case of a limited number of directional measurements [4]. In a next step, the newly interpolated signal is resampled with 312 equidistant directions.

In the following four steps (Block B) we apply the multi-diffusion-tensor approach to the new re-sampled signal. In this way, it is possible to investigate the actual refinement of SR. Both processing blocks will be explained in the following sections.

Spherical ridgelets A proven method to comprehensively represent a measured signal is to reconstruct it via SR [4]. As a prerequirement, the signal is assumed to be representable by a linear combination of basis functions

$$S(\boldsymbol{u}) = \sum_{j \in J} c_j \cdot \psi_j(\boldsymbol{u}) \tag{1}$$

where c_j define the SR coefficients, J contains all indices of possible basis functions ψ_j, and $\boldsymbol{u}$ defines the direction vector. Considering the fact that the set of all basis functions has to be finite, it is fixed to M basis functions ψ_j. The set of M basis functions $\{\psi_j\}_{i=0}^{M}$ is chosen in such a way that all possible shape variations of orientation distribution functions (ODF) can be represented as far as possible [3]. For N measured directions, M basis functions ψ_j are considered and stored in a $N \times M$ matrix $\boldsymbol{A}$. To calculate the SR coefficients $\boldsymbol{c}$

$$\boldsymbol{A} \cdot \boldsymbol{c} = \boldsymbol{y} + \boldsymbol{e} \tag{2}$$

is solved, where $y := [S(u_1), S(u_2), ..., S(u_N)]$ is a vector of all signal values and e is an error vector that contains all measurement and model errors [4]. The applicability of compressed sensing follows from the assumption that the signal is sparsely representable by a set $\{\psi_j\}_{j=0}^M$ of basis functions ψ_j which are incoherent to the diffusion sampling bases [5]. Assuming $\eta \leq ||e||_2$, c satisfies $||Ac - y||_2 \leq \eta$. The compressed SR coefficients c^* are found as

$$c^* = \arg\min ||c||_1 \text{ subject to } ||Ac - y||_2 \leq \eta \tag{3}$$

which represents a convex optimization problem that is solved using Orthogonal Marching Pursuit [3].

Multi-diffusion tensor fitting For voxels containing multiple fibers, the associated signal is split into k single diffusion tensors D_i with eigenvalues $\lambda_1 \geq \lambda_2 \geq \lambda_3 \geq 0$. Now, every single signal $S(g)$ can be described as

$$S(g) = S_0 \cdot \sum_{i=1}^{k} f_i e^{b \cdot g^T D_i g} \tag{4}$$

where S_0 is the B_0 weighted signal, f_i the compartment specific fraction, b the diffusion weighting and g the gradient direction.

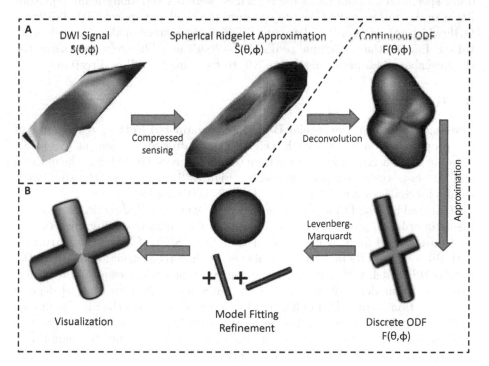

Fig. 1. Combination of Spherical Ridgelets and the Multi-Diffusion-Model.

Schultz et al. [2] proposed an algorithm that is based on this multi diffusion decomposition and can be divided into three steps (Fig. 1, Block B):

In the first step, the ODF $F(\theta', \Phi')$ is reconstructed using spherical deconvolution based on

$$\widehat{S}(\theta, \Phi) = \int_0^{2\pi} \int_0^{\pi} F(\theta', \Phi') R(\gamma') \sin(\theta') \, d\theta' \, d\Phi' \tag{5}$$

where $R(\gamma)$ defines an axially symmetric single-fiber response function, γ the angle between (θ, Φ) and (θ', Φ') and $\widehat{S}(\theta, \Phi)$ the diffusion signal [7, 8].

In a second step, the ODF is discretized using a nonlinear optimization based on 4th-order spherical harmonics, thereby increasing peak sharpness and reducing signal noise [9].

The Ball-and-Stick model is applied in the final step, which requires at least one diffusion tensor to be isotropic ($\lambda_1 = \lambda_2 = \lambda_3$), while the remaining tensors are linear ($\lambda_2 = \lambda_3 = 0$). The assumption that there are n fiber terms implies that there will be at least $k = n + 1$ single diffusion tensors. In our case, n is fixed to 2.

To estimate the actual fiber directions, Schultz et al. substituted $R(\gamma)$ in (5) by adding $S_0 f_{iso} e^{-bd}$ outside the integral [2]. After that a spherical harmonic reconstruction is fit to the residual of the signal from which a predicted isotropic part $S_0 f_{iso} e^{-bd}$ is subtracted [2]; the coefficients are then divided by the nth-order specific rotational harmonic R_n which were derived analytically [2]. Nonlinear optimization is then used to compute the resulting approximated discrete ODF which considers only 15 harmonic coefficients, instead of all measured signal values. Finally, the n maximal peaks of the resulting ODF are refined using the the Levenberg-Marquardt algorithm [10] to to estimate n fiber directions.

3 Results

The angular error of the regular BS model is compared to the angular error of our proposed advanced approach, i.e. BS model after SR refinement (SR+BS). Possible angular error values range from 0 to 90 degrees with 0 being the optimal and 90 being the worst possible result. Figures 2 and 3 show the simulation results for SNRs of 3 and 30, averaged across 500 samples.

It should be noted that the BS model requires at least 15 directional measurements in order to provide a reasonable estimate of intra-voxel fiber directions.

Considering Fig. 2, it can be seen that for a SNR of 3 the reconstruction with SR + BS results in a lower angular error than reconstruction based on the regular BS model, with a minimal angle error of 24.20 degrees at 50 directions, while the BS model performs worse with a minimal angle error of 22.91 degrees at 50 directions. For a SNR of 30, the BS model outperforms the SR+BS model. In this case, the SR+BS model achieves a minimal angle error of 2.97 degrees at 50 directions, while the regular BS model is able to reconstruct the signal with an angle error of 1.90 degrees at 50 directions (Fig. 2).

The results for the second simulated fiber direction show the same trends as for the first fiber direction, but with a higher absolute angle error.

4   Discussion

The comparison shows that the BS model can be improved with SR refinement for low SNR (fig. 2). Also, in case of less than 15 directional measurements, SR refinement makes it possible to obtain reasonable results (Fig. [2,3]). On the other hand, the BS model outperforms the reconstruction with SR+BS for high SNR.

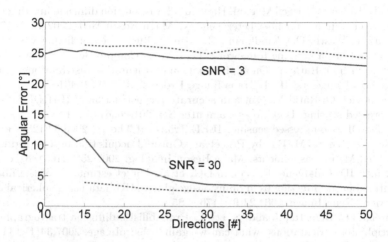

Fig. 2. Angular error for reconstructing the *first* fiber with a SNR = [3,30] and $b = 3000 \frac{s}{mm^2}$, averaged across 500 samples. The dashed line represents the BS model, the solid line shows the SR+BS model.

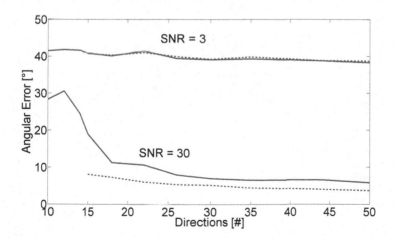

Fig. 3. Angular error for reconstructing the *second* fiber with a SNR = [3,30] and $b = 3000 \frac{s}{mm^2}$, averaged across 500 samples. The dashed line represents the BS model, the solid line shows the SR+BS model.

Overall, we can state that the SR reconstruction is more robust to noise, but offers decreased accuracy for high SNR values. Therefore, the SR+BS model is only suitable if there are less than 15 directional measurements available or if the measurements exhibit very low SNR.

References

1. Tuch D, Reese T, Wiegell M, et al. High angular resolution diffusion imaging reveals intravoxel whitematter fiber heterogeneity. Magn Reson Med. 2002;48(4):577–82.
2. Schultz T, Westin CF, Kindlmann G. Multi-diffusion-tensor fitting via spherical deconvolution: a unifying framework. Lect Notes Comput Sci. 2010;6361:674–81.
3. Michailovich O, Rathi Y. On approximation of orientation distributions by means of spherical ridgelets. IEEE Trans Image Process. 2010;19(2):461–77.
4. Michailovich O, Rathi Y. Fast and accurate reconstruction of HARDI data using compressed sensing. Lect Notes Computer Sci. 2010;6361:607–14.
5. Donoho DL. Compressed sensing. IEEE Trans Inf Theory. 2006;52:1289–306.
6. Cook PA, Symms M, Boulby PA, et al. Optimal acquisition orders of diffusion-weighted MRI measurements. Magn Reson Imaging. 2007;25(5):1051–8.
7. Tournier JD, Calamante F, Gadian DG, et al. Direct estimation of the fiber orientation density function from diffusion-weighted MRI data using spherical deconvolution. NeuroImage. 2004;23(3):1176 – 85.
8. Behrens TE, Berg HJ, Jbabdi S, et al. Probabilistic diffusion tractography with multiple fibre orientations: what can we gain? NeuroImage. 2007;34(1):144–55.
9. Schultz T, Seidel HP. Estimating crossing fibers: a tensor decomposition approach. IEEE Trans Vis Comput Graph. 2008;14(6):1635–42.
10. Deserno-Marquardt D. An algorithm for least-squares estimation of nonlinear parameters. J Soc Indust Appl Math. 1963;11(2):431–41.

Real-Time Resampling of Medical Images Based on Deformed Tetrahedral Structures for Needle Insertion VR-Simulation

Martin Meike[1], Dirk Fortmeier[1,2], Andre Mastmeyer[1], Heinz Handels[1]

[1]Institute of Medical Informatics, University of Lübeck
[2]Graduate School for Computing in Medicine and Life Sciences, University of Lübeck
meike@miw.uni-luebeck.de

Abstract. To provide real-time visualization of deformed volumetric image data for virtual surgery simulation, a resampling algorithm based on deformed tetrahedral structures has been developed. Deformations of the tetrahedral mesh are computed by a soft-tissue simulation. The major advantage of this approach is the possibility to use the resampled image data in different rendering methods such as ray casting, simulated ultrasound or simulated X-ray imaging. To achieve real-time capability, the algorithm was parallelized on the GPU using Nvidia Cuda. Performance measurements have been done on different mesh resolutions. For a subset of 1688 tetrahedrons, short resamplings times of around 2.3 ms are measured on an Nvidia GTX 680, endorsing the algorithm for real-time application.

1 Introduction

Virtual surgery simulation with soft-tissue deformation models based on the finite element method (FEM) is a current field of research. In the special case of needle insertion simulation, fundamental methods were presented by [1] and similar approaches have been applied for example in simulation of brachytherapy [2] where real-time capable models are used for needle insertion simulation.

Apart from a realistic computation of deformations, the visualization of the results is an important part of a VR-surgery simulation system. To be able to provide a realistic and patient-specific simulation, virtual patient models have to be based on medical image data such as CT or MRI. Using direct volume rendering, this data can be displayed to the user without the need of creating surface meshes.

Volume rendering of image data deformed by tetrahedral meshes was done for instance by [3]. Their approach is based on ray casting and limited to standard direct volume rendering. Similar to our algorithm, the idea is to determine the enclosing tetrahedron and the barycentric coordinates for every voxel.

In [4], deformed tetrahedral meshes are used to provide an ultrasound B-mode image simulation of deformed virtual soft-tissue. This resampling method generates a deformed image by computing the inverse transformation of the tetrahedral mesh. With deformed voxel coordinates it is easy to interpolate on a given regular structure in the given undeformed image. Therefore, for every voxel the enclosing tetrahedron has to be computed and then barycentric coordinates give the relative position in a tetrahedron in the deformed and undeformed mesh. To accelerate the determination of the enclosing tetrahedron, an adapted scan-line algorithm is used. The resampling algorithm shows real-time capabilities for medical images of considerable size. In contrast to our algorithm, the resulting image is only two dimensional. An early deformation and resampling model limited to hexaedral grids based on a three dimensional texture was presented by [5]. Their deformation model subdivides the object into sub-cubes and then the deformation is computed by translating vertex coordinates. Similar to the approach presented here, in [6] a tetrahedral mesh is used to resample a volumetric image and render it by conventional volume rendering techniques.

Instead of tetrahedron or other unstructured grid based approaches, methods using regular grids can be used for volume rendering of deformed image data: In [7], a method using finite-difference techniques for computation of deformations as occurring in a needle insertion scenario was presented. Liver biopsy simulation with direct volume rendering and simulation of deformations in an ultrasound simulation caused by needle interaction and breathing was performed by [8].

The motivation of the work present in this paper is to enable direct volume rendering of deformed volume data by different rendering methods without using surface representations of the volumetric data. For this, the approach of [4] was adapted and generalized to resample a 3D sub-volume of a volumetric image. By combining the resampled sub-volume and the original image data, any volume rendering technique that processes volumetric data (ray casting, ultrasound and X-ray simulation, etc.) can be used without modifications, which we consider the major contribution of this work. To ensure real-time capability, the methods were parallelized using Nvidia Cuda. We show the suitability of our method by applying it to deformations occurring in a liver puncture scenario.

2   Materials and methods

The aim of the presented method is to resample a given medical CT image deformed by a given tetrahedral mesh. First, it is described how this tetrahedral mesh is created in an off-line preprocessing step and how deformations are computed, then the resampling algorithm itself is presented.

2.1   Soft-tissue simulation

For every time step, a soft-tissue simulation as a function of external influences (needle insertion to a virtual patient) and inner forces (physical tissue properties) is performed to compute a deformed tetrahedral mesh.

Starting with a segmented volumetric CT image, we used Cleaver [9] to generate the original undeformed mesh for the complete dataset. Since Cleaver generates a mesh with respect to different tissues and homogeneities, tissue boundaries are meshed finely and homogeneous volumes coarser (Fig. 1).

The entire CT image was meshed, giving a large amount of tetrahedral elements. For a needle insertion, it is a valid assumption that deformations are present only close to the shaft of the needle, whereby only a section around the needle tip is extracted from the mesh at run-time. The resulting sub-mesh consists of all tetrahedrons which have at least one vertex inside a cubical region around the needle tip. All vertices outside the tetrahedrons are assumed to be fixed (Fig. 1).

2.2   Initial steps

The structure of the given sub-mesh consists of k = number of mesh points, m = number of tetrahedrons, undeformed mesh points $\mathbf{X}_i$ with $i \in 1...k$, deformed mesh points $\mathbf{x}_i$ and $\mathbf{t}_n$ with $n < m$ containing the information of every tetrahedron, where every $\mathbf{t}_n$ is a tuple of 4 indexes of mesh points. The undeformed voxel image I_0 is also needed to interpolate the image values.

A copy of the undeformed image I_0 is the starting point for the deformed image. The algorithm first cuts out a three dimensional image section P around the mesh, which is now our volume of interest. This image section lies centered around the mesh. The rest of the image is expected to be undeformed.

We now compute an image value for every voxel in P with respect to the deformed mesh $M = (\mathbf{x}, \mathbf{t})$. For all voxels inside the mesh, we search for the inverse transformation $f(*)^{-1}$ of the result of the FE-simulation with the deformed mesh M and undeformed mesh $M_0 = (\mathbf{X}, \mathbf{t})$.

We need to match every voxel $V_{i,j,k}$ in P with their surrounding tetrahedron $e_q, q \in 1, ..., m$ where q is the index of the surrounding tetrahedron. Every voxel $V_{i,j,k}$ lying inside an element of the mesh gets a unique tag, which is the index of the element. After that, it is easy to compute barycentric coordinates of every voxel in its surrounding tetrahedron by its vertices and the voxel coordinates. Because the barycentric coordinates in the deformed and undeformed tetrahedron are the same, we use the barycentric position in the undeformed

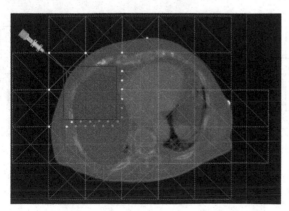

Fig. 1. Schematic overview of the meshing. Based on the full mesh (green), a subset of tetrahedrons is selected around the needle tip. Vertices outside of this region are assumed to be fixed (yellow). The segmented liver is highlighted in red.

tetrahedron converted to image coordinates to interpolate the image value we are searching for in the undeformed image.

2.3 Rasterization and resampling

Marking voxels with their surrounding tetrahedrons is the most complex part of the algorithm. An efficient method was developed, which is split into two steps: In the first step we mark all triangular faces of tetrahedrons by their index, so that all voxels lying between two tetrahedrons and on outer surfaces are marked. After that, we have a rough voxel structure of the tetrahedral mesh with empty tetrahedrons.

To avoid marking a shared triangle of two adjacent tetrahedrons twice, only the plane with a normal showing in positive y-direction is marked. In addition to that, we want to mark all these dividing surfaces with the index of the underlying tetrahedron in y-direction. Vertical surfaces are disregarded. To mark the relevant triangles of all tetrahedrons, every relevant triangle is projected to the x-z plane.

We now iterate over the entire x-z plane and check for every pixel $A(x, z)$ if it lies inside the two dimensional triangle of the three dimensional projected triangle. If a pixel inside is determined, we now compute the y-coordinate of the voxel lying on the 3D-plane. This problem can be reduced to a simple linear equation where only y is unknown.

Tests showed that the result of this method is not unique in case of parallelization on the GPU. If a voxel lies on a vertex or intersection line of more than one tetrahedron, it depends on the program sequence which tetrahedron index finally would be written into the index image matrix. Thus, these conflicting voxels have to handled separately.

Therefore, we use mutual exclusion using Cuda atomics to prevent simultaneous access and test the tetrahedron's location for its plausibility. We now have a nearly complete marked rough structure of the tetrahedral mesh. All the before-mentioned steps are implemented in a single Cuda kernel. It will be referenced in the evaluation as *cuFlag*.

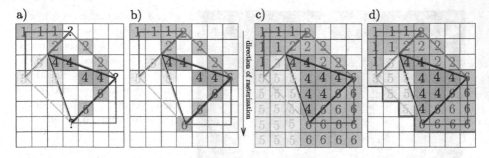

Fig. 2. Rasterization process shown in 2D: a) marking all faces with positive normal, b) handle conflict voxels, c) rasterization through the image top down, d) cut off overhanging marks.

The following kernel (*cuGetUpper*) evaluates and stores the y-coordinate of the lowest mark for each element of the x-z plane for later elimination of "over-hanging" marks.

In a next kernel, the whole cut out image P is rasterized (*cuRaster*) to get a completely marked image. This rasterization is similar to scan-line rasterization of triangles used for surface rendering and proceeds top down in y-direction. This step also includes the processing of conflicting voxels, shown for one slice (x-y plane) in Fig. 2 in 2D.

With given tetrahedron indices, now the barycentric coordinates and thus image coordinates in the undeformed image are computed by the final kernel (*cuInterp*). The overhanging marks (Fig. 2c) are discarded, indicated by the barycentric coordinates and the upper boundary estimated earlier. Finally, image values for P can be computed by interpolation.

2.4 Experiments

A human CT dataset with the resolution of $256 \times 256 \times 236$ voxels and a voxel spacing between and 1.5 and 2 mm was processed with Cleaver in two different downsampled versions, resulting in meshes with (#1) 43,962 tetrahedrons and 7,808 nodes and (#2) 1,522,990 tetrahedrons and 270,438 nodes. Run-time performance of the algorithm is of major interest for real-time capable algorithms. To measure it, the processing times of the four Cuda kernels have been measured for the different resolutions of the tetrahedral mesh. This has been performed for a scenario where the needle is inserted into the virtual liver using a Nvidia GTX 680 with 4CB memory and each measurement was performed $n = 20$ times.

3 Results

Extracting the sub-meshes during run-time resulted in meshes with 1688 and 7091 tetrahedrons. The results of time measurements are shown in Tab. 1. It can be seen that the flagging-kernel is the most time consuming part, especially for large number of tetrahedrons. Fig. 3 shows an exemplary visual result for ray casting.

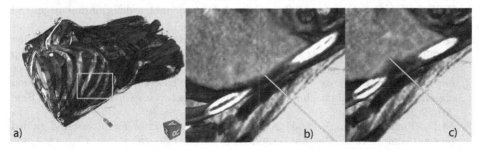

Fig. 3. Exemplary result for ray casting with a clipping plane coplanar to the needle in b) and c). In b), the needle tip is located on the liver capsule, whereas in c) the needle has indented the capsule.

Table 1. Single and total runtime of kernels in ms.

| | Mesh #1 (1688 tetrahedrons) | | | | Mesh #2 (7091 tetrahedrons) | | | |
	min	mean	max	sd	min	mean	max	sd
cuFlag	1.12	1.17	1.34	0.07	4.23	4.88	6.97	0.80
cuGetUpper	0.24	0.27	0.52	0.07	0.25	1.25	4.45	1.32
cuRaster	0.43	0.45	0.64	0.05	0.60	0.83	1.56	0.26
cuInterp	0.38	0.41	0.56	0.05	0.46	0.66	1.12	0.26
Total	2.17	2.31	3.06	0.23	5.54	7.62	14.10	2.63

4 Discussion

We presented a resampling algorithm for medical image data and applied it in a
VR-needle insertion simulation. Based on a subset of a tetrahedral mesh, soft-
tissue deformations are computed to provide a deformed mesh for the resampling.
The resampling shows good real-time capability and thus makes it a reasonable
choice in case different direct volume rendering methods rely on the same image
data in a simulation framework. In a soft-tissue simulation, tetrahedrons can
invert or become very flat. We noticed that this can cause the resampling algorithm to fail to resample parts where tetrahedrons become inverted. This should
be prevented by the soft-tissue simulation in the future. More future work will
include research on speed-up by considering time and spatial coherency.

References

1. DiMaio SP, Salcudean SE. Interactive simulation of needle insertion models. IEEE
   Trans Biomed Eng. 2005;52(7):1167–79.
2. Goksel O, Sapchuk K, Morris WJ, et al. Prostate brachytherapy training with simulated ultrasound and fluoroscopy images. IEEE Trans Biomed Eng. 2013;60(4):1002–
   12.
3. Georgii J, Westermann R. A generic and scalable pipeline for GPU tetrahedral grid
   rendering. IEEE Trans Vis Comput Graph. 2006;12(5):1345–52.
4. Goksel O, Salcudean SE. B-mode ultrasound image simulation in deformable 3-D
   medium. IEEE Trans Med Imaging. 2009;28(11):1657–69.
5. Rezk-Salama C, Scheuering M, Soza G, et al. Fast volumetric deformation on general
   purpose hardware. Proc HWWS. 2001; p. 17–24.
6. Gascón J, Espadero JM, Perez AG, et al. Fast deformation of volume data using
   tetrahedral mesh rasterization. Proc ACM SIGGRAPH/EUROGRAPHICS Symp
   Comput Anim. 2013; p. 181–5.
7. Fortmeier D, Mastmeyer A, Handels H. Image-based soft tissue deformation
   algorithms for real-time simulation of liver puncture. Curr Med Imag Rev.
   2013;9(2):154–65.
8. Ni D, Chan WY, Qin J, et al. A virtual reality simulator for ultrasound-guided
   biopsy training. IEEE Comput Graph Appl. 2011;31:36–48.
9. CIBC; 2014. Cleaver: a multimaterial tetrahedral meshing library and application. scientific computing and imaging institute (SCI), download from:
   http://www.sci.utah.edu/cibc/software.html.

Enhanced Visualization of the Knee Joint Functional Articulation Based on Helical Axis Method

Ricardo Manuel Millán-Vaquero[1], Sean Dean Lynch[2], Benjamin Fleischer[2], Jan Rzepecki[1], Karl-Ingo Friese[1], Christof Hurschler[2], Franz-Erich Wolter[1]

[1]Institut für Mensch-Maschine-Kommunikation, Leibniz Universität Hannover
[2]Labor für Biomechanik und Biomaterialien, Medizinische Hochschule Hannover
rmillan@welfenlab.de

Abstract. Comprehensive descriptions of the motion in articulating joints open new opportunities in biomedical engineering. The helical axis is a established method that describes flexion-extension at joints, which currently lacks an intuitive visualization. In this paper, we present a comprehensive visualization of knee joint motion based on a direct measurement of the helical axis. The proposed approach incorporates the three-dimensional motion of patient-specific bone segments and the representation of helical axes on the bone, facilitating the observation of the flexion-extension motion at the knee joint.

1 Introduction

Within the medical field, the axis of rotation about the knee joint is commonly discussed in order to improve joint functionality and increase prosthesis longevity. The generally adopted method to define this axis depends on anatomical landmarks and is widely considered as a fixed axis throughout motion [1]. However, this practice has proven to have inter- and intra- individual discrepancies [2].

The description of motion based on helical axes has been verified to be superior within the biomechanical engineering field, removing repeatability errors [3, 4]. In contrast to the fixed axis of rotation, the description of a bone motion in three-dimensional space can be more faithfully captured in terms of a temporal sequence of helical axes $HA[t]$ and angles of flexion $\alpha[t]$ with respect to a reference bone (Fig. 1) [5].

Comprehensive 3D representations are needed to further understand methods describing motions, e.g. [1]. However, the existing applications used to calculate helical axes lack an intuitive visualization to analyse states and conditions. Besier et al [3] represent their helical data with 2D graphical plots, i.e. alongside the conventionally captured gait curve. Bogert et al [4] represent helical axes by lines passing through a 2D illustration of a joint model and use a numbering system to depict the temporal evolution of the axes. Until now studies have been realized under these premises. In particular, such approaches lack an interactive

3D visualization to represent the temporal evolution of the helical axes $HA[t]$ together with patient-specific bone segments, which facilitates the understanding of the motion.

In this paper, we present a visualization that enriches the joint motion representation based on a direct measurement of helical axes. We focus on the representation of the knee joint flexion-extension motion. The implemented approach visualizes the three-dimensional motion of patient specific bone segments and the representation of helical axes on the bone, facilitating the description of the knee flexion-extension motion for kinematical studies and surgery applications.

2   Material and methods

We have applied our proposed approach in the context of the experimental work described in [6]. Extending upon this work, in the following subsection we describe the data collection process employed in order to calculate helical axes data from biomechanical experiments applied to specific specimens. Afterwards, in Sec. 2.2 we describe how that data is merged with information obtained in CT scans of the respective specimen in order to visualize the knee joint flexion and helical axes.

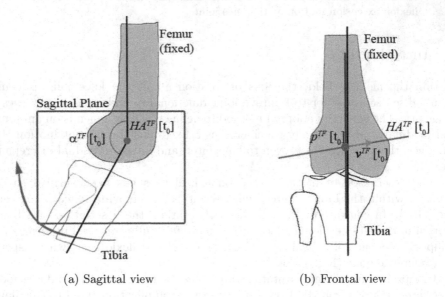

(a) Sagittal view   (b) Frontal view

Fig. 1. Helical axes of tibia with respect to the femur (reference bone) $HA^{TF}[t]$, composed of instantaneous centers of rotation and direction vectors $HA^{TF}[t] = (p^{TF}[t], v^{TF}[t])$, defined in three-dimensional space. The angle $\alpha^{TF}[t]$ is defined between the axes attached to the femur and to the tibia, both of them being contained in the sagittal plane. $HA^{TF}[t]$ and $\alpha^{TF}[t]$ characterize the flexion-extension motion of the tibia with respect to the femur along the time t.

Fig. 2. Helical data collection setup with the tracking coordinate system T_E (a). Landmarks on the bone's surfaces L_V defined in the viewer to obtain the coordinate system T_V (b). 3D Representation of the knee joint flexion and helical axis $HA_V^{TF}[t]$ (c).

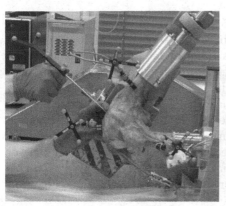 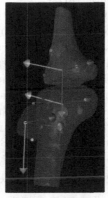 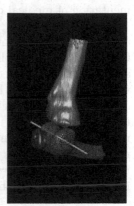

(a) Experimental setup [6]   (b) Defining T_V (c) Knee joint motion

2.1   Helical axes data collection

The data collection was performed with the help of a specifically designed in vitro knee simulator (Fig. 2a). Freshly frozen cadaver knee joints were prepared by removing skin and subcutaneous tissue, whilst keeping the articular capsule intact. The femur was fixed in position and the tibia was fixed to a lever arm that constrains the tibia to flexion-extension but further the tibia has complete freedom of motion. The simulator applied loads to the quadriceps and hamstring tendons, forcing the knee specimen to complete an extension motion.

The tracking of bone motion was performed using a two camera Polaris Optical Tracking System[1], with passive reflective marker tools rigidly fixed to the femur, tibia and patella providing rigid bone motion at an accuracy of 0.35mm at 10Hz. The tracking yields the temporal evolution of the helical axis $HA_E^{TF}[t]$ and angle $\alpha_E^{TF}[t]$ (tibia to femur) as well as $HA_E^{PF}[t]$ and $\alpha_E^{PF}[t]$ (patella to femur) with respect to a fixed tracking coordinate system T_E used in the experiment. We calculate this data by using an adaptation of the algorithm presented in [5] that extracts the centres of rotation $p[t]$ and direction vectors $v[t]$ from the tracked marker positions with accuracy improvements proposed in [7]. This refined adaptation was implemented within the LabVIEW platform[2]. Additionally, a set of standardized characteristic anatomical landmarks L_E found on the bone's surfaces [8] was also acquired (referenced with respect to T_E), which is used in the mapping of coordinate systems of the experiment within the viewer. This acquisition is made manually by touching specific points of the bones with a passive reflective marker pointer device.

---

[1] Polaris Optical Tracking System, Northern Digital Inc., USA
[2] LabVIEW [online] http://www.ni.com/labview/

2.2   Data processing for visualization

Our viewer of the joint motion was implemented in Java using the Java3D API[3]. It constitutes a module for the open platform for 3D visualization and 3D segmentation of medical data YaDiV [9].

Within our viewer, CT images ($512 \times 512 \times 163$) of the considered specimen are accurately segmented, thereby obtaining a 3D segment-visualization of the femur, tibia and patella. Then, a set of significant landmarks L_V is identified according to those used in the experimental setup, on the bone segment surfaces within in the viewer (Fig. 2b). These landmarks can be specified using manual or automated approaches, also on MRI images [10]. Afterwards a matching between L_E and L_V is used to establish the mapping between the experimental reference frame T_E and the reference frame T_V used within in the viewer. Finally, the helical axes data collected in Sec. 2.1 is transformed into the viewer reference system, thereby yielding $HA_V^{TF}[t], \alpha_V^{TF}[t]$ and $HA_V^{PF}[t], \alpha_V^{PF}[t]$. This information can now be directly used to provide a 3D representation (Fig. 2c).

---

[3] Java3D [online] https://java3d.java.net/

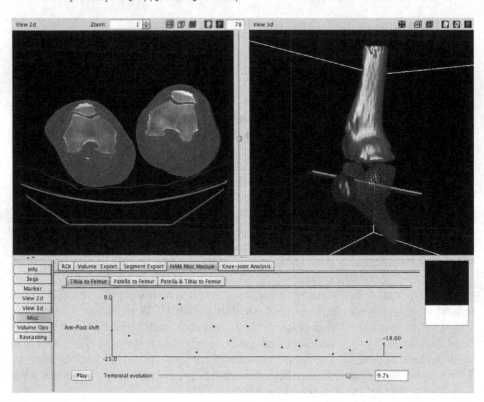

Fig. 3. Visualization of a healthy knee joint completing flexion-extension motion from experimental data, including the helical axes $HA_V^{TF}[t]$ (green) and $HA_V^{PF}[t]$ (blue).

3   Results

The implemented visualization (Fig. 3) has the following functionalities:

- The 3D view (Fig. 3, top right) shows the spatial configuration of helical axes $HA_V^{TF}[t], HA_V^{PF}[t]$, including the centers of rotation $p_V^{TF}[t], p_V^{PF}[t]$ for a fixed time t. By varying t, the view reproduces the patient-specific motion of the knee, according to $\alpha_V^{TF}[t]$ and $\alpha_V^{PF}[t]$.
- The 2D sub-panel views (Fig. 3, bottom) present analytical data concerning the translations of the centers of rotation $p_V^{TF}[t], p_V^{PF}[t]$ (i.e. indicating anterior and posterior shifts). Both 2D and 3D views are synchronized in time, supporting a rapid interpretation of the motion.

4   Discussion

Compared to the previous approaches referenced in Sec. 1, the realistic visualization of bone motion incorporating helical axis data provides a more understandable and precise representation of the knee joint functional articulation. This visualization can facilitate biomechanical engineers to localize the functional flexion axis in terms of anatomical bone motion.

The introduction of the helical axes viewer can be highly beneficial for surgical intervention, as surgeons often try to replicate the joints original and healthy functionality during total knee replacement. Moreover, we expect our approach to be commonly applicable, since optical tracking systems similar to the one utilized here (Sec. 2.1) are already used during total knee replacement surgeries. In our ongoing research, we plan to conduct further data acquisition of knee joint motion related to several surgery techniques and to provide an extended analysis and visualization of helical axis data. This will facilitate the interpretation of diverse states throughout deterioration and the pre-post intervention comparison.

Acknowledgement. This work was supported from the EU Marie Curie ITN Multi-ScaleHuman (FP7-PEOPLE-2011-ITN, Grant agreement no.: 289897). The two first authors R. Millán and S. Lynch have contributed equally to the writing of the paper. The authors would like to thank Dr. med. Calließ for his support in the experimental setup and Dr. Vais for his support in the proof-reading of the manuscript.

References

1. Eckhoff DG, Dwyer TF, Bach JM, et al. Three-dimensional morphology of the distal part of the femur viewed in virtual reality. J Bone Joint Surg Am. 2001;83(2):43–50.
2. Victor J. Rotational alignment of the distal femur: a literature review. Orthop Traumatol Surg Res. 2009;96(5):365–72.

3. Besier TF, Sturnieks DL, Alderson JA, et al. Repeatability of gait data using a functional hip joint centre and a mean helical knee axis. J Biomech. 2003;36(8):1159–68.
4. den Bogert AV, Reinschmidt C, Lundberg A. Helical axes of skeletal knee joint motion during running. J Biomech. 2008;41(8):1632–8.
5. Spoor C, Veldpaus F. Rigid body motion calculated from spatial co-ordinates of markers. J Biomech. 1980;13(4):391–3.
6. Ostermeier S, Hurschler C, Stukenborg-Colsman C. Quadriceps function after TKA: an in vitro study in a knee kinematic simulator. Clin Biomech. 2004;19(3):270–6.
7. Metzger M, Faruk Senan N, O'Reilly O, et al. Minimizing errors associated with calculating the location of the helical axis for spinal motions. J Biomech. 2010;43(14):2822–9.
8. Wu G, Siegler S, Allard P, et al. ISB recommendation on definitions of joint coordinate system of various joints for the reporting of human joint motion-part I: ankle, hip, and spine. J Biomech. 2002;35(4):543–8.
9. Friese KI, Blanke P, Wolter F. -E. YaDiV: an open platform for 3D visualization and 3D segmentation of medical data. Vis Comput. 2011;27(2):129–39.
10. Olender G, Hurschler C, Fleischer B, et al. Validation of an anatomical coordinate system for clinical evaluation of the knee joint in upright and closed MRI. Ann Biomed Eng. 2014;42(5):1133–42.

Panorama Mapping of the Esophagus from Gastroscopic Video

Martin Prinzen[1], Martin Raithel[2], Tobias Bergen[1], Steffen Mühldorfer[3],
Sebastian Nowack[1], Dirk Wilhelm[4], Thomas Wittenberg[1]

[1]Fraunhofer Institute for Integrated Circuits IIS Erlangen
[2]University Medical Center Erlangen
[3]Medical Center Bayreuth
[4]Technical University Munich
martin.prinzen@iis.fraunhofer.de

Abstract. For the examination and clinical assessment of the esophagus, video endoscopy is applied. Video clips and still images are generated along these procedures which are then used for routine documentation. Due to the tight tubular geometry of the esophagus and the constrained field of view of endoscope devices, the provided insight into the esophagus and the relation to contextual information are limited. In this contribution, a shape-from-shading approach for the computation of panorama images of the esophagus wall from gastroscopic video is presented. Furthermore, the content of these panorama images can be mapped back to the original video data which gives the advantages of both panorama-view for improved contextual information and unaltered detail-views for improved examinations.

1 Introduction

Video endoscopy is a common procedure for the visual examination of body cavities such as the esophagus, stomach, colon, airways, or bladder. Along these examination procedures, digital video sequences and still images are acquired, which are used for diagnosis and documentation. Despite its advantages, video endoscopic imaging applied to tubular structures such as the esophagus, bears several challenges including a narrow field of view, limited perception of depth and restricted possibilities for endoscopic movements.

Some approaches have been presented in the field of so-called panoramic endoscopy in order to compensate for the reduced spatial view when dealing with spherical body cavities [1, 2] and tubular cavities, such as the trachea [3], urethra [4] or esophagus [5, 6]. These approaches take endoscopic video sequences and provide some type of panorama or map as output. These maps can be used for enhanced documentation and digital image assessment.

In this contribution we present a shape-from-shading approach to extract such an image map from endoscopic videos of the esophagus. More specifically, our approach extends the work of [5] where endoscopic image data has been acquired from a phantom setup by steadily withdrawing the endoscope in-vitro from an esophagus by using a stepper motor. In contrast to that approach, we use real gastroscopic image sequences which have been obtained from routine clinical examinations of the esophagus. In [5], for each frame a circumference of constant radius and centered around a fixed point with a local intensity minimum are used to detect the circular border of the esophagus, which are then unwound and concatenated consecutively, resulting in a panorama image map. We extend this approach to non-circular shapes of the esophagus and furthermore allow variations of the shape over time, which may be caused by the patients movements due to the swallowing reflex, heartbeat or breathing, as well as by the endoscopes movements. Furthermore, a back-mapping from the resulting panorama image to the unaltered original gastroscopic video is presented, enabling cross referencing of a general-view provided by the panorama image and the unaltered detail-views provided by the frames of the video sequence.

2 Materials and methods

The extraction of a panorama image from a gastroscopic video sequence of the esophagus and the mapping from the resulting panorama image to the original video frames follow a straightforward pipeline shown in Fig. 1.

2.1 Panorama extraction

A gastroscopic video sequence (Fig. 2, left) forms the input to the processing pipeline, supposing the video sequence shows a withdrawal from the esophagus at preferably constant and slow speed, starting from the cardia moving upwards to the larynx. Essentially, a video frame runs through the pre-processing-, unwinding- and concatenation step. This part of the pipeline is repeated for all frames of the input video sequence, thus computing the full panorama image which is then visualized and mapped back to the original input video sequence.

The first step of pre-processing is the optional de-interlacing of the image frame using a linear de-interlacing approach followed by masking the image back ground content, mainly including black borders, leaving only 'valid' gastroscopic image data. For simplicity, the masking area can be manually adjusted once according to the endoscope system prior to the execution of the pipeline. The remaining image is converted from RGB color space to gray level intensities

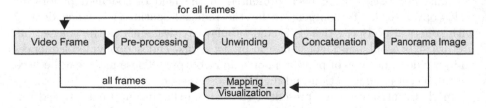

Fig. 1. Processing pipeline for computing a panorama image from gastroscopic video frames and for computing their mapping and visualization.

and a Gauss filter with a large smoothing constant σ is applied to the masked gray scale image.

In the following, a preprocessed frame is unwound by applying a contour filter using a constant border intensity b. This contour filter aims to estimate iso-valued (b-valued) contours of the image with sub-pixel precision by using the marching-squares approach [7]. Hence, the contour is computed from a (strongly smoothed) pre-processed image, Fig. 2(center), given the presumptions that the image shows a tubular geometry, that there exists only one point-light source located at the distal end of the endoscope, and that the esophagus wall shows constant reflectance. Under these presumptions, a b-valued contour approximately describes the esophagus wall at a constant point of depth as a line with matching length and height of one pixel. Taking the spatial coordinates of the resulting contour, its color values are obtained from the original and unaltered color image video frame. The start point of a contour is chosen as the nearest neighbor to its centroid regarding the x-coordinates with greater y-coordinate only. The unwound contours are then concatenated to the panorama images upper horizontal edge, stretched to a fixed length using linear interpolation (Fig. 1, right). After all frames of the given input video have been processed, the panorama image of the esophagus wall is obtained. The overall process is illustrated in Fig. 2.

2.2 Panorama mapping

In order to provide a visual relationship between the extracted panorama image (Fig. 2, right) and the original input video (Fig. 2, left), a back-mapping from the resulting panorama image to the original gastroscopic video sequence has been implemented using a lookup table. This back-mapping enables interaction possibilities and a cross reference between the general overview of the esophagus provided by the panorama image and the unaltered detail-views provided by the frames of the gastroscopic video sequence. The mapping from the panorama image to the related input video frames is exemplary shown in Fig. 3. Each pixel in the panorama image is associated with exactly one pixel of the corresponding video frame. Marking a region of interest in the panorama image thus returns a set of original video frames, each frame again contributing a set of pixels.

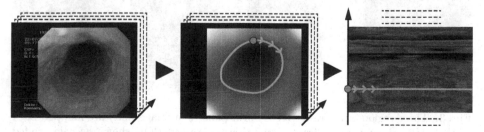

Fig. 2. Computation of a panorama image from a gastroscopic video sequence. Left: input video frame; Center: the pre-processed and unwound frame, Right: the output panorama. The orange dot denotes the starting point of the unwound contour which is depicted as blue line.

458   Prinzen et al.

3   Results

A quantitative evaluation for the matter of assessing accuracy, completeness and robustness of the presented method is challenging as no ground truth information of esophagus wall texture images are available. Hence, experiments for a proof of concept have been performed by using a rigid esophagus model using a pipe and a series of printed textures as interchangeable wall texture. Using an Storz Gastro Pack endoscopy system, a series of video sequences has been acquired by slowly withdrawing the endoscope as smooth and centered as possible. The obtained video sequences have been processed by the proposed method and the resulting panorama images were visually examined. Furthermore, first experiments have been performed using 22 gastroscopic videos of in-vivo examinations of the human esophagus. The videos highly differ in terms of image quality, number of frames, consistency of illumination, steadiness of the endoscopes movement, consistency of withdrawal speed and direction, esophagus wall texture and color, amount and density of contaminates and steadiness of the patients movements. More stable video material tends to provide visually better panorama images as a result, although currently, the parameter optimization has to be applied individually. Some qualitative results are shown in Fig. 3 and 4.

4   Discussion

In this paper, an extended shape-from-shading approach for the computation of a panoramic mapping of the esophagus from gastroscopic video sequences has been presented. The view of the panorama image and its back-mapping to details provided by the input video frames enable an interactive visualization of enriched contextual information. Given the direct connection and visual relationship between the panorama and the unaltered (deinterlaced if applicable) original video frames, this approach provides possibilities for an enhanced documentation of the esophagus, an interactive assessment of depicted lesions in a multi-view approach and new educational possibilities.

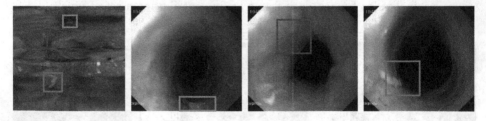

Fig. 3. Three region of interests (ROIs) in a panorama image (left) are mapped back to their related input video frames and their contained ROIs shown as color coded rectangles. From left to right(top to bottom in the panorama image): the green ROI shows a marginal detail, the blue ROI shows a redness of the esophagus wall and the red ROI shows a complete extant detail.

Fig. 4. A panorama image of the esophagus wall (center) showing four color coded ROIs as and their related input video frames. From left to right, top to bottom: The green ROI shows tiny details preserved in the panorama. The red ROI depicts a complete extant vascular structure. The blue ROI shows contamination, whose differing color is identifiable in the panorama image. The cyan ROI shows preserved details.

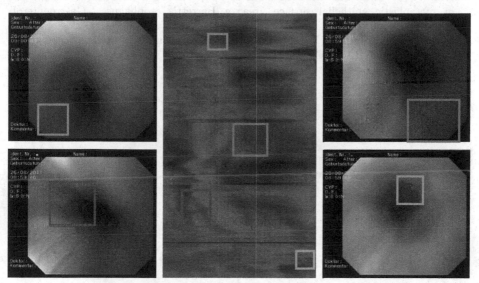

First qualitative experiments on both phantom and real data show promising results, still leaving room for a range of improvements. The parameters of the presented method are mostly constant but vary dependent on the quality and properties of a given input video. Hence, one future goal thereby consists of piecewise elimination of algorithm parameters, as well as their automated or adaptive setting if applicable.

The panorama map is able to provide valuable context information of the esophagus wall texture. Geometrical features, such as cavities or deformations are likely not to be represented. A three dimensional reconstruction of the esophagus can hereby provide an intuitive and effective representation. Given the already unwound contours frame by frame, which approximately describe the esophagus section by section, a first attempt of a three dimensional reconstruction of the esophagus has been implemented.

References

1. Bergen T, et al. A graph-based approach for local and global panorama imaging in cystoscopy. Proc SPIE. 2013;8671:86711K–1.
2. Miranda-Luna R, et al. Mosaicing of bladder endoscopic image sequences: distortion calibration and registration algorithm. IEEE Trans Biomed Eng. 2008;55(2):541–553.
3. Tokgozoglu HN, et al. Color-based hybrid reconstruction for endoscopy. IEEE Conf Comput Vis Pattern Recognit Workshop. 2012; p. 8–15.

4. Ishii T, et al. Urine flow dynamics through prostatic urethra with tubular organ modeling using endoscopic imagery. IEEE J Transl Eng Health Med. 2014;2:1–9.
5. Ishii T, et al. Novel points of view for endoscopy: panoramized intraluminal opened image and 3D shape reconstruction. J Med Imaging Health Inf. 2011;1(1):13–20.
6. Kim R, et al. Quantitative endoscopy: precise computerized measurement of metaplastic epithelial surface area in Barrett's esophagus. Gastroenterol. 1995;108(2):360–6.
7. Lorensen WE, Cline HE. Marching cubes: a high resolution 3D surface construction algorithm. SIGGRAPH Comput Graph. 1987;21(4):163–9.

Dealing with Intra-Class and Intra-Image Variations in Automatic Celiac Disease Diagnosis

Michael Gadermayr[1], Andreas Uhl[1], Andreas Vécsei[2]

[1]Department of Computer Sciences, University of Salzburg, Austria
[2]St. Anna Children's Hospital, Department of Pediatrics, Medical University Vienna, Vienna, Austria
mgadermayr@cosy.sbg.ac.at

Abstract. Computer aided celiac disease diagnosis is based on endoscopic images showing the villi structure in regions of the small bowel. Especially unavoidably variable illuminations and varying viewing angles of the individual villi are a source for high intra-class as well as intra-image variations in the image domain. We clarify that common texture descriptors are unable to compensate such a high degree of variance, which is supposed to be a crucial problem in computer aided diagnosis. In this work, a straight-forward split and merge approach is presented which facilitates the final classification task by reducing the intra-image variance and simultaneously enlarging the training set. Using different well known feature extraction techniques as well as two classifiers, it can be shown that the overall classification accuracies can be increased consistently. Additionally, the proposed approach is compared to the related but more complex bag-of-visual-words method.

1 Introduction

Typically an image texture is associated with a regular, periodic pattern (Fig. 1). However, in real work applications, textured images are often quite non-periodic as well as inhomogeneous. This is especially true in case of computer aided celiac disease diagnosis which relies on images of the mucosa of a part of the small bowel, taken during endoscopy (Fig. 2).

This inhomogeneity could be due to variations in the acquisition conditions. In recent years high effort has been made on developing texture descriptors which are invariant to certain properties such as illumination, scale, affine transformations and rotations. However, in case of endoscopic images the variations often

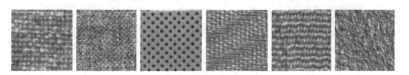

Fig. 1. Periodic texture patches from Kylberg texture database [1].

cannot be effectively described. For example, a slightly different viewing angle leads to a different illumination which might cause totally different image properties. Furthermore, as villi present a three dimensional flexible structure, a varying viewing angle cannot be modeled approximatively for instance by means of an affine transformation.

In case of our image data, image variations occur between different images of one class, which is referred to as intra-class variation. However, even within one image the degree of self similarity is often quite low, which is referred to as intra-image variation (Fig. 2).

Visually it is obvious that the degree of regularity as well as periodicity in case of the endoscopic images is significantly lower compared to the regular patterns (Fig. 1). In Fig. 3(a), this is quantified by computing the average distances of extracted features from the upper-left quarter and the lower-right quarter (64×64 pixels) of the same patch (128×128 pixels). Especially, Local Binary Patterns [2] (the exact setup is given in Sect. 2.1) are used for feature extraction in combination with the squared Euclidean distance. However, with other image descriptors a similar output is generated. It can be seen, that the endoscopic images not only visually present a high degree of intra-image distances. The variations are even preserved if switching to feature domain.

Previous work on computer aided celiac disease diagnosis relies on feature extraction from 128×128 pixel patches [3] or even on 576×576 pixel images [4]. Features which have been declared to be invariant to scale, rotations as well as affine transformations have been investigated in previous work [3, 5]. However, although some of them seem to be beneficial in synthetic scenarios (e.g. if training is based on idealistic and evaluation is based on transformed images), for real world applications highly straight-forward methods such as Local Binary Patterns and derivatives [2, 6, 7] often outperform these more elaborated techniques. This is supposed to be due to the fact that often distinctiveness has to be sacrificed for a higher degree of invariance, which has been particularly discussed in previous work [8].

In this work, we propose a split and merge approach which decreases the degree of intra-image variations by splitting the images into several smaller sub-images. After feature extraction and classification of the sub-images, the deci-

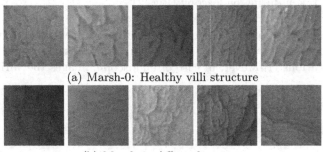

(a) Marsh-0: Healthy villi structure

(b) Marsh-3: Affected mucosa

Fig. 2. Endoscopic images showing the mucosa of the small bowel.

sions are merged in order to get one final decision. Experiments with high performing feature extraction techniques and two well known and commonly used classifiers show that in case of most configurations an improvement is achieved.

2 Split and merge approach

Most highly distinctive texture feature extractors such as Local Binary Patterns and derivatives are based on the assumption that a textured image is homogeneous, which allows a simple global collection of data in histograms. We try to retrieve an increased degree of homogeneity by splitting the original image into several non-overlapping sub-images of equal size and aspect ratio. Theoretically the method could also handle overlapping sub-images, however, in our case this did not significantly improve the overall results. Afterwords, for each sub-image, a texture feature extraction method is performed individually. Based on these computed feature vectors, classification is just as done individually for each sub-image. Classifier training is performed as well based on the sub-images. The final decision for an image is obtained by majority voting of the decisions of all sub-images. Fig. 3(b) schematizes this methodology. The proposed method attends the following potentially beneficial effects:

- By focusing on smaller regions in a textured image, the degree of intra-image variances is reduced as the neighborhood is limited.
- The training stage is also based on the smaller sub-images, which means that the number of images in the training set is multiplied by the split factor. This is especially valuable in case of small training sets.
- A set of decisions is available for acquiring the final decision for one image. This redundancy can be used to increase the accuracy as well as to give a statement on the certainty of the overall decision.

Using the bag-of-visual-words approach [9], in a similar way small sub-images are extracted to introduce a higher degree of invariance. The major difference is that in case of this elaborated technique one final feature is computed per image and not per sub-image.

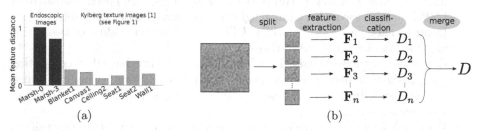

(a)   (b)

Fig. 3. Intra-image feature distances with the Local Binary Pattern descriptor (a) and Schematization of the sequences of the split and merge methodology (b).

2.1 Experimental setup

The image testset used for experimentation contains images of the duodenal bulb and the pars descendens taken during endoscopies at the St. Anna Children's Hospital using pediatric gastroscopes (Olympus GIF N180 and Q165). Prior to processing, all images are converted to gray scale images as the additional use of color information did not lead to continuous improvements. In a preprocessing step, texture patches with a fixed size of 128×128 pixels have been manually extracted. These patches are split into several smaller sub-images. We consider splits into four, nine and 16 equally sized square sub-images. In case of the four and the 16 sub-images split, another (overlapping) patch in the center is extracted to avoid ties during majority voting. To get the ground truth for the texture patches, the condition of the mucosal areas covered by the images has been determined by histological examination of biopsies from corresponding regions. The severity of the villous atrophy has been classified according to the modified Marsh classification [10]. Although it is possible to distinguish between different stages of the disease, we aim in distinguishing between images of patients with (Marsh-3) and without the disease (Marsh-0), as this two classes case is most relevant in practice. Our experiments are based on a data set containing 612 images (306 Marsh-0 and 306 Marsh-3 images) from 171 patients [3]. All overall accuracies computed are based on the mean accuracy of 32 random splits. One distinct split divides the data set into an approximately balanced training (50 %) and evaluation set (50 %), restricting images of one patient to be in the same set to avoid any bias.

To extensively study the effect of the proposed approach on the overall classification accuracy, six different feature extraction techniques which turned out to be appropriate for celiac disease classification are investigated. The chosen parameters turned out to be optimally suited in earlier experiments.

- Local Binary Patterns (LBP) [2]: LBP is deployed with eight circularly neighboring samples and a radius of two pixels.
- Multi-resolution Local Binary Patterns (MRLBP) [2]: This feature vector consists of the concatenation of an LBP vector with a neighborhood radius of one and a radius of two pixels.
- Extended Local Binary Patterns (ELBP) [6]: This edge-based derivative of LBP is as well used with eight neighbors and a radius of two pixels.
- Local ternary patterns [7] (LTP): LTP is used with a radius of two, eight neighbors and a threshold of three.
- Edge Co-occurrence Matrix [11] (ECM): The ECM is achieved by computing the gray-level co-occurrence matrix of the edge-orientation within a specified displacement. In the experiments the matrices for a displacement of one and two pixels are concatenated.
- Wavelet Variance [12] (WAV): After computing a four level two dimensional wavelet packets decomposition, the variance in each sub band is calculated. The final feature vector consists of the concatenation of these values.

For feature discrimination, we deploy the linear support vector classifier [13] (SVM) and the (highly non-linear) nearest neighbor classifier (NN) which are both commonly utilized. The results of the split and merge approach are compared to the traditional classification (i.e. feature extraction is based on original images) and the bag-of-visual-words approach which is similar to our new approach as the descriptors are also extracted from small sub-images. For this, the cluster count has been fixed to seven and a sub-image size of 32 × 32 pixels has been chosen, which turned out to be optimal and corresponds to the 16 sub-images split in our novel approach. Additionally, to get a higher data density, 49 (instead of 16) sub-images have been extracted in an overlapping manner.

3   Results and discussion

The overall classification accuracies are shown in Fig. 4. The wide bars indicate the rates obtained with traditional classification without splitting. The narrow bars indicate the rates achieved with the novel split and merge method and the splitting into four (left bar), nine (center bar) and 16 sub-images (right bar). The dashed line represents the accuracy obtained with the Bag-of-visual-words approach. It can be seen that in each case, except for ELBP in combination with the NN classifier, the traditional classification accuracy (wide bars) can be increased using the split and merge approach. Especially the splitting into nine sub-images (represented by the center bar) mostly corresponds to remarkable improvements. These improvements are slightly more significant if the linear SVM is used. This is supposed to be due to the high flexibility of the non-linear NN classifier (compared to the linear SVM) that helps to compensate the intra-class variations using the traditional method. Considering the performance compared to the bag-of-visual-words approach it can be seen that the new method is highly effective in case of LBP-derivatives. Whereas the computationally more complex bag-of-visual-words approach is rarely ever able to outperform traditional classification, the novel method definitely is. The interruptions of the narrow

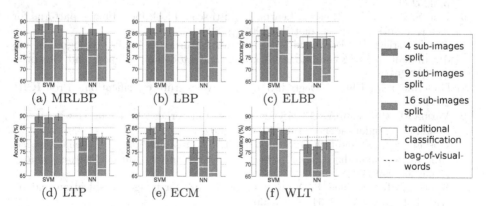

Fig. 4. Classification accuracies of traditional classification (wide bars), split and merge (narrow bars) and bag-of-visual-words based classification (dashed lines). The interruption of the narrow bars indicate the accuracies, achieved with small sub-images without the final decision level fusion.

bars indicate the accuracies achieved with the sub-images without a decision-level fusion. It can be seen that with an increasing size reduction, the error rates rise with varying extent. This effect is more distinct in case of the NN classifier. This shows us that, especially in case of the 16 sub-images split, the final decision fusion has a highly positive effect on the accuracies.

In conclusion, we have proposed a straight-forward split and merge approach for improving the classification of images showing high intra-image and intra-class variations. The intra-image variations are reduced and simultaneously the training set is increased, which helps to handle intra-class variances. Using different well known feature extraction techniques as well as two classifiers, it has been shown that the overall classification accuracies can be increased consistently, although we have concentrated on feature extraction methods which are known to be effective in case of traditional classification. We suppose that other features that are optimized for small image data could lead to even higher overall accuracies.

References

1. Kylberg G. The Kylberg texture dataset v. 1.0. Centre for Image Analysis, Swedish University of Agricultural Sciences and Uppsala University, Uppsala, Sweden; 2011. 35.
2. Ojala T, Pietikäinen M, Harwood D. A comparative study of texture measures with classification based on feature distributions. Pattern Recognit. 1996;29(1):51–9.
3. Hegenbart S, Uhl A, Vécsei A, et al. Scale invariant texture descriptors for classifying celiac disease. Med Image Anal. 2013;17(4):458–74.
4. Ciaccio EJ, Tennyson CA, Lewis SK, et al. Distinguishing patients with celiac disease by quantitative analysis of videocapsule endoscopy images. Comput Methods Programs Biomed. 2010;100(1):39–48.
5. Hegenbart S, Uhl A. A scale-adaptive extension to methods based on LBP using scale-normalized laplacian of gaussian extrema in scale-space. Proc ICASSP. 2014; p. 4352–6.
6. Liao S, Zhu X, Lei Z, et al. Learning multi-scale block local binary patterns for face recognition. Adv Biometrics. 2007; p. 828–37.
7. Tan X, Triggs B. Enhanced local texture feature sets for face recognition under difficult lighting conditions. Analysis and Modelling of Faces and Gestures. 2007;4778:168–82.
8. Gadermayr M, Uhl A. Degradation adaptive texture classification. Proc ICIP. 2014.
9. Varma M, Zisserman A. Classifying images of materials: Achieving viewpoint and illumination independence. Proc ECCV. 2002; p. 255–71.
10. Oberhuber G, Granditsch G, Vogelsang H. The histopathology of coeliac disease: time for a standardized report scheme for pathologists. Eur J Gastroenterology Hepatol. 1999;11:1185–94.
11. Rautkorpi R, Iivarinen J. A novel shape feature for image classification and retrieval. Proc ICIAR. 2004; p. 753–60.
12. Garcia C, Zikos G, Tziritas G. Wavelet packet analysis for face recognition. Image Vis Comp. 2000;18(4):289–97.
13. Fan RE, Chang KW, Hsieh CJ, et al. LIBLINEAR: a library for large linear classification. J Mach Learn Res. 2008;9:1871–4.

Calibration of Galvanometric Laser Scanners Using Statistical Learning Methods

Stefan Lüdtke[1], Benjamin Wagner[1,2], Ralf Bruder[1], Patrick Stüber[1,2], Floris Ernst[1], Achim Schweikard[1], Tobias Wissel[1,2]

[1]Institute for Robotics and Cognitive Systems, University of Lübeck
[2]Graduate School for Computing in Medicine and Life Sciences, University of Lübeck
stefan_luedtke@gmx.net

Abstract. Galvanometric laser scanners can be used for optical tracking. Model-based calibration of these systems is inaccurate and not adaptable to variations in the system. Therefore, a calibration method based on statistical learning methods is presented which directly incorporates the triangulation problem. We investigate linear regression as well as Artificial Neural Networks. The results are validated using (1) the cross-validated prediction accuracy within the calibration space, and (2) plane reconstruction accuracy. All statistical learning methods outperformed the model-based approach leading to an improvement of up to 74 % for the cross-validated 3D root-mean-square error and 70-74 % for the plane reconstruction. While the neural network achieved mean errors below 0.5 mm, the linear regression results suggest a good compromise between accuracy and computational load.

1 Introduction

Galvanometric laser scanners are used in many different applications, like barcode readers [1] and material processing [2]. These systems consist of galvanometric mirrors that deflect a laser beam and can – depending on the application – be of different complexity. A rather complex deflection system is, for example, used in novel approaches for optical head-tracking in radiotherapy [3, 4]. Standard laser scanners cannot be used in this context, because neither the scanner hardware nor the patient can be moved. Laser line scanners are also not applicable, because the setup also measures the tissue thickness by analyzing the backscatter and absorption of the laser spot on the skin. The system used in this context consist of two mirrors deflecting a laser beam. A camera then records the laser spot on the subject's skin surface and extracts features from the images.

As pointed out by Manakov and colleagues, common calibration methods cannot be used, because the used system does not have a single center of projection. Instead, a more elaborated model-based calibration approach needs to be used [5]. Enforced by the hardware setup, this calibration method is very complex and results in optimization problems that are difficult to handle. Furthermore, this method can still not model all influences, such as distortions

Fig. 1. Hardware setup with galvanometric unit (1), triangulation camera (2), and laser source (3).

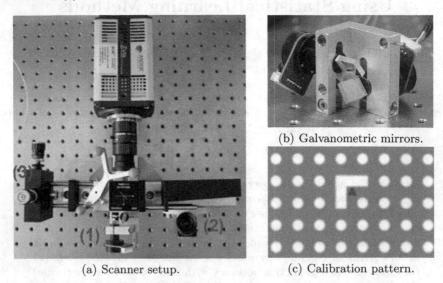

(a) Scanner setup.

(b) Galvanometric mirrors.

(c) Calibration pattern.

caused by non-planar mirrors. On top of that, a mathematical model must be adapted even to small modifications of the setup.

A more flexible approach is not to explicitly develop a model, but use statistical learning methods to approximate a model function. It has already been shown that artificial neural networks (ANNs) are suitable for machine vision calibration tasks [6]. We adapt this computationally rather complex approach to the galvanometric system used for optical tracking [3, 4] and compare to simpler methods based on linear regression (ridge regression and stepwise regression).

2   Materials and methods

2.1   Hardware setup

The optical setup is shown in Fig. 1(a). To track the head motion, it measures the tissue thickness, but is also capable of triangulating the 3D skin surface. Therefore, the systems needs to be calibrated. Fig. 3(a) illustrates all relevant components in a simplified sketch. First, the laser source emits a beam with a central wavelength of 850 nm. The beam is then deflected by two galvanometric mirrors with approximately orthogonal axes (Fig. 1(b)). Using these mirrors, the direction of the laser beam is controlled. The beam then hits the subject's skin surface, where the triangulation camera recognizes the laser spot on the skin surface.

2.2   Data acquisition

The input features $x \in \mathbb{R}^4$ of the training data consist of the 2D coordinates of the laser spot in the camera image and the voltage at the drives of both

Fig. 2. Model for a galvanometric laser scanner (a) and cross validation data (blue) and validation data (red) in 3D space (b).

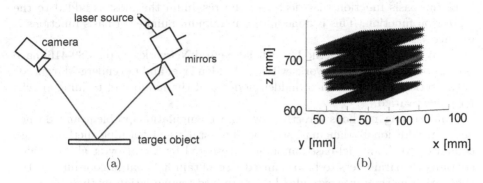

(a)   (b)

galvanometric mirrors. The 3D-coordinates of the laser spot are the target labels $y \in \mathbb{R}^3$ of the training data. The calibration (including triangulation) now tries to model a function $y = f(x)$, with $f : \mathbb{R}^4 \to \mathbb{R}^3$. The labels are acquired in two steps:

First, a camera calibration [7] provides intrinsic and extrinsic camera parameters. For the camera calibration, 40 different poses of the calibration pattern (Fig. 1 (c)) were recorded. With the coordinates of the circle markers in the camera image and on the calibration pattern, a homography that projects coordinates in the camera image to coordinates on the calibration pattern can be obtained.

In a second step, a number of laser spots is projected onto the calibration pattern. Using the homography and the extrinsic camera parameters (the 3D pose of the calibration pattern relative to the camera), we computed the 3D-position of the laser spots. This was done for ten poses of the calibration pattern. In total, we projected 900 laser spots on an equally spaced grid for each board pose. After manually removing outliers (image spots incorrectly assigned to spots on the calibration pattern), the data consisted of $N = 7193$ samples. Note that the data acquisition process was not central for our study and can be optimized in such a way that manual intervention is not necessary. These data samples covered the desired calibration space. The computed 3D target labels are shown in Fig. 3(b) (planes colored in blue).

2.3   Statistical learning methods

Basic methods based on linear regression as well as ANNs were examined. We investigated linear regression with polynomial basis functions. To avoid overfitting, it is necessary to reduce the complexity of the underlying function to a proper level. A common technique to do this is ridge regression [8, pp. 59-64]. The regression function is smoothed by adding a penalty to large coefficients. For this technique, the regularization parameter λ as well as the maximal degree of the basis can be changed.

An alternative method to avoid overfitting is stepwise regression [8, p. 58]. This iterative technique starts with an empty set of basis functions. In each step, the basis function that decreases the residuum the most is added to the regression function. This is done until a maximum number of basis functions is reached.

As a third learning method, Artificial Neural Networks [8, pp. 389-416] have been applied. We used networks with one hidden layer and Levenberg-Marquardt optimization. The number of hidden nodes and the number of training epochs have been varied.

All learning methods directly solve the triangulation problem and do not need an additional triangulation step. The statistical learning methods were compared to the model-based approach presented by Manakov et al. [5], which contains 22 parameters to be optimized. To obtain 3D spatial coordinates, the calibration method was extended by a standard triangulation method based on the direct linear transform (DLT) algorithm [9, p. 88].

2.4 Validation

To measure the performance of the regression methods, we use 10-fold cross validation, which splits the entire data into training and test data to get an unbiased estimate of the triangulation accuracy. In addition, we used a validation set consisting of 900 data points where all labels lie within the same plane. This plane (Fig. 3(b), colored in red) was not part of the remaining data (colored in blue), which was used for training. For this second validation measure, the plane reconstruction error is given by the departure of the predicted labels from an ideal plane, which is measured by the standard deviation along the principal component (PC) with the smallest eigenvalue. To find the optimal parameters with respect to these validation measures, we performed a grid search, investigating every combination of parameters. Once we found these ideal parameters, we investigated the accuracy of the ideal models when only a fraction of the training data is used, as well as the time required for training and testing with each algorithm (Intel Core 2 Duo E6600, 4 GB RAM, Tab. 1).

3 Results

The linear regression-based methods show quite similar results. For ridge regression, the optimum for both validation methods lies at $\lambda = 10^{-4}$ and a polynomial degree of four. The best results for both validation methods in stepwise regression used a maximum of 31 basis functions. Both learning methods have a cross-validated root mean squared error (RMSE) of about 0.77 mm and a plane reconstruction error of about 0.47 mm. ANNs show the best results with 17 inner nodes and 5000 training epochs. For this method, the cross-validated RMSE is only 0.48 mm, while the plane reconstruction RMSE is 0.43 mm. When only a fraction of the training data is used, ANNs still show the lowest error (Tab. 1). The performance of the model-based calibration is clearly inferior to all learning

Table 1. Performance measures [mm], training time and query time [s] of statistical learning based calibration.

	Ridge	Stepwise	ANN
X-axis CV-RMSE	0.044	0.044	0.03
Y-axis CV-RMSE	0.044	0.045	0.03
Z-axis CV-RMSE	0.77	0.78	0.48
3D CV-RMSE	0.77	0.78	0.48
Plane RMSE	0.49	0.46	0.43
Plane RMSE, 50 % training data	0.52	0.57	0.52
Plane RMSE, 25 % training data	0.74	0.59	0.58
Plane RMSE, 10 % training data	0.87	1.06	0.79
Training time	0.048	47.86	2921
Query time	0.0031	0.0030	0.358

methods. We found an overall cross-validated RMSE of 1.83 mm and a plane reconstruction error of 1.61 mm (Fig. 3).

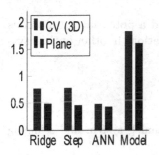

Fig. 3. 3D cross validation RMSE and plane reconstruction RMSE of statistical learning based calibration and model-based calibration.

4 Discussion

We showed that statistical learning methods can be used to calibrate galvanometric laser scanning systems. We validated our methods using cross-validation and a plane-reconstruction error.

The learning methods showed a cross-validated RMSE which was between 57 % and 74 % lower than the model-based calibration. They were even 70 % to 74 % better for the plane-reconstruction error. There are several reasons for the poor performance of the model-based calibration. First, the optimization that is part of the model-based calibration process is not very robust. The result strongly depends on the initial values. Avoiding local minima in the highly non-convex, and high-dimensional optimization problem requires quite a lot of manual intervention. Furthermore, the optimization does not ensure that the rotation matrix that is part of the extrinsic parameters of the model is a valid rotation matrix per definition. On top of that, the model cannot allow for all influences and real world details, such as offsets in the mirror alignment, non-planar mirrors or nonlinear dependencies of the mirror rotation angle from the applied voltage. Statistical methods can express all of these influences without the need of explicitly modeling them. This makes our approach flexible, general and hence easily adaptable to other setups.

ANNs have a better performance than simple learning methods, but they also show a higher computational cost (Tab. 1). Furthermore, the resulting model contains sigmoidal basis functions. Therefore, ANNs are only feasible when powerful hardware can be used for the calibration, which, for example, can easily approximate complex nonlinear functions or at least involves a floating point unit. Ridge regression and stepwise regression, on the other hand, only rely on polynomial basis functions and can therefore also run on a basic microcontroller. While both methods show similar results, they still have different advantages. The stepwise regression model contains fewer basis functions, which makes it faster when processing a query point. It also has a smaller memory footprint. On the other hand, the training process of the ridge regression model is faster (Tab. 1), because there exists a closed-form solution for the training step. With this method, it may therefore be possible to autonomously recalibrate a scanning device, using, for example, only a microcontroller.

Finally, high flexibility, a low calibration error and a potential autonomous recalibration suggest promising adaptations for applications in other optical systems.

References

1. Bridgelall R, Dvorkis P, Goren DP, et al.. Laser scanning system and scanning method for reading 1-d and 2-d barcode symbols; 2000.
2. Gorham EW, Risser CJ, Schultz DW, et al.. Laser material processing system with multiple laser sources apparatus and method; 2001.
3. Wissel T, Stüber P, Wagner B, et al. Tissue thickness estimation for high precision head-tracking using a galvanometric laser scanner: a case study. Proc EMBC. 2014; p. 3106–9.
4. Wagner B, Stüber P, Wissel T, et al. Accuracy analysis for triangulation and tracking based on time-multiplexed structured light. Med Phys. 2014;41(8).
5. Manakov A, Seidel HP, Ihrke I. A mathematical model and calibration procedure for galvanometric laser scanning systems. Proc VMV. 2011; p. 207–14.
6. Smith LN, Smith ML. Automatic machine vision calibration using statistical and neural network methods. Image Vis Comput. 2005;23(10):887–99.
7. Bradski G. The OpenCV Library. Dr Dobb's J Softw Tools. 2000.
8. Hastie T, Tibshirani R, Friedman J. The Elements of Statistical Learning. Springer Series in Statistics. Springer New York Inc.; 2001.
9. Hartley R, Zisserman A. Multiple View Geometry in Computer Vision. 2nd ed. Cambridge University Press; 2004.

Überwachtes Lernen zur Prädiktion von Tumorwachstum

Christian Weber[1,2], Michael Götz[1,2], Franciszek Binczyck[3,4],
Joanna Polanska[3], Rafal Tarnawski[4], Barbara Bobek-Billewicz[4],
Hans-Peter Meinzer[2], Bram Stieltjes[5], Klaus Maier-Hein[1,2]

[1]Medical Image Computing (MIC), DKFZ Heidelberg
[2]Abteilung für Medizinische und Biologische Informatik, DKFZ Heidelberg
[3]Silesian University of Technology, Gliwice, Poland
[4]Maria Skodowska-Curie Memorial Cancer Center and Institute of Oncology, Gliwice,
Poland
[5]Departement Radiologie, Universitätsspital Basel, Schweiz
ch.weber@dkfz.de

Kurzfassung. In der Bestrahlungsplanung bei Hirntumoren wird typischerweise ein Sicherheitsabstand von $2 - 2,5$ cm um das im T2-Flair MR-Bild hyperintense Gebiet eingeplant. Verläßliche Vorhersagen des Tumorwachstums können dazu beitragen, die Strahlendosis noch besser auf gefährdete Regionen zu konzentrieren und gleichzeitig gesundes Gewebe zu schonen. Aktuelle Verfahren aus der Forschung nähern sich diesem Problem mit einer expliziten, generativen Modellierung des Wachstumsprozesses. Wir präsentieren ein alternatives, diskriminatives Verfahren. Mit Hilfe einer annotierten Datenbasis und überwachtem Lernen wird ein Wachstumsmodell trainiert und im nächsten Schritt auf ungesehene Daten angewendet. In allen 6 Testpatienten lieferte der Ansatz genauere Vorhersagen (DICE $0,80 \pm 0,09$) als die bisherige Herangehensweise (DICE $0,56 \pm 0,07$).

1 Einleitung

Maligne Gliome sind eine spezielle Art primärer Hirntumore die durch infiltratives und hochgradig anisotropes Wachstum charakterisiert sind. Tumorzellen können bis zu mehrere Zentimeter tief in das um den Tumor liegende Gewebe eindringen ohne sichtbare Signalveränderungen in MR- oder CT-Aufnahmen zu verursachen. Deshalb wird in der Strahlentherapie typischerweise ein Sicherheitsabstand von $2 - 2,5$ cm um das im T2-Flair MR-Bild hyperintense Gebiet eingeplant. Verläßliche Simulationen der Tumorausbreitung können dabei helfen, die applizierte Strahlendosis auf gefährdete Regionen zu konzentrieren und gleichzeitig gesundes Gewebe zu schonen.

Bisherige Arbeiten zur Wachstumssimulation modellieren mit Hilfe der Diffusions-Reaktions-Gleichung zwei voneinander unabhängige Mechanismen: Zelldiffusion und Proliferation. Swanson et al. modellieren hierbei unterschiedliche Ausbreitungsgeschwindigkeiten von Tumorzellen in weißer und grauer Substanz [1]. Die Diffusionstensorbildgebung (DTI) ermöglicht eine weitere Verfeinerung der Modellierung des Diffusionsprozesses [2, 3, 4]

$$\frac{\partial c}{\partial t} = \nabla(\boldsymbol{D}\nabla c) + p(c) \tag{1}$$

Hier repräsentiert c die Tumorzellkonzentration, $p(\cdot)$ den Proliferationsterm und $\boldsymbol{D}$ den sog. Tumor-Diffusionstensor (TDT), welcher aus dem Wasser-Diffusionstensor abgeleitet wird und die Motilität von Tumorzellen beschreibt.

Grundsätzlich haben generative Herangehensweisen bei der Modellierung den Nachteil, dass sämtliche Einflussgrößen explizit mathematisch formuliert werden müssen. Diese sind jedoch sehr komplex und teils noch gänzlich unverstanden. Wir stellen hier einen diskriminativen Modellierungsansatz vor, der mit Hilfe maschineller Lernverfahren das Verhalten von Gliomen anhand von annotierten Krankheitsverläufen erlernt. Da hierbei keine explizite Modellierung der Zusammenhänge mehr notwendig ist, kann eine Vielzahl zusätzlicher Informationen integriert werden, zum Beispiel um so der Tumorheterogenität besser Rechnung zu tragen.

2 Material und Methoden

2.1 Patientendaten

Das Datenkolletiv bestand aus 6 Glioblastoma Grad IV Patienten. Für jeden Patient existierte ein Paar multimodaler Bilder (Baseline $I^{t=0}$, Follow-up $I^{t=1}$), jeweils bestehend aus T1 MR mit Konstrastmittelgabe, T2-Flair und DTI. Das Gross Tumor Volume (GTV) wurde auf T2-Flair manuell segmentiert ($S^{t=0}, S^{t=1}$). Alle Bilder eines Patienten wurden rigide auf das T2-Flair Bild aus $I^{t=0}$ registriert und auf eine gemeinsame Auflösung gebracht. Die Intensitätswerte in T1, T2-Flair und B0 wurden über den Median der Ventrikel und der weißen Substanz normalisiert. Aus den DTIs wurden die sechs skalaren Kenngrößen fraktionelle/relative/geclusterte Anisotropie sowie mittlere/radiale/axiale Diffusivität jeweils mit und ohne Bereinigung des freien Wasseranteils f berechnet [5].

2.2 Klassifikation

Um beobachtbare Tumorverläufe mit Hilfe maschineller Lernverfahren analysierbar zu machen, wurde die Wachstumsprädiktion als Klassifikationsproblem formuliert. Jedem Voxel $v^{t=0}$ aus der Baselineaufnahme $I^{t=0}$ wird ein Label $y \in \{'gesund', 'tumor'\}$ zugewiesen, welches beschreibt ob dieser Voxel im Follow-up $S^{t=1}$ als Tumor annotiert ist oder nicht. In dieser Arbeit nutzen wir Random Forests für die Klassifikation [6]. Der Klassifikator lernt, welche Merkmale für unterschiedliche Ausbreitungsgeschwindigkeiten, Infiltrationswahrscheinlichkeiten oder regionale Inhomogenitäten in der Aktivität und Agressivität des Tumorgewebes ausschlaggebend sind. Der Random Forest wurde mit 400 Bäumen trainiert, und die maximale Baumtiefe auf 9 begrenzt um eine gute Generalisierung zu gewährleisten. Als Split-Kriterium wurde die Gini-Impurity gewählt.

2.3   Merkmale

Wir unterscheiden drei verschiedene Kategorien von Merkmalen, die einem Voxel v für die Klassifikation zugeordnet werden (Abb. 1). Die erste Kategorie, *lokale Gewebemerkmale*, beinhaltet alle Bildgebungsinformationen, die zu dem Voxel lokal vorliegen. Die zweite Kategorie, *pfadbasierte Merkmale*, repräsentiert Merkmale die entlang des Pfades ausgehenden vom initialen Tumor $S_{t=0}$ erhoben werden. Die dritte Kategorie, *entfernte Tumormerkmale*, steht für Merkmale, die das nächstliegende Tumorrandgebiet repräsentieren. Während die Gewebe- und Tumormerkmale direkt die am Pfadanfang bzw. Pfadende zur Verfügung stehenden Bildinformationen repräsentieren, gehen wir im Folgenden noch näher auf die pfadbasierten Merkmale ein.

2.4   Pfadbasierte Merkmale

Die Kosten entlang eines Pfades ergeben sich aus den Einzelkosten der jeweils aneinander grenzenden Voxeln v_l und v_k. Bei skalaren Bildern spiegelt die Kostenfunktion die Grauwertdifferenz zweier Voxel wieder

$$s_{\text{scal}}(v_l, v_k) = e^{|f(v_k)-f(v_l)|} - 1 \qquad (2)$$

Für tensorwertige Voxel (DTI) wurde ein Distanzmaß definiert, welches diejenige Voxelverbindungen mit niedrigen Kosten versieht, die deutlich über eine Nervenfaser verbunden sind

$$s_{tens}(v_l, v_k) = \frac{c(v_l) \cdot c(v_k)}{\sqrt{\|D_l \cdot r\|_2 \cdot \|D_k \cdot r\|_2}} \qquad (3)$$

Hier beschreibt $\|D \cdot r\|_2$ die Projektion des Pfadrichtungsvektors r von v_l nach v_k auf den Diffusionstensor D. Regionen mit hoher FA werden durch $c(\cdot) = (1 - \text{FA}(\cdot))$ mit niedrigeren Kosten versehen. Eine weitere Kostenfunktion ergibt sich aus der Multiplikation der tensoriellen mit der skalaren Kostenfunktion $s_{tens,scal} = s_{tens}(v_l, v_k) \cdot s_{scal}(v_l, v_k)$. Pfade von nicht-adjazenten Voxeln

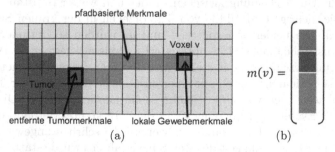

(a)   (b)

Abb. 1. (a) Räumliche Zuordnung der Merkmalsklassen für lokale Gewebemerkmale, pfadbasierte Merkmale (aggregiert über Pfade vom Tumor zum Zielvoxel v) und entfernte Tumormerkmale am Startpunkt des Pfades mit den geringsten Kosten vom Tumor zum Zielvoxel v. (b) Komposition des Merkmalsvektors.

$p : (v_0, v_1, \ldots, v_n)$ erhalten die kummulative Distanz der jeweils benachbarten Voxel. Die finale Distanz $\hat{s}$ für ein Voxel v zum Tumor ergibt sich als Minimum aller möglichen Pfade die im Tumorgebiet beginnen

$$\hat{s}(p) = \arg\min_p \sum_{j=0}^{n-1} s(v_j, v_{j+1}) \tag{4}$$

Die finalen Merkmalsvektoren für die Klassifikation bestanden aus 16 lokalen Gewebemerkmalen, 48 entfernten Tumormerkmalen sowie 33 pfadbasierten Merkmalen, da die Basismerkmale nicht in die tensoriellen Kostenfunktion einfließen. Diese wurden zusammmen mit der euklidschen Distanz zwischen v und der nächstgelegenen Tumorregion zu einem 83-dimensionalen Merkmalsvektor zusammengefasst.

2.5   Evaluation

Die Evaluation basiert auf dem Leave-One-Patient-Out Protokoll. Die Wachstumsprädiktion auf einem bisher ungesehenen Patienten wurde mit dem tatsächlichen Wachstum aus der Follow-up Aufnahme $S^{t=1}$ dieses Patienten verglichen. Hierzu wurden die Sensitivität, der DICE Koeffizient und der quadratische Mittelwertsfehler (RMSE) bezüglich der Tumorkontouren berechnet.

Um die Ergebnisse mit dem Stand der Forschung (SoA) zu vergleichen, wurde ein aktuelles, auf patienten-spezifischen DTIs basierendes Diffusions-Reaktions-Modell implementiert [4]. Der TDT wird wie von Swanson et al. [7] vorgeschlagen gewebeabhängig berechnet und nach Mosayebi et al. [8] im anisotropen Fall aus dem Diffusions-Tensor des Wassers $\boldsymbol{D}_w$ durch Gewichtung mit dem jeweiligen FA Wert des Voxels v berechnet. Der Proliferations-Term $p(c)$ in Gl. 1 wird als logistisches Wachstum modelliert. Für den TDT ergibt sich daraus folgende Formel

$$\boldsymbol{TDT}(v) = \begin{cases} \mathrm{FA}(v) \cdot \boldsymbol{D}_w(v) & \text{für } \mathrm{FA}(v) > \tau \\ d_g \boldsymbol{I} & \text{sonst} \end{cases} \tag{5}$$

wobei τ zur Unterscheidung zwischen grauer und weißer Substanz dient, und durch d_g die niedrigere Motilität von Tumorzellen in der grauen Substanz gesteuert wird. Die beiden Parameter τ und d_g wurden so optimiert, dass die Methode hinsichtlich des RMSE optimale Ergebnisse liefert ($\tau = .19$, $d_g = \frac{1}{9}$). Die Wachstumsgeschwindigkeit stellt einen weiteren freien Parameter dar, der üblicherweise patientenspezisch mit einer zusätzliche Aufnahme vor der Baseline auf den Bobachtungen von $I^{t=-1}$ und $I^{t=0}$ initialisiert wird [4]. Dieser Schritt wurde in der Evaluierung umgangen, da die vorgestellte Methode das Tumorwachstum vorhersagen kann, ohne auf weitere Zeitschritte angewiesen zu sein. Die Wachstumsgeschwindigkeit des Referenzverfahrens wurde stattdessen so eingestellt, dass die Simulation die gleiche Sensitivität wie das vorgestellte Verfahren liefert.

Tabelle 1. Ergebnisse der vorgestellten Methode (neu) im Vergleich zum Stand der Forschung (SoA) bei gleicher Sensitivität.

Patient	Sensitivität	DICE		RMSE[mm]	
		neu	SoA	neu	SoA
Patient 0	0.45	0.83	0.59	2.1	2.3
Patient 1	0.96	0.77	0.50	3.1	4.1
Patient 2	0.63	0.89	0.64	2.4	1.8
Patient 3	0.83	0.69	0.49	2.8	3.1
Patient 4	0.71	0.90	0.63	1.9	2.1
Patient 5	0.83	0.71	0.50	3.2	4.2

3 Ergebnisse

Die Ergebnisse in Tab. 1 zeigen, dass die neue Methode bei gleicher Sensitivität für alle Patienten einen höheren DICE Koeffizient und mit Ausnahme von Fall 2 ebenfalls einen niedrigeren RMSE liefert. Abb. 2 zeigt ein Prädiktionsbeispiel mit erfolgreicher Anpassung der Wachstumsraten entlang verschiedener Richtungen und Anerkennung der Liquorräume als natürliche Wachstumsgrenze.

4 Diskussion

Während bisherige Ansätze zur Tumorwachstumsprädiktion auf generativer Modellierung basierten, haben wir erstmalig einen datengetriebenen Ansatz vorgestellt und an sechs über die Zeit beobachteten malignen Gliomen validiert. Die Experimente zeigen, dass auf Basis bildbasierter Merkmale diverse Aspekte des Tumorverhaltens automatisiert gelernt werden können. Trotz der relativ kleinen Menge an Trainingsdaten lieferte das Verfahren genauere Vorhersagen als bisherige Modellierungsansätze. Der schlechtere RMSE bei Patient 2 kommt hauptsächlich durch eine falsch-positiv vorausgesagte Tumorspitze zustande. Die

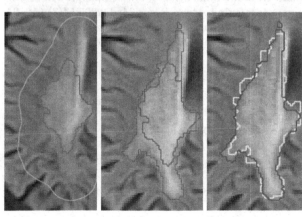

Abb. 2. Beispielergebnis: (a) Gross Tumor Volume (GTV$_{t=0}$, grün) und Illustration des typischen Sicherheitsabstands (orange) (b) Tatsächliches Wachstum (GTV$_{t=1}$, rot). (c) Vorhersageergebnis (gelb). Ausläufer (blaue Pfeile) werden gut vorhergesagt.

(a) Patient 4$_{t=0}$ (b) Patient 4$_{t=1}$ (c) Prädiktion höhere Genauigkeit der Vorhersagen lässt sich teilweise sicherlich durch die viel reichhaltigere Bildinformation erklären, welche dem Lernverfahren zur Verfügung steht. Generative Ansätze beschränken diese bislang auf die Nutzung der DTI Daten sowie einer Segmentierung der weißen und grauen Hirnsubstanz und des Tumors. Weiterhin beinhaltet die diskriminative Modellierung keine Vorannahmen, welche die möglichen Wachstumsmuster apriori einschränken.

Die Limitationen des Verfahrens haben sich in der teilweise recht niedrigen Sensitivität der Vorhersage gezeigt. Ein Grund hierfür könnte die beschränkte Datenbasis sein, welche insbesondere für eine verlässliche Vorhersage der Fälle 0 und 2 unzureichend schien.

Eine weitere Limitation ist die momentane Beschränkung des Verfahrens in seiner jetzigen Form auf die Prädiktion diskreter Zeitintervalle. Generative Modelle benötigen für die Initialisierung zwar eine zusätzliche Aufnahme, um aus dem vergangenen Verlauf eine patientstenspezifische Wachstumsgeschwindigkeit zu schätzen. Dadurch sind diese Modelle aber auch in der Lage, zeitkontinuierlich zu simulieren. In unserer Methode kann auf diese zusätzliche Aufnahme verzichtet werden, jedoch ist die Vorhersage dadurch auf die gelernte Zeitspanne beschränkt. In zukünfigen Arbeiten wird der Fokus auf die Einarbeitung einer Regression für die Wachstumsmodellierung liegen. Eine derartige Vorgehensweise könnte die Vorteile beider Welten vereinen und zeitlich kontinuierliche Simulationen mit hoher Genauigkeit ermöglichen.

Danksagung. Diese Arbeit wurde im Rahmen des von der Deutschen Forschungsgemeinschaft (DFG) geförderten SFB/TRR 125 „Cognition-Guided Surgery" (Projekt R01) erstellt.

Literaturverzeichnis

1. Swanson K, Alvord E, Murray J. A quantitative model for differential motility of gliomas in grey and white matter. Cell Prolif. 2000;33:317–29.
2. Jbabdi S, Mandonnet E, Duffau H, et al. Simulation of anisotropic growth of low-grade gliomas using diffusion tensor imaging. Magn Reson Med. 2005;54(3):616–24.
3. Konukoglu E, Clatz O, Menze BH, et al. Image guided personalization of reaction-diffusion type tumor growth models using modified anisotropic eikonal equations. IEEE TMI. 2010;29(1):77–95.
4. Stretton E, Geremia E. Importance of patient DTI's to accurately model glioma growth using the reaction diffusion equation. Proc ISBI. 2013;1130(32):5–8.
5. Pasternak O, Sochen N, Gur Y, et al. Free water elimination and mapping from diffusion MRI. Magn Reson Med. 2009;62(3):717–30.
6. Breiman L. Random forest. Mach Learn. 1999;45:1–35.
7. Swanson KR, Bridge C, Murray JD, et al. Virtual and real brain tumors: using mathematical modeling to quantify glioma growth and invasion. J Neurol Sci. 2003;216(1):1–10.
8. Mosayebi P, Cobzas D, Murtha A, et al. Tumor invasion margin on the Riemannian space of brain fibers. Med Image Anal. 2012;16(2):361–73.

Classification of Confocal Laser Endomicroscopic Images of the Oral Cavity to Distinguish Pathological from Healthy Tissue

Christian Jaremenko[1], Andreas Maier[1,2], Stefan Steidl[1], Joachim Hornegger[1], Nicolai Oetter[3], Christian Knipfer[3], Florian Stelzle[3], Helmut Neumann[4]

[1]Pattern Recognition Lab, Department of Computer Science, FAU
Erlangen-Nürnberg, Martenstr. 3, 91058 Erlangen, Germany
[2]SAOT Graduate School in Advanced Optical Technologies
[3]Department of Oral and Maxillofacial Surgery, University Hospital Erlangen
[4]Department of Medicine I, University Hospital Erlangen
christian.jaremenko@fau.de

Abstract. Confocal laser endomicroscopy is a recently introduced advanced imaging technique which enables microscopic imaging of the mucosa in-vivo. This technique has already been applied successfully during diagnosis of gastrointestinal diseases. Whereas for this purpose several computer aided diagnosis approaches exist, we present a classification system that is able to differentiate between healthy and pathological images of the oral cavity. Varying textural features of small rectangular regions are evaluated using random forests and support vector machines. Preliminary results reach up to 99.2% classification rate. This indicates that an automatic classification system to differentiate between healthy and pathological mucosa of the oral cavity is feasible.

1 Introduction

Cancer of the oral cavity and pharynx can only be reliably diagnosed by performing biopsies of lesions. These biopsies may lead to unfavorable sequelae such as permanent damage in sensitive areas. Another difficulty is finding an adequate resection margin of the primary tumor site as intraoperative surveillance of the resection margin is complex since it includes histological analysis. Both treatments are influenced by the experience of the physician and may introduce operator dependent errors.

Confocal laser endomicroscopy (CLE) allows intraoperative real time visualization of the mucosa as an optical biopsy with en face view, whereas the histological analysis of biopsies investigates a transverse section through the tissue. To obtain a high contrast visualization of the mucosa, a contrast agent such as fluorescein has to be administered. The resulting images allow a microscopic comparison between inconspicuous epithelium and neoplastic lesions by visualizing the different structural and architectural compositions of cells. The image quality can be enhanced by band-pass filtering [1] to reduce noise and emphasize cell boundaries.

Currently CLE has been successfully used in different diseases such as Ulcerative colitis or Crohn's disease [2]. CLE seems to be a promising technique when it comes to intraoperative analysis of the mucosa and has been rarely used for diagnosis of cancer in the oral cavity e.g. [3]. When it comes to computer aided diagnosis only a few approaches exist, all handling the gastric intestinal tract based on analyzing the arrangement of crypts e.g. [4] by using the Scale-Invariant-Feature-Transform (SIFT). Another approach using SIFT is accomplished by Mualla et al. [5] for automatic cell detection in bright-field microscope images.

This paper investigates whether it is possible to classify the acquired images into two stages *pathological* and *healthy* using textural features and pattern recognition methods.

2   Materials and methods

Three subjects, two patients and one healthy control, were examined using a probe based CLE (pCLE) system from Cellvizio (GastroFlex/UHD, Mauna Kea Technologies, Paris, France) that can be applied via the accessory channel of an endoscope. IRB approval was provided and procedures were performed after written informed consent was obtained from the patients. The 16 bit grayscale images with a resolution of 576×578 are streamed with a frame rate of 12 frames per seconds. The resulting CLE video sequences are separated into n images per second and annotated individually by experts of the Oral and Maxillofacial Surgery. Sequences of the alveolar ridge were acquired and examined leading to a database consisting of 206 images with no pathological characteristics and 45 images being cancerous (Fig. 1). The image on the left hand side visualizes the healthy oral mucosa with flat, uniform, polygonal cells. These have a regular architectural arrangement with alternating dark and light bands. The image on the right hand side shows a cancerous region highlighted by the rectangle. The architectural arrangement of cells is completely lost and cells have varying sizes. Besides this, cell piles with no architectural structures and strong

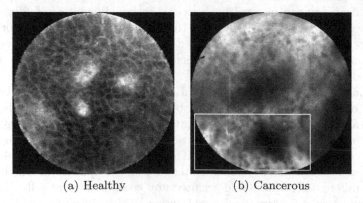

(a) Healthy   (b) Cancerous

Fig. 1. Exemplary pCLE images with different image characteristics.

(white) fluorescein leakage prevail. The circular shape of the pCLE images is a challenge, as the shape itself or its large dark areas may introduce artefacts during the processing of images. Instead of cropping the image to a quadratic region inside the circle and losing large parts of image information, multiple small rectangular regions of the image are extracted and examined separately. To find the coordinates of these patches, the intensity values of their corners are compared with a threshold which is delineated by the dark background. The step length in x and y direction consists of half the edge length leading to an overlap of 50%. Two different patch sizes with an edge length of 80 and 105 pixels are examined, so that a certain amount of structure is comprised within each patch and a symmetrical distribution of patches is accomplished as emphasized by Fig. 2b. This leads to a diverse amount of 110 and 52 processed patches, respectively. Fig. 2 shows a single patch with edge length of 105 pixels as well as the resulting gradually processed image.

To accomplish a classification into images with healthy and pathological characteristics, four different features are computed for every patch:

- *Histogram features:* These features describe the local distribution of gray level values. First order statistics, like mean, standard deviation, coefficient of variance, skewness, kurtosis, and entropy are computed from the histogram to describe a local patch.
- *Homogeneity features:* As images with no pathological characteristics appear more structured than pathological ones, the amount of included edges within a patch may imply the presence or absence of cancerous regions. For this reason the image is filtered with a Sobel operator. As homogeneity features, the mean, standard deviation and variance are computed from the edge image, as well as of the gray level image.
- *Gray level co-occurrence matrices (GLCM):* Haralick et al. [6] propose different indicators to describe an image texture by numerical characteristics called Gray-Level Co-Occurrence Matrices Features. These features are based on a statistical analysis of the frequency of certain gray levels in dependance of their geometrical arrangement to each other. In this study, a

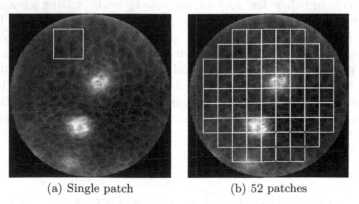

(a) Single patch   (b) 52 patches

Fig. 2. Division of images into patches.

distance of one and two between the pixels as well as the orientations of $0°$, $45°$, $90°$, $135°$ are investigated. This leads to a feature vector including the angular second moment, contrast, correlation, variance, inverse difference moment, entropy, energy, homogeneity and inertia. In addition the recursivity and inverse recursivity introduced by Beraldi et al. [7] are included.

- *Local binary patterns (LBP):* LBP is another approach to describe images by using the distribution of binary patterns in the image [8]. For every pixel a binary pattern is constructed by thresholding the center pixel with its circular neighborhood. If the neighboring pixel has a larger value it is set to one and when connected with the results of all neighboring pixels this leads to a local binary pattern. This approach has been extended to uniform rotation independent local binary patterns. In this version, LBP are bitwise rotated circularly to their minimum code. A uniform pattern is defined by having ≤ 2 1 to 0 or 0 to 1 transitions and represents a certain structure. For instance, the LBP 00001111_2 denotes an edge, and 00000111_2 denotes a corner. These binary patterns are sampled into a histogram describing the image. If a pattern is non-uniform, the reject bin comprising of all non-uniform patterns is assigned. In this study the classical LBP, as well as the rotation invariant uniform LBP are evaluated. Instead of using the histogram itself, the already mentioned first order statistics are computed and used as features.

These features are combined during the processing of the patches leading to two different characteristic vectors. The first one is specified by a concatenation of the features of every patch representing the whole image while preserving local image information. The second feature vector consists of the average (mean, std. deviation and variance) of all features and patches describing the mean or global representation of the patches.

On the previously introduced features, a support vector machine (SVM) [9] classifier as well as a random forest (RF) [10] classifier are trained. Within the SVM approach, a separation between the classes is realized by transforming the feature space to a higher dimension. The optimal hyperplane is then constructed using the critical points next to it as support vectors by solving a maximization problem to increase the margin using a polynomial kernel function. The other approach being applied is the RF. This classifier constructs many unpruned decision trees and includes bagging as well as random selection of features. These random combinations of input data lead to a reduction of correlation between trees. Furthermore, the influence of strong features as chosen predictors is reduced as every feature vector can contain duplicate values or miss features. The final class of the examined feature vector is then assigned by the majority votes of the particular decision trees.

3   Results

The SVM and RF classifier are implemented using WEKA, with a 10 fold cross-validation approach as a result of the small image database. In addition, different

Table 1. Accuracy (acc) and average recall (rec) of the particular features of the concatenated feature vector (Patchsize 105).

Features	Property	SVM		RF	
		Acc	Rec	Acc	Rec
Histogram	256 bins	88.5%	70.4%	90.4%	78.6%
Histogram	512 bins	89.3%	72.7%	92.4%	81.5%
Histogram	768 bins	89.2%	72.6%	89.6%	77.2%
Homogeneity	—	90.8%	77.1%	96.4%	91.7%
GLCM	8 Imglvl	99.2%	97.8%	92.8%	79.8%
GLCM	16 Imglvl	99.2%	97.8%	90.8%	74.5%
GLCM	32 Imglvl	98.8%	97.6%	90.0%	73.1%
LBPc	R1 N8	86.1%	71.6%	89.6%	73.5%
LBPr	R1 N8	85.7%	73.9%	87.3%	65.3%
LBPr	R2 N16	83.7%	65.8%	92.0%	83.0%

settings of the feature types are investigated. For the histogram features varying amounts of bins (256, 512, 768) are used. The GLCM matrices are evaluated with 8, 16, 32 gray value quantization levels. The classical LBP is evaluated with a radius of one and a neighborhood of 8. In case of the rotation invariant uniform LBP, a radius of one and two as well as a neighborhood of 8 and 16 are evaluated.

The recognition rate (acc) as well as the average recall (rec) for the two different investigated patch sizes are illustrated in Tabs. 1 and 2 in case of the non-averaged feature vector. The corresponding results of the averaged feature vector are shown in Tabs. 3 and 4. In both cases the classification rate is illustrated in dependance of the underlying feature types and its adjusted properties. Overall the GLCM based classification reaches the best results with a recognition rate of 99.2% and average recall of 97.8% in case of the SVM with 80px patchsize in the non-averaged classification problem. For the average feature vector a classification rate of 98.0% and an average recall of 95.3% is reached in case of the 80px patchsize using the RF classifier.

4 Discussion and conclusion

The GLCM features achieve the best classification result (99.2%) without strong dependance on the patchsize as they deliver nearly equal classification results. Though the larger patchsize strongly reduces computation time. Even in case of the averaged feature vector, a strong accuracy of 98.0% is reached. This feature vector may be of advantage when a classification between different stages of the disease into hyperplasia, dysplasia or carcinoma is conducted, especially when multiple disease characteristics are apparent on a single image. Besides this, the simple homogeneity features reach a strong accuracy of up to 96.8%. This indicates that the amount of included edges gives insight about the state of

Table 2. Accuracy (acc) and average recall (rec) of the particular features of the concatenated feature vector (Patchsize 80).

Features	Property	SVM		RF	
		Acc	Rec	Acc	Rec
Histogram	256 bins	88.4%	74.7%	92.4%	82.4%
Histogram	512 bins	88.8%	75.0%	91.6%	79.3%
Histogram	768 bins	88.5%	74.7%	92.4%	81.5%
Homogeneity	—	94.8%	87.3%	95.2%	86.7%
GLCM	8 Imglvl	99.2%	98.7%	90.8%	74.5%
GLCM	16 Imglvl	99.2%	98.7%	90.0%	72.0%
GLCM	32 Imglvl	99.2%	98.7%	90.4%	74.2%
LBPc	R1 N8	89.6%	79.8%	86.1%	63.7%
LBPr	R1 N8	88.8%	77.6%	88.4%	74.7%
LBPr	R2 N16	83.3%	65.5%	91.2%	88.5%

Table 3. Accuracy (acc) and average recall (rec) of the particular features of the averaged feature vector (Patchsize 105).

Features	Property	SVM		RF	
		Acc	Rec	Acc	Rec
Histogram	256 bins	82.1%	50.0%	91.2%	85.2%
Histogram	512 bins	82.1%	50.0%	92,0%	83.0%
Histogram	768 bins	82.1%	50.0%	91.2%	83.3%
Homogeneity	—	82.1%	50.0%	94.0%	87.7%
GLCM	8 Imglvl	96.0%	91.5%	96.0%	91.5%
GLCM	16 Imglvl	96.0%	91.5%	95.2%	90.2%
GLCM	32 Imglvl	96.0%	90.6%	96.4%	91.7%
LBPc	R1 N8	84.1%	60.8%	86.9%	74.7%
LBPr	R1 N8	82.1%	50.0%	86.9%	70.3%
LBPr	R2 N16	84.5%	60.2%	90.8%	78.8%

disease. The main drawback of this study is the small patient database and the consequent small image database. Besides this, only preselected images without a high level of noise or image artefacts are investigated, which would decrease the classification process significantly. In addition, only the basic problem, the differentiation between pathological and healthy images is conducted, which leads to the overall very optimistic classification rate. Nevertheless, these results show that a classification in pathological and healthy images can be accomplished with a high accuracy of 99.2%. As the clinical trial is ongoing, the image database is currently increased and in future work a discrimination between different disease stages will be investigated. Therefore, our proposed algorithm may help to improve real time diagnosis of suspicions lesions in the oral cavity to guide subsequent therapy.

Table 4. Accuracy (acc) and average recall (rec) of the particular features of the averaged feature vector (Patchsize 80).

Features	Property	SVM		RF	
		Acc	Rec	Acc	Rec
Histogram	256 bins	82.1%	50.0%	92.0%	83.9%
Histogram	512 bins	82.1%	50.0%	90.8%	84.5%
Histogram	768 bins	82.1%	50.0%	91.2%	83.4%
Homogeneity	—	82.1%	50.0%	93.2%	84.6%
GLCM	8 Imglvl	97.2%	94.8%	95.6%	90.4%
GLCM	16 Imglvl	97.2%	95.7%	94.4%	97.3%
GLCM	32 Imglvl	96.0%	92.4%	98.0%	95.3%
LBPc	R1 N8	82.1%	50.0%	86.1%	70.7%
LBPr	R1 N8	84.9%	64.7%	87.7%	76.9%
LBPr	R2 N16	86.1%	64.6%	90.0%	78.3%

References

1. Mualla F, Schöll S, Bohr C, et al. Epithelial cell detection in endomicroscopy images of the vocal folds. Springer Proc Phy. 2014;154:201–5.
2. Neumann H, Vieth M, Langner C, et al. Cancer risk in IBD: how to diagnose and how to manage DALM and ALM. World J Gastroenterol. 2011;17(27):3184–91.
3. Volgger V, Conderman C, Betz CS. Confocal laser endomicroscopy in head and neck cancer: steps forward? Curr Opin Otolaryngol Head Neck Surg. 2013;21(2):164–70.
4. Couceiro S, Barreto P, Freire P, et al. Machine learning in medical imaging: description and classification of confocal endomicroscopic images for the automatic diagnosis of inflammatory bowel disease. Lect Notes Comput Sci. 2012;7588:144–51.
5. Mualla F, Schöll S, Sommerfeldt B, et al. Automatic cell detection in bright-field microscope images using SIFT, random forests, and hierarchical clustering. IEEE Trans Med Imaging. 2013;32(12):2274–86.
6. Haralick RM, Shanmugam K, Dinstein I. Textural features for image classification. IEEE Trans Syst Man Cybern. 1973;3(6):610–21.
7. Baraldi A, Parmiggiani F. An investigation of the textural characteristics associated with gray level cooccurrence matrix statistical parameters. IEEE Trans Geosci Remote Sens. 1995;33(2):293–304.
8. Pietikainen M, Hadid A, Zhao G, et al. Computer Vision Using Local Binary Patterns. vol. 40 of Computational Imaging and Vision. Springer, London; 2011.
9. Platt J. Sequential minimal optimization: a fast algorithm for training support vector machines. Microsoft Research; 1998.
10. Breiman L. Random forests. Mach Learn. 2001; p. 5–32.

Automatische Tumorsegmentierung mit spärlich annotierter Lernbasis

Michael Götz[1,2], Christian Weber[1,2], Franciszek Binczyck[3,4],
Joanna Polanska[3], Rafal Tarnawski[4], Barbara Bobek-Billewicz[4],
Hans-Peter Meinzer[2], Bram Stieltjes[5], Klaus Maier-Hein[1,2]

[1]Medical Image Computing (MIC), DKFZ Heidelberg
[2]Abteilung für Medizinische und Biologische Informatik, DKFZ Heidelberg
[3]Silesian University of Technology, Gliwice, Poland
[4]M. Skodowska-Curie Memorial Cancer Center and Inst. of Oncology, Gliwice, Poland
[5]Departement Radiologie, Universitätsspital Basel, Schweiz
m.goetz@dkfz-heidelberg.de

Kurzfassung. Die Erstellung von Trainingsdaten für lernbasierte Segmentierungsverfahren ist häufig sehr zeitaufwendig und fehleranfällig. Gleichzeitig muss die Lernbasis an die konkrete Bildgebung einer Klinik angepasst werden, was eine weite Verbreitung solcher automatischer Segmentierungsverfahren in der klinischen Routine verhindert. Wir schlagen daher ein Verfahren vor, welches durch die Verwendung eines Domain Adaption Ansatzes auf spärlichen, leicht anzufertigenden Segmentierungen trainiert werden kann. Wir validieren das vorgestellte System auf einem Kollektiv von 19 Patienten mit malignen Gliomen und zeigen, dass unser Ansatz die benötigte Annotierungszeit deutlich reduziert, während die Klassifikationsergebnisse gegenüber klassisch trainierten Segmentierungsansätzen kaum beeinträchtigt werden. Der vorgestellte Ansatz erhöht die Attraktivität automatischer Segmentierungsverfahren für den klinischen Einsatz. Weiterhin lässt er die Erstellung umfangreicher Datenbanken mit großen Fallzahlen für unterschiedlichste Szenarien in greifbare Nähe rücken.

1 Einleitung

Die Diagnose, Therapie und Verlaufskontrolle von Tumorerkrankungen profitieren von einer vollständigen Segmentierung des Tumors. Diese ist jedoch besonders für maligne Gliome, die häufigsten primären Gehirntumore bei Erwachsenen, sehr zeitaufwendig und fehleranfällig. So veröffentlichten z.B. Mazzara *et al.* Inter-, bzw. Intra-Beobachtervariabilitäten von $20 \pm 15\,\%$ bzw. $28 \pm 12\,\%$ [1]. Mittels einer Automatisierung strebt man daher eine Optimierung des Prozesses an.

Methodisch haben sich in diesem Anwendungsfeld lernbasierte Herangehensweisen, die das Aussehen von Gliomen anhand von Beispieldaten erlernen, bewährt [2]. Derartige Ansätze treffen wenige Annahmen über die Natur der Daten und erlauben es, auf einfache Art, mehrere Informationsquellen, wie z.B. unterschiedliche MR-Sequenzen, zu integrieren.

Nachteil der lernbasierte Ansätze ist jedoch, dass eine Trainingsdatenbank mit bereits segmentierten Bilddaten vorliegen muss. Eine Übertragung einer solchen Trainingsbasis von einer Klinik auf andere Zentren ist aufgrund der Variabilität von MR-Daten im Allgemeinen nicht möglich. Um die vielfältigen Probleme bei der Erstellung von Trainingsdatenbanken zu umgehen, schlagen Verma et al. daher die Nutzung partieller Segmentierungen als Lernbasis vor [3]. Der Ansatz sieht vor, alle eindeutig zuordenbare Regionen zu segmentieren.

Wir erweitern diesen Ansatz, indem wir in der Trainingsdatenbank nur noch wenige kleine und eindeutige Regionen ablegen. Abb. 1 zeigt jeweils ein Beispiel für eine (a) komplette Segmentierung und (b) kleine, eindeutige Regionen. Da das Verhältnis von Merkmalen und Klassen innerhalb der kleinen Regionen nicht dem des gesamten Bildes entspricht, entsteht ein Sampling-Fehler. Wir nehmen an, dass sich der Sampling-Fehler durch einen Covariate-Shift [4] abbilden lässt und korrigieren diesen.

2 Material und Methoden

Wenn nur kleine Regionen innerhalb eines Bildes annotiert werden, führt das zu einem Sampling-Fehler. Manche Gebiete sind innerhalb dieser Regionen über- und andere unterrepräsentiert. Dies gilt sowohl in Bezug auf einzelne Klassen als auch auf die Verteilung der Merkmale innerhalb dieser Klassen. Dadurch ist die Annahme der unabhängigen und gleichmäßigen Verteilung der Trainingsdaten (i.i.d) verletzt.

Konkret bedeutet dies, das Trainingsmaterial spiegelt nicht mehr die Testsituation wieder. Die von Klassifikatoren – direkt oder indirekt – geschätzte Wahrscheinlichkeit $P(x, y)$ von Merkmalen x und Klassen y ist für die Trainings- und Testdaten unterschiedlich. Es liegen also zwei unterschiedliche Domänen vor. Dementsprechend spricht man bei Techniken, die diese Unterschiede korrigieren, von Domain Adaption (DA) Techniken.

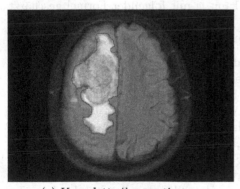
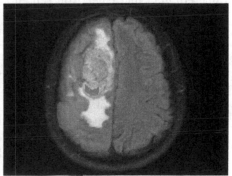

(a) Komplette Segmentierung   (b) Kleine Regionen

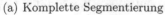

Abb. 1. Eine vollständige Segmentierung (a) ist auch in weiteren Schichten vorhanden, während kleine und eindeutige Regionen (b) meist nur in einer Schicht markiert sind.

Nimmt man an, dass die von den Regionen beinhaltete Merkmale repräsentativ für das gesamte Bild sind, d.h. die Zuordnung von Merkmalen x zu Klassen y der des gesamten Bildes entspricht, dann sind lediglich die Auftretungswahrscheinlichkeiten P für einzelne Merkmale x unterschiedlich

$$P_{\text{Klein}}(y \mid x) = P_{\text{Gesamt}}(y \mid x) \tag{1}$$

$$P_{\text{Klein}}(x) \neq P_{\text{Gesamt}}(x)$$

Diese Situation wird nach Shimodaira als Covariate-Shift bezeichnet [4]. Um sie zu korrigieren schlägt er vor, die einzelnen Datenpunkte mit dem Verhältnis der Auftretungswahrscheinlichkeit der Merkmale zu gewichten

$$w(x) = \frac{P_{\text{Gesamt}}(x)}{P_{\text{Klein}}(x)} \tag{2}$$

Eine anschauliche Deutung bekommt man durch das Einsetzen von (1) und (2)

$$P_{\text{Gesamt}}(x,y) = P_{\text{Gesamt}}(x) \cdot P_{\text{Gesamt}}(y \mid x) = \frac{P_{\text{Klein}}(x)}{P_{\text{Klein}}(x)} \cdot P_{\text{Gesamt}}(x) \cdot P_{\text{Gesamt}}(y \mid x)$$

$$= w(x) \cdot P_{\text{Klein}}(x) \cdot P_{\text{Klein}}(y \mid x) = w(x) * P_{\text{Klein}}(x,y)$$

Der Gewichtungsfaktor w ist in den meisten Anwendungen unbekannt und muss aus den Daten geschätzt werden, wozu verschiedenen Verfahren veröffentlicht wurden [5]. Da in unseren Versuchen die Daten voxelweise klassifiziert werden, fallen große Datenmengen an. Wir haben uns daher entschieden, w mit einem lernbasierten Ansatz zu schätzen. Dieser kann sehr gut mit großen Datenmengen umgehen und wurde bereits in anderen Arbeiten erfolgreich eingesetzt.

Konkret wird für diesen Ansatz ein Logistischer Regressions-Schätzer (LRC) trainiert, der schätzt, ob ein Voxel aus den annotierten Regionen oder dem gesamten Bild stammt. Mit den während dem Training des LRC berechneten Parametern $\theta(x)$ und einer Konstanten c kann w mit folgender Formel geschätzt werden [5]

$$w(x) = c \cdot \exp\left(\theta(x)\right)$$

Die Gewichtung einzelner Datenpunkte haben wir bildweise vorgenommen. D.h., innerhalb jedes Bildes wurden zuerst die kleinen Regionen eingezeichnet. Anschließend wurden für diese die Gewichte berechnet und erst dann diese Daten der Trainingsmenge hinzugefügt. Diese Methode hat gegenüber dem gleichzeitigen Berechnen aller Daten den Vorteil, dass Unterschiede zwischen den einzelnen Bildern in diesem Schritt keine zusätzlichen Fehler einführen.

Als Klassifikatoren werden Random Forests benutzt [6], die bereits erfolgreich für die Segmentierung von Gehirntumoren eingesetzt wurden [2]. Prinzipiell ist dieser Ansatz aber nicht auf eine Art von Klassifikatoren beschränkt. Um eine Überanpassung zu verhindern, wurde die maximale Baumtiefe begrenzt. Weiter wurde die Gini-Impurity $I(V)$ angepasst, um eine Gewichtung der einzelnen Datenpunkte zu ermöglichen. Dafür wird die Klassenwahrscheinlichkeit – anstatt wie bisher über die Anzahl der Punkte – nun über die Summe der Gewichte geschätzt

$$I(V) = 1 - \sum_{y_c \in Y} \left[\frac{1}{\sum w_i} \cdot \sum_{y_j = y_c} w_j \right]$$

Der Ansatz wird mit einer Studie von 19 Patienten mit malignen Gliomen evaluiert. Für jeden Patienten liegen 16 MR-, bzw. MR-abgeleitete Bilder vor, z.B. T2-Flair, T1 mit Kontrastmittel und diffusionsgewichtete Bilder. Der Merkmalsvektor besteht aus den Intensitäten aller Bilder – es werden keine zusätzlichen Merkmale berechnet.

Experten erzeugten für jeden Patienten eine vollständige Segmentierung in die Klassen gesundes und tumoröses Gewebe. Diese wurden iterativ verbessert, um eine ausreichende Qualität zu erreichen. Dazu wurde u.a. der Zeitverlauf der Daten benutzt um Unstimmigkeiten zu finden und zu beheben. Weiter wurden kleine Regionen mit den Klassen „Fluid", „Gesund", „Ödem", „Aktiver Tumor" und „Nekrose" markiert. Im Gegensatz zu den vollständigen Segmentierungen, die immer alle Schichten beinhalten, wurden hier lediglich einzelne, eindeutig einer Gewebeklasse zuordenbare Gebiete ausgewählt. Meistens liegen alle Regionen dabei in einer einzelnen Schicht. Um die Klassen der vollständigen Segmentierungen und die der kleinen Regionen vergleichbar zu machen, wurden die 5 Klassen der Regionen in der Evaluation zu 2 Klassen zusammengefasst.

Basierend auf diesen Daten werden drei unterschiedliche Klassifikatoren trainiert. Der erste Klassifikator wird mit den vollständigen Segmentierungen trainiert, wobei $0,5\%$ aller Voxel zufällig gezogen und für das Training verwendet worden um die Trainingsdauer zu reduzieren. Die beiden anderen Klassifikatoren werden ausschließlich auf den kleinen Regionen trainiert, jeweils einmal mit und einmal ohne eine Anpassung an den Sampling-Fehler.

3   Ergebnisse

3.1   Zeitersparnis

Der Zeitbedarf für die unterschiedlichen Schritte während dieser Versuche ist in Tab. 1 aufgeführt. Sie zeigt, dass eine Trainingsbasis mit kleinen und eindeutigen Segmentierungen deutlich schneller erstellt werden kann. So dauerte das Erstellen der Trainingsbasis mit 19 Patienten für unsere Versuche weniger als 2 Stunden und ist damit schneller als die vollständige Segmentierung eines einzelnen Patienten. Dies ermöglicht auch das prospektive Segmentieren von Patienten während der klinischen Routine.

Die Trainingszeiten bewegen sich alle in einem ähnlichen Rahmen – die Unterschiede sind in der Praxis eher unbedeutend. Das Training ist dann am kürzesten, wenn lediglich kleine Regionen für die Trainingsbasis genutzt werden und am längsten, wenn zusätzlich eine Domänanpassung durchgeführt wird. Ursache hierfür ist die lange Berechnungsdauer von w. Werden mehrere Trainingsvorgänge durchgeführt, ist es deshalb sinnvoll w lediglich einmal pro Patient zu

Tabelle 1. Zeitbedarf für verschiedene Aufgaben.

Methode	Labeling	Training	Prädiktion
Kleine Seg.	< 5 min	12.4 ± 1.1 sec	45.7 ± 4.3 sec
Kleine Seg. mit DA	< 5 min	63.8 ± 14.4 sec	74.4 ± 8.3 sec
Komplett	> 240 min	46.9 ± 1.1 sec	$149.3.4 \pm 16.3$ sec

berechnen und während des eigentlichen Trainings die vorberechneten Werte zu nutzten.

3.2 Segmentierungsqualität

Die Qualität der automatischen Segmentierungen wird anhand des DICE-score bewertet. Die Tumor-Prädikation für jede einzelne Patient/Klassifikator-Kombination wurde mit der manuell erstellten Tumorsegmentierung verglichen. Die Ergebnisse sind in Abb. 2 dargestellt.

Die Resultate, die mit Klassifikatoren der gesamten Segmentierungen erzielt werden, erweisen sich als signifikant (p= .008) besser als die Ergebnisse der Klassifikatoren, die mit kleinen Regionen trainiert werden. Dies ist unserer Ansicht nach hauptsächlich auf zwei Effekte zurückzuführen: Erstens beinhalten die kleinen Regionen weniger Informationen als die kompletten Segmentierungen. Der so trainierte Klassifikator ist deshalb weniger generalisierbar. Das schlägt sich auch in der höheren Varianz der Ergebnisse nieder. Dieses Problem kann durch das Hinzufügen von weiterer Patientendaten behoben werden und ist durch die schnelle Annotierung dieser Daten gut möglich.

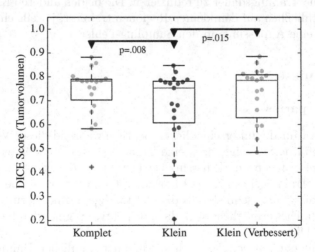

Abb. 2. Die Ergebnisse der Leave-one-out-Experimente mit drei unterschiedlich trainierten Klassifikatoren. Dargestellt wird der DICE-Score zwischen der manuellen und vollständigen Segmentierung gegen die jeweilige automatische Klassifikation für den jeweiligen Patienten. Signifikant unterschiedliche Gruppen sind mit schwarzen Balken verbunden.

Der zweite Grund, der zu einer Verschlechterung der Ergebnisse führt, ist der Sampling-Fehler. Dieser Effekt wird durch DA korrigiert, was zu signifikant ($p = .015$) besseren Ergebnissen führt. Die Leistung ist damit deutlich näher an denen, die mithilfe einer kompletten Segmentierung erreicht werden; zwischen diesen beiden Gruppen ist kein statistisch signifikanter ($p = .10$) Unterschied festzustellen.

4 Diskussion

Wir haben in dieser Arbeit gezeigt, dass Klassifikatoren mit Hilfe von Domain Adaptation erfolgreich auf partiell annotierten Daten trainiert werden können. Der Sampling-Fehler, der dabei während der Erstellung der Trainingsbasis gemacht wird, wird mittels DA korrigiert und der erhaltene Klassifikator weist eine ähnliche Performance auf wie ein Klassifikator, der auf vollständig segmentierten Bilddaten trainiert wird. Dies ist ein wichtiger Schritt, um automatische, lernbasierte Verfahren zur Tumorsegmentierung in die klinische Routine zu integrieren, denn es erlaubt das schnelle Erzeugen und Anpassen einer Trainingsbasis.

Danksagung. Diese Arbeit wurde im Rahmen des von der Deutschen Forschungsgemeinschaft (DFG) geförderten SFB/TRR 125 „Cognition-Guided Surgery" (Projekt I04) erstellt.

Literaturverzeichnis

1. Mazzara GP, Velthuizen RP, Pearlman JL, et al. Brain tumor target volume determination for radiation treatment planning through automated MRI segmentation. Int J Radiat Oncol Biol Phys. 2004.
2. Bauer S, Wiest R, Nolte LP, et al. A survey of MRI-based medical image analysis for brain tumor studies. Phys Med Biol. 2013.
3. Verma R, Zacharaki EI, Ou Y, et al. Multiparametric tissue characterization of brain neoplasms and their recurrence using pattern classification of MR images. Acad Radiol. 2008.
4. Shimodaira H. Improving predictive inference under covariate shift by weighting the log-likelihood function. J Stat Plan Inference. 2000.
5. Sugiyama M, Kawanabe M. Machine Learning in Non-Stationary Environments: Introduction to Covariate Shift Adaptation. MIT Press; 2012.
6. Criminisi A, Shotton J, editors. Decision Forests for Computer Vision and Medical Image Analysis. Springer London; 2013.

3D Tensor Reconstruction in X-Ray Dark-Field Tomography
The First Phantom Result

Shiyang Hu[1,2], Christian Riess[1,3], Joachim Hornegger[1,2], Peter Fischer[1,2],
Florian Bayer[4], Thomas Weber[4], Giesla Anton[4], Andreas Maier[1]

[1]Pattern Recognition Lab, Department of Computer Science, Friedrich-Alexander
University of Erlangen-Nuremberg, Erlangen, Germany
[2]Erlangen Graduate School in Advanced Optical Technologies (SAOT),
Friedrich-Alexander University of Erlangen-Nuremberg, Erlangen, Germany
[3]Department of Radiology, Stanford University, Stanford, California
[4]Erlangen Centre for Astroparticle Physics (ECAP), Friedrich-Alexander University
of Erlangen-Nuremberg, Erlangen, Germany
shiyang.hu@fau.de

Abstract. X-ray dark-field imaging is a novel technique which provides
complementary information on structural variation and density fluctua-
tion. It allows to obtain object structures at micrometer scale and also
contains information on the orientation of these structures. Since it can
be acquired by a conventional X-ray imaging system, dark-field imaging has great potential for medical diagnosis. However, fully recovering
3D orientations in dark-field reconstruction still remains unexplored. In
this paper, we propose an improved reconstruction method based on the
zero-constrained dark-field reconstruction by Bayer *et al.* and a simplified principle axes transformation. A well-defined phantom containing
representative 3D orientations is reconstructed in our experiment. On
average, the structure orientations in the reconstructed volume differ
from the ground truth by 9%. Within the boundaries of an object, the
error drops to 6%. Application of this method in real diagnosis data can
be expected in future.

1 Introduction

X-ray dark-field imaging reveals ultra-small-angle scattering. It has attracted attention in recent years for providing unprecedented information [1]. Such images
are usually obtained by Talbot-Lau grating interferometer with conventional X-
ray tube and detectors [2, 3]. Ultra-small angle scattering is generated by local
orientations of micro-structures in the order of magnitude of the grating period.
Thus dark-field imaging allows reconstruction of structures at length scales below
the resolution of conventional X-ray imaging systems. Dark-field reconstruction
shows great potential for medical diagnosis and specimens in nondestructive materials testing. One promising application is the diagnosis of osteoporosis where
detection of different bone structures is required. Micrometer-sized calcifications

in mammography have been observed in dark-field imaging by Michel et al. [4], which is currently investigated for its suitability for early detection of breast cancer.

Previous work presented experiments in dark-field radiography and observations of periodical dark-field signals caused by structural variation. Several groups partially reconstructed local orientations. Revol t al. exploited prior knowledge on micro-structure orientations to separate isotropic and anisotropic components [5]. Malecki et al. formulated contributions of scattering and sensitivity for each voxel [6]. However, a full 3D reconstruction of vectorial information of the imaging object with separated isotropic and anisotropic contributions is still not available. Bayer et al. [7] successfully reconstructed scalar and vectorial components in dark-field tomography and presented several test specimens. However, the reconstructed local orientation is the projected angle from 3D local orientation and it remains in a 2D plane. In this paper, we present an approach to extend the tensorial information to 3D. This improved method reconstructs two sets of projection data from different imaging coordinate systems and registers them into the same object to acquire fully three-dimensional structures. The proposed method demonstrates that two tomographic scans in different trajectories suffice to recover the microstructure orientation with great accuracy.

2   Materials and methods

1. Reconstruct two sets of dark-field signal by gradient descent method with zero constraints.
2. Register reconstructed results from Step 1 into the same system by center of mass alignment.
3. Calculate 3D local orientation by in-plane angle from Step 1 according to Equation 2.

2.1   Two maging models

Two sets of dark-field projections in different imaging coordinate systems are required for the proposed method. As illustrated in Fig. 1, the object in projection model A is located in the position such that its $\hat{y}$-axis is along y-axis in world coordinate system and is scanned around $\hat{y}$-axis. In projection model B, the $\hat{x}$-axis of the object coordinate system, around which the object is scanned, is aligned with y-axis in world coordinate system.

We reconstruct each set of projections using the gradient descent method with zero constraints proposed in Bayer $et\ al.$ [7]. This computation provides for both image planes the in-plane local orientation as well as its isotropic and anisotropic contributions.

The phantom dimensions are denoted as $M \times N \times L$, $\theta^y, d_{iso}^y, d_{aniso}^y$ denote reconstructed orientations in the $X - Z$ plane and their isotropic and anisotropic contributions to dark-field signal from projection model A, respectively. $d_{iso}^x, d_{aniso}^x, \theta^x$ represent reconstructed isotropic components, anisotropic components and local orientations in $Y - Z$ plane from projection Model B, respectively.

2.2 Registration

Before calculating 3D structures from reconstructed results described above, it is necessary to register both results into the same object due to mechanical instability in the experiments. Therefore, we introduce a simplified principal axes transformation here [8]. In this registration step, we register two sets of data by aligning their center of mass, which is calculated by position (x, y, z) and the isotropic component $d_{\mathrm{iso}}(x, y, z)$ at that position. $d_{\mathrm{iso}}(x, y, z) = d_{\mathrm{iso}}^{y}(x, y, z)$ in projection model A and $d_{\mathrm{iso}}(x, y, z) = d_{\mathrm{iso}}^{x}(x, y, z)$ in projection model B. The center of mass can be expressed as

$$C(d) = [x_c, y_c, z_c] := \frac{\sum_{i=1}^{M} \sum_{j=1}^{N} \sum_{k=1}^{L} d_{iso}(x_i, y_j, z_k) \cdot (x_i, y_j, z_k)}{\sum_{i=1}^{M} \sum_{j=1}^{N} \sum_{k=1}^{L} d_{iso}(x_i, y_j, z_k)} \tag{1}$$

Between the two projection models, we only move the object rigidly. Since we already know the axis around which the object rotates in the two models, only translation needs to be calculated. Thus the center of mass provides sufficient information for our registration. However, we expect that we will require a more sophisticated transform for real data, which is subject to future work.

2.3 3D orientation reconstruction

3D local orientations are calculated from two sets of reconstructed in-plane angles after the registration step. If the unknown orientation is parallel to $\hat{y}$-axis or $\hat{x}$-axis, it will only show isotropic scattering when rotating around the axis it is parallel to. To avoid infinite from tangent, the orientation is set as $(0, 1, 0)$ if $\theta_x = 90°$. A 3D orientation, which is denoted by a unit vector (v_x, v_y, v_z) can be obtained by

$$[v_x, v_y, v_z] = \begin{cases} (1, 0, 0) & \text{if } d_{iso}^x = 0 \\ (0, 1, 0) & \text{if } d_{iso}^y = 0 \\ (0, 1, 0) & \text{if } \theta_x = 90° \\ \frac{(\cos(\theta_y), \sin(\theta_y) \tan(\theta_x), \sin(\theta_y))}{\|(\cos(\theta_y), \sin(\theta_y) \tan(\theta_x), \sin(\theta_y))\|} & \text{otherwise} \end{cases} \tag{2}$$

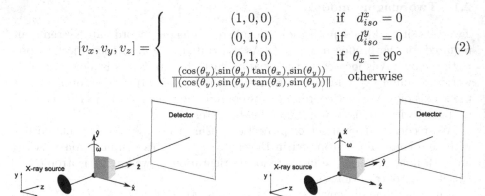

Fig. 1. Two imaging models with different object orientation.

2.4 Experiment

For the tomography scans, 101 projections were taken over 360° for both projection models. For reconstruction, 100 iterative steps have been taken for each projection model.

3 Results

The 3D local orientation dark-field tomography reconstruction was evaluated using a well-defined phantom (Fig. 2, Column A). This phantom was created as a mathematical block of $20 \times 25 \times 30$ pixels in an imaging space of $50 \times 50 \times 50$ pixels. To simulate two imaging models and their mechanical instability, the phantom was positioned differently in each projection model. In projection model A, the center of phantom was located at position $(26, 22, 21)$ in the world system. In projection model B, the center of phantom was positioned at $(28, 25, 16)$ in the world system. The phantom has the isotropic parameter $d_{\mathrm{iso}}(\hat{x}, \hat{y}, \hat{z}) \equiv 1.0$ and anisotropic parameter $d_{\mathrm{aniso}}(\hat{x}, \hat{y}, \hat{z}) \equiv 1.5$. Different local orientations are obtained in five sub-blocks among $\hat{y}$-axis. These orientations are visualized in Fig. 2, Column A1 and Column A2.

From calculation of registration step, center of mass in projection model A is $(26, 22, 21)$ and center of mass in projection model B is $(28, 25, 16)$. This result matches our phantom design.

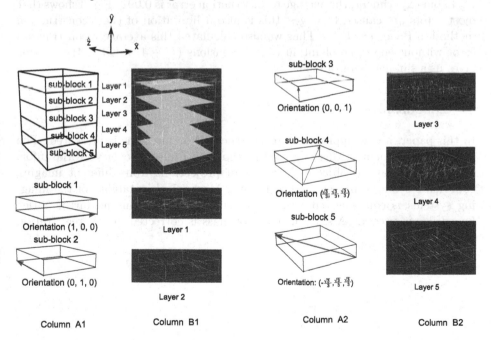

Fig. 2. Orientations from the phantom and reconstructed results. Five representative layers are visualized to show different orientations in each sub-block.

Reconstructed results are visualized in Fig. 2, Column B1 and Column B2. Five representative layers from each sub-block are visualized and compared with the same layer from ground truth in Column A1 and Column A2. Visualization was created using ParaView. The microstructure, which can be represented by $(d_{aniso}v_x, d_{aniso}v_y, d_{aniso}v_z)$ are visualized by lines. The length of each line is the magnitude of its anisotropic component. Orientations are visualized by the line directions. Five representative layers from five sub-blocks are shown in Fig. 2 from top to bottom for both phantom and reconstructed results.

To quantitatively evaluate our algorithm, we calculated the error between reconstructed orientation and ground truth. Error per voxel at position (x, y, z) is defined as

$$e_{pv} = \|(v_x^\star(x,y,z), v_y^\star(x,y,z), v_z^\star(x,y,z)) - (v_x(x,y,z), v_y(x,y,z), v_z(x,y,z))\| \tag{3}$$

where $(v_x^\star, v_y^\star, v_z^\star)$ is a unit vector which denotes local orientation in ground truth.

Fig. 3 shows error per voxel from the five representative layers by color legend of magnitude. Empty space in this visualization implies zero error.

To measure the average error of reconstructed result, we introduce average reconstruction error as

$$e_v = \frac{\sum_{x,y,z} \|(v_x^\star, v_y^\star, v_z^\star) - (v_x, v_y, v_z)\|}{N \cdot M \cdot L} \tag{4}$$

In our experiment, the average reconstruction error is 0.091. Fig. 3 shows that most errors are caused by edges, this is also a limitation of the reconstruction method in Bayer *et al.* [7]. Thus we also calculated this average reconstruction error without edges, i.e phantom with dimensions $(N-4) \times (M-4) \times L$, this gives us a smaller error of 0.059.

4   Discussion

In this paper, a new approach to reconstruct 3D orientations is presented. The major improvement of this proposed method is to fully recover vectorial information in a scanned object. Two sets of projections from different imaging coordinate systems are required as inputs. Mechanical instability of the imaging systems is compensated by a registration step and thus no further prior knowledge is needed. A shift in center of mass is corrected in this registration

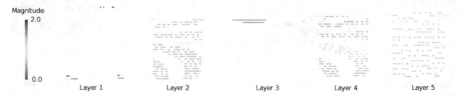

Fig. 3. Visualization of error per voxel at five representative layers according to equation 3. Empty space denotes zero.

step. Visualized microstructure of the well-defined phantom showed that this method is able to reconstruct 3D local orientations. Error measurement shows orientations from reconstructed results have error by 9% from orientations of the phantom and 6% if we omitted edges.

This algorithm shows great potential of dark-field imaging by its ability of providing unique information using a conventional X-ray imaging system. Real data will be examined in our future work. Furthermore, we will investigate how much the axes must deviate to reconstruct a correct image.

Acknowledgement. The authors acknowledge funding of the Erlangen Graduate School in Advanced Optical Technologies (SAOT) by the German Research Foundation (DFG) in the framework of the German excellence initiative. Furthermore, we acknowledge support from the RTG 1773 by the German Research Foundation.

References

1. Kaeppler S, Bayer F, Weber T, et al. Signal decomposition for x-ray dark-field imaging. Lect Notes Computer Sci. 2014;8673:170–7.
2. Pfeiffer F, Bech M, Bunk O, et al. Hard-x-ray dark-field imaging using a grating interferometer. Nat Mater. 2008;7(2):134–7.
3. Yashiro W, Terui Y, Kawabata K, et al. On the origin of visibility contrast in x-ray talbot interferometry. Opt Express. 2010;18(16):16890–1.
4. Michel T, Rieger J, Anton G, et al. On a dark-field signal generated by micrometer-sized calcifications in phase-contrast mammography. Phys Med Biol. 2013;58(8):2713.
5. Revol V, Kottler C, Kaufmann R, et al. Orientation-selective x-ray dark field imaging of ordered systems. J Appl Phys. 2012;112(11):114903.
6. Malecki A, Potdevin G, Biernath T, et al. X-ray tensor tomography. Europhys Lett. 2014;105(3):38002.
7. Bayer FL, Hu S, Maier A, et al. Reconstruction of scalar and vectorial components in x-ray dark-field tomography. Proc Natl Acad Sci USA. 2014;111(35):12699–704.
8. Modersitzki J. Numerical Methods for Image Registration. OUP Oxford; 2003.

Towards 3D Thyroid Imaging Using Robotic Mini Gamma Cameras

Tobias Lasser[1], José Gardiazabal[1,2], Matthias Wieczorek[1], Philipp Matthies[1],
Jakob Vogel[1], Benjamin Frisch[1], Nassir Navab[1,3]

[1]Computer Aided Medical Procedures (CAMP), Technische Universität München
[2]Department of Nuclear Medicine, Klinikum Rechts der Isar, Technische Universität
München
[3]Robotics, Vision & Graphics, Johns Hopkins University
lasser@in.tum.de

Abstract. Thyroid imaging using radioactive tracers is a common task
in clinics and is usually performed using 2D gamma cameras (scintigraphy). In this work we present a setup for 3D imaging of the thyroid
using a mini gamma camera mounted on a robotic arm. Several images
are acquired moving the mini gamma camera along a trajectory around
the thyroid. Afterwards, a tomographic reconstruction computes a 3D
SPECT-like image of the thyroid. First results are shown of a thyroid
phantom using a conventional statistical reconstruction scheme (MLEM)
and using a sparse regularization approach based on total variation.

1 Introduction

The thyroid is a very commonly imaged organ in nuclear medicine. For this, radioactive tracers are injected systemically into the patient (one common tracer
is ^{99m}Tc-Pertechnetat), and then the thyroid is imaged using a 2D gamma camera (this process is called scintigraphy, see [1]). Additional imaging is also often
performed with ultrasound [2]. It has been indicated that three-dimensional nuclear imaging (SPECT) can improve the diagnosis over planar scintigraphy [3, 4].
Doing a SPECT scan however loses the advantage of easy patient handling and
fast imaging times compared to planar scintigraphy.

It has been shown in the last few years that localized SPECT-like reconstructions can be performed using a mobile, hand-held single pixel detector (called
freehand SPECT [5]), while keeping the ease of patient handling and fast imaging times of planar scintigraphy. Recent developments employing a mini gamma
camera held by a robotic arm have shown significant increases in imaging quality [6], while still using a fairly mobile setup.

In this work we show the application of a mobile, robotic mini gamma camera
to the thyroid imaging case, allowing for easy patient handling and fast imaging
times. We demonstrate first results using a thyroid phantom and reconstructing
with the standard statistical reconstruction method (MLEM [7]). As the thyroid typically contains some homogeneous areas with a sparse gradient, we also
demonstrate total variation regularized reconstructions (similar to [8]) in order
to show if image quality improves for this application.

2   Materials and methods

2.1 Hardware setup

We use a 16×16 pixel gamma camera (CrystalCam, Crystal Photonics, Germany) with a CdZnTe crystal ($4 \times 4\,cm^2$) and a lead/tungsten collimator, mounted on a robotic arm (UR5, Universal Robots, Denmark) using a custom-printed mount (Fig. 1(a)). The robotic arm moves the mini gamma camera around the object to be measured, a custom-printed thyroid phantom (Fig. 1(b)).

2.2 Thyroid phantom

The phantom was designed to mimick a regular thyroid, with embedded nodules to simulate hot and cold regions of the thyroid. The thyroid (with a width, height and depth of 52 mm, 48 mm and 13 mm, respectively) is contained in a rectangular water-tight box (dimensions $63 \times 69 \times 24\,mm^3$). Three nodules have spherical shapes (with diameters of 6 mm, 8 mm and 8 mm), while the fourth nodule is shaped like an elongated capsule (height 20 mm and width 8 mm), as illustrated in Fig. 1(b).

The thyroid shape in the phantom was filled with a solution of ^{99m}Tc (total activity 7 MBq). 3.5 MBq of activity was deposited in three of the four nodules, while the remaining 3.5 MBq was deposited as background throughout the thyroid (yielding a foreground to background ratio of 10:1). The rectangular box around the thyroid shape was filled with water.

2.3 Data acquisition

For data acquisition the robot moved the mini gamma camera around the thyroid phantom in three half-circular trajectories at different areas on the phantom, stopping at 9 positions each for 10 s exposure time to record an image, for a total of 27 images. Total acquisition time was thus 4.5 minutes.

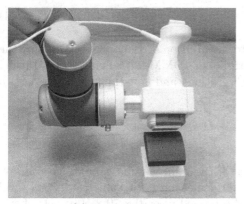 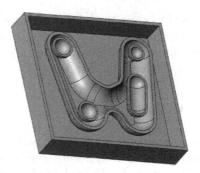

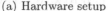

(a) Hardware setup   (b) Thyroid phantom

Fig. 1. Photo of experimental setup with robotic arm holding mini gamma camera and phantom (a) and illustration of the phantom by cutting through its middle (b).

2.4   Tomographic reconstruction

For tomographic reconstruction we consider the radioactivity distribution in the object $V \subset \mathbb{R}^3$ as a non-negative signal $f : V \to \mathbb{R}$. We discretize this signal using an expansion of voxel basis functions $b_i : V \to [0, \infty)$

$$f(\cdot) \approx \sum_i x_i b_i(\cdot) \tag{1}$$

where $\mathbf{x} = (x_i) \in \mathbb{R}^n$ denotes the vector of unknown values to be reconstructed, describing the amount of radioactivity in each voxel location.

To model the detection process, we measure the response of the mini gamma camera to a point-like source at various locations in V (see [6] for details). We denote the resulting detection probabilities as $p(i, j)$, the probability of a detector j detecting emissions from voxel i. The detector readings $\mathbf{m} = (m_j) \in \mathbb{R}^m$ can be interpreted as independently distributed Poisson random variables with expectation

$$E(m_j) = \sum_i x_i \cdot p(i, j) \tag{2}$$

The traditional way of doing reconstruction for emission tomography is now to maximize the likelihood [7]

$$L(\mathbf{x}|\mathbf{m}) = m_j \log \left(\sum_i x_i \cdot p(i, j) \right) - \sum_i x_i \cdot p(i, j) \tag{3}$$

which we do by employing the maximum likelihood expectation maximization (MLEM) approach as outlined in [7].

Alternatively, we can interpret equation (2) as a linear system of equations using the matrix $\mathbf{A} = \left(p(i, j) \right)_{i,j} \in \mathbb{R}^{m \times n}$. We can then compute a regularized least squares approximation to the solution of

$$\arg\min_{\mathbf{x}} \|\mathbf{A}\mathbf{x} - \mathbf{m}\|_2^2 + \lambda \|\mathrm{TV}(\mathbf{x})\|_1 \tag{4}$$

where $\mathrm{TV}(\mathbf{x})$ denotes the anisotropic total variation of $\mathbf{x}$. For this we employ the Alternating Direction Method of Multipliers (ADMM [9]) solving method using three linear conjugate gradient inner iterations and soft-thresholding (see [10] for implementation details).

3   Results

The data was acquired at 27 positions of the mini gamma camera with an exposure time of 10 s, resulting in $m = 6912$ measurement values. (280683 total counts detected). The volume V was discretized into $70 \times 70 \times 50$ voxels of size $1 \times 1 \times 1\,\mathrm{mm}^3$ (yielding $n = 245000$ voxels).

The data was reconstructed twice, once using 50 iterations of the MLEM algorithm maximizing the likelihood (3), the result is shown in Fig. 2(a). The time for reconstruction on an Intel i7-3720QM system with 16GB RAM was 73 s. The second time the data was reconstructed using 50 iterations of the ADMM algorithm computing a TV-regularized least squares approximation (4), the result is shown in Fig. 2(b). The time for reconstruction on the same system was 753 s. The regularization parameter λ was chosen manually.

The same images are shown again in Fig. 2(c),2(d) with the typical SPECT approach of post-smoothing with a 2D Gaussian filter ($\sigma = 1\,mm$). All images are showing a projection of the central slices (slice 20 to 30) of V, windowed to the intensities $[0.00075, 0.06]$.

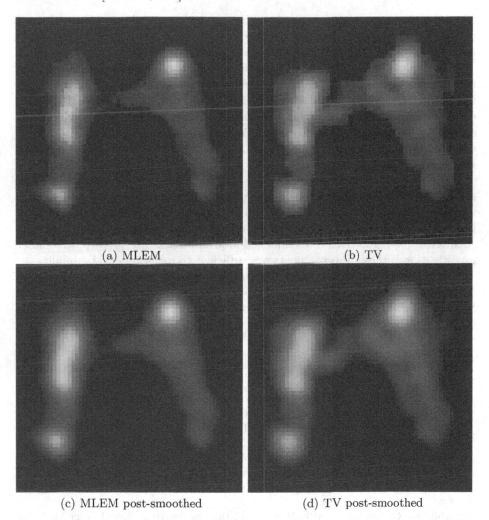

(a) MLEM   (b) TV

(c) MLEM post-smoothed   (d) TV post-smoothed

Fig. 2. Results of thyroid phantom reconstructions. Top row: without post-smoothing; Bottom row: with post-smoothing (projection of central slices, windowed to $[0.00075, 0.06]$).

The MLEM approach shows a smoother image of the thyroid, but catches less of the radioactive background of the thyroid phantom. The TV shows more of the radioactive background, however there are more artifacts compared to the MLEM result (particularly outside the central slices, images not shown for brevity). The cold nodule at the bottom right is not visible in either reconstruction.

4 Discussion

The MLEM reconstruction manages to display the hot nodules inside the thyroid phantom quite nicely. However, the radioactive background is not completely reconstructed, and the cold nodule is not visible either.

In comparison, the TV reconstruction shows the hot nodules quite well too, reconstructs somewhat more of the radioactive background, but also fails to reconstruct the cold nodule. It also shows more artifacts than the MLEM reconstruction, owing to the relatively unsuited least squares approach (4). It should be advantageous to also use a Poisson likelihood approach here, which together with the TV regularization should yield improved results (this is a work in progress).

Overall, however, image quality does not quite reach the diagnostic levels of regular SPECT yet. Improvements are possible in many aspects, for example a more sensitive mini gamma camera, longer integration times, more acquisition positions or better angular coverage as well as improved reconstruction methods, such as a TV-regularized Poisson likelihood approach. It is currently under investigation if these improvements are sufficient to reach diagnostic quality.

In summary, we have presented a simple, low-cost mobile setup to quickly acquire 3D nuclear images of the thyroid, without the complications of a full SPECT scan. First results on a thyroid phantom show a potential for this approach to be clinically useful.

References

1. Meller J, Becker W. The continuing importance of thyroid scintigraphy in the era of high-resolution ultrasound. Eur J Nucl Med Mol Imaging. 2002;29(2):S425–38.
2. Gühne F, Winkens T, Mothes H, et al. Differential diagnosis of thyroid nodules via real-time PET/ultrasound (US) fusion in a case of co-existing medullary thyroid cancer and adenoma. J Clin Endocrinol Metab. 2013;98(11):4250–1.
3. Avram AM. Radioiodine scintigraphy with SPECT/CT: an important diagnostic tool for thyroid cancer staging and risk stratification. J Nucl Med. 2012;53(5):754–64.
4. Abikhzer G, Keidar Z. SPECT/CT and tumour imaging. Eur J Nucl Med Mol Imaging. 2014;41(1):67–80.
5. Wendler T, Herrmann K, Schnelzer A, et al. First demonstration of 3D lymphatic mapping in breast cancer using freehand SPECT. Eur J Nucl Med Mol Imaging. 2010;37(8):1452–61.

6. Matthies P, Gardiazabal J, Okur A, et al. Mini gamma cameras for intra-operative nuclear tomographic reconstruction. Med Image Anal. 2014;18(8):1329–36.
7. Shepp LA, Vardi Y. Maximum likelihood reconstruction for emission tomography. IEEE Trans Med Imaging. 1982;1(2):113–22.
8. Panin VY, Zeng GL, Gullberg GT. Total variation regulated EM algorithm SPECT reconstruction. IEEE Trans Nucl Sci. 1999;46(6):2202–10.
9. Boyd S. Distributed optimization and statistical learning via the alternating direction method of multipliers. FNT Mach Learn. 2011;3(1):1–122.
10. Wieczorek M, Vogel J, Lasser T. CampRecon. TUM Tech. Rep.; 2014.

Investigation of Single Photon Emission Computed Tomography Acquired on Helical Trajectories

Maximilian P. Oppelt, James C. Sanders, Andreas Maier

Pattern Recognition Lab, FAU Erlangen-Nuremberg
maximilian.oppelt@fau.de

Abstract. This study compares the quality of single photon emission computed tomography images obtained using step-and-shoot and helical trajectories. Monte Carlo simulations of an extended phantom on both trajectories were performed using a parallel hole collimator. Standard filtered-backprojection was used for reconstruction. Both trajectories collected data for the same amount of time. Corresponding to equivalent useful acquisition times, the background signal-to-noise ratios and sphere to background contrasts were roughly equivalent in both reconstructions. However, the helical trajectory requires 20% less true acquisition time due to the elimination of delay due to detector repositioning. Helical trajectories in SPECT can thus reduce overall acquisition time while having negligible effects on image quality.

1 Introduction

Single photon emission computed tomography (SPECT) is a nuclear imaging modality that provides three-dimensional functional information of different tissues. It utilizes distribution properties of radioactive tracers injected into the human body to image processes such as blood perfusion and metabolism and aid in the detection of tumors or other pathologies. During a tomographic scan, the detector is rotated about the patient in discrete steps, with time loss between projections during which no data are acquired. Additionally, a translation of the bed between circular rotations is required if the anatomical region of interest exceeds the detector's axial field of view.

This procedure, referred to as step-and-shoot here, is standard in clinical applications and has several limitations. The most obvious of these is the time loss between projections, which may approach three seconds in a commercial system. Another drawback is the overlap required by adjacent bed positions to limit artifacts that may occur during the connection, or *zipping*, of neighboring reconstructions. This overlap requires extra rotations, and, together with the time loss between projections, requires the patient to endure a longer time within in the imaging device.

In 1993, Weng et al. originally introduced an approach for reconstructing helical cone-beam SPECT images [1], the primary motivation for which was the fulfillment of data sufficiency conditions. Despite the utility of cone-beam SPECT, most of the clinical imaging systems use parallel projection geometry and thus circumvent the data sufficiency issues associated with cone-beam collimation. Subsequent work focused on the sister modality of Positron Emission Tomography (PET), where groups such as Townsend et al. in [2] and Braun et al. in [3] proposed whole body spiral PET with continuous bed motion and extension to PET/MR, respectively. Both authors showed equivalent to slightly better statistical properties due to improved axial uniformity, and indicated that time savings were possible due to elimination of discrete bed translations. Braun et al. also concluded that continuous bed motion brings a higher flexibility in simultaneous PET and MR whole-body data acquisition. In SPECT imaging, a variant of continuous detector rotation was proposed by Cao et al. in [4], where a rough equivalence between it and standard step-and-shoot was shown.

The goal of this work is to investigate the feasibility of using continuous detector and bed motion in SPECT imaging to provide equivalent image quality in less total acquisition time. To accomplish this, we employ a novel helical acquisition trajectory and compare it to step-and-shoot using Monte Carlo simulations. The results of these simulations, as well as a discussion and outlook, are presented below.

2   Materials and methods

2.1   Experimental data and simulation

A voxelized cylinder phantom with radius 22 pixels and axial length 192 pixels was created, and two sets of six spheres with diameters of 6.5, 5.2, 4.1, 3.2, 2.6, 2.1 pixels in a hexagonal formation were centered in axial planes 96 and 160 (Fig. 1). The spheres were given a contrast of 5:1 relative to the rest of the cylinder to emulate hot objects in a warm background. With a virtual pixel size of 4.8 mm, they represent respective volumes of 16, 8, 4, 2, 1 and 0.5 ml found in the commonly used Jaszczak phantom.

We used the SIMIND Monte Carlo simulation program to generate SPECT projection data [5], where the detector was rotated, and the phantom shifted

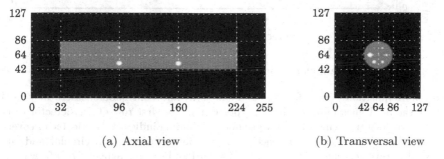

(a) Axial view   (b) Transversal view

Fig. 1. Transversal and axial view of the phantom source density map.

between projections to emulate various acquisition trajectory parameters. The detector had axial and transverse dimensions of 64 and 128 pixels, respectively, and the pixel size was matched to the phantom's at 4.8 mm. A single detector head outfitted with a low energy high resolution, parallel hole collimator was simulated, and all orbits were circular with a radius of 25 cm. Projections were scaled and Poisson noise incorporated to achieve realistic noise levels that would be obtained if the phantom were loaded with 700 MBq of ^{99m}Tc and acquired for dwell times discussed below. The effects of scatter and attenuation were neglected in this preliminary investigation

2.2 Acquisition trajectories

Our proposed acquisition trajectory in Fig. 2(a) consists of one circular continuous rotation with no bed movement followed by a pair of continuous helix rotations with a constant forward bed speed. This is then followed by a second circular rotation at the opposite end of the phantom and concludes with two continuous helix rotations with a constant reverse bed speed. The rotation speed is constant, and each complete orbit lasts 900 seconds, throughout which data are acquired, thus yielding a total useful acquisition time of 90 minutes. Our

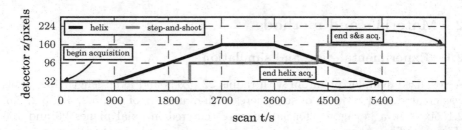

(a) Detector position versus true acquisition time

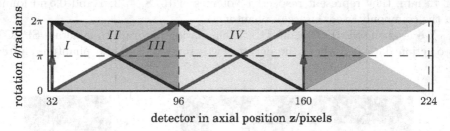

(b) Angular sampling for continuous camera motion

Fig. 2. Acquisition details for step-and-shoot (a) and continuous camera motion (b), where the bold lines indicate the axial position of the first row of the detector (green: circle, red: forward helix, blue: reverse helix). Shading indicates the degree of coverage for each position in sinogram space. (*I*): circular rotation, (*II*): circular and either forward or reverse helical, (*III*) circular, forward and reverse helical, (*IV*) forward and reverse helix.

simulated projection duration was 2.5 seconds, which provided 360 projections for each rotation.

Fig. 2(b) shows the resulting coverage in sinogram space. The white areas *I)* are only scanned once with a circular trajectory, lightly shaded areas (*II* and *IV*) are scanned twice with either a combination of circular and helical or two helical rotations, respectively. Darkly shaded regions (*III*) are scanned three times, with a circular and both forward and reverse helical orbits.

In order to compare the results of our helical scan to the standard step and shoot case, we performed a second simulation incorporating orbits of 120 projections over a 360 degree arc at three axial positions. The projection time was set to the 15 seconds often used in clinical situations, yielding a total useful acquisition time equivalent to the helix case. In practice, roughly three seconds is spent rotating the camera between projections, leading to the longer total acquisition time reflected by the light gray curve in Fig. 2(a). The overlap between axial positions used in clinical situations was neglected.

2.3 Reconstruction and evaluation

To reconstruct our helical trajectory, we rebinned the acquired data into a pseudo-step and shoot sinogram. Our sinogram is binned in 360 steps for a full rotation, and for each angle in the sinogram the columns of the detector are interpolated to a 128x64 pixel gird. If one pixel is measured multiple times, the average is computed. Reconstruction of the sinograms was carried out using the standard filtered-backprojection method with a ramp filter [6].

For evaluation, we computed the contrast in the spheres relative to a region in the center of the phantom. We also computed the signal to noise ratio (SNR) in each homogeneous phantom slice. This was defined as follows: $SNR = \frac{\mu_{sig}}{\sigma_{bg}}$.

3 Results

The reconstructed results are shown in Fig. 3. Visual inspection indicates the image quality within the phantom to be roughly equivalent, although streaking artifacts outside the cylinder are more apparent in the step-and-shoot case.

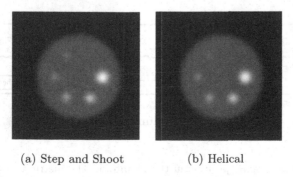

(a) Step and Shoot   (b) Helical

Fig. 3. Filtered backprojection of slices with spheres within volume.

Table 1. Sphere to background contrasts for source map (C_{src}), helix (C_{helix}) and step-and-shoot ($C_{S\&S}$) acquisition trajectories. The average value for a given sphere size over the two sets is reported.

D(pixels)	C_{src}	C_{helix}	$C_{S\&S}$
6.5	5.0	4.36	4.21
5.2	5.0	3.64	3.56
4.1	5.0	2.91	2.91
3.2	5.0	2.25	2.26
2.6	5.0	1.77	1.75
2.1	5.0	1.19	1.27

Sphere contrast appears equal, and the smaller spheres suffer from partial volume effects caused by the collimator's point spread function. Visual impressions in the spheres are confirmed by the contrasts reported in Tab. 1, which show no significant difference between the two methods.

The SNR is shown for each axial position in Fig. 4, where the helix acquisition yields slightly better noise characteristics, potentially corresponding to a reduction in streaking artifacts within the phantom. Nevertheless, this difference is very small and subjectively difficult to discern in the images. A slight dip in helix acquisition's SNR is visible at both ends of the phantom corresponding to the areas of single coverage indicated in Fig. 2(b).

4 Discussion

We have shown that for an acquisition on helical trajectories with both continuous bed and detector motion, the image quality is approximately equivalent to the case of an analogous step-and-shoot trajectory. Both acquisitions yield the same *useful* acquisition time for acquiring data, but the step-and-shoot case requires approximately 20% more *true* acquisition time for detector repositioning. In practice, axial overlap is required by step-and-shoot methods to prevent reconstruction artifacts, leading to even more time losses relative to our proposed helix acquisition.

This time saving could be further increased by using statistical iterative reconstruction methods like Maximum Likelihood Expectation Maximization,

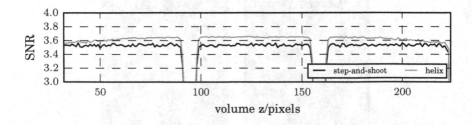

Fig. 4. SNR at each axial position in the phantom. The metric was not computed in slices containing spheres, hence the pair of dips in the curves.

which circumvent the angular sampling requirement of filtered backprojection and would allow one to shorten the circular rotations at the ends of the phantom. We can also think of varying the speed of axial and rotational motion during the acquisition to have more control over the temporal resolution and statistical properties of the acquisition.

However, the study is not without limitations. Specifically, our simulation method assumed a stationary volume during each 2.5 second projection. However, for a true acquisition with continuous bed and detector motion, the volume would be translated by 0.85 mm, and rotated by one degree during this time, leading to a finite amount of blurring. In SPECT imaging, resolution loss due to relatively large detector pixel sizes and wide point spread functions (both on the order of several millimeters) may dominate this blurring, but its characterization would become important for higher-resolution systems or faster acquisition trajectories. Additionally, we did not consider the physical effects of scatter and attenuation, which are a further image quality impediment in SPECT imaging.

4.1 Conclusion

Using helical trajectories in SPECT saves *true* acquisition time, while maintaining the image quality of traditional step-and-shoot protocols. In this experiment, we observed no adverse effects of a helical trajectory, but this conclusion must be qualified by our exclusion of physical factors such as detector movement during the projection, attenuation, and scatter. Nevertheless, our results motivate further investigation of SPECT acquisition on helical trajectories and a more thorough characterization of the aforementioned effects excluded here.

References

1. Weng Y, Zeng G, Gullberg G. A reconstruction algorithm for helical cone-beam SPECT. IEEE Nucl Sci Symp Conf Rec. 1993;40(4):1092–101.
2. Townsend DW, Reed J, Newport DF, et al.; IEEE. Continuous bed motion acquisition for an LSO PET/CT scanner. IEEE Nucl Sci Symp Conf Rec. 2004;4:2383–7.
3. Braun H, Ziegler S, Lentschig MG, et al. Implementation and performance evaluation of simultaneous PET/MR whole-body imaging with continuous table motion. J Nucl Med. 2014;55(1):161–8.
4. Cao Z, Maunoury C, Chen CC, et al. Comparison of continuous step-and-shoot versus step-and-shoot acquisition SPECT. J Nucl Med. 1996;37(12):2037–40.
5. Ljungberg M, Strand SE. A Monte Carlo program for the simulation of scintillation camera characteristics. Comput Methods Programs Biomed. 1989;29(4):257–72.
6. Bracewell RH, Riddle AC. Inversion of fan beam scans in radio astronomy. Astrophys J. 1967;150:427–34.

Blind Sparse Motion MRI with Linear Subpixel Interpolation

Anita Möller, Marco Maaß, Alfred Mertins

Institute for Signal Processing, University of Lübeck
moeller@isip.uni-luebeck.de

Abstract. Vital and spontaneous motion causes major artifacts in MRI. In this paper a method is presented which reduces subpixel motion artifacts via computational post processing on a complete MR scan without additional data. On the compressed sparse MRI representation, translational subpixel motion is estimated iteratively from a fully sampled, but motion corrupted k-space, and motion free images are reconstructed by linear interpolation. Motion adjusted results are presented for the Shepp-Logan phantom and brainweb data.

1 Introduction

In MRI, patient motion causes artifacts like ghost replications of the object. Therefore, spontaneous and unavoidable motion like heart beating or breathing causes problems in clinical diagnosis. Regularly applied methods such as motion avoidance through extended breath holding significantly reduces patient comfort. On the other hand, a reconstruction including motion correction is a complex task, due to the fact that each k-space point is related to two degrees of freedom in two dimensional rigid motion.

In compressed sensing, the data compressibility is used to reduce the amount of measurements that are necessary to reconstruct an image from the k-space [1]. The time needed for an MRI scan and consequently the possibility of patient motion is reduced, but it can not be excluded. Other approaches use navigators which are additionally recorded information used to calculate the motion which is included in reconstruction [2].

A sparsity based algorithm was proposed in [3]. The sparsity of MR images in the wavelet domain and the redundancy of a fully sampled k-space are used to estimate rigid motion. However, the phase-based motion model used in this approach is not suitable for realistic subpixel movement. Subpixel frequency interpolation causes ringing artifacts in the image which has to be avoided.

2 Materials and methods

The method proposed in this paper introduces a linear subpixel motion interpolation model in the image domain. The motion used for reconstruction is blindly estimated on a fully sampled k-space without additional measurements.

The sparsity-based estimation used in [3] is applied and extended for subpixel movement: a translational movement of the object during an MRI scan occurs as a circular shift of the object in the image domain. Let $X \in \mathbb{R}^{m,n}$ be an arbitrary discrete image. A circular shift in one image dimension by $b = n + d$, $n \in \mathbb{N}$, $d \in (0,1]$ with linear interpolation between adjacent pixels can be formulated using convolution matrices of the form

$$
C_d = \begin{bmatrix}
1-d & d & 0 & 0 & \cdots & & 0 \\
0 & 1-d & d & 0 & \cdots & & 0 \\
\vdots & \ddots & \ddots & \ddots & \ddots & & \vdots \\
0 & \cdots & 0 & 1-d & d & & 0 \\
0 & \cdots & \cdots & 0 & 1-d & & d \\
d & 0 & \cdots & \cdots & 0 & & 1-d
\end{bmatrix}
\tag{1}
$$

A two dimensional positive image shift $S_b[X]$ with $b = (b^y, b^x)$ is calculated as

$$
S_b[X] = C_{d^y} C_1^{n^y} X \left(C_1^{n^x} \right)^T C_{d^x}^T
\tag{2}
$$

where $n^x, n^y \in \mathbb{N}$ denote the numbers of full pixel shifts in both directions and d^x, d^y denote subpixel shifts (upper indices x, y denote directions). Due to circularity, negative shifts are realized as large positive shifts.

2.1 Recording of k-space

In MR imaging, the k-space $K \in \mathbb{R}^{m,n}$ is recorded. More exactly, one line of the k-space denoted by $K(k^y, \cdot)$, $k^y = 1, ..., m$ is generated at one measurement read-out. Assuming that the movement during one measurement is constant due to short recording time, one line of the recorded k-space $\hat{K}$ gained from a shifted image $S_{b_{k_y}}[X]$ can be modeled as

$$
\hat{K}(k^y, \cdot) = e_{k^y}^T \mathcal{F}^y S_{b_{k_y}}[X] \mathcal{F}^x
\tag{3}
$$

by applying the Fourier transform matrices $\mathcal{F}^y, \mathcal{F}^x$ in x- and y-direction, respectively and selecting one line with the unit vector e_{k^y}. Let $F[X]$ be an operator which applies the Fourier transform to X in the way $F[X] = \mathcal{F}^y X \mathcal{F}^x$. Then, the whole k-Space is gained as

$$
\hat{K} = F_B[X] = \left[e_{k^y}^T F \left[S_{b_{k_y}}[X] \right] \right]_{k^y=1}^m \quad \text{with} \quad B = [b_{k^y}^y, b_{k^y}^x]_{k^y=1}^m
\tag{4}
$$

A further reformulation step uses the property that the multiplication of two convolution matrices stays a convolution matrix. Also, $\mathcal{F}C = D\mathcal{F}$, $C^T\mathcal{F} = \mathcal{F}D$ holds for a convolution matrix C and a corresponding $D = \mathcal{F}C\mathcal{F}^H$ with $\mathcal{F}$ being a one-dimensional Fourier matrix and D a diagonal matrix. Now, (4) yields

$$
\hat{K} = F_B[X] = \left[e_{k^y}^T D_{k^y} [F[X]] \right]_{k^y=1}^m =: Q_B[F[X]]
\tag{5}
$$

2.2   Reconstruction algorithm

It is assumed that an MR image without motion artifacts has the highest sparsity compared to images gained from the same but moved object [3]. This assumption is founded in MRI artifacts being shifted ghost replications of the object. Using the wavelet transform as sparsifying transform, the problem is formulated similar to [4] as

$$\arg\min_{X,B} \left\| \hat{K} - Q_B\left[F\left[X\right]\right]\right\|_F \text{ subject to } \left\|\mathcal{W}X\right\|_1 \leq c, \, B \in \mathcal{D}_B \qquad (6)$$

The sparsifying constant $c > 0$ has to be determined experimentally in the later given algorithm with a few propositions [4]. The space $\mathcal{D}_B$ defines motion constraints. For each point in one k-space line, the same translational motion should be estimated and also subpixel motion is permitted as advantage to [3].

The iterative motion estimation is divided into three steps [3]. At first, a sparse representation $\tilde{X}$ of $\hat{X} = F^{-1}[\hat{K}]$ is found. Secondly, the motion between $\tilde{X}$ and $\hat{X}$ is calculated. At the third step, the estimated motion is used to find a better $\tilde{K}$ as approximation of $\hat{K}$ to reconstruct the corresponding new $\tilde{X}$ with which the algorithm is started again.

3   Results

The presented algorithm was tested on the Shepp-Logan phantom and human brain images [5]. As different sizes of the images were tested with similar results, representatives of 256×256 pixels for the Shepp-Logan phantom and of 217×181 pixels for the brain images were chosen (Fig. 1).

Starting from the assumptions $\tilde{B} = 0$ and $\tilde{K} = \hat{K}$, the subproblem

$$\tilde{X} = \arg\min_{X} \left\| \tilde{K} - Q_{\tilde{B}}\left[F\left[X\right]\right]\right\|_F \text{ subject to } \left\|\mathcal{W}X\right\|_1 \leq c \qquad (7)$$

is solved by an algorithm proposed in [3], which keeps the largest entries in $\mathcal{W}F^{-1}[\tilde{K}]$, so that $\left\|\mathcal{W}F^{-1}[\tilde{K}]\right\|_1 \leq c$, and sets all other entries to zero ($\mathcal{W}$ denotes the wavelet transform). This step solves the subproblem

$$\tilde{B} = \arg\min_{B} \left\| \tilde{K} - Q_B\left[F[\tilde{X}]\right]\right\|_F \text{ subject to } B \in \mathcal{D}_B \qquad (8)$$

Fig. 1. Shepp-Logan phantom (left) and human brain image (right).

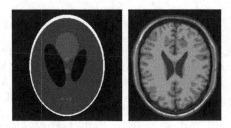

As the properties of the Fourier transform deliver, the relation of the k-space $K \in \mathbb{R}^{m,n}$ of an unmoved object and $\hat{K}$ is found in the phase and written as

$$\hat{K}(k^y, k^x) = \exp\left(-i2\pi\left(\frac{k^y}{m}b_{y_{k^y}} + \frac{k^x}{n}b_{x_{k^y}}\right)\right) K(k^y, k^x) \qquad (9)$$

as explained in [4]. This property is used for motion estimation based on [2]. For each k-space line, the motion is calculated separately between $\mathcal{F}\tilde{X}$ as motion corrected k-space approximation and $\tilde{K}$. As derived in [2], the motion in x-direction by $b_{k^y}^x$ can be calculated as index of the maximal cross-correlation of $\mathcal{F}\tilde{X}(k^y, \cdot)$ and $\tilde{K}(k^y, \cdot)$. To extend this for subpixel motion, a parabola is generated with the correlation maximum and its both neighbors. The index of the parabola maximum approximates the shift $b_{k^y}^x$. The shift $b_{k^y}^y$ is calculated from the phase of the maximal correlation [2].

To update $\hat{K}$ with the estimated $\tilde{B}$ in order to find a better approximation for the motion free k-space, the shift operation has to be revoked. Starting with the shifts b^x in x-direction and (3), the following recursion is derived

$$\hat{K}(k^y, \cdot) = e_{k^y}\mathcal{F}^y\hat{X}\mathcal{F}^x \qquad (10)$$

$$\Leftrightarrow \qquad \hat{K}\left(k^y, \cdot \mathcal{F}^{x^{-1}}\right) = e_{k^y}\mathcal{F}^yC_{d^y}C_1^{n^y}X(C_1^{n^x})^TC_{d^x}^T \qquad (11)$$

$$\Leftrightarrow \underbrace{\hat{K}(k^y, \cdot)\mathcal{F}^{x^{-1}}C_{-d^x+1}^T\left(C_0^{n^x+1}\right)^T}_{\hat{K}_y} = e_{k^y}\mathcal{F}^yC_{d^y}C_1^{n^y}X \qquad (12)$$

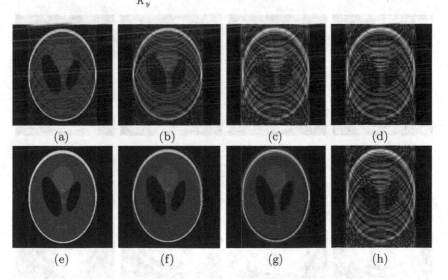

Fig. 2. Moved Shepp-Logan phantom with maximal motion of (a): 2, (b): 5, (c),(d): 8 pixels in all k-space lines. Related reconstructed images gained by the presented algorithm (e)-(g) and gained by reconstruction algorithm from [3] (h).

Applying $\tilde{b}^x$ with (12) to the current approximation $\tilde{K}$ delivers an estimate $\tilde{K}_y$ that is motion free in x-direction. With (9) follows

$$\hat{K}_y\left(k^y, \cdot\right) = \exp\left(-i2\pi \frac{k^y}{m} b_{k^y}^y\right) K_y\left(k^y, \cdot\right) \tag{13}$$

and the recursion is given by

$$\exp\left(i2\pi \frac{k^y}{m} b_{k^y}^y\right) \hat{K}_y\left(k^y, \cdot\right) = K_y\left(k^y, \cdot\right) \tag{14}$$

The full k-space is $K = \mathcal{F}\mathcal{F}^{y^{-1}} K_y$. Applying $\tilde{b}^y$ in this way to $\tilde{K}_y$ results in a new estimation for $\tilde{K}$, which is used as starting point for the next iteration.

The algorithm stops if no significant motion higher than a threshold (here selected as 0.1 pixels) is estimated anymore.

As the repeated application of the convolution matrix in the x-directional reconstruction could constitute a low pass filtering a global motion variable $G \in \mathbb{R}^{m,2}$ is defined to avoid blurring. It starts at $G = 0$ and $\tilde{B}$ is added in each iteration. The final estimation $\tilde{K}$ is generated by applying G in an extra reconstruction step to $\hat{K}$ at the algorithm end.

Randomly chosen k-space lines were calculated directly from moved images of the object. The motion was simulated in the image domain by a circularly shift of up to 8 pixels independently in both directions. This simulation is similar to the random k-space line recording order in MRI. In some simulations, only half

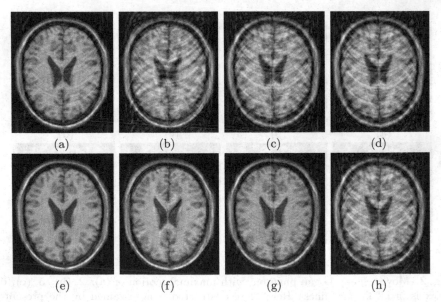

(a)   (b)   (c)   (d)

(e)   (f)   (g)   (h)

Fig. 3. Moved brain image with maximal motion of (a): 2, (b)-(d): 5 pixels in all ((a),(c),(d)), half (b) of the k-space lines. Related reconstructed images gained by the presented algorithm (e)-(g) and gained by reconstruction algorithm from [3] (h).

of the k-space lines were chosen randomly and calculated from shifted images, the remaining ones were calculated from the original. The images gained from the inverse Fourier transform of so produced k-spaces are shown in the upper lines of Figs. 2 and 3.

The sparsifying step was tested with different wavelets (Daubechies and Symlets), and due to its good results, the Haar wavelet was selected. For the calculation of the sparsifying constant, a variable $a \in \mathbb{R}^+$ was chosen with $c = a \, \|\mathcal{W}X\|_1$. For the test environment, $a \in [0.4, 0.6]$ turned out to be suitable.

The results gained by reconstruction with the proposed blind motion compensation are shown in Fig. 2 (e)-(g), 3 (e)-(g). Even for large motion shifts, an excellent reconstruction of image details is achieved. Image structures that were not even noticeable before get revealed. Only a small amount of noise remains. As reference, reconstruction results gained by [3] are shown in 2 (h), 3 (h). With under 30 seconds, the enhanced algorithm is much faster than [3] on a similar computer. In addition to motion interpolation via convolution matrices, the approach was tested for a cubic translational motion interpolation in the image domain, for which the same quality of results was achieved.

4 Discussion

The proposed approach offers a promising and fast MRI motion correction with subpixel accuracy without collecting additional data. MRI reconstruction gets more stable. For a clinician, a diagnostic of in distorted images not noticeable structures gets possible. In future works, the aim is to extend the algorithm to more general non-rigid motion. New methods for motion estimation need to be tested, and an adaption rule for the sparsifying constant has to be found. A noise reduction step could be inserted to erase remaining small artifacts.

References

1. Lustig M, Donoho DL, Santos JM, et al. Compressed sensing MRI. IEEE Signal Process Mag. 2008;25:72–82.
2. Lin W, Huang F, Börnert P, et al. Motion correction using an enhanced floating navigator and GRAPPA operations. Magn Reson Med. 2009;63:339–48.
3. Yang Z, Zhang C, Xie L. Sparse MRI for motion correction. Proc IEEE Int Symp Biomed Imaging. 2013; p. 962–5.
4. Yang Z. Analysis, Algorihms and Applications of Compressed Sensing. Nanyang Technological University. Singapore; 2013.
5. Cocosco CA, Kollokian V, Kwan RKS, et al. BrainWeb: online interface to a 3D MRI simulated brain database. NeuroImage. 1997;5(4):425.

Truncation Robust C-Arm CT Reconstruction for Dynamic Collimation Acquisition Schemes

Thomas Kästner[1], Joachim Hornegger[1], Andreas Maier[1], Yan Xia[1], Sebastian Bauer[2]

[1]Friedrich-Alexander Universität Erlangen-Nürnberg
[2]Siemens AG, Forchheim, Germany
thom.kaestner@gmail.com

Abstract. Volume-of-interest (VOI) C-arm computed tomography (CT) imaging is a promising approach to acquire anatomical information in a pre-defined target volume at low dose, using both axial and trans-axial collimation. However, also the region outside the target volume, below referred to as peripheral region (PR), could contain some valuable information for image guidance. The potential use of a fast dynamically changing collimator would allow for new acquisition schemes, that acquire projection data in a way that allows for both a high-quality reconstruction of the diagnostic VOI and a low-quality reconstruction of the peripheral region, still at a low overall dose. In this paper, we present a novel reconstruction algorithm for an acquisition scheme that acquires a large portion of the projections in a collimated manner, while acquiring a small portion of the projections in a non-collimated manner. Experimental results indicate that few non-truncated projections can help to improve the image quality compared to a conventional VOI acquisition, while simultaneously providing valuable information about the peripheral region.

1 Introduction

Reducing dose while maintaining image quality has become an emerging field in CT imaging and a general rule for any practical medical X-ray imaging application. In some clinical applications, in particular in image guided therapy, only a small portion of the patient is required to be examined. A promising approach is Volume of Interest (VOI) computed tomography (CT). In order to reduce the field of view (FOV) to the region-of-interest (ROI), an X-ray beam collimator is deployed to laterally and axially block the radiation during the scan. As a consequence, VOI imaging results in truncated projections which pose a challenge to conventional 3D cone beam reconstruction algorithms. Furthermore, no information of the region outside the VOI, the peripheral region (PR), is provided. However, some knowledge about the PR could be helpful in image-guided therapy and interventional procedures. Certain procedures require a high image quality of the VOI, while a low image quality of the PR might be sufficient. Even though that would involve the acquisition of a sparse set of non-truncated projections, the overall applied dose would remain well below the amount of a conventional scan. When it comes to the deployment of an implant for instance, not only the VOI but also the PR may contain relevant information. This information might be helpful in image guided procedures in order to reach the target location. Another application could be in cancer or tumor treatment, where the PR covers organs-at-risk, holding valuable information to optimize the treatment plan.

Leary and Robar [1] demonstrated the acquisition of multiple volumes, an inner VOI and a nested VOI. In particular, they performed one acquisition and modified the collimation during the scan. The projection data was processed using the conventional FDK [2] algorithm in combination with an extrapolation [3] of the truncated projection data, followed by an additional normalization of relative image intensity of the inner and the nested VOI. However, as stated in the paper, the approach does not preserve HU values compared to the FDK reconstruction of non-truncated data.

In this paper, we performed a simulation study of a new acquisition scheme that provides truncated and non-truncated projections within one scan. To our knowledge, no reconstruction algorithms have been developed so far that are specifically dedicated to this kind of acquisition scheme. This work introduces a novel algorithm that is capable to reconstruct such data, yielding both a high-quality VOI reconstruction and a low-quality PR reconstruction.

2 Materials and methods

2.1 Acquisition scheme

In this work, which is a simulation study, we made use of the concept of a dedicated acquisition scheme (Fig. 1). It acquires two sets of different projections, non-truncated and truncated projections. In practice, this would require a fast dynamic collimator that blocks the radiation both axially and laterally during a C-arm CT acquisition and that is capable of changing its size dynamically over the entire possible range, while the C-arm is rotating from one angular position to another. While the FOV is collimated to the ROI for most projection angles, every n-th frame the collimator opens completely to acquire a non-truncated projection. This results in a sparse number of full FOV projections and a dense number of ROI projections, within one single scan. In this context, let us introduce the term sparsity, referring to the frequency of full projections. For instance,

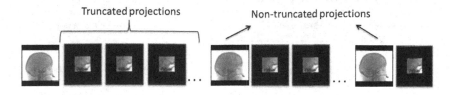

Fig. 1. Schematic illustration of the acquisition scheme.

a sparsity of $k = 10$ corresponds to an acquisition protocol where every 10-th projection is a full projection. The parameter k is calculated by dividing the total number of acquired projections by the number of acquired full projections.

2.2   FDK reconstruction

From our simulated acquisition scheme we obtain two data sets, a dense set of truncated projections and a sparse set of non-truncated projections. In a first step, we perform an initial reconstruction of the sparse set of non-truncated projections. To this end, we use an iterative total-variation (iTV) based algorithm [4] to obtain acceptable reconstruction results from such sparse data. In a second step, we perform a forward projection of the initial reconstruction to de-truncate the subset of truncated projections. The forward projections are being adapted by using the unprocessed truncated projection data. That way, we obtain a full set of non-truncated data, consisting of a dense set of detruncated projection data as well as the sparse set of non-truncated projection data, being eventually backprojected along the lines of a conventional FDK algorithm [2]. An illustrative overview of the algorithm is given in Fig. 2. Below, we elaborate on the individual processing steps.

Adaption and transition weighting We perform a transformation of the forward projection values in order to handle incorrect values in the transition region. We choose $(v_2 - v_1) \times u_t$ to be the size of the transition region, where $(v_2 - v_1)$ is the size of the ROI in v-direction and u_t corresponds to the number

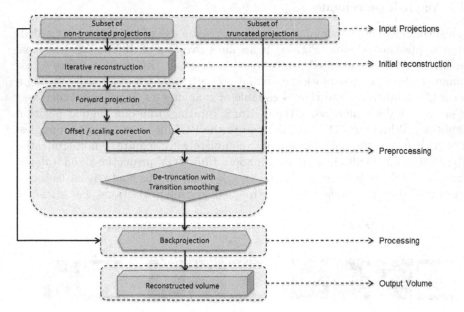

Fig. 2. Flowchart of the reconstruction approach.

of columns in the u-direction, e.g. $u_t = 60$. Similar to the suggested method described in [5], we designed two 2D parameter masks $A(\lambda_T, u, v)$ and $B(\lambda_T, u, v)$ (1) for each projection of the set of forward projections that correspond to the same angular position as a truncated projection. We used these filter masks to perform the scaling and offset correction of the forward projections

$$A = \frac{\sigma_{TR}}{\sigma_{FP}} \quad \text{and} \quad B = \mu_{TR} - A \cdot \mu_{FP} \tag{1}$$

where σ_{TR} and σ_{FP} correspond to the standard deviations, and μ_{TR} and μ_{FP} to the mean values of the transition region of the truncated projection $g_{TR}(\lambda, u, v)$ and the corresponding forward projection $g_{FP}(\lambda, u, v)$, respectively.

As a first step, the mean values and the standard deviations are calculated for each pixel (u, v) in the transition region over the entire column in u-direction and over the entire row in v-direction of the forward projection and the truncated projection. Filter values outside the transition region are obtained by constant extrapolation of the most outer filter values of the transition region in u-direction. Finally, the actual transformation of each pixel is achieved according to

$$g_{C,FP}(\lambda_T, u, v) = A(\lambda_T, u, v) \cdot g_{FP}(\lambda_T, u, v) + B(\lambda_T, u, v) \tag{2}$$

where $g_{C,FP}(\lambda_T, u, v)$ describes the corrected forward projection at rotation angle λ_T, which corresponds to the rotation angle of a truncated projection from the proposed acquisition scheme. The filter mask A is employed as the scaling correction parameter, while the filter mask B is used to compensate the offset problem.

Cosine filtering and combination By applying a cosine filtering step, we handle sudden changes of values at the boundary of the ROI and provide a smooth transition region in the combined projection data. Finally, the reconstruction is carried out by a standard FDK algorithm [2].

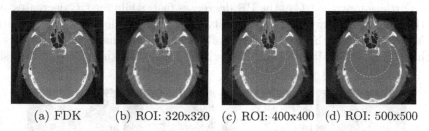

(a) FDK   (b) ROI: 320x320   (c) ROI: 400x400   (d) ROI: 500x500

Fig. 3. Transversal slices of the reconstruction results. The grayscale window is [-1000 HU, 2500 HU]. Slice thickness is 0.4 mm and volume size is $512 \times 512 \times 350$. The sparsity-level is $k = 10$. (a) Ground truth reconstruction (FDK on non-truncated data), (b) proposed reconstruction on partially truncated projection data from the proposed acquisition scheme at a small ROI size, (c) a medium ROI, (d) a large ROI.

3   Experiments

The developed algorithm is evaluated in a qualitative and quantitative manner using a clinical data set (data courtesy of St. Luke's Episcopal Hospital, Houston, TX, USA). It holds a full set of non-truncated projections. We used virtual truncation to simulate the collimator and to generate the truncated projections. The experiments were performed for different sparsity levels ($k \in \{1, 2, 4, 6, 8, 10\}$) as well as for three different collimation sizes (320×320 px, 400×400 px, 500×500 px). The VOI and the PR were evaluated separately and were visually compared to the ground truth (FDK on full set of non-truncated projection data). Standardized image quality metrics (correlation coefficient (CC), root mean square error (RMSE), both with respect to the FDK reconstruction on full set of non-truncated projection data) were used for a quantitative evaluation.

3.1   Results

Fig. 3 shows the reconstruction results for three different ROI sizes, which are visually compared to the ground truth. In Fig. 3(b), we observed slight streak artifacts at the bone structures of the head, which are decreasing with an increasing ROI size (Fig. 3(d)). Fig. 4 shows a rather comparable image quality in the PR for different levels of sparsity, indicating that the dose reduction associated with increasing sparsity levels comes with a much less pronounced degradation of image quality in the PR. Only a slight increase in streak artifacts can be observed in the PR at a higher sparsity level. In summary, both, for a decreasing ROI size (Fig. 3) as well as for an increasing sparsity level (Fig. 4), the degradation in image quality in the PR is rather low. In addition, details in the VOI are well preserved and no additional artifacts could be observed. Furthermore, a smooth transition region between the VOI and the PR is observed (Sec. 2.2).

In Fig. 5(a) and Fig. 5(b), quantitative results are shown for three different ROI sizes. For all ROI sizes, we notice that the RMSE of the PR is increasing rapidly with a higher sparsity, while the RMSE of the VOI increases substantially less. Furthermore, the CC of the PR decreases fast, while the CC decreases slow for the VOI even at an increasing sparsity level. The previous visual observation is also confirmed by the quantitative evaluation. Additionally, better results for both, the CC and RMSE are achieved within the VOI with increasing ROI size.

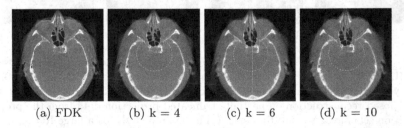

(a) FDK   (b) k = 4   (c) k = 6   (d) k = 10

Fig. 4. Same slice and volume information as in Fig. 3. The ROI is 400×400 px.(a) Ground truth, (b) proposed reconstruction at different sparsity levels.

Fig. 5. RMSE (a) and CC (b) of the PR and VOI from the reconstruction result at a medium ROI size of 400×400 px.

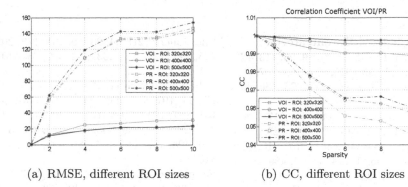

(a) RMSE, different ROI sizes   (b) CC, different ROI sizes

4   Discussion

We presented an algorithm that is tailored to dynamically collimated acquisitions and were able to obtain reconstruction results with a high image quality in the VOI, while promising results for the PR were achieved. By incorporating the sparse set of full FOV projections, we were able to not only improve the image quality of the VOI but also to obtain additional information in the PR region, while keeping the total radiation dose low. Furthermore, we showed that our algorithm is robust in terms of different ROI sizes as well as for an increasing level of sparsity.

Acknowledgement. The concepts and information presented in this paper are based on research and are not commercially available.

References

1. Leary D, Robar JL. CBCT with specification of imaging dose and CNR by anatomical volume of interest. Med Phys. 2014;41(1):011909.
2. Feldkamp L, Davis L, Kress J. Practical cone-beam algorithm. J Opt Soc Am A. 1984;1(6):612–9.
3. Robar JL, Parsons D, Berman A, et al. Volume-of-interest cone-beam CT using a 2.35 MV beam generated with a carbon target. Med Phys. 2012;39(7):4209–18.
4. Ritschl L, Bergner F, Fleischmann C, et al. Improved total variation-based CT image reconstruction applied to clinical data. Phys Med Biol. 2011;56(6):1545.
5. Kolditz D, Kyriakou Y, Kalender WA. Volume-of-interest (VOI) imaging in c-arm flat-detector CT for high image quality at reduced dose. Med Phys. 2010;37(6):2719–30.

Kategorisierung der Beiträge

Kardiovaskuläres System, 23, 53, 65, 95, 137, 161, 191, 257, 293, 305, 329, 377, 425
Respiratorisches System, 107, 227, 245, 317, 329, 335, 425
Gastrointestinales System, 41, 173, 221, 365, 413, 455, 461
Muskoloskeletales System, 35, 101, 323, 335, 449

Primärfunktion des Verfahrens
Bilderzeugung und -rekonstruktion, 35, 47, 59, 113, 119, 131, 143, 149, 155, 167, 173, 197, 215, 221, 233, 251, 257, 269, 335, 437, 455, 467, 492, 498, 504, 510, 516
Bildverbesserung und -darstellung, 35, 59, 83, 113, 131, 137, 173, 203, 221, 263, 269, 311, 317, 401, 413, 437, 443, 449, 455, 510, 516
Bildtransport und -speicherung, 275
Merkmalsextraktion und Segmentierung, 11, 29, 65, 77, 95, 101, 107, 119, 143, 155, 161, 167, 209, 239, 263, 281, 287, 293, 305, 329, 341, 347, 353, 359, 377, 389, 407, 413, 419, 461, 479, 486
Objekterkennung und Szenenanalyse, 5, 23, 77, 119, 143, 185, 197, 209, 227, 263, 281, 287, 299, 359, 407

Quantifizierung von Bildinhalten, 41, 77, 125, 131, 143, 191, 257, 293, 323, 365, 377, 401, 407, 425, 479
Multimodale Aufbereitung, 149, 245, 407, 486

Art des Projektes
Grundlagenforschung, 17, 47, 125, 185, 215, 251, 269, 371, 377, 383, 401, 431, 449, 510
Methodenentwicklung, 5, 11, 29, 35, 41, 47, 89, 101, 107, 113, 119, 125, 131, 137, 143, 149, 161, 167, 173, 185, 191, 197, 203, 215, 221, 227, 233, 239, 245, 251, 257, 269, 281, 287, 293, 299, 305, 311, 317, 329, 335, 341, 347, 353, 359, 389, 407, 413, 419, 425, 431, 437, 455, 461, 467, 473, 479, 486, 498, 504, 510, 516
Anwendungsentwicklung, 59, 65, 71, 77, 95, 125, 131, 137, 149, 155, 185, 197, 203, 209, 215, 227, 239, 263, 281, 311, 341, 389, 401, 419, 425, 437, 467, 504
Klinische Diagnostik, 17, 41, 173, 257, 365, 407, 449, 455

Autorenverzeichnis

Stichwortverzeichnis